The newborn brain

The development of the human brain is one of the most important concerns of contemporary biology, with profound implications for medicine and society. In this book a distinguished international team of clinicians, neuroscientists and geneticists presents recent findings about the basic mechanisms of brain development and the pathophysiology of the infant brain.

The book follows the major milestones of brain development, from formation of the neural tube, through neurogenesis, neuronal migration, and the organization of brain wiring. Neurotrophic factors, transmitters, glial cell biology, cerebral circulation and the development of sensory functions are all described in detail, and the authors emphasize the clinical applications of basic neuroscience. Coverage extends from the normal to the disordered brain in preterm and full-term infants

At a time of rapid and exciting advances in developmental neurobiology, this book provides a uniquely authoritative survey for scientists and clinicians alike.

Hugo Lagercrantz is Professor of Pediatrics at the Karolinska Institute and Director of the Neonatal Unit at the Astrid Lindgren Children's Hospital in Stockholm.

Mark Hanson is Professor at the Centre for Fetal Origins of Adult Disease at the University of Southampton.

Philippe Evrard is Professor of Neuropediatrics at the Faculté de Médecine Xavier-Bichat and Chief of Neuropediatrics at the Hôpital Robert-Debré in Paris.

Charles H. Rodeck is Professor of Obstetrics and Gynaecology and Director of the Fetal Medicine Unit at the Obstetric Hospital, University College London.

The newborn brain

Neuroscience and clinical applications

Edited by

Hugo Lagercrantz
Karolinska Institute and Astrid Lindgren Children's Hospital, Stockholm, Sweden

Mark Hanson
University of Southampton, UK

Philippe Evrard
Faculté de Médecine Xavier-Bichat and Hôpital Robert-Debré, Paris, France

Charles H. Rodeck
Obstetric Hospital, University College London, UK

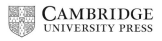

CAMBRIDGE
UNIVERSITY PRESS

BS

PUBLISHED BY THE PRESS SYNDICATE OF THE UNIVERSITY OF CAMBRIDGE
The Pitt Building, Trumpington Street, Cambridge, United Kingdom

CAMBRIDGE UNIVERSITY PRESS
The Edinburgh Building, Cambridge CB2 2RU, UK
40 West 20th Street, New York, NY 10011–4211, USA
477 Williamstown Road, Port Melbourne, VIC 3207, Australia
Ruiz de Alarcón 13, 28014 Madrid, Spain
Dock House, The Waterfront, Cape Town 8001, South Africa

http://www.cambridge.org

First published 2002

Printed in the United Kingdom at the University Press, Cambridge

Typeface Adobe Minion 10.5/14pt   *System* QuarkXPress™   [SE]

A catalogue record for this book is available from the British Library

Library of Congress cataloguing in publication data

The newborn brain: neuroscience and clinical applications / edited by Hugo Lagercrantz
. . . [et al.]
    p.   cm.
Includes bibliographical references and index.
ISBN 0 521 79338 6 (hardback)
1. Developmental neurobiology.   2. Brain – Growth.   I. Lagercrantz, Hugo, 1945–
[DNLM: 1. Brain – embryology.   2. Brain – growth and development – Child.   3.
Brain – growth and development – Infant.   4. Brain Chemistry – Child.   5. Brain
Chemistry – Infant.   6. Brain Diseases – Child.   7. Brain Diseases – Infant. WL 300 N5318 2001]
QP363.5. N496   2001
612.8′2–dc21   2001025510

ISBN 0 521 79338 6 hardback

3/28/04

Contents

Contributors

Monique André
Service de Médecine et Réanimation
    Néonatales – Génétique,
Maternité Regionale A Pinard,
10, rue de Dr Heydenreich,
BP 4213,
F-54042 Nancy,
France

A. James Barkovich
Department of Radiology,
University of California,
Box 0628,
L-371505 Parnosses Avenue,
San Francisco,
CA 94143
USA

Harm-Gerd K. Blaas
National Center for Fetal Medicine,
    Women's Hospital RiT,
N-7006 Trondheim
Norway

Jean-Pierre Bourgeois
Laboratoire de Neurobiologie Moléculaire,
Département des Biotechnologies,
Institut Pasteur,
75724 Paris Cedex 15,
France

Verne S. Caviness, Jr.
Department of Neurology,
Massachusetts General Hospital,
25 Fruit Street,
Boston,
MA 02114, USA

Jean-Pierre Changeux
CNRS URA 1284,
Neurobiologie Moléculaire,
Institut Pasteur,
25 rue du Docteur Roux,
75724 Paris Cedex 15,
France

S. Allen Counter
Neurology Department,
The Biological Laboratories,
Harvard Medical School,
16 Divinity Avenue,
Cambridge,
MA 02138,
USA

Anne Marie D'Allest
Service de Pédiatrie et Réanimation
    Néonatales
Hôpital Antoine Béclère,
157 rue de la Porte de Trivaux,
92141 Clamart,
France

A. David Edwards
Weston Laboratory,
Division of Paediatrics, Obstetrics and
    Gynaecology,
Imperial College School of Medicine,
Hammersmith Hospital,
du Cane Road,
London W12 0NN,
UK

Sturla H. Eik-Nes
National Center for Fetal Medicine,
    Women's Hospital RiT,
N-7006 Trondheim,
Norway

Olof Flodmark
Department of Pediatric Neuroradiology
    Research,
Karolinska Institute,
S-171 76 Stockholm,
Sweden

Hans Forssberg
Department of Women and Child Health,
Karolinska Institute,
Astrid Lindgren Children's Hospital
S-171 76 Stockholm,
Sweden

Pierre Gressens
Service de Neurologie
Pédiatrique and INSERM CRI 97-01,
Hôpital Robert-Debré,
48 BD Sérurier,
F-75019 Paris,
France

Mijna Hadders-Algra
Department of Medical Physiology,
University Hospital Groningen,
CMC IV, 3rd floor,
Hanzeplein 1,
9713 GZ Groningen,
The Netherlands

Henrik Hagberg
Perinatal Center,
Department of Obstetrics and Gynecology,
Sahlgrenska University Hospital, Östra,
S-416 85 Göteborg,
Sweden

Lena Hellström-Westas
Department of Paediatrics,
University Hospital,
SE-221 85 Lund,
Sweden

Eric Herlenius
Department of Women and Child Health,
Karolinska Institute,
Neonatal Unit,
Astrid Lindgren Children's Hospital
S-171 76 Stockholm,
Sweden

Hugo Lagercrantz
Department of Women and Child Health,
Karolinska Institute,
Neonatal Unit,
Astrid Lindgren Children's Hospital
S-171 76 Stockholm,
Sweden

Urban Lendahl
Department of Cell and Molecular Biology,
Medical Nobel Institute,
Karolinska Institute,
S-171 77 Stockholm,
Sweden

Stephen G. Matthews
Department of Physiology,
Faculty of Medicine,
University of Toronto,
Medical Sciences Building,
1 King's College Circle,
Toronto M5S 1A8,
Canada

Huseyin Mehmet
Weston Laboratory,
Division of Paediatrics,
Obstetrics and Gynaecology,
Imperial College School of Medicine,
Hammersmith Hospital,
du Cane Road,
London W12 0NN,
UK

Richard S. Nowakowski
Department of Neuroscience and Cell
    Biology,
UMDNJ-Robert Wood Johnson Medical
    School,
Piscataway,
NJ 08854,
USA

William J. Pearce
Department of Physiology,
Center for Perinatal Biology,
Loma Linda University,
Loma Linda,
CA 92350,
USA

Anna A. Penn
Department of Neonatology and
    Developmental Medicine
Lucille Salter Packard Children's Hospital at
    Stanford
750 Welch Road, Suite 315
Palo Alto, CA 94304, USA

Nilima Prakash
Department of Cell and Molecular Biology,
Medical Nobel Institute,
Karolinska Institute,
S-171 77 Stockholm,
Sweden

John Rawson
Department of Anatomy and Cell Biology,
The University of Melbourne,
Parkville,
Victoria 3052,
Australia

Sandra Rees
Department of Anatomy and Cell Biology,
The University of Melbourne,
Parkville,
Victoria 3052,
Australia

Thomas Ringstedt
Department of Women and Child Health,
Karolinska Institute,
Neonatal Unit,
Astrid Lindgren Children's Hospital
S-171 76 Stockholm,
Sweden

Arne Schousboe
NeuroScience PharmaBiotec Research
    Center,
Department of Pharmacology,
Royal Danish School of Pharmacy,
Universitetsparken 2,
DK-2100 Copenhagen,
Denmark

Carla J. Shatz
Department of Neurobiology,
Harvard Medical School,
220 Longwood Avenue,
Boston,
MA 02115,
USA

Takao Takahashi
Department of Pediatrics,
Keio University School of Medicine,
Tokyo 160,
Japan

Marianne Thoresen
Division of Child Health,
University of Bristol Medical School,
Southmead Hospital,
Bristol BS10 5NB,
UK

Helle S. Waagepetersen
NeuroScience PharmaBiotec Research
  Center,
Department of Pharmacology,
Royal Danish School of Pharmacy,
Universitetsparken 2,
DK-2100 Copenhagen,
Denmark

Michael Weindling
Neonatal Unit,
Liverpool Women's Hospital,
Crown Street,
Liverpool L8 7SS,
UK

Andrew Whitelaw
Division of Child Health,
University of Bristol Medical School,
Southmead Hospital,
Bristol BS10 5NB,
UK

John S. Wyatt
Department of Paediatrics,
Royal Free and University College Medical
  School,
5 University Street,
London WC1E 6JJ,
UK

Preface

For ages philosophers have discussed how the brain and the mind are created. Descartes and Kant thought that true ideas are innate, while Locke and Hume claimed that the brain is a blank slate at birth. William Harvey opposed the idea that the organs, e.g. the brain are preformed and maintained that the organs develop successively – epigenesis. Sigmund Freud who can be regarded as determinist wrote that our ideas and psychology are based on small substructures (genes). The mapping of the human genome has reinitiated a debate on the concept of preformation – today genetic determinism vs. environmental instructionism. A third alternative is the idea of selectionism or neuronal darwinism. The premature brain is a jungle according to Gerald Edelman with redundant neurons and pathways and due to environmental influences only the most suitable neuronal circuits survive (see chapter by Changeux). 'Cells that fire together wire together – those that don't won't.' (Penn & Shatz, p. 207).

The busy obstetrician scanning the fetal brain by ultrasound or the neonatologist monitoring the newborn brain may have limited time to ponder these eternal questions. The main reason for publishing this book is to present the state of the art on how the brain is formed. The recent breakthroughs in our understanding of the development of the brain originate from studies of invertebrates like fruit-flies or nematodes, mice or ferrets. It is difficult for the hard-working clinician attending the delivery, neonatal or neuropediatric ward to grasp this literature. On the other hand, the basic scientist may have only a vague idea of the clinical expression of mutations or disorders of neuronal migration and synaptogenesis, preterm birth or perinatal asphyxia.

Jean-Pierre Changeux commences the book with some reflections on the origin of the human brain. The chapters then follow the major milestones of brain development: formation of the neural tube, neurogenesis, migration of neurons, synaptogenesis and organization of the brain wiring. Special chapters are devoted to neurotrophic factors, neurotransmitters, glial cell biology and cerebral circulation. Then the development of sensory functions is described.

The second part of the book deals with more clinical aspects, particularly methods

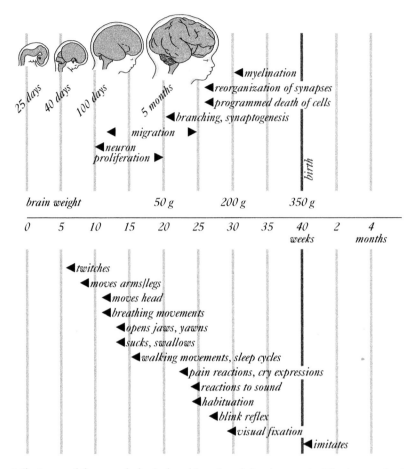

Fig. 1.   Milestones of the morphological and functional development of the human brain.
(Drawing by Stig Söderlind, based on an idea by H. Lagercrantz.)

to investigate the infant brain by imaging and electrophysiological techniques. Two chapters deal with clinical aspects of the brain of the full-term infant and one with the preterm infant. The authors have specially emphasized how the knowledge from basic science can be applied in clinical practice.

We hope that this book is of interest for a broad readership from the more theoretical biologist, molecular geneticist and the biophysicist to the clinical fellow in obstetrics, neonatology or neuropediatrics as well as the neuropsychologist. The book can also be recommended as a textbook for graduate courses.

Stockholm, Paris and London Dec. 30, 2000
The Editors

Reflections on the origins of the human brain

Jean-Pierre Changeux

Neurobiologie Moléculaire, Institut Pasteur, Paris, France

Introduction

Human beings belong to the biological species *Homo sapiens*. The definition of the species includes the description of the characteristic anatomy of the body, as well as of the functional organization of the brain. It also deals with the multiple facets of a behaviour unique to human beings. The human brain is thus an outstanding object of scientific investigation.

The aim of this chapter is to debate the origins of the human brain. This raises an overwhelming challenge. First of all, one should attempt to delineate what makes the human brain human, even in the newborn, and to identify the features which distinguish it from its fossil antecedents and from the presently living primates. It is intriguing to find ways of specifying 'human nature' in objective terms. On the other hand, the broad diversity existing between individuals, in particular as a consequence of their past and recent personal and/or cultural history, raises a second challenge. Does such diversity break the unity of the human brain within the human species?

A tension thus exists in the neurosciences, as well as in the humanities, between two main lines of research: one that aims at defining the universal characteristics of the human species, for instance, at the level of the infant brain, and the other that stresses the variability of adults' cognitive abilities, such as the language they speak and the social conventions they adopt. It is a formidable task to deal with these contrasting approaches with the aim of achieving a meaningful scientific understanding of the human brain, its learning capacities, and its higher functions. Nevertheless, it appears plausible that a realistic picture of the human brain will require the synthesis of these divergent approaches. I shall therefore consider successively these two aspects of research on the human (and non-human) brain.

Universality within complexity

An often-quoted source of problems in the study of the human brain is the complexity of its organization (Tononi & Edelman, 1998; Koch & Laurent, 1999). René

Thom, in a thoughtful essay (1990), critically analysed the ambiguity of the notion of complexity applied to a biological object. According to him, the word complexity 'too often serves as an excuse for intellectual laziness in front of a system that we neither understand nor master' (p.220). Thom further distinguishes two distinct views in the attempt to evaluate the complexity of a system. One is essentially analytical: the idea is to dissociate the system into elementary components – here the neurons and their constitutive molecules – which, when canonically recombined, will allow the reconstruction of the system. Then, the length of the operations necessary for such reconstruction will be a measure of the complexity of the object. In theory, this is a most valid scientific approach which might be referred to as a 'fair reductionism'. It has been successful in past decades (or even centuries) in the life sciences, leading, in particular, to remarkable progress in our understanding of the molecular biology of the cell (Watson, 1976). This approach equally applies to the elementary components of the brain, such as the nerve cell, its synapses and especially to the molecular mechanisms of intercellular communications by neurotransmitters (Changeux, 1998). Does it follow from these steps that soon we should be able to 'reconstruct' the human brain and evaluate its complexity in scientific terms? In theory, this is a horizon towards which brain research should tend. On practical grounds, to describe objectively brain complexity in scientifically acceptable terms appears out of reach, if ever possible, with the presently available methods and concepts because of the immense number of connections and their variability from neuron to neuron and from individual to individual.

The alternative view discussed by Thom is to approach the complexity of the brain from a strictly functional, holistic evaluation of its functions and their dynamics. This approach, frequently adopted by cognitive psychologists, linguists or philosophers, does not refer to, and even sometimes denies, the relevance of brain organization. It relies upon strictly behavioural (or introspective) investigations of the brain (together with the debated validity of subjective reports from phenomenal consciousness) and has led to useful descriptions of brain functions – often in algorithmic terms. Diagrams and models with multiple connected boxes, each one with a defined 'function', have proliferated in past decades (Shallice, 1988), always with the appropriate mention that a given box cannot be identified with an anatomically defined brain area. Yet, such a functionalist approach, while necessary, is in my opinion insufficient and even becomes erroneous when one further attempts to posit that 'the functional organization of the nervous system crosscuts its neurological organizations' (Fodor, 1976). According to these views, it suffices to investigate behaviour (and psychology in particular) independently of any scientifically observable neural constraint. The consequences of such an attitude are, in practice, particularly harmful: it broadens the already existing gap between the brain and what is currently called the mind and thus overlooks the consequences of the neural organization of the brain on its psychological functions.

A third approach to deal with brain complexity aims at bridging these two lines of research by the deliberate attempt to relate concomitantly (i) given anatomical structures in the brain, (ii) the dynamic processes and activities demonstrated by a particular neural network, and (iii) a defined behavioural action upon the outside world (or within the organism itself). This approach is certainly not straightforward. It proceeds, in a progressive manner, by testing models (see Changeux & Connes, 1989) that bridge anatomy, physiology, and behaviour in 'neurorealistic', experimentally testable terms. Multidisciplinary and convergent experimental approaches will result in either their validation or (more often!) their rejection. Such a trial-and-error approach to brain complexity is nevertheless intrinsically limited in its scope by several obvious difficulties.

A first difficulty raised by the philosopher John Searle (1995) concerns the notion of function, particularly psychological function. One should never underestimate the conceptual and experimental difficulties of any attempt to singularize a behavioural or mental trait. Searle even suggests that functions are not intrinsic, but are assigned to, or imposed upon living objects or organisms, and in particular the human brain, by the observer. This problem must be taken seriously. Even though, since Darwin, attempts have been made to eliminate teleology from the life sciences, one has to be aware of a possible observer bias in the definition of a function. In my opinion, Searle's criticism may go beyond the definition of function and apply equally to the description of the anatomy or to the dynamics of the electrical and chemical activities that take place within the brain. The theoretical models aimed at resolving brain complexity include the concerned function but go beyond this definition since my view is that relevant models about the human brain have to systematically bring together defined and delimited anatomical, physiological, and behavioural data (see Changeux et al., 1973). In any case, the aim of the modelling enterprise is not to give an exhaustive description of brain reality: it will always be limited by its scope and by its formalization. One should never forget that the modelling process involves the selection of theoretical representations by the brain of the model builder!

Another difficulty resides in the very attempt to establish an appropriate link between the structural elements of the system and the function considered. The reductionist approach, as mentioned, has to be 'fair', in contrast to statements one frequently encounters, such as 'the gene(s) of intelligence' or the 'neurotransmitters of schizophrenia'! Such simplistic and incorrect proposals bypass one essential feature of brain organization, namely the parallel and hierarchical levels of organization nested within each other and with abundant cross-connections. These levels develop from the molecule to the cell, from elementary circuits to populations (or

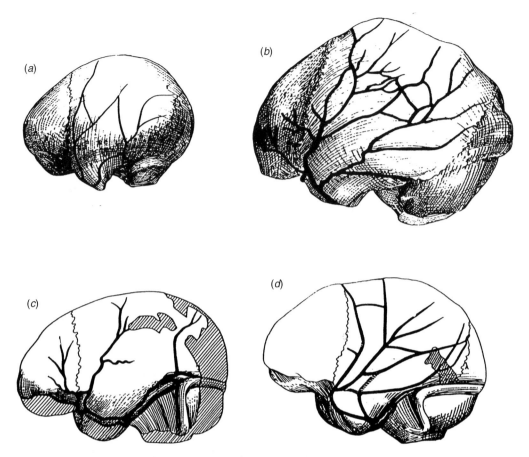

Fig. 1.1.   Comparison of the impression of the meningeal vessels on endocranial casts of 40-day-old infant (*a*) and 1-year-old infant (*b*) with the endocranial casts of *Australopithecus gracilis* (*c*) and *Homo habilis* (*d*). (From Saban, 1995.)

assemblies) of neurons, up to complex global patterns engaged in higher cognitive functions. The definition of these relevant parallel and hierarchical levels is by itself a theoretical problem and should be rendered explicit (Changeux & Connes, 1989). A critical conceptual step will thus be to specify the selected hierarchical level (or, more probably, levels) of organization at which a relevant causal link can be established between anatomy, activity and behaviour, together with the massive parallelism and strong lateral interactions which potentially contribute to a coherent unitary brain process.

Last but not least, the investigations on the human brain – in particular, that of the newborn – have to be kept within the framework of biological evolution (Fig. 1.1). This requirement is obviously beneficial, since it tentatively legitimizes for instance, the commonly adopted (sometimes erroneously) utilization of animal models for human diseases. But the evolutionary perspective raises difficulties. Take, for instance, the anatomy of the brain. No simple apparent logic explains simultaneously the actual morphology, distribution and interrelation of the multiple areas or (nuclei) from which it is made up (see Changeux, 1985). The simultaneous occurrence, for instance, of archeo-, paleo- and neocortices within human brain anatomy cannot be understood without considering that they have been derived by evolutionary 'tinkering' (Jacob, 1981) from prior ancestral brains. The older structures have not been eliminated, but rather incorporated and rested within the novel ones. Millions of years of evolutionary history under extremely variable environmental conditions thus introduce, indirectly, contingencies in the anatomy such that the intrinsic logic of the functional organization of the brain may no longer be apparent by simple inspection. This situation frequently invalidates attempts to infer anatomy from function. It also illustrates why the most adequate models may neither necessarily be the simplest nor the minimal ones. Theoretical model building thus has to be 'neurorealist' and to rely upon concrete observational approaches, and it becomes a particularly difficult, though necessary, task to understand the human brain.

Finally, one should not limit the evolutionary perspective to the context of biological – or genetic – origins of the human brain. Rather, as discussed in the following sections, the brain of a human subject may be more appropriately viewed as the synthesis of multiple nested evolutions by variation selection (Changeux, 1983a,b). These evolutions include the past genetic evolution of the species, but also the epigenetic development of the brain of each individual, within the framework of his or her personal history, as well as the more recent social and cultural evolution of the social environment with which the newborn interacts. The data are scarce, but the potential outcomes of future research could be richly rewarding.

Genes and the newborn brain

The brain of the newborn is often taken as holding the innate features that characterize 'human nature'. In reality, many more characteristics proper to the human brain develop after birth, in particular, through postnatal development and learning which is one of the longest known among the living species. Even though, as we shall see, epigenetic regulations may take place which involve specific interactions with the environment, strictly innate, DNA encoded mechanisms contribute, in a definite manner, to the pre- and postnatal development of the adult brain. But, these genes are not expressed all at once in either the egg, the embryo or the newborn, as postulated by the extreme views of the eighteenth-century preformationists, views that assumed that the adult organism was already present in a miniaturized form in the sperm and in the egg. On the contrary, they are activated (or suppressed) throughout embryogenesis and postnatal development in a sequential and combinatorial manner.

The straightforward inspection of the genetic endowment of the species compared with the organization of the brain raises, however, two apparent paradoxes (Changeux, 1983a, b; Edelman, 1987; Miklos & Rubin, 1996). The total amount of DNA present in the haploid genome comprises approximately 3 billion base pairs, but no more than 30 000–40 000 structural genes (Lander et al., 2001; Venter et al., 2001). On the other hand, the total number of neurons in the brain ranges from 50 to 100 billion, each neuron possessing its particular connectivity – or 'singularity' (Changeux, 1983a). There is thus a striking parsimony of genetic information to code for brain complexity.

Another paradox is raised by the relationship between the total number of genes and the evolution of brain organization. The 97 million bases that constitute the total sequence of the genome of a small invertebrate, the nematode *Caenorhabditis elegans* (Miklos & Rubin, 1996; Hodgkin et al., 1998), with its humble 302 neuron nervous system, contains a predicted 18 266 protein-coding genes. *Drosophila* possesses a much larger nervous system, with about 250 000 neurons, but with a similar number of genes (13 338; Rubin et al., 2000). Even more striking, the gene number from bony fish, through laboratory mouse to human is roughly constant. Yet, notwithstanding the increase of cell numbers (from about 40 million in the mouse to 50–100 billion in humans), mammalian brain anatomy has evolved dramatically from a poorly corticalized lissencephalic brain with about 10–20 identified cortical areas to a brain with a very high relative cortical surface, multiple gyri and sulci and possibly as many as 100 identified cortical areas (Mountcastle, 1998). Thus, there exists a remarkable non-linearity between the evolution of brain anatomy and that of the total number of genes (Changeux, 1983a, b; Edelman, 1987; Miklos & Rubin, 1996).

The molecular genetics of the early stages of embryonic development in *Drosophila*, *Xenopus*, chick, and mouse offers at least one major perspective on resolving these paradoxes. For example, in *Drosophila*, a variety of genes have been identified that control the Cartesian coordinates of the embryo, the segmentation of the body, and the identity of its segments (Nüsslein Volhard, 1990; Lawrence, 1992). A significant fraction of these genes, which are also found in *C. elegans* (Ruvkun & Hobert, 1998) are absent in bacteria and yeast but conserved throughout the evolution of higher animal species and may plausibly act in equivalent regulatory cascades in mammals. In the course of embryonic and postnatal development, these developmental genes become expressed according to well-defined spatio-temporal patterns, in a hierarchical and parallel manner with cross regulatory interactions and reutilizations. Such a view of morphogenesis, as a developing network of gene interactions, may account, at least in part, for the parsimony paradox. An enormous diversity, indeed, may arise from such combinatorial expression of a limited number of genes.

Moreover, at critical stages of development, the symmetry of the embryo changes. Symmetry breaking (Turing, 1952; Meinhardt & Gierer, 1974) is manifest, for example, by the development of anteroposterior and dorsoventral polarities, of sharp boundaries between territories, and/or of patterns of stripes. On formal grounds, such defined and reproducible patterns might be generated from a set of chemical substances, or morphogens, which cross-react and diffuse throughout the organism (Turing, 1952). For instance, gradients of diffusible morphogens are thought to contribute to the unfolding of developmental gene expression resulting in anteroposterior polarity (Meinhardt & Gierer, 1974). The main factors (but not the only ones) are the products of the developmental genes: regulatory proteins referred to as transcription factors that control gene transcription at the level of the core RNA polymerase II transcription complex (see Mannervik et al., 1999). These protein molecules may have played a critical role in the evolution of the body form. They bind to DNA elements (enhancers or silencers) that lock or unlock the transcription of adjacent structural genes and are themselves often conserved across species. Interplay between morphogens and transcription factors (coactivators and/or corepressors) builds up intracellular networks of gene regulation, together with membrane receptors and the relevant second messengers. Such sets of molecules may contribute to the 'reading' of a gradient of morphogen by some kind of all-or-none switch in both a non-cellularized (Kerszberg & Changeux, 1994) and a cellularized embryo (Kerszberg, 1996) (Fig. 1.2). It has even been proposed that such reading may require particular kinds of molecular interconnections at the level of the transcription factors: the assembly of molecular partners into hetero-oligomers between, for instance, one morphogen molecule from the gradient and a transcriptional coregulator now coded by a gene expressed in the embryonic nuclei. Non-linear relationships between transcription factor concentration and morphogenesis may thus emerge from these combinations. Such a concept of non-linear networks of transcription factors (Kerszberg & Changeux, 1994) has been recently documented with particular reference to *Drosophila* (Mannervik et al., 1999) and may plausibly contribute to morphogenesis, together with receptors, kinases, phosphatases, G-proteins and second messengers (Lisman & Fallon, 1999) within and between the developing embryonic cells. Along these lines, one may note that what makes the main difference in sequence between yeast and the nematode as a 'minimal' multicellular organism are genes coding for transcription factors (e.g. 270 nuclear hormone receptors), protein–protein interaction domains (e.g. 156 POZ domains) or signal transduction domains (e.g. 11 phosphotyrosine binding domain) (Chervitz et al., 1998). As a consequence, minute variations in morphogen, transcription factor, or signalling molecule con-

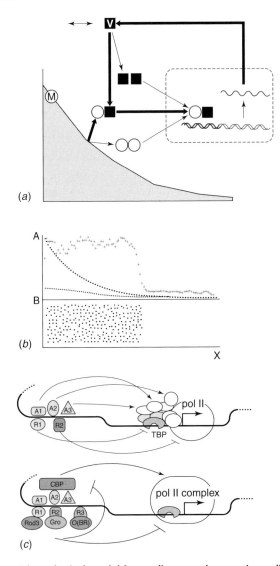

Fig. 1.2.   A hypothetical model for reading morphogenetic gradients underlining the importance of protein–protein interaction and combinational information between transcription factors at the gene level. (*a*) A morphogen M (circles) is initially distributed along a smooth anteroposterior gradient; a 'vernier' molecule V (square) is coded by a gene present in the embryonic nucleus (broken line). Morphogen and vernier may form heterodimers but may also exist as homodimers. These various dimers form transcription factors which diffuse in the cytoplasm and bind to a promoter element regulating, in *cis*, the transcription of the vernier gene. Each dimer contributes to activation/inactivation of the vernier gene transcription thus yielding autocatalysis and competition and, as a consequence, sharp boundaries (*b*) and/or stripes (from Kerszberg & Changeux, 1994; see also Smolen et al., 2000). (*c*) Plausible schemes for the integration of combinatorial information from various transcription activators and repressors (various letters) at the level of the RNA polymerase (pol II) transcription complex (from Mannervick et al., 1999).

centrations may dramatically shift boundaries and thus the relative surface of embryonic territories. Such a possibility offers plausible, although of course still hypothetical, explanations for the non-linear relationships observed in the evolution of the complexity of the anatomical organization of the body, and in particular of the brain, compared to that of the genome (see Kerszberg & Changeux, 1994; Smolen et al., 2000).

Many developmental genes are expressed in the nervous system. They are parts of a still largely uncharacterized population of genes concerned with brain morphogenesis: its segregation into definite patterns of areas and nuclei and even the differentiation of asymmetric hemispheres. The concepts mentioned for embryonic development may also apply to brain morphogenesis, in particular to the very early stage referred to as neurulation (see Kerszberg & Changeux, 1998). The process of neurulation differs strikingly in invertebrates and vertebrates. In the former case, the neuroblasts delaminate from the neural ectoderm to form progressively the solid ganglion chain of the adult (which may reach up to 520 million neurons in *Octopus*). In the latter, the neural plate invaginates *en bloc* to form a hollow neural tube which, as such, may facilitate a dramatic growth of the central nervous system through a surface expansion. This is observed from cyclostomes to mammals, primates and humans.

Such a decisive evolutive step is not fully understood. Yet, on strictly formal grounds, one may propose the hypothesis that it does not require a large number of molecular changes at the gene transcription level. These molecular transitions may, for instance, affect transcription factor switches which themselves regulate cell motion (Kerszberg & Changeux, 1998), as well as cell adhesion (see Edelman, 1987). As a consequence, either the whole neural plate infolds into a tube (in vertebrates) or individual neuroblasts delaminate, yielding a solid nervous system (in invertebrates). This illustrates hypothetically how only a few gene changes may contribute to the critical transition between the invertebrate and vertebrate nervous system.

Another example, even less well understood, is that of the fast expansion of the cerebral cortex that took place in the course of vertebrate brain evolution (see Changeux, 1983a,b; Mountcastle, 1998). The number of neurons per cortical column is uniform throughout vertebrates (Rockwell et al., 1980). Thus, the surface area of the cortex, i.e. the number of columns, appears as the primary target of the evolutionary changes (Rakic, 1988). One may further speculate that the fast expansion of the frontal lobe and parieto-temporal areas which contributed to the evolutionary origins of *Homo sapiens'* brain have resulted from the exceptionally prolonged action of some developmental genes (or of slight variation of concentration of morphogens) (Changeux, 1983a,b), the genomic evolution underlying this process engaging a rather small set of genes.

In the course of the subsequent development of the cellular organization of the nervous system, large populations of cells project into other large ensembles of neurons, and neural maps develop in regular species-specific patterns. The molecular mechanisms governing the formation of ordered connections of neural maps are progressively being understood and, again, a few molecular events are anticipated to modify dramatically the developmental patterns (for review see Tessier-Lavigne & Goodman, 1996; Drescher et al., 1997).

Many important anatomical features of our brain have been inherited from our direct ancestors (see Mountcastle, 1998; Changeux, 1983a,b). The soft parts of their brains may be lost forever, but comparison of the endocranial casts for modern man and fossil ancestors provides interesting information. It reveals striking analogies between the various stages of the phylogenetic evolution of the ancestors of *Homo sapiens* and the ontogenetic development of the brain in the modern human (Saban, 1995). The observations are limited to the impression of the meningeal veins and thus yield only limited information. Yet, the simplified topography of the human newborn meningeal system strikingly resembles the arrangement in *Australopithecus robustus* (who lived about 3–2 million years ago). With *Homo habilis*, who lived two million years ago (cranial capacity 700 ml) the meningeal topography is rather similar to that of a modern 40-day-old infant. *Homo erectus*, who lived one million years ago (cranial capacity of about 1000 ml), has a meningeal system topography similar to that of a modern 1-year-old child. Neanderthals (brain volume about 1500 ml, larger than modern *H. sapiens*) retained many archaic features of *H. erectus*. Recent DNA studies indeed suggest that they were only our cousins (Krings et al., 1997).

It is a highly controversial issue to infer from these rather scarce paleontological data how spoken language emerged. Chimpanzees use tools, have intricate social lives and show rudiments of self-awareness (Hauser, 1999). They utilize a number of vocalizations, but lack rapid manipulation of symbolic representations, as well as the capacity to form and organize abstract concepts. Monkeys have been claimed to possess the equivalent of Broca and Wernicke areas, although without the rich connectivity that characterizes language processing in humans (Aboitiz & Garcia, 1977; Deacon, 1997). Analysis of fossil skulls supports the view that the early evolution of the hominoid brain has included three major reorganizations (Holloway, 1995): a relative enlargement of the inferior parietal lobe, an expansion of the frontal lobe, and a greater hemispheric specialization occurring before major increases of brain volume. Similar conclusions are reached from a neuroanatomical perspective (Aboitiz & Garcia, 1997). This study more specifically points to the development of strong cortico-cortical cross-modal interactions in the postrolandic cortex, providing the basis of a semantic neural device that converges into a prospective Wernicke area in which concepts acquire their specific link with sound. These phonological representations project into inferoparietal areas which connect to Broca's area and the premotor representations of orofacial movements. Finally, a fundamental element in the evolution of linguistic capacity would be the coordinated operations of these networks which are required to generate higher levels of syntax and discourse associated with the expansion of prefrontal cortex, together with the development of its interconnections with the above-mentioned cortical (and subcortical) areas.

The morphology of the face and skull, as well as many body characteristics of human adults, resembles those of newborn chimpanzees (Stark & Kummer, 1962). It has thus been suggested that neoteny, i.e. access to sexual maturity at early stages of development and/or persistence of embryonic or fetal characters in the adult, together with prolonged development and increase of brain size after birth, contributed to the evolution of the human brain (see Gould, 1977). In any case, the intrinsic changes in the cellular organization of the brain that make us human are already present before birth and cannot be derived exclusively from neoteny; the proliferation of nerve cells largely (but not definitively) stops around 8 months of prenatal development (except in the hippocampus and cerebellum). Without doubt, in the newborn the brain already possesses a highly organized neuronal architecture determined by an envelope of genetically coded processes.

This conclusion has important medical consequences, since more than 3000 genetic diseases are known in man that correspond to gene mutations or defects. Many of them affect brain functions in one way or another (including some dyslexias) and are already expressed in the infant brain (see Mandel, 1995). At variance with the commonly accepted 'empiricist' point of view, the brain of the newborn is not a tabula rasa but a richly organized structure.

Individual variability of the human brain and the activity-dependent epigenesis of neuronal networks

Recent studies on human genomes carried out at the level of individuals have revealed an important inherent variability that may not systematically result in disease phenotypes. Indeed, about one base pair in 400–500 is polymorphic in the nuclear genome. Thus, two copies of the genome from different individuals will show about 1×10^6–2×10^6 sequence differences. The vast majority of these differences are selectively neutral but others may, as discussed, alter in a subtle way the function, or regulation, of a gene. Most of the polymorphism of the HLA region was already present in the ancestors of chimpanzees and gorillas before the separation of the human lineage (Gyllensten & Erlich, 1989). Heredity is thus often stated to be a major source of individual variability in the human brain. It may possibly account for significant variations in the precise topology of defined Brodman areas noticed among the few brains of different individuals investigated with the required anatomical accuracy (see Mountcastle, 1998). A significant variability also exists at the functional level. Joint positron emission tomography (PET) and magnetic resonance imaging (MRI) reveal significant intersubject variability of functional areas in the visual cortex in the range of 5 mm (Hasnain et al., 1998).

To analyse further the relative contribution of genetic vs. 'epigenetic' or environmental factors in this variability, a series of anatomical (see Steinmetz et al., 1995; Traino et al., 1998) and behavioural (see Kee et al., 1998) investigations were carried out with genetically identical monozygotic twins who were discordant for handedness. Both the in vivo measurements of the planum temporale by MRI and the results of behavioural tasks (e.g. finger tapping with anagram load) collected with left- and right-handed monozygotic co-twins yielded convergent results. The right handers showed leftward hemispheric asymmetry, whereas the left handers lacked symmetry. Early epigenetic events taking place during early embryogenesis may thus contribute significantly to variability in the development of the anatomo-functional laterality of the cerebral hemispheres in genetically identical twins. In other words, 'cloned' individuals are not anticipated to be neurally identical.

Another rather important cause of variability originates from the way the entire network of connections becomes established between neurons during embryonic and postnatal development. The million billion (10^{15}) synapses that form the human brain network do not assemble like the parts of a computer according to a plan which defines precisely the disposition of all individual components. If this were the case, the slightest error in the details for carrying out this programme could have catastrophic consequences. The mechanism appears, on the contrary, to rely on the progressive setting of robust interneuronal connections through trial-and-error mechanisms that, even though they are typically non-genetic, i.e. epigenetic, formally resemble an evolutionary process by variation selection (Changeux et al., 1973; Changeux & Danchin, 1976; Edelman, 1978, 1987).

Information about synaptogenesis in the developing brain may be provided by examining in the adult the variance of the synaptic phenotype of genetically identical individuals. The analysis has to be carried out at the level of the single nerve cell and of the exact topology of all the synaptic contacts it establishes with its partners. Such an analysis was achieved by serial sectioning the brain of parthenogenetic animals such as the water flea *Daphnia magna* and the fish *Poecilia formosa* (see Levinthal et al., 1976). At the electron microscope level, there exists a fringe of variability – a 'graininess' – in the details of the axonal or dendritic branching of an identifiable neuron, the variability between left and right arborisation being smaller than that found from one individual to another.

In a mammal such as the mouse – the situation might be even more extreme in humans – the number of cells is much greater and there are no longer identifiable single cells recognizable from one individual to another. Despite common principles in gross architectural features delimited by a species specific genetic envelope,

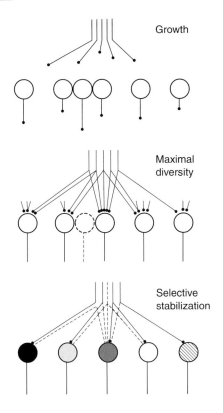

Fig. 1.3.   A simple representation of the model of epigenesis by selective stabilization of synapses (from Changeux, 1983b). An interesting outcome of the formal model is that after selection different patterns of connections may yield the same behavioural input–output relationship. The different shadings of the cell bodies indicate different neuron individualities or singularities.

the individual variability of the fine anatomy observed between individuals from genetically homogeneous strains increases dramatically, to the extent that one wonders how such an apparently scrambled connectivity may result in reproducible behaviour, even in identical twins!

One plausible solution (among many others) is that the state of activity of the developing nervous system contributes to the organization of the adult network by trimming up synapse formation at sensitive periods of development. The formal model suggested (Changeux et al., 1973; Changeux & Danchin, 1976; Edelman, 1978, 1987; Purves & Lichtman, 1980; Changeux, 1983a, b) relies on the observation that synapses do not form *en masse*, at once, but progressively, through exuberance followed by pruning steps, under the control of the state of activity of the developing network (Fig. 1.3). Throughout the overall development of the cortical mantle in primates and humans, several distinct phases may be recognised (Bourgeois et al.,

2000 and this volume). For instance, quantitative measurements of mean synaptic density in the developing human neocortex reveal that synaptogenesis begins before 27 weeks of gestation and continues actively during the first two postnatal years. The mean density reaches a maximum which differs between cortical regions: near post-natal age 3 months in the auditory cortex but after age 15 months in the late-maturing middle frontal gyrus (Huttenlocher & Dabholkar, 1997). A phase of net increase in mean synaptic density occurs late in childhood, where it ends earlier in auditory cortex (until 12 years) than in prefrontal cortex (until mid-adolescence). Most likely, this global evolution of mean synaptic density represents the summation of 'nested' waves of synapse outgrowth and elimination, the later process becoming dominant and thus visible for the evolution of the net density later in development (Huttenlocher & Dabholkar, 1997; Bourgeois, this volume). Examination of synaptogenesis in simpler systems, at the single cell (or even single synapse) level, for instance, in the cerebellum confirms this interpretation.

Concomitant phases of proliferation and regression already take place in the generation of the nerve cell layers of the spinal cord, or of the cerebral cortex. The classical observation of Hamburger (1975) that about 40% of the motor neurons die in the chick embryo between the 6th and the 9th days of embryonic life is now further documented in the mouse for the cerebral cortex. Enzymes such as caspase 3 and caspase 9 must be expressed for a cell to die. Interestingly, inactivating their genes in the mouse reduces apoptosis, increases the number of founder and precursor cells, of radial cortical units and thus of cortical neurons. As a result, the cortical surface expands and even forms the beginnings of sulci and microgyri in this lissencephalic brain (Kuida et al., 1996, 1998). The extent to which the state of activity of the developing nervous system controls such proliferative vs. apoptotic steps is still debated. Yet, correlations have been established between cell death and neuronal activation, a well-documented case being that caused by calcium entry mediated by glutamate NMDA receptors (Nicotera et al., 1999). The example of the neuromuscular junction is particularly simple since only a single synaptic contact persists in the adult. On the other hand, in the newborn rat, each muscle fibre receives four or five active motor axon terminals. As the rat begins to walk, the number of these functional terminals progressively decreases until for the adult only one is left and the state of activity of the innervated muscle controls this elimination (e.g. Benoit & Changeux, 1975, 1978, see Sanes & Lichtman, 1999). Similar regressive phenomena have also been documented at the synaptic level in other systems such as the sympathetic ganglia (Purves & Lichtman, 1980) or the climbing fibre Purkinje cell synapse in the cerebellum (for review, see Crépel, 1982; Changeux & Mikoshiba, 1978; Kano et al., 1997). For the latter, a mutation which inactivates a specific neurotransmitter receptor (the type 1 metabotropic glutamate receptor mGluR1) delays the regression of supernumerary climbing fibre innervation (Kano et al., 1997).

The contribution of synaptic activity (evoked and/or spontaneous) in the formation of cortical circuits has been well documented since the classic experiments of Wiesel and Hubel (1963), which demonstrated the important role of visual experience in fixing the organization of ocular dominance columns (for review, see Katz & Shatz, 1996). The exuberant sprouting and proliferation of axon branches, accompanied by limited though critical elimination of collaterals, has been visualized at different locations along the visual pathway (retinogeniculate, thalamocortical, and pyramidal cell arbours) (see Stretavan & Shatz, 1986; Katz & Shatz, 1996) at sensitive periods of development. The state of activity of the developing cortical circuits controls synaptic evolution by more than simply validating preformed circuits (Wiesel & Hubel, 1963). Such epigenetic regulation may concern the overall development up to elementary social experience (see Hadders-Algra et al., 1996).

The model suggested (Changeux et al., 1973; Changeux, 1983a, b; see also Harris et al., 1997; Elliott & Shadbolt, 1998; Miller, 1998) posits that during synapse formation the genetic envelope controls, in addition to the division, migration and differentiation of cell categories, the behaviour of the growth cone, the outgrowth and formation of widespread connections, the recognition of the target cells and the onset of spontaneous activity; it also determines the structure of the molecules that enter into the architecture of the synapse, the rules governing their assembly, and the evolution of this connecting link by the activity of the network. Yet, at sensitive periods of circuit development, the phenotypic variability of nerve cell distribution and position, as well as the exuberant spreading and the multiple figures of the transiently formed connections originating from the erratic wandering of growth cone behaviour, introduce a maximal diversity that is then reduced by the selective stabilization of some of the labile contacts and the elimination (or retraction) of the others. The crucial hypothesis of the model is that the evolution of the connective state of each synaptic contact is governed globally, and within a given time window, by the overall 'message' of signals experienced by the cell on which it terminates. In other words, the activity of the postsynaptic cell regulates the stability of the synapse in a retrograde manner (Changeux et al., 1973).

Among the various consequences of the modelling approach, a simple one has been to look for the molecular mechanisms of the regulation of synaptic outgrowth, stabilization and elimination by neural activity. At the presynaptic level, neurotrophins like NGF, BDNF, NT4 and several others (for review, see Levi-Montalcini, 1987; Barde, 1990) have become plausible candidates for retrograde signals in activity-dependent synaptic outgrowth and selection (Thoenen, 1995; Katz & Shatz, 1996; Zhang et al., 1998). For instance, in vivo intracortical infusion of diverse neurotrophins prevents the shift of ocular dominance in favour of the eye which has not been deprived of visual experience (Maffei et al., 1992; Carmignoto et al., 1993) on the formation of ocular dominance columns (Cabelli et al., 1995). Also, rapid and opposite effects of BDNF and NGF have been demonstrated on the whisker barrel representation of the rat somatosensory cortex. Moreover, neurotrophins modulate synaptic strength within minutes in vitro at cultured neuromuscular synapses (Lohof et al., 1993) and GDNF overexpression in the mouse delays the elimination of supernumerary motor axons and causes hyper-innervation of neuromuscular junctions (Nguyen et al., 1998). Additional evidence for a contribution of neurotrophins in epigenetic regulation of synapse development is the observation that their synthesis and release from dendrites are regulated by neuronal activity (Thoenen, 1995). Formal models of synapse-selective stabilization based on competition for limited stocks of trophic factors have been developed (Gouzé et al., 1983; Harris et al., 1997; Elliott & Shadbold, 1998; Miller, 1998), giving plausibility to the theory.

On the postsynaptic side, the molecular mechanisms involved in the development of the postsynaptic domain and in the respective role played by factors released by the afferent nerve and by electrical activity are becoming progressively understood, in particular in the simple case of the neuromuscular junction (Duclert & Changeux, 1995; Sanes & Lichtman, 1999). The methods of recombitant DNA technology have led to the demonstration that, within the multinucleated adult muscle fibre, only the nuclei located under the afferent motor nerve express the subjunctional molecules such as the nicotinic acetylcholine receptor subunits. On the other hand, in the extrajunctional nuclei, the receptor genes that were transcribed in the non-innervated myotubes become repressed by electrical activity in the adult. Denervation that silences the muscle fibres causes a reactivation of transcription in the extrajunctional nuclei.

The DNA regulatory elements and transcription factors which bind to these elements and are selectively involved in the transcriptional regulation of acetylcholine receptor genes in the junctional and extrajunctional compartments have been identified, together with the intracellular second messenger systems, establishing the membrane-to-gene link (Schaeffer et al., 1998). Trophic factors released from the motor nerve (such as ARIA-heregulin) bind to a tyrosine kinase receptor and initiate a cascade of signals including a MAP kinase. On the other hand, electrical activity propagated in the extrajunctional domain causes the entry of Ca^{2+} ions, and activates a serine/threonine kinase (see Schaeffer et al., 1998). In both cases, a differential phosphorylation/dephosphorylation of distinct transcription factors takes place (Altiok et al., 1997; Schaeffer et al., 1998). Post-transcriptional regulatory mechanisms involving molecules from both the basal lamina and the cytoskeleton also contribute to the targeting, clustering and stabilization of the receptor molecules that compose the postsynaptic domain (see Duclert & Changeux, 1995; Sanes & Lichtman, 1999). These post-transcriptional mechanisms become predominant in the formation and stabilization of neuronal synapses (Betz, 1998; Xia et al., 1999). As mentioned, the genes that make the difference between worm and yeast include, among other numerous copies of tyrosine kinase, protein phosphatase and transcription factor genes (Ruvkun & Hobert, 1998). A molecular biology of the epigenetic regulation of synapse formation has emerged.

Brain epigenetic capacities to store stable representations of the outside world give human beings the opportunity to create an artificial world of cultural objects at the social level. The considerable increase of synapse numbers and multiple nested processes of synapse stabilization, which take place postnatally in the human brain, makes possible the acquisition of spoken and written language, among many other social representations. But this epigenetic evolution has another consequence: the diversification of the cultures that human beings have developed throughout their recent history. In other words, the postnatal epigenetic evolution of brain connectivity opens the way to cultural evolution.

Representations, reward and consciousness in the infant brain

Wittgenstein, in his *Philosophical Investigations*, wondered how human beings can understand each other despite so many language differences. He suggested that the identity of the representations we build up in our mind (I would say in our brain) develops from shared 'language games' or 'experiments' that we play as infants, but also continuously throughout our lives as adults. For him the final criterion when somebody else possesses this representation is 'what he says and what he does' in other words what use he makes in his current life of this particular representation. For the neurobiologist, Wittgenstein raises a serious issue. Will it ever be possible to identify the postulated 'common element' in the brain of social partners who understand each other. We know, from the previous chapter, that the detailed connectivity of the brain may vary considerably from one individual to the other, even among identical twins.

A first reassuring statement comes from the mathematical formalization of the synapse selection model. It is the theorem that within a developing network 'the same afferent message may stabilize different arrangements of connections which nevertheless result in the same input-output relationship' (Changeux et al., 1973; Changeux, 1983a,b). This may explain why the variability of the connectivity found between isogenic animals and *a fortiori* between non-isogenic ones may be behaviourally tolerable for the organism. This contrasts with Edelman's (1998) claim that because of such variability there should not be any code or representation in the stored traces of past experience. The way memories are stored in the brain is not expected to resemble those of our computer devices. But, some code nevertheless has to exist which allows reproducible behaviours and, even, shared understanding within the social group (with a common semantic) between individuals possessing anatomically variable brains. What might constitute such codes?

It has been widely accepted since Hebb (1949) that the representations, images, ideas or mental states which form in our brain spontaneously, or as a consequence of interactions with the outside world (including the sociocultural one), can be identified as the physical state created by the correlated (or coherent) transient and dynamic activity, both electrical and chemical, in a defined distributed population (or assembly) of neurons (see Gray et al., 1992; Vaadia et al., 1995). The graph of the neurons mobilized together with the frequency and coherence of the impulses flowing in the graph is anticipated to carry the 'meaning' or, following de Saussure, the 'signifié' (signified). How does a shared, neurally coded, *signifié* emerge? First of all, the commonality of meaning between different individuals may simply result from shared hard-wired species-specific circuits of the infant brain. These are the 'conspecs' of Johnson and Morton (1991) which, for instance, account in the infant brain for recognition of conspecific faces or speech sounds, in addition to elementary behaviours such as grasping or sucking. On the other hand, very early on, the newborn learns features, for instance those unique to the mother's voice or face. These are the 'conlerns' of Johnson and Morton. Within the framework of learning by selection (see Changeux, 1983a, b; Dehaene & Changeux, 1989), such learned *signifiés* would result from the selective stabilization of fleeting prerepresentations spontaneously produced by the infant's brain.

The conjecture is that the brain would generate 'crude', transient and labile prerepresentations – or hypotheses – that vary from one instant to the other. The infant brain would thus operate in a projective way (see Changeux, 1983a, b; Berthoz, 1997) constantly testing hypotheses on the outside world and later on its own inner world. Several plausible mechanisms may lead to the selection of the relevant prerepresentation and to its storage as a stable synaptic and/or neuronal but also semantic trace in the brain. A simple one (Dehaene & Changeux, 1989; Edelman & Tononi, 1996; Montague et al., 1996, Schütz et al., 1997) is based on the reward (or punishment) received from the outside world that would ultimately result in the release of reward substances, e.g. dopamine, acetylcholine or serotonin. Accordingly, the efficacies of the synapses concerned would change if, for instance, the reward neurotransmitter reached the surface of the neurons at the moment (or after a defined delay) they were actively mobilized by the relevant prerepresentation. Such a reading of time coincidence could be accomplished, for instance, by 'multihead' molecules, named allosteric proteins, which include neurotransmitter receptors (see Dehaene & Changeux, 1989, 1991; Changeux & Edelstein, 1998). Those receptors are known to undergo slow regulatory transitions of potentiation and/or desensitization, which can be regulated by a variety of effectors, in particular phosphorylation (see Changeux & Edelstein, 1998). Yet, at this stage, their precise contribution to the storage of 'meaningful' representations remains to be documented.

At a higher social level, what could be the actual mechanisms that result in a shared representation within the brains of different social partners? One possible mechanism in the case, for instance, of mother and child, could involve a 'shared attention' toward a common object or referent which would accompany its designation by eye movements, gestures, and finally verbal utterances (De Brysson-Bandis, 1998). The *signifiant–signifié* link would progressively become established, first by selection of the *signifiés* via 'cognitive games' which, subsequently, would develop in authentic 'language games' between the child and his parents, partners or teachers. Then, another distinction has to be made. The same referent resulting in the same neurally stored *signifié* may plausibly be viewed as shared by all members of the human species, in other words be universal, but this is not to be anticipated for the arbitrary *signifiants* which are known to vary from one language to another.

Recent brain imaging experiments support this distinctive point of view. In bilingual individuals who learned their second language after the age of 7, the first language production (or listening) systematically activated a similar set of areas, while the production (or listening) of the second language activated partially different and individually variable areas (Kim et al., 1997; Dehaene et al., 1997). Secondly, when subjects are presented with pictures and the corresponding words in letters, modality specific activation occurs in different areas for words (left inferior parietal lobule) and for pictures (right middle occipital gyrus), while a semantic network common to both words and pictures extends, in a distributed manner, from the occipital and temporal cortex to the frontal lobe (Vandenberghe et al., 1996; see also Gorno Tempini et al., 1998). Moreover, different regions of the brain are mobilized by different semantic knowledge, such as knowledge about the body parts or about numbers (Le Clerc et al., 2000). Such distributed category-specific activation of the cerebral cortex appears largely reproducible from individual to individual at the macroscopic (centimetric scale) level. Yet, a significant variability is anticipated at the microscopic synaptic level. A plausible scheme which simultaneously accommodates macroscopic constancy, local variability, and universality of the semantic representation relies on the notion that it is not the precise anatomical connectivity between identifiable neurons which counts (as it does in *Caenorhabditis* nervous system). Rather a common 'functional pattern' of connections, as opposed to a precise geometry, is selected by 'shared' learning. The functional pattern of the connections as, for instance, a common menu of neurons sampled from a variety of brain areas, would then neurally implement the semantic code. It is an important issue for further studies to define to what extent such neural anatomy of semantics displays (or not) analogies with the semantic networks postulated by linguists.

The newborn infant is an emotionally reactive sentient being. But he (or she) must still develop what makes human beings rational and self-conscious. These psychological functions progressively build up, in the following years, together with the memories of the semantic lexicon. The prefrontal cortex becomes accessible to delayed response tasks by 12 months (Diamond, 1991). A working memory and global workspace (see below) starts to contribute to cognitive tasks, for instance those which are no longer automatic and demand a conscious mental effort. Global regulatory circuits that provide, in particular, reward and vigilance inputs (such as the mesocortical catecholaminergic neurons and cholinergic pathways) progressively develop their adult pattern of connections.

The neural bases of consciousness have been, in recent years, the subject of intense debates (Baars; Crick; Posner; Edelman; Llinas; Damasio; in Dehaene et al., 1998) (Fig. 1.4), which are outside the scope of this review (see Searle, 2000). I will only mention recent modelling studies aimed at elaborating neural architectures able successfully to carry conscious effort demanding tasks. Accordingly, in simplified, formal terms, two main computational spaces can be distinguished in the brain (Dehaene et al., 1998).

The first is a processing network composed of parallel, distributed and functionally encapsulated processors ranging from primary (or even heteromodal) sensory processors and which include motor processors. A second is what can be referred to as a global workspace (Baars, 1989) consisting of a distributed set of cortical neurons characterized by their ability to receive impulses from, and send them back to, homologous neurons in other cortical areas by horizontal projections through long-range excitatory axons. Pyramidal cells from layers 2 and 3, which are particularly abundant in dorsal lateral prefrontal and inferoparietal cortical structures, may be postulated to contribute to this workspace in a privileged manner.

The model posits (Dehaene et al., 1998) that, in a 'conscious' task, workspace neurons become spontaneously coactivated forming discrete, though variable, spatiotemporal patterns (some kinds of global prerepresentations) subject to modulation by vigilance signals and to selection by reward signals. Such workspace activation interconnects multiple brain processors (and suppresses the contribution of others), which would otherwise be mobilized (or extinguished) independently. As a consequence, the organism performs cognitive tasks requiring cross-modal processing such as the Stroop task (which involves the distinction between the colour words and the colour of the ink used to print the word). Such a scheme accounts in particular for the brain imaging data. In particular, it predicts the active, though transient, mobilization of the dorsolateral prefrontal cortex and anterior cingulate areas, which are known to contain a very high proportion of layer 2 and 3 long range excitatory neurons.

The model is still at a primitive stage of formalization and suffers from shortcom-

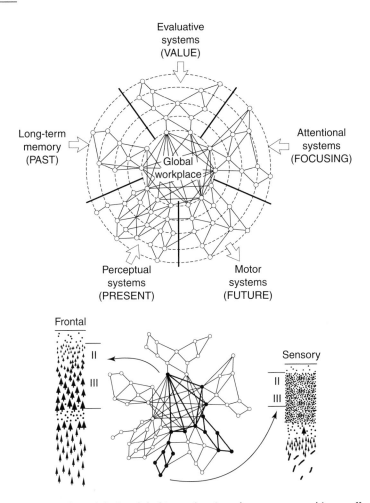

Fig. 1.4.   A neuronal model of a global 'conscious' workspace engaged in an effortful cognitive task. The global workspace is composed of distributed and heavily interconnected neurons with long range axons originating, principally, from layers two and three from the cerebral cortex. The multiple processors (here 5) are modular and informationally encapsulated. Workspace neurons (abundant in frontal type cortex) are mobilized in effortful, multimodal, tasks for which the specialized processors do not suffice and regulate in a top-down manner the activity of specific processor neurons (from Dehaene et al., 1998).

ings. It should integrate, in the future, the connection to the workspace of self-representations that might allow the simulated organism to reflect on its own internal processes. Longer-term research should also include the more elaborate dynamic organization of nested workspace units (Dehaene & Changeux, 1997) and auto-evaluation loops (Dehaene & Changeux, 1991). Modelization of the linguistic proposition and of rational reasoning in terms of neural network is still a far-fetched enterprise. Yet, in any case, imaging of the infant brain and of its postnatal development is anticipated to bring essential information on the development of the neural bases of higher brain functions including thought and consciousness!

Conclusions

These reflections on the origins of the human brain are still fragmentary and rather speculative. They nevertheless illustrate the urgent need for adequate theories (or models) which establish neurally plausible links between the anatomy and molecular biology, the physiology and biochemistry and the actual behaviour with the world as well as the 'tacit' mental states which arise in the infant brain.

Aware that the whole sequence of the human genome is known, the overall philosophy of the neurosciences is anticipated to shift from a strictly 'reductionist' point of view to a 'reconstructionist' approach. Knowing all the genes which serve as building blocks of the human being, the emphasis will be to understand the molecular and cellular networks of interaction which yield the so-called 'complexity' of the human brain. The task is immense and may not yield a unique answer. The 'epigenetic' internalization of the personal history of each individual, together with the social and cultural environment in which he/she developed, raises tremendous problems of analysis and formalization. In any case, the brain of each human individual will meld, in a singular manner, multiple nested evolutions by variation selection: the genetic evolution of the species, together with the many epigenetic evolutions of the experiences and memory traces stored within the brain but also outside the brain as a cultural heritage of civilizational history.

Still promising, but increasingly difficult, will thus be the scientific understanding (in neuronal terms) of particularly elaborate cognitive functions such as those involved in aesthetic judgement (see Changeux, 1994) and the genesis of moral norms. These functions include, for instance, the attribution of mental state to others (theory of mind), the so-called moral emotions such as sympathy and/or violence inhibition and, of course, the ability to integrate past memories and present information into a decision-making process leading to action in a social world (see Changeux & Ricoeur, 1998 for references). Yet, one should not forget that all these elaborate cognitive processes become established in the human brain under conditions in which the infant and the child are never in social isolation but, on the contrary, constantly interacting with other human beings. If the spontaneous tendency exists for the biologist to consider the human brain as an independent and autonomous object of science, this is a misleading endeavour. First of all, during postnatal development, interaction with parents, playmates and classmates leads to the spontaneous acquisition of the maternal oral language. Subsequently, but then with considerable effort, the child acquires written language. The deep traces left in the human brain by alphabetization underlines the dramatic importance of early training (Castro-Caldas et al., 1998) in the connectivity and performance of the adult brain.

Pedagogy, according to Premack, is a unique attribute of human beings, and the early social environment in which the child is embedded also marks each infant brain by the particular culture and thus the history of the social community to which his or her parents belong. This constitutes, by its diversity, an unlimited source of innovation (Levi-Strauss, 1961). But, on a world scale, it may also be a source of ethnic conflict. In-between the universality of the human species and the diversity of cultures, the brain makes the synthesis. It is a wish of neuroscientists that a better understanding of our brain will help to reconcile these opposing tensions.

Acknowledgments

We thank Professor Stuart Edelstein and Matilde Cordero-Erausquin for their suggestions about the manuscript.

This work was supported by grants from the Collège de France, Centre Nationale de la Recherche Scientifique (CNRS), l'Association Française contre les Myopathies, and EEC Biotech program.

REFERENCES

Aboitiz, F. & Garcia, R. (1997). The evolutionary origin of the language areas in the human brain. A neuroanatomical, perspective. *Brain Research Reviews*, 25, 381–96.

Altiok, N., Altiok, S. & Changeux, J-P. (1997). Heregulin-stimulated acetylcholine receptor gene expression in muscle: requirement for MAP kinase and evidence for a parallel inhibitory pathway independent of electrical activity. *EMBO Journal*, 16, 717–25.

Baars, B. J. (1989). *Cognitive Theory of Consciousness*. Cambridge: Cambridge University Press.

Barde, Y. A. (1990). The nerve growth factor family. *Progress in Growth Factor Research*, 2, 237–48.

Benoit, P. & Changeux, J-P. (1975). Consequences of tenotomy on the evolution of multiinnervation on developing rat soleus muscle. *Brain Research*, 99, 354–8.

Benoit, P. & Changeux, J-P. (1978). Consequences of blocking the nerve with a local anaesthetic on the evolution of multiinnervation at the regenerating neuromuscular-junction of the rat. *Brain Research*, 149, 89–96.

Berthoz, A. (1997). Parietal and hippocampal contribution to topokinetic and topographic memory. *Philosophical transactions of the Royal Society of London*, Série B, 352, 1437–48.

Betz, H. (1998). Gephyrin a major player in GABAergic postsynaptic membrane assembly. *Nature Neuroscience*, 1, 541–43.

Bourgeois, J. P., Goldman-Rakic, P. S. & Rakic, P. (2000). Formation, elimination and stabilization of synapses in the primate cerebral cortex. *The Cognitive Neurosciences*, ed. M. Gazzarriga. Cambridge, MA: MIT Press.

Cabelli, R. J., Hohn, A. & Shatz, C. J. (1995). Inhibition of ocular dominance column formation by infusion of NT4/5 or BDNF. *Science*, **267**, 1662.

Carmignoto, G., Canella, R., Candeo, P., Cornelli, M. C. & Maffei, L. (1993). Effects of nerve growth factor on neuronal plasticity of the kitten visual cortex. *Journal of Physiology*, **464**, 343–60.

Castro Calds, A., Petersson, K. M., Reis, A., Stone-Elander, S. & Ingvar, M. (1998). The illiterate brain: learning to write and read during childhood influences the functional organization of the adult brain. *Brain*, **121**, 1053–63.

Changeux, J-P. (1983a). Concluding remarks on the 'singularity' of nerve cells and its ontogenesis. *Progress in Brain Research*, **58**, 465–78.

Changeux, J-P. (1983b). '*L'Homme neuronal*'. Fayard: Paris. English translation: (1985). '*Neuronal man*'. Princeton University Press.

Changeux, J-P. (1985). Genetic determinism and epigenesis of neuronal network: is there a biological compromise between Chomsky and Piaget? In *Language and Learning: The Debate Between Jean Piaget and Noam Chomsky*, ed. M. Piattelli-Palmarini, pp. 184–202.

Changeux, J-P. (1994). *Raison et plaisir*. Paris: Odile Jacob, 1994.

Changeux, J-P. (1998). Drug and abuse. *Journal of the American Academy of Arts and Sciences, Daedalus*, **127**, 145–65.

Changeux, J-P. & Connes, A. (1989). *Matière à pensée*. Paris: Odile Jacob. [English translation: Conversations on mind, matter and mathematics, 1991. Princeton University Press.]

Changeux, J-P. & Danchin, A. (1976). Selective stabilization of developing synapses as a mechanism for the specification of neuronal networks. *Nature*, **264**, 705–12.

Changeux, J-P. & Edelstein, S. (1998). Allosteric receptor after 30 years. *Neuron*, **21**, 959–80.

Changeux, J-P. & Mikoshiba, K. (1978). Genetic and epigenetic factors regulating synapse formation in vertebrate cerebellum and neuromuscular junction. In *Maturation of the Nervous System*, ed. M. A. Comer et al., *Progress in Brain Research*, **48**, pp. 43–64.

Changeux, J-P. & Ricoeur, P. (1998). *La nature et la règle*. Paris: Odile Jacob.

Changeux, J-P., Courrège, P. & Danchin, A. (1973). A theory of the epigenesis of neural networks by selective stabilization of synapses. *Proceedings of the National Academy of Sciences, USA*, **70**, 2974–8.

Chervitz et al. (1998). Comparison of the complete protein sets of worm and yeast: orthology and divergence. *Science*, **282**, 2022–8.

Crépel, F. (1982). Regression of functional synapses in the immature mammalian cerebellum. *Trends in Neuroscience*, **5**, 266–9.

Deacon, T. (1997). *The Symbolic Species*. New York: W.W. Norton & Co.

De Brysson-Bardis, B. (1998). Comment la parole vient aux enfants. Paris: O. Jacob.

Dehaene, S. & Changeux, J-P. (1989). A simple model of prefrontal cortex function in delayed-response tasks. *Journal of Cognitive Neuroscience*, **1**, 244–61.

Dehaene, S. & Changeux, J-P. (1991). The Wisconsin card sorting test: theoretical analysis and simulation of a reasoning task in a model neuronal network. *Cerebral Cortex*, **1**, 62–79.

Dehaene, S. & Changeux, J-P. (1997). A hierarchical neuronal network for planning behavior. *Proceedings of the National Academy of Sciences of the USA*, **94**, 13293–8.

Dehaene, S., Dupoux, E., Mehler, J. et al. (1997). Anatomical variability in the cortical representation of first and second language. *NeuroReport*, **17**, 3775–8.

Dehaene, S., Kerszberg, M. & Changeux, J-P. (1998). A neuronal model of a global workspace in effortful cognitive tasks. *Proceedings of the National Academy of Sciences, USA*, **95**, 14529–34.

Diamond, J. (1991). Neurophysical insights into the meaning of object concept development. In *The Epigenesis of Mind: Essays on Biology and Cognition*, ed. S. Carey & R. Gelman, pp. 67–110, Erlbaum Ass.

Drescher, U., Bonhoeffer, F. & Muller, B. K. (1997). The Eph family in retinal axon guidance. *Current Opinion in Neurobiology*, **7**, 75–80.

Duclert, A. & Changeux, J-P. (1995). Acetylcholine receptor gene expression at the developing neuromuscular junction. *Physiological Reviews*, **75**, 339–68.

Edelman, G. (1978). *The Mindful Brain: Cortical Organization and the Group-selective Theory of Higher Brain Function*. Cambridge MA: MIT Press.

Edelman, G. (1987). *Neural Darwinism. The Theory of Neuronal Group Selection*. New York: Basic Books.

Edelman, G. (1998). Building a picture of the brain. *Journal of the American Academy of Arts and Science, The Brain*, **127**, 37–69.

Edelman, G. & Tononi, G. (1996). *Selection and Development: The Brain as a Complex System. Behavioral, Neurobiological and Psychosocial Perspectives*, ed. T. G. D. Magnusson, L. G. Nilsson, B. Windbald, T. Hökfelt & L. Terenius, pp. 107–38. Cambridge: Cambridge University Press.

Elliott, T. & Shadbolt, N. R. (1998). Competition for neurotrophic factors: mathematical analysis. *Neural Computation*, **10**, 1939–81.

Fodor, J. (1976). *The Language of Thought*. Hassocks, UK: The Harvester Press.

Gorno Tempini, M. L., Price, C. J., Josephs, O. et al. (1998). The neural systems sustaining face and proper name processing. *Brain*, **121**, 2103–18.

Gould, S. J. (1977). *Ontogeny and Phylogeny*. Cambridge MA: Harvard University Press.

Gouzé, J. L., Lasry, J. M. & Changeux, J-P. (1983). Selective stabilization of muscle innervation during development: a mathematical model. *Biological Cybernetics*, **46**, 207–15.

Gray, C. M., Engel, A. K., König, P. & Singer, W. (1992). Synchronisation of oscillatory neuronal responses in cat striate cortex: temporal properties. *Visual Neuroscience*, **8**, 337–47.

Gyllensten, U. B. & Erlich, H. A. (1989). Ancient roots for polymorphism at the HLA-D Q alpha locus in primates. *Proceedings of the National Academy of Sciences of the USA*, **86**, 9986–90.

Hadders-Algra, M., Brogren, E. & Forssberg, H. (1996). Ontogeny of postnatal adjustments during sitting in infancy, variation, selection and modulation. *Journal of Physiology*, **493**, 273–88.

Hamburger, V. (1975). Cell death in the development of the lateral motor column of the chick embryo. *Journal of Comparative Neurology*, **160**, 535–46.

Harris, A. E., Bard Ermentront, G. & Small, S. L. (1997). A model of ocular dominance column development by competition, for trophic factors. *Proceedings of the National Academy of Sciences of the USA*, **94**, 9944–9.

Hasnain, M. K., Fox, P. T. & Woldorff, M. (1998). Intersubject variability of functional areas in the human visual cortex. *Human Brain Mapping*, **6**, 301–15.

Hauser, M. (1999). *Wild Minds*. Cambridge MA: Harvard University Press.

Hebb, D. O. (1949). *The Organization of Behavior: A Neuropsychological Theory*. New York: Wiley.

Hodgkin, J., Horvitz, H. R., Jasny, B. R. & Kimble, J. (1998). *C. elegans*: sequence to biology. *Science*, **282**, 2011–46.

Holloway, R. (1995). Toward a synthetic theory of human brain evolution. In *Origins of the Human Brain*, ed. J-P. Changeux and J. Chavaillon, pp 42–60. Oxford: Oxford University Press.

Huttenlocher, P. & Dabholkar, A. (1997). Regional difference in synaptogenesis in human cerebral cortex. *Journal of Comparative Neurology*, **387**, 167–78.

Jacob, F. (1981). *Le jeu des possibles*. Fayard: Paris.

Johnson, M. & Morton, J. (1991). *Biology and Cognitive Development. The Case of Face Recognition*. Oxford: Blackwell.

Kano, M., Hashimoto, K., Kurihara, H. et al. (1997). Persistent multiple climbing fiber innervation of cerebellar Purkinje cells in mice lacking mGluR. *Neuron*, **B18B**, 71–9.

Katz, L. C. & Shatz, C. J. (1996). Synaptic activity and the construction of cortical circuits. *Science*, **274**, 1133–8.

Kee, D. W., Cherry, B., McBride, D. & Segal, N. (1998). Multi task analysis of cerebral hemisphere specialization in monozygotic twins discordant for handedness. *Neuropsychology*, **12**, 468–78.

Kerszberg, M. (1996). Accurate reading of morphogen concentrations by nuclear receptors: a formal model of complex transduction pathways. *Journal of Theoretical Biology*, **183**, 95–104.

Kerszberg, M. & Changeux, J-P. (1994). A model for reading morphogenetic gradients: autocatalysis and competition at the gene level. *Proceedings of the National Academy of Sciences of the USA*, **91**, 5823–7.

Kerszberg, M. & Changeux, J-P. (1998). A simple molecular model of neurulation. *BioEssays*, **20**, 758–70.

Kim, K., Relkin, N., Lee, K. M. & Hirsch, J. (1997). Distinct cortical areas associated with native and second languages. *Nature*, **388**, 171–4.

Koch, C. & Laurent, G. (1999). Complexity of the nervous system. *Science*, **284**, 96–8.

Krings, M., Stone, A., Schmitz, R.W., Krainitzki, H., Stoneking, M. & Paabo, S. (1997). Neanderthal DNA sequences and the origin of modern humans. *Cell*, **90**, 19–30.

Kuida, K., Zheng, T., Na, S. et al. (1996). Decreased apoptosis in the brain and premature lethality in CPP32-deficient mice. *Nature*, **384**, 368–72.

Kuida, K., Haydan, T., Kuan, C. et al. (1998). Reduced apoptosis and cytochromic-mediated caspase activation in mice lacking caspase 9. *Cell*, **94**, 325–37.

Lander, E. S., Linton, L. M., Birren, B. et al. (2001). International Human Genome Sequencing Consortium. Initial sequencing and analysis of the human genome. *Nature*, **409** (6822), 860–921.

Lawrence, P. (1992). *The Making of a Fly*. Oxford: Blackwell.

Le Clerc', H., Dehaene, S., Cohen, L. et al. (1999). Category specific representation of words independent of language and input modality. *Proceedings of the National Academy of Sciences, USA*, (in press).

Levi-Montalcini, R. (1987). The nerve growth factor: thirty five years later. *Science*, **237**, 1154–62.

Levi-Strauss, C. (1961). *Race et histoire*. Gonthiers: UNESCO.

Levinthal, F., Macagno, E. & Levinthal, L. (1976). Anatomy and development of identified cells in isogenic organisms. *Journal of Theoretical Biology*, **40**, 321–31.

Lisman, J. & Fallon, J. F. (1999). What maintains memories. *Science*, **283**, 339–40.

Lohof, A. M., Ip, N. Y. & Poo, M. M. (1993). Potentiation of developing neuromuscular synapses by the neurotrophins NT-3 and BDNF. *Nature*, **363**, 350–3.

Maffei, L., Berardi, N., Domenici, L., Parisi, V. & Pizzorusso, T. (1992). Nerve growth factor (NGF) prevents the shift in ocular dominance distribution of visual cortical neurons in monocularly deprived rats. *Journal of Neuroscience*, **12**, 4651–62.

Mandel, J. L. (1995). The human genome. In *Origins of the Human Brain*, ed. J-P. Changeux and J. Chavaillon, pp. 42–60. Oxford: Oxford University Press.

Mannervik, M., Nibu, Y., Zhang, H. & Levine, M. (1999). Transcriptional coregulators in development. *Science*, **284**, 606–9.

Meinhardt, H. & Gierer, A. (1974). Application of a theory of biological pattern formation based on lateral inhibition. *Journal of Cell Science*, **15**, 321–46.

Miklos, G. L. & Rubin, G. M. (1996). The role of the genome project in determining gene function: insights from model organisms. *Cell*, **86**, 521–9.

Miller, K. (1998). Equivalence of a sprouting-and-retraction model and correlation-based plasticity models of neural development. *Neural Computation*, **10**, 529–47.

Montague, P. R., Dayan, P. & Sejnowski, T. J. (1996). A framework for mesencephalic dopamine systems based on predictive Hebbian learning. *Journal of Neuroscience*, **16**, 1936–47.

Mountcastle, V. (1998). *Perceptual Neuroscience: The Cerebral Cortex*. Cambridge, MA: Harvard University Press.

Nguyen, Q. T., Parsadanian, A. S., Snider, W. D. & Lichtman, J. (1998). Hyperinnervation of neuromuscular junctions caused by GDNF overexpression in muscle. *Science*, **279**, 1725–9.

Nicotera, P., Leist, M. & Manzo, L. (1999). Neuronal cell death: a demise with different shapes. *Trends in Pharmacology*, **20**, 46–51.

Nüsslein Volhard, C. (1990). Axis determination in the *Drosophila* embryo. *Harvey lecture*, **86**, 129–148.

Purves, D. & Lichtman, J. (1980). Elimination of synapses in the developing nervous system. *Science*, **210**, 153–7.

Rakic, P. (1988). Specifications of cerebral cortical areas. *Science*, **241**, 170–6.

Rockwell, A., Hiorns, R. & Powell, T. (1980). The basic uniformity in structure of the neocortex. *Brain*, **103**, 221–4.

Rubin, G. M., Yandell, M. D., Wortman, J. R. et al. (2000). Comparative genomics of the eukaryotes. *Science*, **287** (5461), 2204–15.

Ruvkun, G. & Hobert, O. (1998). The taxonomy of developmental control in *Caenorhabditis elegans*. *Science*, **282**, 2033–40.

Saban, R. (1995). Image of the human fossil brain: endocranial casts and meningeal vessels in young and adult subjects. In *Origins of the Human Brain*, ed. J-P. Changeux and J. Chavaillon, pp. 11–41. Oxford: Oxford University Press.

Sanes, J. R. & Lichtman, J. W. (1999). Development of the vertebrate neuromuscular junction. *Annual Review of Neuroscience*, **22**, 389–42.

Schaeffer, L., Duclert, N., Huchet, M. & Changeux, J-P. (1998). Implication of an Ets and Notch related transcription factor in synaptic expression of the nicotinic acetylcholine receptor. *EMBO Journal*, **17**, 3078–90.

Schütz, W., Dayan, P. & Montague, R. A. (1997). A neural substrate of prediction and reward. *Science*, **275**, 1593–9.

Searle, J. (1995). *The Construction of Social Reality*. New York: Free Press.

Searle, J. (2000). Consciousness. *Annual Review of Neuroscience*, **23**, 557–79.

Shallice, T. (1988). *From Neuropsychology to Mental Structure*. New York: Cambridge University Press.

Smolen, P., Baxter, D. & Byrne, J. (2000). Mathematical modeling of gene networks. *Neuron*, **26**, 567–80.

Stack, D. & Kummer, B. (1962). Zur Ontogenese des Schimpanzenschädels. *Anthropologie Anz*, **25**, 204–15.

Steinmetz, H., Hergoz, A., Schlang, G., Huang, Y. & Jäncke, L. (1995). Brain asymmetry in monozygotic twins. *Cerebral Cortex*, **5**, 296–300.

Stretavan, D. W. & Shatz, C. J. (1986). Prenatal development of retinal ganglion cell axons: segregation into eye-specific layers within the cat's lateral geniculate nucleus. *Journal of Neuroscience*, **6**, 234–51.

Tessier-Lavigne, M. & Goodman, C. S. (1996). The molecular biology of axon guidance. *Science*, **274**, 1123–33.

Thoenen, H. (1995). Neurotrophins and neuronal plasticity. *Science*, **270**, 593–8.

Thom, R. (1990). *Apologie du Logos; Ambiguïté de la Complexité en Biologie*. Paris: Hachette.

Tononi, G. & Edelman, G. (1998). Consciousness and complexity. *Science*, **282**, 1846–51.

Traino, M. J., Loftus, W. C., Stukel, T. A., Green, R. L., Weaver, J. B. & Gazzaniga, M. S. (1998). Brain size, head size and intelligence quotient in monozygotic twins. *Neurology*, **50**, 1246–52.

Turing, A.M. (1952). The chemical basis of morphogenesis. *Philosophical Transactions of the Royal Society London B*, **237**, 37–72.

Vaadia, E., Haalman, I., Abeles, M. et al. (1995). Dynamics of neuronal interactions in monkey cortex in relation to behavioural events. *Nature*, **373**, 515–18.

Vandenberghe, R., Price, C., Wise, R., Josephs, O. & Frackowiak, R. S. J. (1996). Functional anatomy of a common semantic system for words and pictures. *Nature*, **383**, 254–6.

Venter, J. C., Adams, M. D., Meyers, E. W. et al. (2001). The sequence of the human genome. *Science*, **291** (5507), 1304–51.

Watson, J. (1976). *Molecular Biology of the Gene*. Volumes I and II, 4th edn. The Benjamin/Cummings Publishing Company Inc.

Wiesel, T. & Hubel, D. (1963). Effects of visual deprivation on morphology and physiology of cells in the cat's lateral geniculate body. *Journal of Neurophysiology*, **26**, 978–93.

Xia, J., Zhang, X., Staudinger, J. & Huganir, R. L. (1999). Clustering of AMPA receptors by the synaptic PDZ domain-containing protein PiCK1. *Neuron*, **22**, 179–87.

Zhang, L. I., Tao, W. W., Holt, C. E., Harris, W. A. & Poo, M. M. (1998). A critical window for cooperation and competition among developing retinotectal synapses. *Nature*, **395**, 37–44.

2

Molecular mechanisms for organizing the developing central nervous system

Nilima Prakash and Urban Lendahl

Department of Cell and Molecular Biology, Medical Nobel Institute, Karolinska Institute, Stockholm, Sweden

The aim of this chapter is to discuss how the central nervous system (CNS) is generated during development, and the rapid progress that is made in deciphering the underlying molecular programmes for this process. Particular emphasis is placed on the discussion of genes which are directly relevant for human CNS malformations.

The morphology of the developing CNS

In the human and in other vertebrates, the early aspects of nervous system development proceed through a set of stereotypical intermediate steps. The first evidence of the formation of a nervous system appears at the dorsal side of the gastrula-stage embryo where, in a process called neural induction, the chordamesoderm makes the overlaying ectoderm form the neural plate or neuroectoderm, which may comprise as much as 50% of the ectoderm. The neural induction process is only partly understood, but at least in lower vertebrates it appears that formation of the neuroectoderm is the default choice, and that formation of non-neural ectoderm at either side is achieved by blocking signalling through the bone morphogenetic protein (BMP) receptor system. BMP signalling can be blocked by expression of the BMP antagonists noggin, chordin and follistatin (Chitnis, 1999). The bending of the neural plate to form the neural groove is accomplished by forces exerted through both the neural plate cells and the surrounding epidermis (Fig. 2.1). The notochord induces these cells to decrease in height and to become wedge shaped, giving rise to the neural groove (van Straaten et al., 1988; Smith & Schoenwolf, 1989). Shortly thereafter, the edges of the neural plate thicken and move upward to form the neural folds. The cells in the regions formed near the ectoderm boundaries increase in height and become wedge-shaped as well. At the same time, the surface ectoderm pushes towards the centre of the embryo, providing another motive force for the bending of the neural plate (Alvarez & Schoenwolf, 1992). Eventually, the neural folds adhere to each other and the cells from the two folds merge, closing the neural

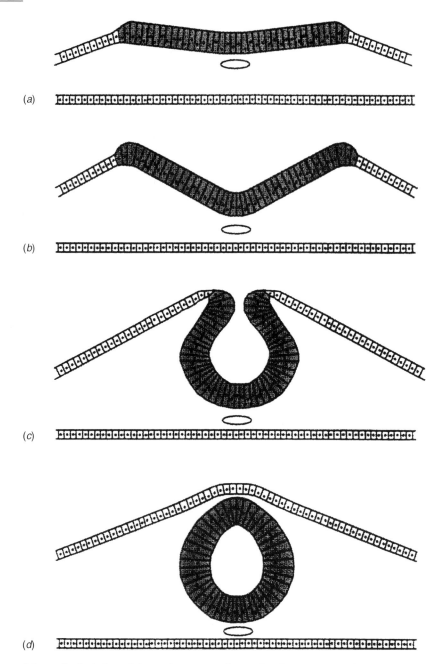

(a)

(b)

(c)

(d)

Fig. 2.1.   Schematic depiction of the early aspects of CNS development, seen in a cross-section of a
mammalian embryo. (*a*) The first sign of nervous system formation is the appearance of
the neural plate at the dorsal side of the embryo. The notochord is located beneath the
neural plate in the midline. (*b*, *c*) The neural plate folds and forms the neural groove.
(*d*) The neural folds fuse and the neural tube is generated. It is then pinched off from the
dorsal ectoderm, which fuses and forms the epidermis. (Reprinted with permission from
Frisén et al., 1998, Birkhauser Publishers Ltd.)

groove to the neural tube (Fig. 2.1). Thus, formation of the neural tube is mainly accomplished by changes in cell shape and cell–cell interactions of committed ectodermal cells, whereas cellular proliferation contributes up to this point only to a minor extent. The cells in the junctional region of the neural folds and later of the neural tube form the neural crest cells, which will migrate away and generate the peripheral nervous system, the pigment cells of the skin and several other cell types.

In mammals, including man, neural tube closure is initiated at several positions along the anterior–posterior axis. Failure to close the neural tube results in neural tube defects. Lack of closure of the rostral neural pore leads to anencephaly, while failure to close the caudal pore results in spina bifida. The frequency of neural tube defects is affected both by chemical compounds such as the antiepileptic drug valproic acid and by genetic determinants, i.e. neural tube defects are more common in certain human populations. We are only beginning to understand which genes are important for neural tube closure, but mutations in the Pax 3 gene (see below) can cause neural tube defects and also result in Waardenburg's syndrome, which affects neural crest derivatives (Baldwin et al., 1992). Furthermore, functional inactivation of certain genes in 'knock out' mice similarly results in neural tube defects, which provides further molecular insights into this process. Examples of such genes are Hes 1 (Ishibashi et al., 1995) and Twist (Chen & Behringer, 1995). Mutations in the human TWIST gene cause the Saethre–Chotzen syndrome, an autosomal dominant craniosynostosis disorder (Howard et al., 1997).

The newly closed neural tube is composed of a single layer of highly proliferative cells. Cell lineage experiments, both in vivo and in primary culture, reveal that these proliferating cells can, in addition to self-renewal, give rise to all major classes of cell types in the CNS, i.e. both neurons and glial cells (McKay, 1997). They are therefore called CNS stem cells, in contrast to developmentally more committed CNS progenitor cells that give rise to either neurons or glial cells and may constitute the majority of proliferating cells later in embryonic development (Williams & Price, 1995). The CNS stem cells are organized as a pseudostratified columnar epithelium of neuroectodermal cells spanning from the inner, ventricular, to the outer, pial, side of the neural tube (Fig. 2.2). They typically have a bipolar morphology and undergo complex morphogenetic changes called interkinetic movements as they progress through the cell cycle: their elongated nuclei lie in the luminal half of the ventricular zone during the G1 phase of the cell cycle, and migrate into the pial half during the S phase, when replication of DNA occurs (Fig. 2.2). They translocate back again toward the ventricular surface in the G2 phase. Simultaneously, cells detach from the pial side and the pial processes collapse; they then divide at the ventricular surface of the neural tube. After completion of mitosis, the pial process is re-extended toward the basal surface by both daughter cells or, alternatively, one cell differentiates to a neuron and migrates out from the columnar neuroepithelium (see below) (Sauer, 1935; for review, see Jacobson, 1991).

CNS stem cells can proliferate either by symmetric or asymmetric cell division. Symmetric cell division often generates two new stem cells. In contrast, asymmetric cell division generates one stem cell and one cell that can undergo differentiation. CNS stem cells are thought to proliferate predominantly by symmetric cell divisions, which builds up a population of stem cells, and later more by asymmetric cell divisions, to generate differentiated progeny (Huttner & Brand, 1997). Thus, the initial single cell layer of the neural tube is converted to a multilayer structure where the CNS stem cells are confined to the inner, ventricular layer, and the newly formed daughter cells migrate outwards to specified layers of the developing cortical plate and spinal cord. During this migratory phase, the young postmitotic neurons are guided by specialised cells, the radial glial cells. Radial glial cells are very elongated cells which traverse the thickened neural tube from the ventricular to the outer pial side (Rakic, 1988). These cells are anchored by endfeet structures to both surfaces of the neural tube, and they retain their extended morphology throughout the cell cycle (Fig. 2.2).

Sustained proliferation of the CNS stem cells in the germinal epithelium of the neural tube, which is then called ventricular zone (and, later, ependymal layer), leads to more and more committed progeny as development of the nervous system proceeds. These daughter cells migrate out of the ventricular zone and form a second layer around the original neural tube, which becomes progressively thicker as more cells are added to it, and is called the mantle or intermediate zone. Postmitotic neurons residing in this zone will establish a pattern of axonal connections among themselves. Eventually, glial cells will cover many of these axons in myelin sheaths. This cell-poor region containing the axonal network of the underlying neurons is called the marginal zone and constitutes the outmost layer of the developing brain and spinal cord. In the spinal cord and medulla, this basic pattern of three layers is retained throughout development. In the brain, however, the three-layer arrangement is modified later in development. After their final mitosis, most of the newly generated neurons migrate radially along the glial processes out from the ventricular zone and establish the highly organized structure of the mammalian neocortex consisting of six vertical layers (ventricular or ependymal, subventricular and intermediate zone, subplate, cortical plate, and marginal zone). Those neurons that were born first form the layers closest to the ventricular zone. Neurons that are born subsequently migrate through these regions to form the more superficial layers of the cerebral cortex. Formation of the mammalian neocortex therefore follows an 'inside-out' gradient of development (Rakic, 1974). Exceptions to this general pattern of cortical development are found in the cerebellum and the hippocampus, where cohorts of progenitor cells migrate away from the ventricular zone, later to form neurons and glial cells.

Formation of the various layers in the cortex is a delicate process which, when

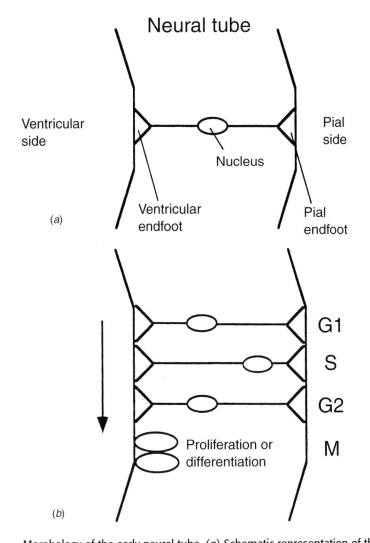

Fig. 2.2.   Morphology of the early neural tube. (*a*) Schematic representation of the early neural
              tube, which at this stage consists of a single-cell layer organized as a columnar
              neuroepithelium. The bipolar neuroepithelial cells are attached at the ventricular and pial
              sides by endfeet structures. (*b*) The process of interkinetic movements, in which the
              nucleus of the neuroepithelial cell relocates during the cell cycle. During the G phase, the
              nucleus is located closer to the ventricular side, whereas during the S phase it is located
              closer to the pial side. During the M phase, the cell detaches from the pial side and
              undergoes cell division close to the ventricular side. The cell progeny can then remain as
              undifferentiated cells in the neural tube or, alternatively, migrate out from the
              neuroepithelium to differentiate into a neuron. (Reprinted with permission from Frisén et
              al., 1998, Birkhauser Publishers Ltd.)

disturbed, leads to CNS malformations in humans. The genetic disease X-linked lissencephaly, or double-cortex, causes a disruption of the structure of the six-layered cortex. The gene causing X-linked lissencephaly was recently cloned and named doublecortin, and it encodes a putative intracellular signal transduction protein (Gleeson et al., 1998; des Portes et al., 1998). There is also a mouse mutant, Reeler, which exhibits impaired cortical layering. The corresponding gene, reelin, encodes an extracellular matrix protein, reelin, which plays a role for neurons to exit from radial glial cells (Goffinet, 1997). A second protein acting downstream in the reelin signalling pathway, mouse disabled 1 (mdabl1), shows some structural similarities to doublecortin, indicating the possibility of a conserved intracellular signalling system for formation of cortical layers.

Patterning in the early CNS

At the same time as the cytoarchitecture of the future brain and spinal cord is being established, the different CNS regions will gradually acquire spatial identities. Morphological changes reflect in the generation of the anlagen of fore-, mid- and hindbrain, including the rhombomeres along the rostro-caudal (or anterior–posterior) axis (for review, see Lumsden & Krumlauf, 1996). Patterning is defined as the subdivision into distinct territories by the expression of certain genes or combinations of genes. In mammals, it is clear that a first crude pattern along the rostro-caudal axis of the emerging neuroectoderm is already established during neural induction in the gastrula-stage embryo, although the precise molecular mechanisms underlying it remain unclear. However, it appears that the prechordal mesoderm, which is the rostralmost continuation of the notochord, specifies rostral, head-specific features, while the notochord itself induces only more caudal neural tissue (for review, see Lumsden & Krumlauf, 1996; Rubenstein & Beachy, 1998). As formation of the neural tube is completed, patterning is seen along the rostro–caudal axis as well as along the dorsal–ventral axis. Some of the genes that will be discussed below are summarized in Fig. 2.3.

The rostral–caudal axis

Along the rostro-caudal axis, patterning is most conspicuous for the expression of various transcription factors, in particular for members of the clustered homeobox-containing genes of the Hox family (capitalized as HOX genes in humans). The four Hox gene clusters (A-D) in the mouse and human genome, consisting of 39 genes in total, are homologous to the homeotic gene complex (HOM-C) in *Drosophila*, which controls parasegment identity in the fly. These gene clusters show a remarkable evolutionary conservation in both flies and mammals, in that structurally equivalent genes are arranged in the same order on the respective chromosomes and show similar expression patterns along the rostro-caudal axis of the

Rostro-caudal axis   *Dorso-ventral axis*

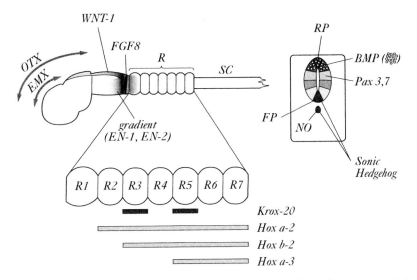

Fig. 2.3.   Schematic representation of a mammalian embryo seen along the rostro-caudal axis (left) or along the dorsal–ventral axis (right). Some genes important for the patterning along these two axes are depicted in the figure. These genes are also discussed in the text. T, telencephalon; D, diencephalon; M, midbrain; R, rhombomeres; SC, spinal cord; RP roof plate; NT, neural tube; FP, floor plate; NO, notochord.

embryo. This has led to the assumption that the four mammalian Hox complexes have evolved from the fly complex through gene duplications and deletions (Hunt & Krumlauf, 1992). Hox genes are expressed throughout the developing neural tube from the anterior boundary of the hindbrain to the tail, including neural crest, paraxial mesoderm, surface ectoderm and their derivatives. Strikingly, the order in which the genes of each cluster are positioned along the respective chromosomes is largely colinear with the order of their expression domains along the rostro-caudal axis of the embryo. The role of Hox gene expression has been best studied in the rhomberic patterning of the chick and mouse hindbrain and at somite boundaries further caudally in the embryo (Wilkinson et al., 1989; Kessel & Gruss, 1991; for review see Mark et al., 1997).

The highly defined expression pattern of the murine Hox genes has led to the formulation of the 'Hox code' hypothesis, whereby particular combinations of Hox genes would specify the segmental identity along the rostro-caudal axis. Support for a Hox code comes from different approaches. First, gene targeting experiments, in which a single Hox gene has been knocked out in mouse embryos, show that the loss of function of a Hox gene generally results in anteriorization of the corresponding region in which this gene is normally expressed, i.e. structures that are normally observed in this region are lacking or replaced by structures corresponding to more rostrally located segments (for reviewed, see Krumlauf, 1994). However, comparison of the defects observed in null mutants in which Hox genes with overlapping expression domains have been deleted, and analysis of double mutants lacking two genes of paralogous set reveal that there are extensive functional synergies between paralogous Hox genes (Gavalas et al., 1998).

Secondly, exposure of mouse embryos in utero to excess doses of retinoic acid (RA) results in posteriorization of the regional fate in the developing hindbrain, i.e. anterior rhombomeres assume the identity of more posterior rhombomeres (Marshall et al., 1992). This is caused by the induction of anterior expression of Hox genes that are normally expressed only in more posterior domains along the rostro-caudal axis. A similar posteriorizing effect is observed when Hox genes are expressed ectopically in the hindbrain or after injection of a constitutively active RA receptor (RAR) into the embryo (Zhang et al., 1994; Blumberg et al., 1997). The opposite effect, i.e. the anteriorization of the regional fate, is observed after injection of a dominant-negative RAR. These results are consistent with a direct induction of Hox gene expression by binding of ligand/RAR complexes to RA response elements in the upstream regulatory regions of some Hox genes (Studer et al., 1994; Gould et al., 1998), and provide a molecular explanation to the teratogenic effects observed after exposure to RA. Thirdly, comparison of Hox gene expression in different types of vertebra among different species reveals that the pattern of Hox gene expression predicts the type of vertebra that will be formed (Burke et al., 1995).

Taken together, these findings pose the question: which are the upstream regulators of Hox gene expression setting up this highly ordered expression pattern? So far, it has been shown that Krox-20, a zinc finger transcription factor expressed in two stripes of the neural plate that will become rhombomeres 3 and 5 (Wilkinson et al., 1989), can directly regulate the expression of Hoxa-2 and Hoxb-2 in these two rhombomeres (Nonchev et al., 1996). Targeted disruption of the Krox-20 gene results in embryos lacking rhombomeres 3 and 5 and showing a partial fusion of rhombomeres 2, 4 and 6 in the hindbrain region (Schneider-Manoury et al., 1993). Long-range signalling from the isthmic constriction, a region located close to the junction of the mesencephalon (midbrain) and rhombencephalon (hindbrain) may also play a role in regulating Hox gene expression. Signalling from this region is mainly controlled by a secreted molecule, fibroblast growth factor 8 (FGF8). FGF8 is first expressed in the axial mesoderm underlying the presumptive isthmic region of the neural plate and later in transverse stripe within the isthmus (Crossley & Martin, 1995). FGF8 can directly induce expression of its own gene and two other genes involved in midbrain patterning, Wnt-1 and En-2 (Crossley et al, 1996; Lee, 1997), homologues to the *Drosophila* genes Wingless and Engrailed, respectively. Wnt-1 is expressed in the neural plate in a region corresponding to the future midbrain and later in a ring of cells lying immediately anterior to the FGF-8-secreting cells of the isthmus. Secretion of Wnt-1 is required for maintenance but not induction of En-1 and En-2 gene expression (McMahon et al., 1992), which is critically involved in the specification of rostro-caudal polarity in the midbrain/hindbrain junctional region. The two Engrailed (En) genes of the mouse, En-1 and En-2, are expressed in a gradient that decreases both rostrally and caudally from the isthmus region and are required for formation of the tectum (dorsal midbrain) and the cerebellum (anterior hindbrain) (for review, see Joyner, 1996).

Patterning of the rostralmost neural tube corresponding to the forebrain region is less well understood, but involves the localized expression of specific homeobox-containing transcription factors (Shimamura & Rubenstein, 1997). In the mouse embryo, Emx-1, Emx-2, Otx-1 and Otx-2, which are homologues of the *Drosophila* homeobox-containing genes Ems (empty spiracles) and Otd (orthodenticle), respectively, are expressed in a similar nested array in the forebrain and midbrain region, as are the Hox genes in more posterior regions (Boncinelli et al., 1993). Evidence for a role of the Otx genes in brain development comes from gene targeting experiments in which the mouse Otx-1 and Otx-2 genes have been deleted. The Otx-2 null mutants lack forebrain and midbrain structures, consistent with an anterior patterning function during early neurulation stages (Acampora et al., 1995). Otx-1 knockout mice, in contrast, show no early phenotype (Acampora et al., 1996) but Otx1$^{-/-}$; Otx2$^{+/-}$ compound mutants lack midbrain and caudal forebrain structures and have a rostrally expanded cerebellum, coincident with a rostrally extended expression boundary of FGF8 from the isthmus region (which would normally delimit the posteriormost expression domain of Otx genes) (Acampora et al., 1997; Suda et al., 1997). The developmental distortions after targeted mutation of the two Emx genes in mice are restricted to the dorsal telencephalon (the rostralmost part of the forebrain), corresponding to their restricted expression domain (Yoshida et al., 1997; Boncinelli et al., 1993). In keeping with this, mutations in the human EMX-2 gene lead to severe defects in the structure of the cerebral cortex, a condition that is known as schizencephaly (Faiella et al., 1997). In conclusion, the currently available data suggest that rostro-caudal patterning of the early CNS is accomplished by a strict temporally and spatially regulated expression of: (i) transcription factors; and (ii) diffusible factors such as retinoids and FGF8, which in turn affect either directly or indirectly the transcription of other genes. The sequential action of induced and repressed genes subsequently confers a specific identify to each region of the developing neural tube.

The dorsal–ventral axis

The dorsal–ventral patterning events are similar along the entire neuraxis, and will therefore be largely referred here to the developing spinal cord. Generation of dorsal cell types is controlled by signals from the dorsal (epidermal) ectoderm at the lateral borders of the neural plate, whereas generation of ventral cell types is triggered by signals from the notochord and prechordal mesoderm underlying the midline of the neural plate. Two secreted signalling molecules with opposing activities play a crucial role in the first steps of dorso-ventral identity specification in the neural tube: bone morphogenetic proteins (BMPs) and Sonic Hedgehog (Shh). BMPs are members of the transforming growth factor-β (TGF-β) superfamily and are produced by cells located at the boundary between the neuroectoderm of the neural plate and the lateral epidermal ectoderm (for review, see Mehler et al., 1997). After neural tube closure, several BMPs are expressed in overlapping domains along the dorsal midline ectoderm (Liem et al., 1995). Although BMPs initially block the neural cell fate during gastrulation, they induce dorsal cell types in the neural tube by promoting the expression of Pax and Msx genes. These genes encode transcription factors, and expression of the Pax3 and Pax7 genes is required for specification and differentiation of neural crest cells (a 'dorsal' cell type) in the mouse (for review, see Mansouri et al., 1996). Although the precise mechanism of BMP action in the dorsal neural tube is still unknown, it is thought that BMPs control the sequential generation of dorsal cell types (neural crest cells, roof plate cells and dorsal sensory relay interneurons) by contact-mediated induction of both BMP and other regulatory genes in responsive neural cells, thus achieving a long-range patterning action in this region (Liem et al., 1995). Recent evidence suggests that, on the other hand, inhibition of BMP signalling in the ventral neural tube by one of its antagonists, Noggin, is essential for maintenance of Shh-induced (see below) ventral cell types (McMahon et al., 1998).

Shh is one of three members of the vertebrate Hedgehog family of secreted glycoproteins that were identified by their structural similarity to the *Drosophila* segment polarity gene Hedgehog (for review, see Hammerschmidt et al., 1997). Shh is initially expressed throughout the axial mesoderm, i.e. notochord and prechordal plate, and later also in floor plate cells lying at the ventral midline of the neural tube (Ericson et al., 1996). Shh may be secreted from both notochord and floor plate cells and subsequently diffuse from this site, thereby establishing a concentration gradient within the ventral neural tube. Ectopic expression of Shh can induce ventral cell types, and mouse Shh null mutants show a loss of ventral structures throughout the CNS (Echelard et al., 1993; Chiang et al., 1996). These results are consistent with a pivotal role of Shh for specification of the ventral fate in the neural tube. Shh appears to act through repression and induction of specific transcription factors in a concentration-dependent manner along the dorso-ventral axis of the neural tube (for review, see Tanabe & Jessell, 1996). Among the transcription factors directly controlled by Shh are the paired box containing proteins of the Pax family, which in turn control specification of cell fates in the neural tube. The Pax 3 and Pax7 genes, for example, are expressed initially along the mediolateral region of the neuroectoderm, but are rapidly repressed in the medial neural plate by a Shh-mediated signal. After neural tube closure, the Pax3 and Pax7 expression domain is restricted to proliferating cells in the dorsal neural tube (Liem et al, 1995; Ericson et al., 1996). Repression of Pax 3 and Pax7 in the ventral neural tube seems to be a condition necessary for specification of ventral cell types, such as floor plate cells, motor neurons and ventral interneurons. The final generation of motor neurons and ventral interneurons, however, requires a second phase of Shh signalling, during which the Pax6 gene product plays a key role in specifying the identities of these cells (Ericson et al., 1996, 1997).

Although most of the previously discussed roles of Shh signalling were discerned in the part of the neural tube corresponding to the future spinal cord, recent evidence also stresses the importance of Shh signalling from the prechordal mesoderm for formation of the ventral forebrain (for review, see Rubenstein & Beachy, 1998). The defects observed in Shh knock-out mice include absence of ventral forebrain structures and a failure to subdivide the eye field, which results in the formation of a cyclopic eye, while the remainder of the forebrain develops as a single, undivided vesicle (Chiang et al., 1996). A similar phenotype is observed in the most severe form of human holoprosencephaly (for review, see Ming & Muenke, 1998) and, indeed, mutations in the coding region of the human Shh gene are associated with an autosomal dominant form of human holoprosencephaly in several pedigrees (Roessler et al., 1996). Mutations in several other loci are also associated with human holoprosencephaly and other developmental disorders, and it appears that they affect genes located in the Shh downstream signalling pathway (Ming et al., 1998).

The vertebrate Hedgehog proteins are synthesized as larger precursors that undergo autoproteolytic cleavage to generate the biologically active amino-terminal fragments (Porter et al., 1995). During the autocatalytic processing, cholesterol is covalently attached to the carboxy-terminus of the amino-terminal fragment of the Shh protein, resulting in an increased hydrophobicity that tethers the molecule to the cell membrane (Porter et al., 1996a). This, in turn, may restrict the diffusibility of the biologically active Shh protein, so that the vast majority of Shh synthesized by the notochord and floor plate cells remains associated with the surface of these cells (Roelink et al., 1995). On the other hand, the incomplete transfer of the cholesterol moiety during the autocatalytic reaction or a postprocessing cleavage of the cholesterol adduct from the active Shh molecule may render a diffusible form of this protein with teratogenic effects (Porter et al., 1996b). Recently, mutations in the carboxy-terminal fragment of the Shh protein, responsible for the autocatalytic cleavage and cholesterol transfer to the amino-terminal fragment, have been associated with several cases of familial and sporadic human holoprosencephaly (Roessler et al., 1997). Moreover, perturbations of the cholesterol metabolism in pregnant rats, ewes and in humans all lead to development of holoprosencephalic phenotypes in the offspring, suggesting that these perturbations affect the Shh signalling pathway (for review, see Rubenstein & Beachy, 1998). Transduction of the Shh signal appears to involve the transmembrane proteins Patched and Smoothened (for review, see Ingham, 1998). Recent studies have revealed the presence of a sterol-sensing domain in the Patched protein (Loftus et al., 1997). Thus, disorders in the cholesterol metabolism, in addition to mutations of the Shh gene, may affect either the synthesis and secretion of active Shh or the ability of target tissues to sense and transduce the Shh signal. Support for the latter view comes from a study showing that late-acting inhibitors of cholesterol biosynthesis do not prevent the sterol modification of Shh (Cooper et al., 1998). Another recent report, however, reveals that the teratogenic effects of cyclopamine, a steroidal alkaloid from the plant *Veratrum californicum*, rely most likely on a cholesterol-independent, direct inhibition of Shh signal transduction (Incardona et al., 1998).

Conclusions

Rapid progress is currently being made in deciphering the molecular programmes that control the early aspects of CNS development. As discussed in the review, many of these molecular programmes are evolutionarily highly conserved, which means that questions can constructively be approached in a wide range of species, including flies, nematodes, mice and man. The accumulation of new data about neural tube closure, formation of layers in the cortex and patterning along the two major body axes has led to the identification of some of the genes involved in human CNS malformations, and it is likely that the next few years will provide us with many more exciting discoveries in this area.

REFERENCES

Acampora, D., Mazan, S., Lallemand, Y. et al. (1995). Forebrain and midbrain regions are deleted in Otx2−/− mutants due to a defective anterior neuroectoderm specification during gastrulation. *Development*, **121**, 3279–90.

Acampora, D., Mazan, S., Avantaggiato, V. et al. (1996). Epilepsy and brain abnormalities in mice lacking the Otx1 gene. *NatureGenetics*, **14**, 218–22.

Acampora, D., Avantaggiato, V., Tuorto, F. & Simeone, A. (1997). Genetic control of brain morphogenesis through Otx gene dosage requirement. *Development*, **124**, 3639–50.

Alvarez, I. S. & Schoenwolf, G. C. (1992). Expansion of surface epithelium provides the major extrinsic force for bending of the neural plate. *Journal of Experimental Zoology*, **261**, 340–8.

Baldwin, C. T., Hoth, C. F., Amos, J. A., da-Silva, E. O. & Milunsky, A. (1992). An exonic mutation in the HuP2 paired domain gene causes Waardenburg's syndrome. *Nature*, **355**, 637–8.

Blumberg, B., Bolado, J. J., Moreno, T. A., Kintner, C., Evans, R. M. & Papalopolu, N. (1997). An essential role for retinoid signaling in anteroposterior neural patterning. *Development*, **124**, 373–9.

Boncinelli, E., Gulisano, M. & Broccoli, V. (1993). Emx and Otx homeobox genes in the developing mouse brain. *Journal of Neurobiology*, **24**, 1356–66.

Burke, A. C., Nelson, A. C., Morgan, B. A. & Tabin, C. (1995). Hox genes and the evolution of vertebrate axial morphology. *Development*, **121**, 333–46.

Chen, Z-F. & Behringer, R. R. (1995). Twist is required in head mesenchyme for cranial neural tube morphogenesis. *Genes and Development*, **9**, 686–99.

Chiang, C., Litingtung, Y., Lee, E. et al. (1996). Cyclopia and defective axial patterning in mice lacking *Sonic hedgehog* gene function. *Nature*, **383**, 407–13.

Chitnis, A. B. (1999). Control of neurogenesis – lessons from frogs, fish and flies. *Current Opinions in Neurobiology*, **9**, 18–25.

Cooper, M. K., Porter, J. A., Young, K. E. & Beachy, P. A. (1998). Teratogen-mediated inhibition of target tissue response to Shh signaling. *Science*, **280**, 1603–7.

Crossley, P. H. & Martin, G. R. (1995). The mouse Fgf8 gene encodes a family of polypeptides and is expressed in regions that direct outgrowth and patterning in the developing embryo. *Development*, **121**, 439–51.

Crossley, P. H., Martinez, S. & Martin, G. M. (1996). Midbrain development induced by FGF8 in the chick embryo. *Nature*, **380**, 66–8.

des Portes, V., Pinard, J. M., Billuart, P. et al. (1998). A novel CNS gene required for neuronal migration and involved in X-linked subcortical laminar heterotopia and lissencephaly syndrome. *Cell*, **92**, 51–61.

Echelard, Y., Epstein, D. J., St-Jacques, B. et al. (1993). Sonic hedgehog, a member of a family of putative signaling molecules, is implicated in the regulation of CNS polarity. *Cell*, **75**, 1417–30.

Ericson, J., Morton, S., Kawakami, A., Roelink, H. & Jessell, T. (1996). Two critical periods of *Sonic hedgehog* signaling required for the specification of motor neuron identity. *Cell*, **87**, 661–73.

Ericson, J., Rashbass, P., Schedl, A. et al. (1997). Pax6 controls progenitor cell identity and neuronal fate in response to graded Shh signaling. *Cell*, **90**, 169–80.

Faiella, A., Brunelli, S., Granata, T. et al. (1997). A number of schizencephaly patients including two brothers are heterozygous for germline mutations in the homeobox gene EMX2. *European Journal of Human Genetics*, **5**, 186–90.

Frisén, J., Johansson, C. B., Lothian, C. & Lendahl, U. (1998). Central nervous system cells in the embryo and adult. *Cellular and Molecular Life Sciences*, **54**, 935–45.

Gavalas, A., Studer, M., Lumsden, A., Rijli, F. M., Krumlauf, R. & Chambon, P. (1998). Hox a1 and Hox b1 synergise in patterning the hindbrain, cranial nerves and second pharyngeal arch. *Development*, **125**, 1123–36.

Gleeson, J. G., Allen, K. M., Fox, J. W. et al. (1998). Doublecortin, a brain-specific gene mutated in human X-linked lissencephaly and double cortex syndrome, encodes a putative signaling protein. *Cell*, **92**, 63–72.

Goffinet, A. M. (1997). Unscrambling a disabled brain. *Nature*, **389**, 668–9.

Gould, A., Itasaki, N. & Krumlauf, R. (1998). Initiation of rhombomeric Hoxb4 expression requires induction by somites and a retinoid pathway. *Neuron*, **21**, 39–51.

Hammerschmidt, M., Brook, A. & McMahon, A. P. (1997). The world according to hedgehog. *Trends in Genetics*, **13**, 14–21.

Howard, T. D., Paznekas, W. A., Green, E. D. et al. (1997). Mutations in TWIST, a basic helix–loop–helix transcription factor, in Saethre–Chotzen syndrome. *Nature Genetics*, **15**, 36–41.

Hunt, P. & Krumlauf, R. (1992). Hox codes and positional specification in vertebrate embryonic axes. *Annual Review of Cell Biology*, **8**, 227–56.

Huttner, W. B. & Brand, M. (1997). Asymmetric division and polarity of neuroepithelial cells. *Current Opinion in Neurobiology*, **7**, 29–39.

Incardona, J. P., Gaffield, W., Kapur, R. P. & Roelink, H. (1998). The teratogenic Veratrum alkaloid cyclopamine inhibits sonic hedgehog signal transduction. *Development*, **125**, 3553–62.

Ingham, P. W. (1998). Transducing Hedgehog: the story so far. *EMBO Journal*, **17**, 3505–11.

Ishibashi, M. Ang, S-L., Shiota, K., Nakanishi, S., Kageyama, R. & Guillemot, F. (1995). Targeted disruption of mammalian *hairy* and *Enhancer of split* homolog-1 (HES-1) leads to up-regulation of neural helix–loop–helix factors, premature neurogenesis, and severe neural tube effects. *Genes and Development*, **9**, 3136–48.

Jacobson, M. (1991). *Developmental Neurobiology.* New York: Plenum Publishing Corp.

Joyner, A. L. (1996). Engrailed, Wnt and Pax genes regulate midbrain–hindbrain development. *Trends in Genetics*, **12**, 15–20.

Kessel, M. & Gruss, P. (1991). Homeotic transformations of murine vertebrae and concomitant alteration of hox codes induced by retinoic acid. *Cell*, **67**, 89–104.

Krumlauf, R. (1994). Hox genes in vertebrate development. *Cell*, **78**, 191–201.

Lee, J. E. (1997). Basic helix–loop–helix genes in neural development. *Current Opinion in Neurobiology*, **7**, 13–20.

Liem, K. F., Tremml, G., Roelink, H. & Jessell, T. M. (1995). Dorsal differentiation of neural plate cells induced by BMP-mediated signals from epidermal ectoderm. *Cell*, **82**, 969–79.

Loftus, S. K., Morris, J. A., Garstea, E. D. et al. (1997). Murine model of Niemann-Pick C disease: mutation in a cholesterol homeostasis gene. *Science*, **277**, 232–5.

Lumsden, A. & Krumlauf, R. (1996). Patterning the vertebrate neuraxis. *Science*, **274**, 1109–15.

McKay, R. (1997). Stem cells in the central nervous system. *Science*, **276**, 66–71.

McMahon, A. P., Joyner, A. L., Bradley, A. & McMahon, J. A. (1992). The mid-brain-hindbrain phenotype of Wnt-1/$^-$/Wnt-1$^-$ mice results from stepwise deletion of engrailed-expressing cells by 9.5 days postcoitum. *Cell*, **69**, 581–95.

McMahon, J. A., Takada, S., Zimmerman, L. B., Fan, C. M., Harland, R. M. & McMahon, A. P. (1998). Noggin-mediated antagonism of BMP signaling is required for growth and patterning of the neural tube and somite. *Genes and Development*, **15**, 1438–52.

Mansouri, A., Hallonet, M. & Gruss, P. (1996). Pax genes and their roles in cell differentiation and development. *Current Opinion in Cell Biology*, **8**, 851–7.

Mark, M., Rijli, F. M. & Chambon, P. (1997). Homeobox genes in embryogenesis and pathogenesis. *Pediatric Research*, **42**, 421–9.

Marshall, H., Nonchev, S., Sham, M. H., Muchamore, I., Lumsden, A. & Krumlauf, R. (1992).

Retinoic acid alters hindbrain Hox code and induces transformation of rhombomeres 2/3 into a 4/5 identity. *Nature*, **360**, 737–41.

Mehler, M. F., Mabie, P. C., Zhang, D. & Kessler, J. A. (1997). Bone morphogenetic proteins in the nervous system. *Trends in Neuroscience*, **20**, 309–17.

Ming, J. E. & Muenke, M. (1998). Holoprosencephaly: from Homer to Hedgehog. *Clinical Genetics*, **53**, 155–63.

Ming, J. E., Roessler, E. & Muenke, M. (1998). Human developmental disorders and the Sonic Hedgehog pathway. *Molecular Medicine Today*, **4**, 343–9.

Nonchev, S., Vesque, C., Maconochie, M. et al. (1996). Segmental expression of Hoxa-2 in the hindbrain is directly regulated by Krox-20. *Development*, **122**, 543–54.

Porter, J. A., von Kessler, D. P., Ekker, S. C. et al. (1995). The product of hedgehog autoproteo-lytic cleavage active in loca and long-range signalling. *Nature*, **375**, 363–6.

Porter, J. A., Young, K. E. & Beachy, P. A. (1996*a*). Cholesterol modification of Hedgehog signaling proteins in animal development. *Science*, **274**, 255–9.

Porter, J. A., Ekker, S. C., Park, W. J. et al. (1996*b*). Hedgehog patterning activity: role of a lipophilic modification mediated by the carboxy-terminal autoprocessing domain. *Cell*, **86**, 21–34.

Rakic, P. (1974). Neurons in rhesus visual cortex: systematic relation between time of origin and eventual disposition. *Science*, **183**, 425–7.

Rakic, P. (1988). Specification of cerebral cortical areas. *Science*, **241**, 170–6.

Roelink, H., Porter, J. A., Chiang, C. et al. (1995). Floor plate and motor neuron induction by different concentrations of the amino-terminal cleavage product of Sonic Hedgehog autoproteolysis. *Cell*, **81**, 445–55.

Roessler, E., Belloni, E., Gaudenz, K. et al. (1996). Mutations in the human Sonic Hedgehog gene cause holoprosencephaly. *Nature Genetics*, **14**, 357–60.

Roessler, E., Belloni, E., Gaudenz, K. et al. (1997). Mutations in the C-terminal domain of Sonic Hedgehog cause holoprosencephaly. *Human Molecular Genetics*, **6**, 1847–53.

Rubenstein, J. L. & Beachy, P. A. (1998). Patterning of the embryonic forebrain. *Current Opinion in Neurobiology*, **8**, 18–26.

Sauer, F. C. (1935). Mitosis in the neural tube. *Journal of Comparitive Neurology*, **62**, 377–405.

Schneider-Manoury, S., Topilko, P., Seitanidou, T. et al. (1993). Disruption of Krox-20 results in alteration of rhombomeres 3 and 5 in the developing hindbrain. *Cell*, **75**, 1199–1214.

Shimamura, K. & Rubenstein, J. L. (1997). Inductive interactions direct early regionalization of the mouse forebrain. *Development*, **124**, 2709–18.

Smith, J. L. & Schoenwolf, G. C. (1989). Notochordal induction of cell wedging in the chick neural plate and its role in neural tube formation. *Journal of Experimental Zoology*, **250**, 49–62.

Studer, M., Popperl, H., Marshall, H., Kuroiwa, A. & Krumlauf, R. (1994). Role of a conserved retinoic acid response element in rhombomere constriction of Hoxb-1. *Science*, **265**, 1728–32.

Suda, Y., Matsuo, I. & Aizawa, S. (1997). Cooperation between Otx1 and Otx2 genes in developmental patterning of rostral brain. *Mechanisms of Development*, **69**, 125–41.

Tanabe, Y. & Jessell, T. M. (1996). Diversity and pattern in developing spinal cord. *Science*, **274**, 1115–23.

van Straaten, H. W. M., Hekking, J. W. M., Wiertz-Hoessels, E. J. L. M., Thors, F. & Drukker, J.

(1988). Effect of the notochord on the differentiation of a floor plate area in the neural tube of the chick embryo. *Anatomy and Embryology*, **177**, 317–24.

Wilkinson, D. G., Bhatt, S., Cook, M., Boncinelli, E., & Krumlauf, R. (1989). Segmental expression of Hox-2 homeobox-containing genes in the developing mouse hindbrain, *Nature*, **341**, 405–9.

Williams, B. P. & Price, J. (1995). Evidence for multiple precursor cell types in the embryonic rat cerebral cortex. *Neuron*, **14**, 1181–8.

Yoshida, M., Suda, Y., Matsuo, I. et al. (1997). Emx1 and Emx2 functions in development of dorsal telencephalon. *Development*, **124**, 101–11.

Zhang, M., Kim, H. J., Marshall, H. et al. (1994). Ectopic Hoxa-1 induces rhombomere transformation in mouse hindbrain. *Development*, **120**, 2431–42.

The discovery of the neuronal organizer

Differentiation of cells in the embryo to become particular tissues is dependent on a stimulus from adjacent tissues. This was first discovered by the German zoologist, Hans Spemann, just before the First World War. To further explore this finding, he suggested that one of his students, Hilde Mangold, should conduct some seminal transplantation experiments between salamander embryos. Mangold was born in 1898 in Thuringa in Germany and studied arts and philosophy and then zoology in Frankfurt. She heard a lecture by Spemann, which impressed her sufficiently to move to Freiburg, where Spemann just had taken a Chair. She wanted to do a PhD thesis, but the first study failed when Spemann suggested that she transplant dorsal blastopore lip material into another embryo. She then discovered that some of these embryos developed two heads, sometimes with only a rudimentry brain but also sometimes with two complete brains (Fig. 1). She submitted her thesis in February 1923 and was examined in philosophy by Edmund Husserl, who found her performance very satisfactory. One year later she died tragically. As a German wife she had to devote her life to *Kinder und Küche*. When warming up food for her baby, she caught herself alight after refuelling a spirit stove and died.

Hans Spemann received the Nobel Prize in physiology or medicine in 1935 mainly for this discovery of the organizer, later called Spemann's organizer. After the Nazis had taken over in Germany, Spemann resigned and went to inner exile. His most successful disciple, Victor Hamburger, left Germany and started a new career in Saint Louis. He became mentor for Rita Levi-Montalcini (see p. 135). It is interesting to note that the great philosopher Martin Heidegger became a member of the Nazi party and was appointed as the president of the same university as Spemann. In retrospect, Spemann's (and Mangold's) contributions to understanding the brain and the mind seem to supervene the much more famous Heidegger.

Reference

Sander, K., ed. (1997). *Landmarks in Developmental Biology 1883–1924*, pp. 66–75, Berlin: Springer-Verlag.

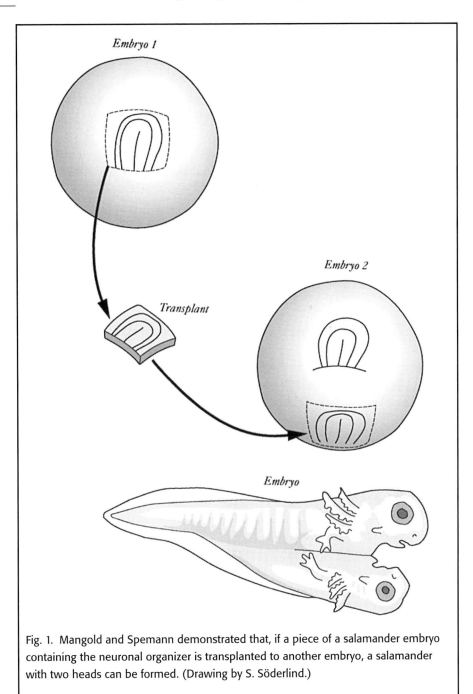

Fig. 1. Mangold and Spemann demonstrated that, if a piece of a salamander embryo containing the neuronal organizer is transplanted to another embryo, a salamander with two heads can be formed. (Drawing by S. Söderlind.)

3

Neocortical neuronogenesis: the G1 restriction point as master integrative mechanism

Verne S. Caviness, Jr.[1], Takao Takahashi[2] and Richard S. Nowakowski[3]

[1]Department of Neurology, Massachusetts General Hospital, Boston, USA
[2]Department of Pediatrics, Keio University School of Medicine, Tokyo, Japan
[3]Department of Neuroscience and Cell Biology, Robert Wood Johnson Medical School, Piscataway, NJ, USA

Introduction

Histogenesis of the neocortex is initiated with neuronogenesis, the formation of neurons, which occurs in the pseudostratified ventricular epithelium (PVE) of the dorsolateral embryonic cerebral wall (Fig. 3.1) (Sidman & Rakic, 1982; Takahashi et al., 1995). Once they become postmitotic, young neurons migrate away from the epithelium across the intervening cerebral wall to become assembled into the neocortex (Sidman & Rakic, 1973). Subsequently, a substantial proportion of the neurons is eliminated by histogenetic cell death (Ferrar et al., 1992; Finlay & Pallas, 1989; Finlay & Slattery, 1983; Spreafico et al., 1995; Verney et al., 1999). Those which survive continue to grow and differentiate as they become integral to neural circuitry.

The transcriptional activity within cells which drives neuronogenesis, migration and postmigratory cortical differentiation is modulated, at least in part, by interactions among cells, but also by a host of other influences which converge upon the cellular environment. Perturbations in this transcriptional activity, arising either from genetic pathology or from an unfavourable cast of the cellular environment, plague this histogenetic sequence with mild or catastrophic consequences for the organism's adaptive capacity (Caviness et al., 1989, 1995a; Caviness & Williams, 1979). The quality of these consequences and their scale reflect complexly both the character of the perturbation and the stage of the histogenetic sequence through which they act. The final phenotype, when not normal, may be of a character which tells something of the cell biological story of the disruption. Thus, disorders affecting principally the proliferative process may be characterized most saliently by an impoverishment of those cell types normally formed in the blighted phase of proliferation. Those which disrupt migration characteristically leave large populations of neurons stranded as heterotopias in the cerebral wall between PVE and cortex.

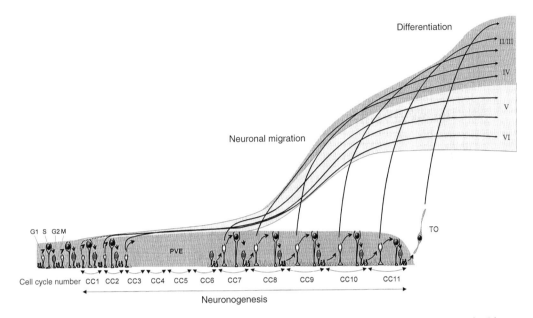

Fig. 3.1.   The neocortical histogenetic sequence. Histogenesis of the neocortex is initiated with
cell proliferation in the pseudostratified ventricular epithelium (PVE) which is
approximately coextensive with the ventricular zone (VZ) at the margin of the lateral
ventricle. The founder population proliferates exponentially through an extended series
of cycles of the preneuronogenetic phase during which no cells exit the cycle ($Q=0$,
$P=1.0$). Proliferative cells of the PVE are attached at the ventricular margin. Their shape
correlates with phase of the cell cycle. Cells undergo mitosis (M) in a rounded
configuration at the ventricular margin. Postmitotic cells in G1 phase progressively
elongate as the nucleus ascends to initiate S phase in the outer half of the PVE. As cells
move through S and G2 phases they shorten and the nucleus descends to undergo
mitosis at the ventricular margin. The onset of the neuronogenetic phase corresponds to
the initial cycle (CC_1) in which Q is greater than 0 and P correspondingly is less than 1.0.
That is, CC_1 is the first cycle from which postmitotic cells exit the cycle as young
neurons. The cells of the PVE then execute a series of integer cycles (CC_1–CC_{11} in
mouse) during which Q ascends to 1.0 (and P descends to 0.0). The PVE then becomes
the cuboidal ependyma. As young neurons of the Q fraction of each CC exit their
respective cycles (Q_{CC1}–Q_{CC11} and terminal output), they migrate across the intervening
subventricular (SVZ) and intermediate zones (IZ) of the embryonic cerebral wall to attain
the cortical plate (CP) at its interface with the neocortical marginal or plexiform layer
(ML) at the surface of the hemisphere. The earliest formed are destined for the deepest
level of the cortex while later formed cells will find positions at progressively more
superficial levels. At the conclusion of migration, a substantial proportion of young
neurons are eliminated by cell death while surviving neurons grow, differentiate and
become integrated into cortical circuitry.

Those expressed later may impair cortical growth and derange the function of the cortex. Thus, normal and pathological neocortical development are the opposite sides of a coin where phenotype is the final expression of a dynamic dialogue between the developmental environment of cells and organisms and intrinsic cellular mechanisms which are the genetic birth right of the organism. The course of this dialogue may be friendly or hostile.

In the present review we focus upon the earliest of the stages of neocortical histogenesis, that is, upon neuronogenesis. The proliferative process through which neurons arise, viewed casually, may appear relatively uncomplicated in that the proliferative epithelium is more or less nonedescript in its appearance, more or less uniform throughout its extent and more or less invariant in its operation as cells proliferate and then migrate away from the epithelium over the neuronogenetic interval (NI) (Caviness et al., 1999). This apparent simplicity of the cytology and cellular structure of the epithelium is highly deceptive with respect to the complexity of the operation of the proliferative process. Our intent here, as an initial objective, is to introduce a more detailed, and at the same time coherent, account of the workings of the proliferative process, which will much enlarge upon the reader's sense of the true complexity of epithelial operation in the conduct of the process. The second and more theoretical objective is to extract from this complexity the essential regulatory principles which drive the overall process. In practice, this exercise will have three layers. The first layer is a presentation of the structure, modes of operation of the epithelium and the parameters which determine its neuronal output behaviour. These parameters, we will see, operate in both the time and the output domains, that is both with respect to cell cycle kinetics and the number of cells that arise with successive cell cycles. The second objective is to restructure our view of the overall operation of the proliferative process, encountered in our first layer as a process encumbered by much detail. In this second layer we consolidate this detail into two domains of proliferative operation. One relates to the neuronogenetic sequence as it unfolds in all regions of the PVE and will be considered to operate in the output domain. The other relates to the coordinated activity of the full expanse of the epithelium and will be considered to operate in the spatiotemporal domain. In the third layer we press beyond this two tiered reduction to postulate a single cell internal master mechanism which integrates neuronogenetic sequence as it operates across the full face of the epithelium. We will offer the hypothesis, and arguments for it , that this mechanism occurring in a single phase of the cell cycle plays the 'master' integrative role as the determinant of the pace, scale and histogenetic output of the overall neocortical neuronogenetic process.

The neuroepithelium: cellular organization and operation

The proliferative epithelium which gives rise to neurons of the neocortex is pseudostratified, and this determines two complex features of its operation which are common to all proliferative pseudostratified epithelia (Fig. 3.1, 3.2(*a*)). First, its cells, attached at the ventricular margin, vary systematically in their form with progression through the cell cycle (Sauer, 1936, 1937; Takahashi et al., 1995). M phase occurs with the cell in rounded configuration at the ventricular margin. The cell elongates through G1 phase and enters S phase in maximally elongated configuration with the nucleus in the outer half of the epithelium. It shortens again with progression through S and G2 phases. Secondly, proliferative activity in the PVE is asynchronous, i.e. the cells in the PVE are relatively evenly distributed in all phases of the cell cycle (Cai et al., 1997). This asynchrony has the critical implication, to which we return later, that proportionate representation of the sequential phases of the cell cycle will correspond to the duration of that phase as a fraction of the duration of the total cell cycle.

A sequence of investigations over recent decades has revealed two systematic operational properties of the neocortical PVE which may be peculiar to the overall integrated operation of this epithelium. The first is that neurons are produced from any given region of the PVE over an extended period of time and that neuron production is sequentially more or less in an inside-out order with respect to their ultimate position in the cortex (Bisconte & Marty, 1975b; Caviness & Sidman, 1973; Fernandez & Bravo, 1974; Hicks & D'Amato, 1968; Luskin & Shatz, 1985; Rakic, 1974; Takahashi et al., 1999b). That is, the neurons of neocortical layer VI are the first to arise while neurons of successive, overlying layers arise more or less in order. We have referred to the period of time during which neurons are produced as the NI and will refer to the sequence of neuron origin with respect to laminar destiny as the neuronogenetic sequence. In the mouse, the NI is 6 days, in monkey it is 60 days and in human it is about 100 days. The second of these properties is that the proliferative process does not proceed synchronously across the face of the epithelium. On the contrary it is initiated at the far rostrolateral margin of the PVE where the neocortical PVE is continuous with that of the ganglionic eminence (Bayer & Altman, 1991; Bisconte & Marty, 1975a, b; Caviness & Sidman, 1973; Fernandez & Bravo, 1974; Hicks & D'Amato, 1968; McSherry, 1984; McSherry & Smart, 1986; Miyama et al., 1997; Rakic, 1974; Smart & McSherry, 1982; Smart & Smart, 1982). Neuronogenesis, once initiated propagates from rostrolateral to caudomedial (the principal axis of the PVE) (Fig. 3.3). At any time the progression of the neuronogenetic sequence will be spatiotemporally graded according to this axis, an operational aspect of the proliferative process in the PVE referred to as the transverse neurogenetic gradient (TNG). In the mouse, the TNG is about 36 hours 'wide', i.e. the time of production of the first neurons rostrolaterally occurs about 36 hours prior to the time of production of the first neurons dorsomedially (Caviness et al., 1999; McSherry, 1984). In ferret, by comparison, the initial width of the TNG may be as much as 5 days (McSherry, 1984).

Output domain

Spatiotemporal domain

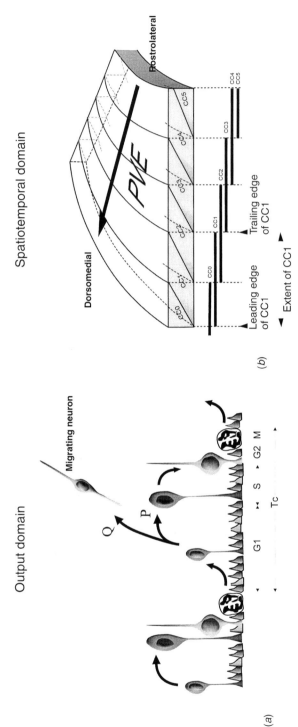

(a)

(b)

Fig. 3.2. The PVE as cell cycle domains. (a) The proliferative cells of the pseudostratified epithelium are attached at the ventricular margin. The cells elongate through G1 phase and those which continue to proliferate (P) enter S phase with the nucleus in the outer half of the epithelium. Those which exit the cycle (Q) following a terminal cell division migrate away from the epithelium. Cells of the P fraction shorten as they progress through S and G2 phases. They undergo mitosis in a rounded configuration at the ventricular margin. The process is asynchronous throughout the epithelium such that at any point there will be cells present which are in each phase of the cell cycle. (b) The distribution of cell cycle domains across the murine neocortical PVE approximately 40 h after the onset of neuronogenesis. Cycle domains are distributed in descending order, CC_{5-1}, from origin along the major axis of the transverse neuronogenetic gradient. The leading edge (LE) of a given domain corresponds to the trailing edge (TE) of the cycle that is two cycles ahead. Thus, in this diagram each domain has the form of a parallelogram, reflecting the idea that at all positions throughout the expanse of the PVE, cells will be mixed systematically such that at any point there will be cells representative of two CC. The size of a given domain, corresponding to the width of each parallelogram, is the distance between the LE and TE (shown with horizontal thick lines for CC_1–CC_5 at the bottom of the figure), and the height is proportional to the relative prevalence of the cells of that CC. The distance between LE and TE of a given domain will increase with increasing T_C. This progression is not actually illustrated in this schematic representation of the domains of the initial five cycles where TC is not great.

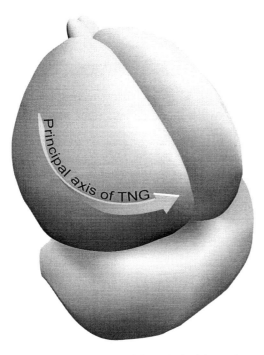

Fig. 3.3.   A schematic projection of the principal (rostrolateral to caudomedial) axis of the transverse neurogenetic gradient (TNG) upon the murine cerebral surface.

Cell cycle, Q and neuron production: experiments in mouse

The cell cycle is the engine that drives the proliferative process and is the cell biological function in which control mechanisms are vested (Fig. 3.2(a)) (Caviness et al., 1999). It is to be emphasized at the outset that the cell cycle of histogenetic systems operates in two domains. First, there is the time domain with reference to the duration of the cell cycle (T_C) and the durations of its successive G1, S, G2 and M (T_{G1}, T_S, T_{G2+M}) phases. Secondly, there is the output domain. During the NI at each pass through the cell cycle some daughter cells quit proliferating to become postmitotic cells(Q) and other daughter cells re-enter the S-phase to continue to proliferate (P, Fig. 3.2(a)). This decision to exit the cell cycle is crucial to the pace of neuron production, and the neurons which exit the cycle are the 'output' of the PVE. Thus, we use the term 'output domain' with reference to the fraction of postmitotic cells which exits at each pass through the cell cycle (Q) as opposed to that fraction which returns to S phase (P; $P + Q = 1.0$). Our investigations into the operation of the PVE, conducted in mouse, have revealed that there are significant changes in the PVE both in terms of the time domain (Tc) and in the output domain (Q/P decision) and that these changes are systematic and apparently tightly constrained. We will approach the evidence for these assertions from the vantage of a larger discussion of the cellular organization and the proliferative operation of the epithelium.

The number of integer cycles

During the course of the NI essentially all of the cells of the PVE are proliferating (Takahashi et al., 1992, 1995). The output of the PVE during the NI will depend on how many times each of its cell lineages divides and the proportion of the daughter cells that becomes postmitotic after each division (Fig. 3.1).

The average number of cell cycles executed over the NI by proliferative cells in a given region of the PVE is calculated from T_C, as sampled experimentally on each day of the NI in that region (Takahashi et al., 1995). Proliferative cells of the PVE, continuously exposed to the thymidine analogue BUdR will incorporate this marker into DNA as they traverse S phase. The proportion of cells labelled with the marker (LI: labelling index) increases with time of exposure until all proliferating cells are labelled. The LI at saturation corresponds to the growth fraction (GF: proportion of cells which are cycling). If LI is plotted as a function of time of exposure to BUdR, the Y-intercept and slope of the line corresponds to $T_S/T_C \times GF$, and GF/T_C, respectively. The interval required for all mitotic figures at the ventricular margin to become labelled corresponds to T_{G2+M}. Thus, the method of cumulative labeling with BUdR provides values for all parameters requisite to estimation of the Tc as well as the duration of the cell cycle phases and GF. Moreover, measurements based upon the method of cumulative labelling taken together with measurements based upon the method of labelled percent mitosis, sensitive, respectively, to the longest and shortest T_C in a population, indicate that the variation in the cell cycle length is small, i.e. about $+/-5$–7% in any small area of the PVE at any time (Cai et al., 1997). That is, the estimate derived for mean T_C is a reasonable estimate for TC for the entire population.

The dorsomedial PVE where these experimental determinations in the mouse embryo were executed initially, is relatively 'down' the TNG. These experiments established that the GF in the dorsomedial region is essentially 1.0 throughout the NI which extends from early E11–early E17. T_C in that region increases from just over 8 h to approximately 20 h (Fig. 3.4(a)). There is no systematic change in T_{G2+M} or T_S. That is, the doubling of T_C is due entirely to a prolongation of T_{G1}, which nearly quadruples over the neurogenetic interval. In other words, the G1 phase is the only phase of the cycle whose duration is regulated in the course of murine neocortical neuronogenesis. It is of interest that this experiment demonstrates that time *per se* is not sufficient to represent the proliferative activity of the PVE. For example, early in the NI when Tc is short there are almost three full cell cycles in a single 24-hour period. In contrast, at the end of the NI when Tc is maximal there is only enough time for just over one cell cycle.

The pattern of progression of T_C, taken together with the observation that T_C is minimally variant in the population, allows the calculation (Takahashi et al., 1992, 1995) that the NI in mouse is constituted uniformly of 11 integer cycles (Fig. 3.1, CC_1 through CC_{11}; Fig. 3.4). That is, the founder population of the dorsomedial murine neocortical PVE and its progeny execute a total of 11 cell cycles over a 6-day period. Virtually identical findings were obtained when the experiment was later repeated in the lateral region of the PVE, i.e. in a location that is relatively 'up' the TNG (Miyama et al., 1997). That is, in the PVE of the lateral cerebral wall there are also 11 cell cycles and the patterns of changes in T_C and T_{G1} are identical to dorsomedial cortex except that they are shifted in time by approximately 24 hours. Overall, therefore, the proliferative behaviour of the cells in the PVE changes both in time (during the NI) and in space (along the TNG) but importantly it seems that the progression and sequence of advance of the proliferative population in the PVE is identical at each point in the PVE. The number of cell cycles in the neocortical NI of various species is different and probably contributes significantly to neocortical development in a species-specific manner (Caviness et al., 1995b; Kornack & Rakic, 1998).

The Q and P fractions

Qualitative and quantitative analyses of the neuronal 'birthdays' in various species suggest that the number of neurons produced increases progressively with advance of the NI (Bayer & Altman, 1991; Hicks & D'Amato, 1968; Luskin & Shatz, 1985; McSherry, 1984; Rakic, 1974; Takahashi et al., 1999b). The change in the number of cell cycles executed per day is not necessarily the sole contributor to this phenomenon, and, in fact, since neuronal production increases at the end of the NI, but the number of cell cycles per day decreases, the output domain, i.e. the Q/P decision must also contribute significantly to total neuronal output per day.

The experimental basis for the determination of Q and P has been a double labelling technique using two S-phase markers: an initial exposure to ^{3}H-TdR followed 2 h later by exposure to BUdR to mark a '2 h cohort' as ^{3}H-TdR only labelled cells (Takahashi et al., 1996). The initial labelling sequence is followed by continued exposure to BUdR for one set of animals (set 1) but no further exposure to the tracer for a second set (set 2). At an interval corresponding to $T_C - T_S$, the number of cells labelled only with ^{3}H-TdR in set 1 corresponds to the number of cells of the Q fraction (N_Q) for the 2 h cohort, while that of the set 2 corresponds to the number of cells of the combined $Q + P$ fractions (N_{Q+P}). Q is calculated as N_Q/N_{Q+P} and P as $1 - Q$.

We have determined Q and P of the dorsomedial neocortical PVE daily in mouse over the 6-day NI. Then, by interpolation, we have reconstructed both Q and P values for the full set of 11 integer cycles (Miyama et al., 1997; Takahashi et al.,

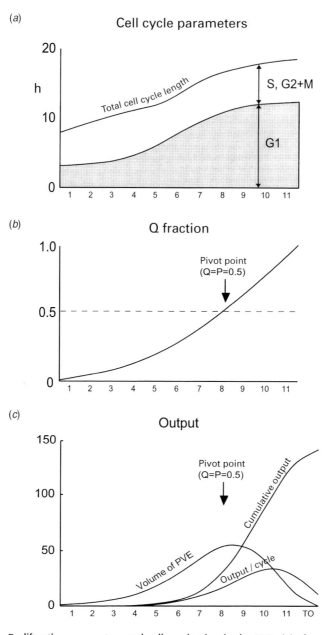

Fig. 3.4.   Proliferative parameters and cell production in the PVE. (*a*) The neuronogenetic interval of
the murine PVE continues 6 days independently of region and lies within the interval,
embryonic day 11–17. In each region total cell cycle length increases from approximately
8 to 18 h corresponding to an 11 cell cycle sequence. The advance in cell cycle length
(ordinate) as a function of cycle (abscissa) is attributable entirely to a near quadrupling of
the duration of the G1 phase. There is no systematic variation in the combined duration of
the S phase and the G2 and M phases. (*b*) The progression of Q, plotted as a function of
the number of elapsed cell cycles, is low at first and the 'pivot point' of the system where

1996) (Fig 3.4(b)). Again the progressions of Q and P in both dorsomedial and lateral regions are identical when plotted as a function of the number of elapsed cell cycles (Miyama et al., 1997; Takahashi et al., 1996)(Fig. 3.4(b)). The increment in Q per cycle is low at first and the 'pivot point' of the system where the number of postmitotic cells leaving the cycle is the same as the number returning to S phase ($P=Q=0.5$) is achieved only during the 8th cycle (CC_8), that is, only at a point nearly 75% of the way through the full set of 11 cycles. The continued advance of the two parameters, Q to 1.0 and P to 0.0, is much more rapid over the terminal three cycles. These changes in Q and P are not accompanied by any overt alteration in the histological appearance of the PVE which remains remarkably unchanged except for a small increase in thickness and a much greater increase in its area in approach to the pivot point where $P=Q=0.5$. After passing the pivot point, the number of cells in the PVE is reduced with each cell cycle. PVE involutes, becoming progressively thinner, and at the end of the 11th cell cycle is eventually transformed to the non-proliferative ependyma, a cuboidal epithelium (Fig. 3.1).

Neuron production

The combined effects of cell cycle lengthening and changes in Q can be determined from a mathematical analysis of the fates of daughter cells integrated with cell cycle progression across time. We have formulated elsewhere equations for the neuronal production from a founder population where P, Q and cell cycle number are variable parameters. Because the rate of cell death among proliferating cells within the PVE, as estimated by reliable methods (Thomaidou et al., 1997) is only a few per cent and within the standard error of our experimental methods, cell death is not entered as a parameter into our equations. The output for each cell cycle is expressed as a function of Q and the size of the PVE for that cycle and the total output is the sum of output of the succession of individual cycles (Fig. 3.4(c)). The PVE increases approximately 50-fold in volume over the initial eight cycles which is observed to occur with only a two-fold increase in its height. This implies that the PVE increases approximately 25 times in area (five times in each of its two tangential dimensions) between the beginning of the NI, i.e. CC_1 and CC_8. As a correlate

Caption for fig. 3.4 (*cont.*)

the number of postmitotic cells leaving the cycle is the same as the number returning to S phase ($P=Q=0.5$) is achieved only during the eighth cycle (CC_8). The continued advance of Q to 1.0 is much more rapid over the terminal three cycles. (c) The PVE increases approximately 50 fold in volume over the initial eight cycles. The initial rate of neuron production per cycle is low but it rises steadily to a peak around CC_8 and then drops. With respect to the founder cell, i.e. a proliferating cell present at the outset of the 11 cell cycle NI, the average total cumulative output is approximately 140 cells.

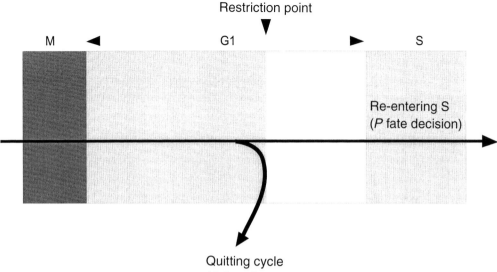

Fig. 3.5.   The restriction point. Postmitotic cells may either quit the cycle (*Q* fate decision) or re-enter S phase (*P* fate decision). The probability that a cell will make the *Q* vs. *P* fate choice is determined by mechanisms which operate at the G1 restriction point.

of the slow initial rise of Q, the initial rate of neuron production per cycle is low but it rises steadily to a peak around CC_8. Afterwards, the rate of cell production drops even though Q continues to increase because there is a marked reduction in the size of the PVE as Q is now greater than 0.5. With respect to the founder cell, i.e. a proliferating cell present at the outset of the 11 cell cycle NI, the average total cumulative output is approximately 140 cells. Of these, approximately 30% are formed through the first seven cycles but 70% are formed at cell cycle 8 and afterwards, i.e. after Q has become greater than 0.5. These estimates of neuron production based upon parameters measured experimentally in the murine neocortical PVE accord well with numbers which have been based on direct counts (Caviness et al., 1999; Rhee et al., 1998; Tan et al., 1998; Vaccarino et al., 1999). The mathematical analysis of neuron number and neuron production works well to explain the developmental parameters of neocortical development in several species, including humans (Caviness et al., 1995b).

Two domains of neuronogenetic operation

The foregoing sections have introduced the cellular structure of the PVE and its modes of operation and have provided the parameters which determine its proliferative behaviour. Amidst this detail we discern two coordinate domains of regulation. That is, internal to this overall complexity of proliferative operation are two separate and distinct, simplifying regulatory principles. Locally, there is the neuronal output domain encompassing the parameters which determine neuronal output from a founder population over the entire NI in that region. Globally, there is the spatiotemporal domain which encompasses those parameters which govern the operation of the TNG.

Output domain

Neuronal output from a founder population is the expression of an iterative proliferative sequence. In the prior section we have seen that Q ascends with each successive cycle and determines the output for each respective cycle. Total output is the sum of output for the set of cycles. That is, only two parameters, the number of cell cycles and the ascent of Q with each cycle, determine the output of the proliferative process from a founder population. It will be appreciated that time, in *sensu strictu*, is not directly a parameter governing output (Caviness et al., 1995b; Takahashi et al., 1996).

The proliferative sequence is initiated from a population that is proliferating exponentially. It terminates when there is no further proliferative activity in the epithelium which is then transformed into the simple cuboidal ependyma (Takahashi et al., 1995). In the course of the intervening interval, the progeny of the founder population will execute a mean number of integer cycles (Takahashi et al., 1996). Precisely then the proliferative sequence corresponds to the number of cycles required for Q to traverse its obligatory path from $Q=0$ to $Q=1.0$. We have seen the experimental finding that this path ascends systematically in non-linear fashion such that the relationship between Q and cell cycle at any moment has the form

$$Q = k \times CC^{1.97}$$

where k is a constant corresponding to the proportionate advance of Q with each cycle (Caviness et al., 1999; Takahashi et al., 1997). The constant is dimensionless and there is no factor with time dimension in the equation. Independently of region of PVE, k is approximately 0.009 in mouse.

Read abstractly, this formulation states a best-fit relationship between the progression of Q and cell cycle. When we consider the biology represented by Q more closely, however, we realize that this formulation carries a substantially deeper significance. This is that the number of cycles which constitutes the neuronogenetic sequence is determined by those molecular biological mechanisms which determine the probability at each successive cycle that postmitotic daughter cells will exit the proliferative process. In other words, the molecular mechanism which sets the probability of cycle exit for each cycle is the mechanism which regulates the output domain of the proliferative process. We will revisit further implications of this regulatory mechanism in the final section of our discussion where we consider integrative mechanisms of the proliferative process.

Spatiotemporal domain

Whereas the output domain is governed by parameters which are without time dimension, global coordination of the neuronogenetic sequence across the expanse of the PVE is strictly regulated in terms of systematic spatiotemporal order (Caviness et al., 1999; Miyama et al., 1997). Specifically, the initiation of the neuronogenetic sequence as it occurs with respect to the principal (rostro-lateral to caudomedial) axis of the PVE (Fig. 3.5) is strictly regulated in time. Regulation is monotonic, we suggest, under the control of the parameter T_C. Consider the constraints imposed on spatiotemporal progression of the advance of Q from 0 to >0 with the initiation of cell cycle 1 (CC_1) by the operating properties of the PVE in which cells proliferate asynchronously. Thus, in all regions of the PVE, there will be cells in all phases of the cell cycle (Fig. 3.2(a)) (Sauer, 1936; Sauer & Walker, 1959; Takahashi et al., 1995) and the proportional representation of cells by phase will correspond to the duration of that phase as a fraction of T_C.

We begin with initiation of CC1 at origin of the TNG in the rostro-lateral PVE (Figs. 3.2(b)). CC1 is initiated in G1 progeny of the founder cycle which we will designate as CC_0 (Caviness et al., 1999). We will refer to the narrow region of the PVE where cells now operate in CC1 as the CC1 domain. The leading edge of this domain will advance spatially within the PVE along the principal axis of TNG at an hourly rate which corresponds to the rate that cells along the leading edge exit CC_0 ($1/T_{C\_}CC_0$). The trailing edge of the CC_1 domain will not move away from origin until all cells at origin have completed CC_1 to be succeeded by progeny in CC_2. This will correspond to the time required for the last cell in CC_1 to complete its cycle plus the time elapsed after the CC1 domain is initiated before the last cell to enter CC_1 can do so. It follows that the extent of CC domains (distance between the leading and trailing edges) will progressively enlarge due to the approximate doubling in T_C through the 11 cycle sequence. The rate of enlargement will obviously reflect also the massive increase in the extent of the PVE observed over the first 7 cycles before P falls below 0.5.

An implication of this wave-like sequence of progression of CC domains through the PVE is that the PVE is, at any given time, an overlapping mosaic pattern of cell cycle domains where the borders of each domain are continuously shifting. The number of domains active across the PVE at any given time has not been determined but, from considerations we have elsewhere estimated from proliferative parameters, this number will be approximately 5 at the time when the LE of the CC1 domain has travelled the full extent of the principal axis and when TC is shortest. This number is estimated to be only 1.2 domains when the TE of CC11 advances from origin at the termination of the NI at that origin.

In consideration of this mode of operation of the PVE and its implications for spatiotemporal priority of neuronogenetic sequence in the epithelium, we begin to engage the true complexities of this epithelium and its operations, so disarmingly simple to casual glance. The first level of complexity is the requirement that at all times the population of the PVE will include cells engaged in two consecutive cell cycles, those entering and advancing through the advancing cycle intermixed with those winding up and completing the retreating cycle. The proportion of cells in the retreating as opposed to the advancing cycle at any point within a domain will change as a function of P of the retreating cycle. The exchange will be 1 for 1 only in the CC_8 domain where P becomes 0.5, so that each cell leaving the retreating cycle will be replaced by a cell entering the advancing cycle. For the earlier cycles, the population shift will be non-linear in favour of the advancing cycle where the magnitude of disparity will decrease with successive cycles. For the later cycles, it will be non-linear in favour of the retreating cycle where the disparity will be increasingly greater with successive cycles.

The second level of complexity is that the proliferative parameters at which cells of each successive cycle operate will distribute across the face of the epithelium as the cells in the respective cycle distribute. This is significant principally for the graded distribution of T_{G1}, which advances in non-linear fashion along the principal axis of the epithelium.

A master integrator

The two domains of proliferative process are coordinated within the overall complexity of the proliferative activity of the PVE. To recapitulate, these are the output domain as it operates locally in all regions of the PVE and the spatiotemporal gradient which reflects a global systematic coordination of output operations along the principal axis of the PVE. Each of these domains represents a complex and coordinated subroutine of the total proliferative process. Each, we have seen, is regulated in its dynamic progression by a single elementary proliferative parameter. In the case of those mechanisms which determine the number of cycles in the output domain, this parameter is the output function Q. In the case of those mechanisms which determine the pace of advance of the cycle domains along the principal axis it is the kinetic parameter T_C. T_C, in turn, advances systematically with cycle as T_{G1} is regulated. In this final section of the discussion, we propose that there is yet a further level of reduction at which the greatly complex operations of the proliferative epithelium is coordinated and integrated. Specifically, we propose that the G1 restriction point is the cell biological mechanism which is integrative to those mechanisms regulated by the parameters Q and T_{G1}.

The G1 restriction point (Pardee, 1989) is an obvious candidate for the 'master' integrative mechanism from its functions which are well established in general cell biology. It is widely accepted that the 'choice' to leave or not to leave the cell cycle is made in the G1 phase of the cell cycle in proliferative vertebrate cells (Fig. 3.5) (Roberts et al., 1994; Sherr, 1993; Sherr & Roberts, 1995). The cycling vertebrate cell passes through two regulatory transitions or 'checkpoints' as it traverses the G1 phase. These are the restriction point and the G1/S phase transition (Murray & Hunt, 1993; Roberts et al., 1994; Sherr, 1993; Sherr & Roberts, 1995). It is probable that, of these two, it is the restriction point which is of principal interest regarding mechanisms regulating Q and, in particular, the operation of cell external influences which modulate Q and also of other domains of proliferative behaviour. Restriction point is a shorthand designation for a complex sequence of molecular actions involving multiple molecular agents (Pardee, 1989; Zetterberg et al., 1995; Coats, 1996). These molecular actions determine whether a cell in G1 phase will leave the cycle or advance to the G1/S transition. If a cell passes the restriction point, its passage through the G1/S transition is assured. Thus, from the perspective of a population of postmitotic cells entering G1 phase of a given cell cycle, Q corresponds to the probability that the cell will not pass the restriction point for that cycle. P for that cycle, the complement of Q, corresponds, therefore, to the probability that the cell will pass the restriction point.

The molecular operators acting at the restriction point of vertebrate cells in general partition into one set whose actions serve to drive the cell through the restriction point. These are represented by the cyclin-dependent kinases Cdk4 and 6 and their regulatory subunit cyclin D (Massague & Polyak, 1995; Roberts et al., 1994; Sherr, 1993, 1994). A second set, working in opposition to the kinases, are the inhibitors represented by p27 and p21 (Massague & Polyak, 1995; Sherr & Roberts, 1995). The inhibitors act to block the passage through the restriction point and in this way force the cell to leave the cycle.

Whether or not a cell passes the restriction point will be determined by the relative balance of facilitatory and inhibitory actions acting at the restriction point (Massague & Polyak, 1995; Roberts et al., 1994; Sherr, 1993, 1994). This balance appears to be subject to modulation by a heterogeneous array of cell external factors, which are both positive (physiological mitogens) and negative (physiological antimitogens) in effect with respect to restriction point passage. It has been established in non-neural cell lines maintained in vitro that one of the actions of physiological mitogens is to upregulate expression and activity of the elements of Cdk4/6–cyclin D complexes and to down regulate the actions of the inhibitors (Koff et al., 1993; Massague & Polyak, 1995; Roberts et al., 1994; Sherr & Roberts, 1995). The physiological antimitogens acting in G1 phase are opposite in effect.

Mechanisms which regulate the length of G1 phase are less completely explored. Nevertheless the restriction point remains the plausible control point, in that variations in Q are closely coordinated with variations in T_{G1}. For example, over-expression of cyclin E in diploid fibroblasts not only drives Q to near 0 but also decreases T_{G1} (Ohtsubo & Roberts, 1993; Ohtsubo et al., 1995). Moreover, when dissociated cells of the PVE are cultured with the mitogen FGF, not only is Q driven downward toward 0 but T_{G1} is shortened to what is essentially its minimal duration observed in the earliest cycles in vivo (Cavanagh et al., 1997). The fabric of the hypothesis is not complete, however, in that we are not aware of complementary studies which have considered whether upward pressure on Q is associated with a corresponding prolongation of G1 phase. Nor has it been clarified in terms of molecular mechanisms how G1 phase becomes shortened in the models mentioned above.

Is the restriction point, established as an integrative mechanism general to proliferative vertebrate cells (indeed to proliferative eukaryotic cells) a mechanism known explicitly to operate in the proliferative cells that form the neocortical PVE? Such evidence that has accumulated in this regard, thus far limited to in vitro analyses, is reassuring. Thus, check points, which arrest the cycle of the PVE, operate adaptively within both the G2 and G1 phases of cells of the PVE and do so according to patterns consistent with the operations of these checkpoints in other proliferative vertebrate cells (Takahashi et al., 1999a). The principal regulatory operators including the kinase cdk2, its regulatory subunit cyclin E, indispensable to the G1/S transition, and the cycle progression inhibitors, p27 and p21, known to operate at the restriction point of vertebrate cells, also have established activity in the PVE (Fero et al., 1996; Kiyokawa et al., 1996; Lee et al., 1996; Nakayama et al., 1996; Tsai et al., 1993). Moreover, the patterns of expression of these operators across the NI are closely in accord with what would be predicted from the progression of the proliferative process itself (Delalle et al., 1999). Specifically, in the course of the early cycles when Q is low and T_{G1} is short, levels of cyclin E expression are maximum and those of p27 are minimum. Subsequently, as the pivot point is approached where $Q = P = 0.5$, the expression of cyclin E plummets, while that of p27 surges to its peak levels of expression, to decline only modestly thereafter as the epithelium involutes and the NI ends.

The restriction point: is there a larger role?

Our emphasis in this discussion has been neuronal output, how it is regulated within a region and throughout all regions of the PVE. Though certainly an important issue in histogenesis, it is in a real sense a secondary one. Thus, the most critical mechanisms of histogenesis are those of specification, specification of cell class and regional specification (Caviness et al., 1999), i.e. cells are produced by class in appropriate numbers; cells are assigned by class to the separate neocortical fields in appropriate numbers. A fuller consideration of proliferative mechanisms fundamental to histogenetic specification is beyond the scope of this discussion and would become heavily theoretical. However, the restriction point may serve an even more elaborate master control mechanism than we have thus far postulated, because the mechanisms determining cell number may at the restriction point become coordinated with those of class and regional specification. The argument for this is, in part, circumstantial not only in that the events of specification of both class and region are in effect within the proliferative epithelium but also that cell enumeration is precisely coordinated with these events of specification. The argument is drawn from the inference that a principal consequence of a cell passing the restriction point is that master transcription factors, in particular the transcription E2F, are activated (Follette & O'Farrell, 1997; Lees & Harlow, 1995; Sherr, 1994). Among the consequences of such activation is the set of events which implement the passage through the G1/S transition. It remains for future investigations to determine whether included among the other consequences are some that are fundamental to histogenetic specification.

Acknowledgements

Supported by NIH grants NS12005 and NS33433, NASA grant NAG2–750 and a grant from Pharmacia-Upjohn Fund for Growth & Development Research. T.T. was supported by a fellowship of The Medical Foundation, Inc., Charles A. King Trust, Boston, MA.

REFERENCES

Bayer, S. A. & Altman, J. (1991). *Neocortical Development*. New York: Raven Press.

Bisconte, J-C. & Marty, R. (1975a). Analyse chronoarchitectonique du cerveau de rat par radio-autographie. I. Histogenese du telencephale. *Journal für Hirnforschung*, **16**, 55–74.

Bisconte, J-C. & Marty, R. (1975b). Etude quantitative du marquage radioautographique dans le systeme nerveux du rat. II. Caracteristiques finales dans le cerveau de l'animal adulte. *Experimental Brain Research*, **22**, 37–56.

Cai, L., Hayes, N. & Nowakowski, R. (1997). Local homogeneity of cell cycle length in developing mouse cortex. *Journal of Neuroscience*, **17**, 2079–87.

Cavanagh, J., Mione, M., Pappas, I. & Parnavelas, J. (1997). Basic fibroblast growth factor prolongs the proliferation of rat cortical progenitor cells *in vitro* without altering their cell cycle parameters. *Cerebral Cortex*, **7**, 293–302.

Caviness, V. S., Jr. & Sidman, R. L. (1973). Time of origin of corresponding cell classes in the cerebral cortex of normal and reeler mutant mice: an autoradiographic analysis. *Journal of Comparative Neurology*, **148**, 141–52.

Caviness, V. S., Jr. & Williams, R. S. (1979). Cellular pathology of developing human cortex. *Research Publications of the Association for Research in Nervous and Mental Disease*, **57**, 69–98.

Caviness, V. S., Jr., Misson, J-P. & Gadisseux, J-F. (1989). Abnormal neuronal patterns and disorders of neocortical development. In *From Reading to Neurons*, ed. A. M. Galaburda, pp. 405–13. Cambridge: MIT Press.

Caviness, V. S., Jr., Hatten, M. E., McConnell, S. K., & Takahashi, T. (1995a). Epilepsy of childhood: perspectives from neurobiology. In *Brain Development and Epilepsy*, ed. P. A. Schwartzkroin, S. L. Moshe, J. L. Noebels, & J. W. Swann, pp. 94–121. Oxford: Oxford University Press.

Caviness, V. S., Jr., Takahashi, T. & Nowakowski, R. S. (1995b). Numbers, time and neocortical neuronogenesis: a general developmental and evolutionary model. *Trends in Neuroscience*, **18**, 379–83.

Caviness, V. S., Jr., Takahashi, T. & Nowakowski, R. (1999). Neuronogenesis and the early events of neocortical histogenesis. In *Development of the Neocortex*, ed. A. Goffinet & P. Rakic, pp. 107–43. Berlin: Springer Verlag: in press.

Coats, S., Flanagan, W. H., Nourse, J. & Roberts, J. M. (1996). Requirement of p27^{Kip1} for restriction point control of fibroblast cell cycle. *Science*, **272**, 877–80.

Delalle, I. T. T., Nowakowski, R., Tsai, L-H. & Caviness, V. S., Jr. (1999). Cyclin E – p27 Opposition and regulation of the G1 phase of the cell cycle in the murine neocortical PVE: a quantitative analysis of mRNA in situ hybridization. *Cerebral Cortex*, **9**, 824–32.

Fernandez, V. & Bravo, H. (1974). Autoradiographic study of the cerebral cortex in the rabbit. *Brain Behavior and Evolution*, **9**, 317–32.

Fero, M., Rivkin, M., Tasch, M. et al. (1996). A syndrome of multiorgan hyperplasia with features of gigantism, tumorigenesis, and female sterility in p27^{Kip1}-deficient mice. *Cell*, **85**, 733–44.

Ferrar, I., Soriano, E., Del Rio, J. A., Alcantara, S. & Auladell, C. (1992). Cell death and removal in the cerebral cortex during development. *Progress in Neurobiology*, **39**, 1–43.

Finlay, B. L. & Pallas, S. L. (1989). Control of cell number in the developing mammalian visual system. *Progress in Neurobiology*, **32**, 207–34.

Finlay, B. L. & Slattery, M. (1983). Local differences in the amount of early cell death in neocortex predict adult local specializations. *Science*, **219**, 1349–51.

Follette, P. & O'Farrell, P. (1997). Connecting cell behavior to patterning: lessons from the cell cycle. *Cell*, **88**, 309–14.

Hicks, S. P. & D'Amato, C. J. (1968). Cell migration to the isocortex in the rat. *Anatomic Record*, **160**, 619–34.

Kiyokawa, H., Kineman, R., Manova-Todorava, K. et al. (1996). Enhanced growth of mice lacking the cyclin-dependent kinase inhibitor function of p27^{Kip1}. *Cell*, **85**, 721–32.

Koff, A., Ohtsuki, M., Polyak, K., Roberts, J. M. & Massague, J. (1993). Negative regulation of G1 progression in mammalian cells; inhibition of cyclin E-dependent kinase by TGF-β. *Science*, **260**, 536–9.

Kornack, D. & Rakic, P. (1998). Changes in cell-cycle kinetics during the development and evolution of primate neocortex. *Proceedings of the National Academy of Sciences, USA*, **95**, 1242–6.

Lee, M-H., Nikolic, M., Baptista, C., Lai, E., Tsai, L-H. & Massague, J. (1996). The brain-specific activator p35 allows Cdk5 to escape inhibition by p27[Kip1] in neurons. *Proceedings of the National Academy of Science, USA*, **93**, 3259–63.

Lees, E. & Harlow, E. (1995). Cell cycle progression and cell growth in mammalian cells: kinetic aspects of transition events. In *Cell Cycle Control*, ed. C. Hutchison & D. Glover, pp. 228–63, Oxford: Oxford University Press.

Luskin, M. B. & Shatz, C. J. (1985). Neurogenesis of the cat's primary visual cortex. *Journal of Comparative Neurology*, **242**, 611–31.

Massague, J. & Polyak, K. (1995). Mammalian antiproliferative signals and their targets. *Current Opinions in Genes and Development*, **5**, 91–6.

McSherry, G. M. (1984). Mapping of cortical histogenesis in the ferret. *Journal of Embryology and Experimental Morphology*, **81**, 239–52.

McSherry, G. M. & Smart, I. H. M. (1986). Cell production gradients in the developing ferret iso-cortex. *Journal of Anatomy*, **144**, 1–14.

Miyama, S., Takahashi, T., Nowakowski, R. S. & Caviness, V. S., Jr. (1997). A gradient in the duration of the G1 phase in the murine neocortical proliferative epithelium. *Cerebral Cortex*, **7**, 678–89.

Murray, A. & Hunt, T. (1993). *The Cell Cycle*. New York: W. H. Freeman and Co.

Nakayama, K., Ishida, N., Shirane, M. et al. (1996). Mice lacking p27[Kip1] display increased body size, multiple organ hyperplasia, retinal dysplasia, and pituitary tumors. *Cell*, **85**, 707–20.

Ohtsubo, M. & Roberts, J. M. (1993). Cyclin-dependent regulation of G1 in mammalian fibroblasts. *Science*, **259**, 1908–12.

Ohtsubo, M., Theodoras, A. M., Schumacher, J., Roberts, J. M. & Pagano, M. (1995). Human cyclin E, a nuclear protein essential to the G1-to-S phase transition. *Molecular and Cell Biology*, **15**, 2612–24.

Pardee, A. B. (1989). G1 events and regulation of cell proliferation. *Science*, **246**, 603–8.

Rakic, P. (1974). Neurons in rhesus monkey visual cortex: systematic relation between time of origin and eventual disposition. *Science*, **183**, 425–7.

Rhee, J., Raballo, R., Schwartz, M. & Vaccarino, F. (1998). Lineage and non-lineage specific effects of fibroblast growth factor (FGF2) on progenitor cells in the developing cerebral cortex. *Society for Neuroscience Abstracts*, **24**, 281.

Roberts, J., Koff, A., Polyak, K. et al. (1994). Cyclins, cdks and cyclin kinase inhibitors. *Cold Spring Harbor Symposia on Quantitative Biolology*, **59**, 31–8.

Sauer, F. C. (1936). The interkinetic migration of embryonic epithelial nuclei. *Journal of Morphology*, **60**, 1–11.

Sauer, F. C. (1937). Some factors in the morphogenesis of vertebrate embryonic epithelia. *Journal of Morphology*, **61**, 563–79.

Sauer, M. E. & Walker, B. E. (1959). Radioautographic study of interkinetic nuclear migration in the neural tube. *Proceedings of the Society for Experimental Biology (NY)*, **101**, 557–60.

Sherr, C. J. (1993). Mammalian G1 cyclins. *Cell*, **73**, 1059–65.

Sherr, C. J. (1994). G1 phase progression: cycling on cue. *Cell*, **79**, 551–5.

Sherr, C. J. & Roberts, J. M. (1995). Inhibitors of mammalian G1 cyclin-dependent kinases. *Genes and Development*, **9**, 1149–63.

Sidman, R. L. & Rakic, P. (1973). Neuronal migration, with special reference to developing human brain: a review. *Brain Research*, **62**, 1–35.

Sidman, R. L. & Rakic, P. (1982). Development of the human central nervous system. In *Histology and Histopathology of the Nervous System*, ed. W. Haymaker & R. D. Adams, pp. 3–145. Springfield, IL: Charles C. Thomas.

Smart, I. H. M. & McSherry, G. M. (1982). Growth patterns in the lateral wall of the mouse telencephalon. II. Histological changes during and subsequent to the period of isocortical neuron production. *Journal of Anatomy*, **131**, 415–42.

Smart, I. H. M. & Smart, M. (1982). Growth patterns in the lateral wall of the mouse telencephalon. I Autoradiographic studies of the histogenesis of the iso-cortex and adjacent areas. *Journal of Anatomy*, **134**, 273–98.

Spreafico, R., Frassoni, C., Arcelli, P., Selvaggio, M. & De Biasi, S. (1995). In situ labelling of apoptotic cell death in the cerebral cortex and thalamus of rats during development. *Journal of Comparative Neurology*, **363**, 281–95.

Takahashi, T., Nowakowski, R. S. & Caviness, V. S., Jr. (1992). BUdR as an S-phase marker for quantitative studies of cytokinetic behaviour in the murine cerebral ventricular zone. *Journal of Neurocytology*, **21**, 185–97.

Takahashi, T., Nowakowski, R. S. & Caviness, V. S., Jr. (1995). The cell cycle of the pseudostratified ventricular epithelium of the murine cerebral wall. *Journal of Neuroscience*, **15**, 6046–57.

Takahashi, T., Nowakowski, R. S. & Caviness, V. S., Jr. (1996). The leaving or Q fraction of the murine cerebral proliferative epithelium: a general computational model of neocortical neuronogenesis. *Journal of Neuroscience*, **16**, 6183–96.

Takahashi, T., Nowakowski, R. S. & Caviness, V. S., Jr. (1997). The mathematics of neocortical neuronogenesis. *Developmental Neuroscience*, **19**, 17–22.

Takahashi, T., Bhide, P., Goto, T., Miyama, S. & Caviness, V. S., Jr. (1999a). Proliferative behavior of the murine cerebral wall in tissue culture: cell cycle kinetics and checkpoints. *Experimental Neurology*, **156**, 407–17.

Takahashi, T., Goto, T., Miyama, S., Nowakowski, R. S. & Caviness, V. S., Jr. (1999b). Sequence of neuron origin and neocortical laminar fate: relation to cell cycle of origin in the developing murine cerebral wall. *Journal of Neuroscience*, **19**, 10357–71.

Tan, S-S., Kalloniatis, M., Sturm, K., Tam, P. & Reese, B. (1998). Separate progenitors for radial and tangential cell dispersion during development of the cerebral cortex. *Neuron*, **21**, 295–304.

Thomaidou, D., Mione, M., Cavanagh, J. & Parnavelas, J. (1997). Apoptosis and its relation to the cell cycle in the developing cerebral cortex. *Journal of Neuroscience*, **17**, 1075–85.

Tsai, L.-H., Takahashi, T., Caviness, V. S., Jr. & Harlow, E. (1993). Activity and expression pattern of cyclin-dependent kinase 5 in the embryonic mouse nervous system. *Development*, **119**, 1029–40.

Vaccarino, F., Schwartz, M., Raballo, R. et al. (1999). Changes in the size of the cerebral cortex are governed by fibroblast growth factor during embryogenesis. *Nature Neuroscience*, **2**, 246–253.

Verney, C., Takahashi, T., Bhide, P. G., Nowakowski, R. S. & Caviness, V. S., Jr. (1999). Independent controls for neocortical neuron production and histogenetic cell death. *Devopmental Neuroscience*, **22**, 125–38.

Zetterberg, A., Larsson, O. & Wiman, K. (1995). What is the restriction point? *Current Opinions in Cell Biology*, 7, 835–42.

The neuron doctrine and proliferation of new neurons before and after birth

Although the cell theory was established in the middle of the nineteenth century, the nerves were assumed to be fused with each other in a reticular network by Camillo Golgi. This view was challenged by the great Spanish neuoroanatomist Santiago Ramon y Cajal (1852–1934). who vigourously claimed that each neuron consititutes its own entity – the neuron doctrine. Golgi and Cajal debated this issue for decades. Ironically, these two strong antagonists shared the Nobel Prize in physiology or medicine in 1906.

The human brain contains 100 billion neurons. Besides the neurons there are about tenfold more glial cells, thus there are totally about 10^{12} cells in the human adult brain. It has been a dogma that all of them are generated during prenatal or early postnatal life (Rakic, 1985). By analysing DNA in the brains of aborted fetuses, Dobbing and Sands (1970) found that most of the neurons are formed between the 10th and the 20th gestational week. After 20 weeks mainly glial cells are generated up to about 2 years. By labelling newly formed neurons with (^{3}H)thymidine in the rhesus monkey Rakic (1985) demonstrated that no new neurons are formed after the early postnatal period. He concluded that 'a stable population of neurons in primates including humans, may be important for the continuity of learning and memory over lifetime'. This idea was challenged by Fernando Nottebohm, who demonstrated the proliferation of new neurons in the singing centre of the adult canary bird (Nottebohm, 1981). Furthermore, he could demonstrate that the number of neurons correlated with the singing repertoire. At a meeting in New York in 1984 he claimed that new neurons can also be formed in the human brain. Rakic responded that, if he were able to change his neurons in his Broca's speech area like the canary birds, he should have got rid of his Croatian accent.

It took more than a decade before the proliferation of new neurons could be demonstrated in the adult human. By chance, a neuroscientist (Peter Eriksson) doing his clinical residency talked coincidently with an oncologist about treating terminally ill cancer patients with bromodeoxyuridine (BrdU). Subsequently, a postmortem study was performed on these patients. Since BrdU is also a marker of DNA, a few hundred new neurons could be detected in the hippocampus (Eriksson & Gage, 1998). Whether these new neurons function or not can be questioned.

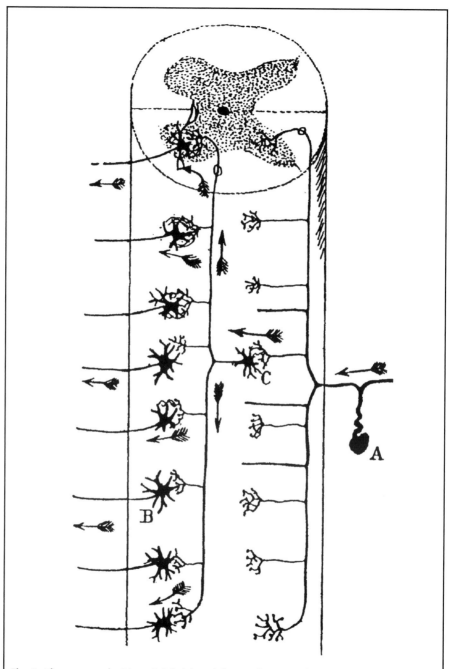

Fig. 1. The neuron doctrine. Cajal claimed that each neuron is separate in contrast to the previous view that the nervous system is a reticulum. (Original drawing published with permission from the Nobel Foundation.)

References

Dobbing, J. & Sands, J. (1970). Timing of neuroblast multiplication in developing human brain. *Nature*, **226**, 639–70.

Eriksson, P. & Gage, F. H. (1998). Neurogenesis in the adult human hippocampus. *Nature Medicine*, **4**, 1313–17.

Nottebohm, F. (1981). A brain for all seasons: cyclical anatomical changes in song control nuclei of the canary brain. *Science*, **214**, 1368–70.

Rakic, P. (1985). Limits of neurogenesis in primates. *Science*, **227**, 1054–6.

4

Neuronal migration

Pierre Gressens

Service de Neurologie Pédiatrique, Hôpital Robert-Debré, Paris, France

Introduction

During brain development, all neurons derive from the primitive neuroepithelium and migrate to their appropriate position in the cerebral mantle including the cortical plate (or prospective neocortex). In humans, migration of neurons destined to the neocortex occurs mostly between the 12th and the 24th weeks of gestation. In laboratory rodents, including mice, rats and hamsters, this ontogenic step extends roughly between embryonic day 12 (the gestation period being around 20 days in these species) and the first postnatal days. The first postmitotic neurons produced in the periventricular germinative neuroepithelium[1] will migrate to form a subpial preplate or primitive plexiform zone (for a review, see Marin-Padilla, 1998) (Fig. 4.1). Subsequently produced neurons, which will form the cortical plate, migrate into the preplate and split it into the superficial molecular layer (layer I or marginal zone containing Cajal–Retzius neurons) and the deep subplate (or cortical layer VIb). The successive waves of migratory neurons will pass the subplate neurons and end their migratory pathway below layer I. These migrating neurons will form successively cortical layers VIa, V, IV, [II and III], following the inside-out pattern of cortical ontogenesis discovered by the pioneering autoradiographic study of Angevine and Sidman (1961).

The analysis of neuronal migration disorders occurring in humans (Table 4.1) and in animal models has provided a large amount of knowledge concerning migratory mechanisms (for reviews, see Evrard et al., 1989, 1992; Gressens, 1998; Caviness et al., 1989; Barkovich et al., 1992, 1996). Neuronal heterotopias can be focal (nodular heterotopias) and located at all levels of the radial migratory corridor, from the lateral ventricle (as in Aicardi syndrome) up to the cortical plate itself. Sometimes, overmigration is observed with neurons present in the molecular layer (as in status verrucosus deformans) or even in the meninges (as in fetal alcohol syndrome). On the other hand, migratory disorders can appear as diffuse band

---

[1] For convenience and clarity, we use the word 'germinative zone' or 'germinative neuropithelium' without discriminating between its parts, the ventricular and subventricular zones.

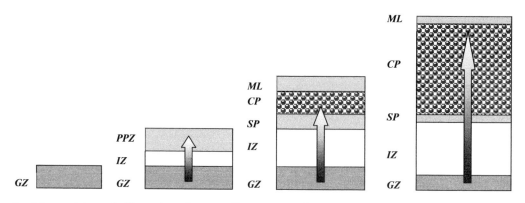

Fig. 4.1.   Schematic illustration of mammalian neocortical formation. GZ, germinative zone; IZ, intermediate zone (prospective white matter); PPZ, primitive plexiform zone; SP, subplate; CP, cortical plate; ML, molecular layer. Arrows indicate migrating neurons.

heterotopias in the white matter as observed in pachygyrias/lissencephalies or in double cortex syndrome.

Radial glia and neuronal–glial units

A central hypothesis of current developmental neurobiology (for a review, see Caviness et al., 1989; Rakic, 1988; Evrard et al., 1992) is that the migrating neuron finds its way on its journey from the germinative zone to the cortical plate by climbing the radially ascending process of a specialized glial cell, the radial glial cell, according to the seminal discovery of Rakic (1971). However, it is now largely accepted that migrating neurons can adopt different types of trajectories (Fig. 4.2). (i) A large proportion of neurons do migrate radially, along radial glial guides, from the germinative zone to the cortical plate. Rakic (1988) has postulated that the radially arranged glial guides keep a topographical correspondence between a hypothesized protomap present in the germinative zone and the cortical areas. In vitro studies (Arimatsu et al., 1992; Ferri & Levitt, 1993), showing an early regional specification of neuronal precursors in the absence of extrinsic stimuli support the protomap hypothesis. Integrin receptors, which are located on radial glia and on migrating neurons, seem to play a critical role in the gliophilic neuronal migration (Anton et al., 1999). (ii) An important group of neuroblasts initially adopts a tangential trajectory at the level of the periventricular germinative zone (Fishell et al., 1993) before adopting a classical migrating pathway along radial glia to reach the emerging cortical plate. The role of this tangential migration could be to permit some dispersion at the level of the cortical plate of neurons originating from a single

Table 4.1. Syndromes and conditions associated with human neuronal migration disorders

Metabolic syndromes	Chromosomal syndromes
Zellweger's syndrome	Trisomy 13
Neonatal adrenoleukodystrophy	Trisomy 18
Glutaric aciduria II	Trisomy 21
Menke's kinky hair disease	Deletion 4p
Gm2 gangliosidosis	Deletion 17p13.3 (LIS1 gene)[a]
	Deletion Xq22.3–q23 (XLIS or DCX gene)[a]
Neuromuscular syndromes	
Walker–Warburg syndrome	**Other CNS dyplasias**
Fukuyama's congenital muscular dystrophy	Aicardi syndrome
Myotonic dystrophy	Joubert syndrome
Anterior horn arthrogryposis	Idiopathic lissencephaly sequence
	Hemimegalencephaly
Neurocutaneous syndromes	
Incontinentia pigmenti	**Twin syndromes**
Type I neurofibromatosis	Parabiotic twin syndrome
Hypomelanosis of Ito	
Tuberous sclerosis	**Infection**
Epidermal nevus syndrome	Cytomegalovirus
	Toxoplasmosis
Multiple congenital anomalies syndromes	
Smith–Lemli–Opitz syndrome	**Toxic exposures**
Potter syndrome	Ethanol
Cornelia De Lange syndrome	Cocaine
Meckel–Gruber syndrome	Methyl mercury poisoning
Oro-facio-digital syndrome	Carbon monoxide poisoning
Coffin–siris syndrome	Isoretinoic acid exposure
Bergeron syndrome	
Short small bowel syndrome	**Ionizing radiation**

Skeletal dysplasias
Thanatophoric dysplasia

Note: [a] Mutations in these two genes also produce neuronal migration disorders.
Source: Adapted and modified from Barkovich et al., (1992).

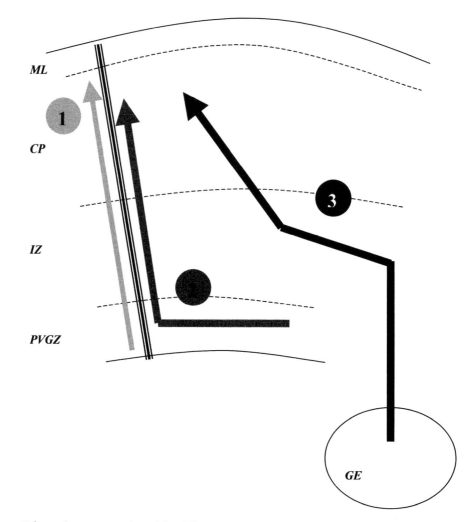

Fig. 4.2.   Schematic representation of the different migratory pathways adopted by neocortical neurons from the petriventricular germinative zone (PVGZ) or from the ganglia eminence (GE). **1**: radial migration along glial fascicles. **2**: tangential migration in the germinative zone followed by a radial migration along glial guides. **3**: tangential migration in the intermediate zone (IZ) CP, cortical plate; ML, molecular layer.

clone in the germinative neuroepithelium; this developmental mechanism would increase the neuronal diversity within a given cortical area (Austin & Cepko, 1990). Recent studies using retroviruses (Austin & Cepko, 1990; Walsh & Cepko, 1992, 1993) and sliced tissue cultures (Fishell et al., 1993) support the hypothesis of a glial-independent horizontal migration of some neurons in the periventricular germinative zone, inducing ultimately a cortical dispersion of clonally related neurons. Tan and Breen (1993), using a transgenic approach permitting one to label roughly half of the brain precursors, propose that both radial and tangential dispersion of neurons occur during corticogenesis; the extent of each phenomenon seems to be 2/3 vs. 1/3, respectively, although their data do not permit exclusion of the reverse proportion. (iii) Tangentially migrating neurons have also been described at the level of the intermediate zone (prospective white matter) (O'Rourke et al., 1992). Recent studies (Anderson et al., 1997; Tamamaki et al., 1997; Zhu et al., 1999) suggest that most of these neuronal cells displaying a migrating pathway orthogonal to radial glia originate in the lateral ganglia eminence (and not in the periventricular germinative zone). Although some of these tangentially migrating cells could end their migrating trajectory in the intermediate zone and not in the cortical plate (Tamamaki et al., 1997), numerous neocortical interneurons including GABA-expressing cells, seem to be produced by this mechanism (Anderson et al., 1997; Zhu et al., 1999).

From the appearance of the cortical plate, the radial glial fibres (RGFs) are grouped in fascicles of five to eight in the intermediate zone (Gadisseux & Evrard, 1985; Gressens & Evrard, 1993; Kadhim et al., 1988; Evrard et al., 1989) (Fig. 4.3). In the mouse, the first appearance of these glial units was observed at 9.5 embryonic days (Gressens et al., 1992a). The final cortical location of the neurons, which is determined by the guiding glial fascicle, partly determines the connections the neuron will be able to establish. It is not known if this fascicular organization of the radial glial guides influences the vertical organization of the cortical neurons and has to act as a module in the Rakic hypothesis or if the glial fasciculation has only an influence on the migratory corridors without shaping the vertical columns at the end of the corridors. The fascicles of glial fibres, filled with glycogen, can also be corridors of energy supply for migrating neurons. Along their migratory pathway, most neurons are far away from developing blood vessels which are sparse during angiogenesis. The glial fascicle unit therefore seems to be an ontogenic mechanism by which the mammalian brain is able to transfer neurons from the germinative zone to their distant sites of function over a pathway that is comparatively avascular during neuronal migration (Kuban & Gilles, 1985). Different ontogenic links between the germinative zone and the cortical plate have been described (Table 4.2 or for a review, see Purves et al., 1992; Kennedy & Dehay, 1993). The developmental units represent an interesting methodological tool for investigating the formation of cortical areas and the genesis of superior functions and for interpreting developmental disturbances.

The phenotype of radial glia seems to be determined both by migrating neurons (Culican et al., 1990) and by intrinsic factors expressed by glial cells. Among the latter, Götz et al. (1998) recently demonstrated that the transcription factor *Pax6*, which is specifically localized in radial glia during cortical development, is critical for the morphology, number, function and cell cycle of radial glia.

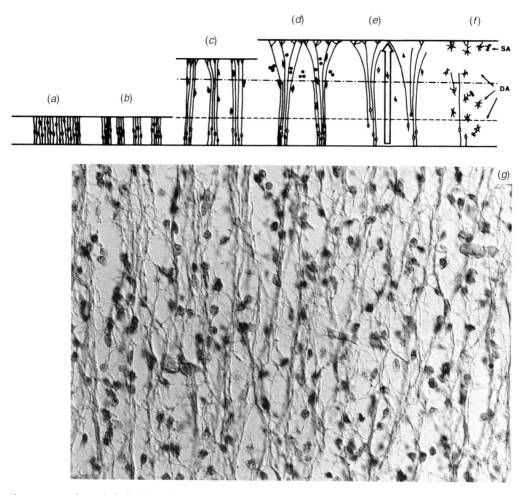

Fig. 4.3.   The radial glial fascicle. (*a*)–(*f*). Schematic representation of the glial fascicle in the
mammalian developing neocortex. Broken line: limit between the intermediate zone and
the cortical plate; dashes–dots: limit between the infragranular cortical layers and the
supragranular cortical layers; v shape: lateral ventricle. (*a*) After neurulation, glial cells are
distributed throughout the entire neuroepithelium (NE) (prospective germinative zone –
GZ). (*b*) Before the onset of any neuronal migration, the radial glial cells are organized in
regularly spaced fascicles, separated by clusters of neurons. (*c*) Migration of neurons
destined for the infragranular layers: from the germinative zone to their final cortical area,
these neurons are guided by radial glial fibres which are fasciculated along their whole
trajectory. (*d*) Migration of supragranular neurons which pass over the vertical columns of
infragranular neurons already in place and defasciculate the radial glial guides in the
cortical plate. This defasciculation is promoted by the resorption of many apical
intracortical processes of radial glial fibres. The defasciculation of the radial glial fibres
could allow some cortical dispersion of the neurons in the supragranular layers: the
neurons that have migrated along the same glial fascicle could be distributed in several
adjacent vertical columns, sometimes mixing with neurons of neighbouring neuronal–glial

The ontogenic neuronal–glial unit made of the radial glial fascicle and of its affiliated migrating neurons is very similar in the mouse, rat, hamster, cat, and in the human (Gressens & Evrard, 1993). Rakic (1988) has suggested that the increase in the number of symmetrical divisions of the neuronal precursors in the germinative zone could explain the evolution-linked increase of the cortical surface. We suggest a more precise and specific expansion with a limitation of Rakic's hypothesis. Because the neuronal–glial unit constituted by the glial fascicle and affiliated neurons is so constant throughout the mammalian species studied, it could represent the basic developmental module of the developing cortex: the unit remains stable while the number of adjacent units gradually increases to permit brain expansion in the evolution of mammalian species. Knowledge of the genetic and environmental factors that control the organization, number and function of these glial fascicles could, therefore, improve our understanding of cortical development and evolution of brain.

Effects of neurotransmitters and growth factors on neuronal migration

The role of neurotransmitters, including GABA and glutamate, in several ontogenic events has been suspected or demonstrated during the last decade. For what concerns neuronal migration, Komuro and Rakic (1993) first reported in tissue culture that the glutamatergic system was involved in the modulation of migration of cerebellar granule neurons. They showed that addition of specific inhibitors of the N-methyl-D-aspartate (NMDA) glutamate receptor subtype slowed down the rate of neuronal migration. The regulation of migration speed by NMDA receptors could be linked to the control of intracellular calcium concentration (Komuro & Rakic, 1992). Further demonstration that glutamate plays a role in neuronal migration was given by Marret et al (1996). They performed focal injections of ibotenate, a glutamate analog mainly acting on NMDA receptors, into the brain of hamsters on the day of birth, a stage where neurons destined for the superficial cortical layers are migrating. The resulting pattern was a laminar band heterotopia (see below) observed in 12% of the pups while ibotenate induced focal periventricular nodular heterotopias and intracortical arrest of migrating neurons in the remaining

Caption to fig. 4.3 (*cont.*)

units. (*e*), (*f*). After the end of neuronal migration, radial glial cells gradually transform into astrocytes which will be located mostly in the infragranular cortical layers and in the underlying white matter (DA : deep astrocytes). The superficial astrocytes (SA) derive from the late multiplication and migration (hollow arrow) of glial cells from the germinative zone (Gressens et al., 1992*d*). (*g*) Coronal section of a embryonic rabbit neocortex showing the glial fascicles and the affiliated migrating neurons.

Table 4.2. Possible ontogenic and phylogenic links between the germinative zone, the angiogenetic corridors, the early gap junctions, the synaptic stabilization, and the neocortical architecture

Perivascular neuronal units (Kuban & Gilles, 1985)
Neuronal unit supported by a radial vessel and its horizontal branches: possible role in morphogenesis through metabolic gradients within the perivascular units

Neuronal domains coupled by gap junctions (Yuste et al., 1992)
Early coupling of postmigrational neurons by gap junctions define cortical domains of spontaneously active neurons.

Protomap of cytoarchitectonic areas (Rakic, 1988)
Radially arranged glial guides keep a topographical correspondence between the proliferative units of the germinative zone and the cortical vertical columns.

Dispersed clonally related neurons (Austin & Cepko, 1990; Fishell et al., 1993; O'Rourke et al., 1992). Cortical spatial dispersion of clonally related neurons: temporary horizontal migration independent from RGCs and vertical migration along the non-perfectly radially arranged glial guides.

Radially and tangentially distributed neurons (Tan & Breen, 1993)
Based on early random labelling of half of the neural progenitors, two-thirds (or one-third) of neurons seem to be radially distributed while the remaining neurons (one-third or two-thirds, respectively) are tangentially dispersed.

The pyramidal cell and its local-circuit interneurons (Marin-Padilla, 1990)
A constant structural and functional unit throughout the mammalian species. It suggests to us a developmental mechanism based on migratory units and/or upon mechanisms of synaptic stabilization.

Glial fascicles (Gadisseux & Evrard, 1985; Kadhim et al., 1988; Gressens & Evrard, 1993)
Neuronal migration along regularly spaced and early formed glial fascicles: guiding role, energy corridors during neuronal anaerobiosis, and organization of cortical neurons. This unit is constant throughout the mammalian species.

Vertical physiological column (Mountcastle, 1957)
Radially organized basic module of a constant amount of neurons responsive to a specific modality of stimulation. It has been suggested that this unit developed from neurons that have migrated along a radial glial cell.

Neuropsychological unit (Changeux & Danchin, 1976; Edelman, 1981)
Functionally but not structurally redundant cortical units; the function is produced by the association of units according to their final connections shaped by synaptic stabilization.

Source: Adapted and modified from Gressens et al., (1993).

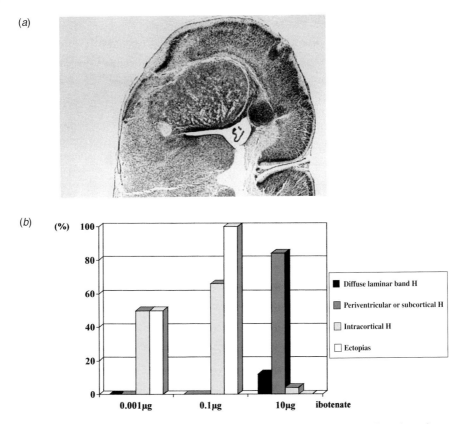

Fig. 4.4.   Ibotenate-induced neuronal migration disorders. (*a*) Cresyl-violet-stained section of a hamster brain injected with 10 μg at birth and showing periventricular heterotopia. (*b*) Frequency of neuronal migration disorders induced by different doses of ibotenate injected in hamster brain at birth (H, heterotopia).

animals (Fig. 4.4). The reasons for the occurrence of focal vs. diffuse migration disorders in this model are still unknown. Ibotenate, a unique molecular trigger of the excitotoxic cascade, produces a wide spectrum of abnormal neuronal migration patterns recognized in mammals, including the neocortical deviations encountered in the human brain such as nodular heterotopias, lissencephalies and double cortex syndromes. Excess release of glutamate during brain development has been described in human conditions and/or in experimental models following several pathological conditions including hypoxia–ischemia, hemorrhagic accidents, hypoglycemia, traumas or viral infections. Furthermore, lack of glutamate recapture by glial cells could also increase extracellular glutamate. The recent description of the glutamate transporter GLAST on radial glia (Shibata et al., 1997) is a further step towards understanding the role of glutamate in neuronal migration.

Among neurotransmitters, GABA also seems to be involved in neuronal migration modulation as it stimulates, in tissue culture, neuronal migration via calcium-dependent mechanisms (Behar et al., 1996, 1998 and 1999). Chemotactic effects of GABA were observed at fentomolar concentrations and involved the three classes of GABA receptors while GABA-induced chemokinesis required micromolar concentrations and involved only $GABA_B$ and $GABA_C$ receptors. Furthermore, the relative contribution of GABA-mediated chemotaxis and chemokinesis was highly dependent upon the stage of neocortical development.

Growth factors have been recently shown to be involved in the control of neuronal migration. Intraventricular injection of neurotrophin-4 (NT-4) (Brunstrom et al., 1997) or overexpression of brain-derived neurotrophic factor (BDNF) (Ringstedt et al., 1998) during mouse brain development produces heterotopic accumulation of neurons in the molecular layer (layer I). The lesion pattern mimics some aspects observed in human status verrucosus deformans. Furthermore, transgenic mice overexpressing BDNF had a decreased Reelin expression and displayed abnormal cortical lamination similar to the reeler phenotype (see below). In the context of trophic factors, two separate studies (Rio et al., 1997; Anton et al., 1997) have shown that neuregulin, a member of the epidermal growth factor (EGF) family, is critical for the interactions between migrating neurons and radial glia: blockade of the neuregulin receptor erbB on radial glia impairs migration of cultured cerebellar granule cells which express neuregulin.

These experimental data demonstrate that several growth factors and neurotransmitters play a critical role in the control or modulation of neuronal migration. The potential implications of these recent discoveries for the understanding and classification of human disorders should arise in the near future.

X-linked periventricular heterotopia: disturbance of the motility control

The X-linked dominant periventricular heterotopia is characterized by neuronal nodules lining the ventricular surface. Hemizygous males die during the embryonic period and affected females have epilepsy which can be accompanied by other manisfestations such as patent ductus arteriosus and coagulopathy. The gene responsible for this disease has been recently identified (Fox et al., 1998): filamin 1 (FLN1) encodes an actin-cross-linking phosphoprotein which transduces ligand-receptor binding into actin reorganization. Filamin 1 is necessary for locomotion of several cell types and is present at high levels in the developing neocortex (Fox et al., 1998). Rakic et al (1996) had previously shown the polarity of microtubule assemblies during migration of rodent cerebellar neurons and proposed that the dynamics of slow polymerization combined with fast disintegration of oriented microtubules was critical for displacement of the nucleus and cytoplasm within the membrane cylinder of the leading process of the migrating neuron.

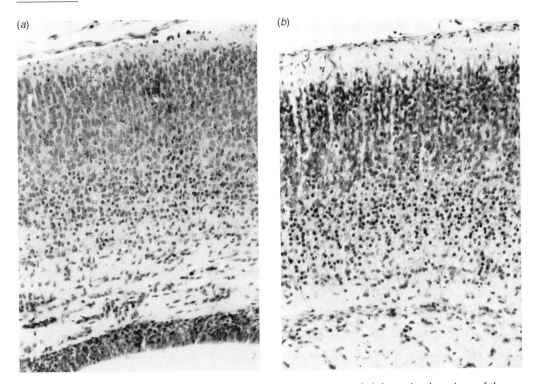

Fig. 4.5.   Migration disorders in murine Zellweger syndrome. Cresyl violet stained sections of the
neocortex of transgenic mice devoid of peroxysomes (*a*) and control mice (*b*) at birth
showing the decreased thickness of the cortical plate and the increased neuronal density
in the underlying intermediate zone (prospective white matter) in the 'Zellweger' mice.

Human Zellweger syndrome and mouse models

The Zellweger cerebro-hepato-renal syndrome is a fatal autosomic recessive disease
caused by an absence of functional peroxysomes. One hallmark of this human
disease is the presence of heterotopic neurons in the neocortex, the cerebellum and
the inferior olivary complex. Patients are characterized by the absence of psychomotor development or a rapid regression, a dysmorphic facies and a severe
hypotonia. Patellar calcifications, ocular abnormalities, cystic kidneys and
hepatomegaly are frequent. Patients generally die within a few months.

Two different animal models of this human disease have been produced by inactivation of a gene critically involved in peroxysome assembly (Baes et al., 1997;
Faust & Hatten, 1997). In both models, animals homozygous for the gene inactivation have no functional peroxysomes, die around birth and display heterotopic
neurons in the subcortical white matter (Fig. 4.5) and dysplastic olivary complex.
The study of radial glia cells and of neocortical astrocytes did not reveal any signifi-

cant morphological change in these glial populations although the available data do not permit exclusion of a functional defect of glial cells in mutant mice. Analysis of mutant mice revealed that the migration defect was caused by altered N-methyl-D-aspartate (NMDA) glutamate receptor-mediated calcium mobilization (Gressens et al., 2000). This NMDA receptor dysfunction was linked to a deficit in PAF, a phenomenon related to peroxysome impairment. These findings confirm NMDA receptor and PAF involvement in neuronal migration and suggest a link between peroxysome metabolism and NMDA receptor efficacy.

Type I lissencephaly and role of platelet-activating factor (PAF) in neuronal migration

Lissencephaly and agyria–pachygyria are the terms used to describe brains with absent or poor sulcation. Agyria refers to brains or portions of brains with absence of gyri and sulci whereas pachygyria refers to brains or portions thereof with few broad, flat gyri and shallow sulci. Lissencephaly ('smooth brain') is another term used to describe such brains. Complete lissencephaly is synonymous with agyria, whereas incomplete lissencephaly refers to brains with shallow sulci and a relatively smooth surface; incomplete lissencephaly is often used synonymously with agyria-pachygyria.

Type I lissencephaly usually has both agyric and pachygyric regions (for a review see Barkovich et al., 1992). The histological appearance of the cortex varies according to the brain area; the majority of the neocortex is that of a 'four-layered' cortex, composed of a molecular layer, a disorganized outer cellular layer, a cell sparse layer, and an inner cellular layer (probably composed of neurons whose migration has been prematurely arrested). The migratory defect is postulated to occur between 12 and 16 gestational weeks. Other gross pathological features of lissencephaly Type I include dilatation of the trigones and occipital horns of the lateral ventricles and hypogenesis of the corpus callosum. Clinically, patients with Type I lissencephaly often have bitemporal hollowing, prominence of the occiput, and micrognathia. The head size is normal to small at birth, but progressive microcephaly is common. Patients are hypotonic at birth, but develop progressive spasticity. Seizures generally begin within the first few months of life. Miller–Dieker syndrome is a malformative syndrome associating classical type I lissencephaly and a characteristic facies.

Miller–Dieker syndrome and up to 40% of cases of isolated lissencephaly sequence (Lo Nigro et al., 1997; Pilz et al., 1998) result from a hemideletion or mutations of the LIS1 gene. LIS1 encodes the beta subunit of a brain acetylhydrolase which degrades the platelet-activating factor (PAF). Accordingly, in vitro stimulation of PAF receptor disrupts neuronal migration (Bix & Clarck, 1998). PAF is an ether phospholipid acting in the brain on receptors present on synaptic endings and intracellular membranes. As PAF increases intracellular calcium concentration and stimulates excitatory amino acid neurotransmission, it is tempting to speculate that some brain abnormalities observed in Miller–Dieker syndrome are secondary to an excess of glutamatergic transmission, potentially linking the hamster model of migration disorder described above to human lissencephaly.

Studying human fetuses, Clarck and colleagues (1997) have shown that LIS gene products are localized in Cajal–Retzius neurons, some subplate neurons, thalamic neurons and in the periventricular germinative zone. The expression of LIS in Cajal–Retzius cells strongly supports the previously suspected role of these cells in the neuronal migration and in the cytoarchitectonic organization of the cortical plate. Cajal–Retzius also synthesize and release the extracellular matrix protein reelin which is lacking in reeler mutant mice. These reeler mice are characterized by an abnormal cortical lamination probably secondary to defects in stop signals for migrating neurons (for a review, see Frotsher, 1997). Previous studies have suggested that subplate neurons are also involved in the control of neocortical lamination (Shatz et al., 1988; Kostovic & Rakic, 1990). Furthermore, growing thalamocortical axons reach the cortical plate before the completion of neuronal migration and remain blocked for a while in the subplate where they temporarily establish connections with subplate neurons. The expression of LIS gene in subplate and thalamic neurons is further evidence of the potential role of these neuronal populations in the modulation of neuronal migration. The presence of LIS gene product in the germinative zone is in agreement with other studies which have shown that laminar distribution of cortical neurons is influenced by events occurring during the mitotic cycle of neuronal precursors in the germinative zone (McConnell & Kaznowski, 1991; Chae et al., 1997; Chevassus-Au-Louis et al., 1998; Gilmore et al., 1998).

Double cortex syndrome and animal models

Diffuse subcortical laminar heterotopias have been described pathologically and on a clinical and imaging basis under the names of 'double cortex', 'bicortical lissencephalies', 'partial lissencephalies', 'laminar heterotopias', 'band heterotopias' (for a review, see Barkovich et al., 1992). The key cytoarchitectonic data is the 'true double cortex'. It seems to us that different conditions have been reported under these names and different clinical pictures have been described. We previously reported a case with a clinical picture suggesting atypical type 1 lissencephaly but a cousin was affected with a clinical and imaging picture suggesting type 2 lissencephaly (Evrard et al., 1989). Friede (1989) reported laminar heterotopias and mentioned that this condition is not inconsistent with social adaptation and mild clinical manifestations. The other patients reported usually had moderate to severe developmental delay and an early onset of medically refractory seizures but other patients showed relatively mild clinical manifestations indicating some variability in clinical presentation. Des Portes et al (1998a, b) and Gleeson et al (1998) have recently identified a novel gene (DCX or XLIS gene) involved in X-linked neuronal migration disorder where females display subcortical laminar heterotopia (or double cortex syndrome) while lissencephaly is found in males. Preliminary reports suggest that, in some affected families, females could have corpus callosum agenesis, arguing for some phenotypic diversity in this genetic syndrome. The gene encodes a predictive protein, doublecortin, which is a microtubule-associated protein expressed by migrating and differentiating neurons (Francis et al., 1999; Gleeson et al., 1999). From a clinical point of view, a recent report has proposed that deletions or mutations of DCX and LIS1 genes account for 76% of isolated type I lissencephalies (Pilz et al., 1998).

Two animal models of laminar band heterotopias are currently available: the ibotenate-induced laminar heterotopias in the newborn hamster (see above) and the tish (telencephalic internal structural heterotopia) rat. The tish rat is a spontaneously mutant animal exhibiting a bilateral laminar band heterotopia which predominates in the frontal and parietal cortex (Lee et al., 1997). The heterotopic cortical plate could be secondary to the combination of abnormal neuronal migration and heterotopic neurogenesis (Lee et al., 1998). The cortical abnormality is inherited in a recessive autosomic manner and affected rats exhibit spontaneous recurrent electrographic and behavioural seizures.

Type II lissencephaly: a mesenchymal disorder?

Type II lissencephaly is characterized by a thickened and severely disorganized unlayered cortex, which is disrupted by penetrating vessels and fibro-glial bundles (for a review, see Barkovich et al., 1992). The neurons are sometimes grouped in large poorly established vertical columns that are out of register with the neighbouring columns. Subcortical heterotopias are not rare. The meninges are thickened and densely adherent to the cortex, obliterating the subarachnoid space and resulting in hydrocephalus. The entire cerebral hemispheres and cerebellum are involved. Furthermore, the cerebellar cortex displays a diffuse microgyric aspect. Associated anomalies include microphthalmia with retinal dysplasia, callosal dysgenesis, cerebellar cortical dysplasia, cerebellar vermian hypoplasia, and hypomyelination of the white matter. Classically, the clinical presentation of patients with Type II lissencephaly is that of the Walker–Warburg syndrome. These patients are almost always severely abnormal at birth and may have severe congenital eye mal-formations, posterior cephaloceles, congenital hydrocephalus, or congenital hypo-tonia. The hypotonia is usually profound and unchanging, with most patients dying in the first year of life. The relationships between agyria-pachygyria, Fukuyama disease and other muscular diseases are discussed elsewhere (Voit, 1998).

The literature contains hypotheses of genetic causes and of a destructive process in the second half of the second trimester (for a review, see Barkovich et al., 1992; Evrard et al., 1989, 1992). A mesenchymal abnormality is evidently present either as a causative agent with secondary migration disorder or as an accompanying factor (Lyon et al., 1993). A provocative etiological discussion has arisen to explain the high intrafamilial recurrence rate. The vulnerability to a viral or teratogenic process during successive pregnancies could explain more features of this clinico-pathological entity than the metabolic or genetic hypothesis, but there is no way to close this debate with the available data.

Effects of environmental factors on neuronal migration

Neuronal migration disorders have been described in humans and in animal models following in utero exposure to several environmental factors, including cytomegalovirus infection, ethanol, cocaine, isoretinoic acid or ionizing radiation. In most cases, the mechanisms by which these factors disturb neuronal migration remain unclear. However, prenatal cocaine administration to pregnant mice or monkeys induces abnormal addressing of neurons in the neocortical plate (Gressens et al., 1992b; Lidow, 1995). This abnormal neuronal migration pattern is probably linked to the observed abnormalities of radial glia density and distur-bances of neuronal proliferation in the germinative zone (Fig. 4.6) (Gressens et al., 1992b). Similarly, ethanol administration to pregnant mice severely alters the ontogeny of radial glia and neocortical astrocytes (Gressens et al., 1992c): these glial abnormalities could participate in the formation of neuronal ectopias frequently observed in the fetal alcohol syndrome.

Conclusions

Neocortical neuronal migration appears as a complex ontogenic step occurring early during embryonic and fetal development. Control of neuronal migration involves different cell populations including Cajal–Retzius, subplate and thalamic neurons, periventricular neuronal precursors or radial glia. The integrity of multi-ple molecular mechanisms, such as cell cycle control, cell-cell adhesion, interac-tion with extracellular matrix protein, neurotransmitter release, growth factor

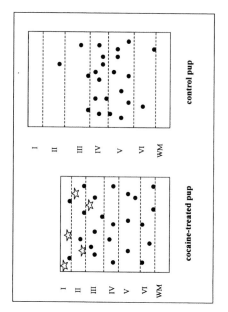

(c)

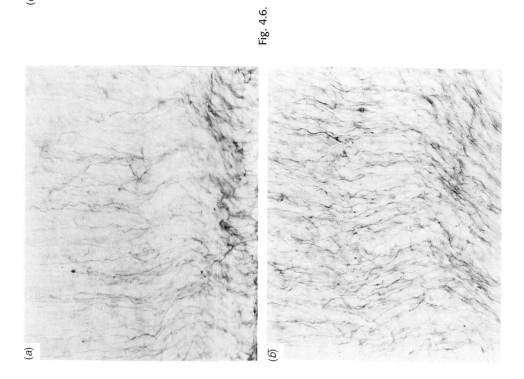

(a)

(b)

Fig. 4.6.

Effects of cocaine on neuronal migration. (*a,b*) Coronal sections through the intermediate zone (prospective white matter) of a mouse embryo treated with cocaine (*a*) and a control embryo (*b*) showing the cocaine-induced lower density of glial fascicles labelled at embryonic day 17 with the specific 'radial cell 2' antibody. (*c*) *Camera lucida* drawings of the distribution of neurons (dots) and glial cells (stars) intensely labelled with ³H-thymidine in murine dorsolateral frontal cortex. ³H-thymidine was injected into pregnant dams at embryonic day 14, and pups sacrificed on postnatal day 5. The layer IV–V predominance of neural distribution in controls is contrasted with a more random laminar distribution evident in drug-exposed mice. WM: white matter; I to VI: cortical layers.

Table 4.3. Summary of the established or hypothetical links between genes and gene products and neuronal migration disorders in human and rodent neocortex

LIS1 gene, PAF and PAF acetylhydrolase	Miller–Dieker syndrome and some isolated type I lissencephalies
DCX or XLIS gene	X-linked subcortical laminar heterotopia and lissencephaly syndrome (or double cortex syndrome)
filamin 1 (FLN1)	X-linked dominant periventricular heterotopia
tish gene	Laminar band heterotopias, double cortex syndrome
reelin	Inverted cortical layers
p35/cdk5 kinase	Inverted cortical layers
neurotrophins	Status verrucosus, molecular ectopias, inverted cortical layers
GABAergic system	Neuronal migration disorders
glutamatergic system	Neuronal heterotopias, molecular ectopias
peroxysomal apparatus	Zellweger syndrome
Pax6 gene	Abnormalities of radial glia

Source: Adapted and modified from Gressens, (1998).

availability, PAF degradation or transduction pathways seems to be critical for permitting a normal neuronal migration. The complexity and the multiplicity of these mechanisms probably explain the clinical, radiological and genetic heterogeneity of human disorders of neuronal migration.

A few human and rodent genes and factors linked to neuronal migration disorders have been recently identified (Table 4.3). The elucidation of their function should help to clarify the mechanisms of neuronal migration as well as the pathophysiology of some brain malformations. Furthermore, patients with these diseases can now benefit from a genetic diagnosis which can also be applied in some instances to prenatal cases. Improvement of imaging techniques has also permitted new classifications of neuronal migration disorders to be proposed as well as their diagnosis very early during fetal brain development. On the other hand, basic research has led to the identification of some critical molecular factors involved in normal and abnormal neuronal migration and has also emphasized the critical interactions between genetic and environmental/epigenetic factors. The long-term consequences in terms of behaviour, learning and motor abilities or electrophysiological properties of animals with migration disorders are being extensively studied, opening new avenues in the understanding of human disorders such as epilepsy, learning disabilities, mental retardation and some psychiatric diseases.

REFERENCES

Anderson, S. A., Eisenstat, D. D., Shi, L. & Rubenstein, J. L. (1997). Interneuron migration from basal forebrain to neocortex: dependence on Dix genes. *Science*, **278**, 474–6.

Angevine, J. B. & Sidman, R. L. (1961). Autoradiographic study of cell migration during histogenesis of the cerebral cortex. *Nature*, **192**, 766–8.

Anton, E. S., Marchionni, M. A., Lee, K. F. & Rakic, P. (1997). Role of GGF/neuregulin signaling in interactions between migrating neurons and radial glia in the developing cerebral cortex. *Development*, **124**, 3501–10.

Anton, E. S., Kreidberg, J. A. & Rakic, P. (1999). Distinct functions of α_3 and α_V integrin receptors in neuronal migration and laminar organization of the cerebral cortex. *Neuron*, **22**, 277–89.

Arimatsu, Y., Miyamato, M., Nihonmatsu, I. et al. (1992). Early regional specification for a molecular neuronal phenotype in the rat neocortex. *Proceedings of the National Academy of Sciences, USA*, **89**, 8879–83.

Austin, C. P. & Cepko, C. L. (1990). Cellular migration patterns in the developing mouse cerebral cortex. *Development*, **110**, 713–32.

Baes, M., Gressens, P., Baumgart, E. et al. (1997). Peroxisome deficiency induces abnormal brain development and intrauterine growth retardation in Zellweger mice. *Nature Genetics*, **17**, 49–57.

Barkovich, A. J., Gressens, P. & Evrard, P. (1992). Formation, maturation, and disorders of neocortex. *American Journal of Neuroradiology*, **13**, 423–46.

Barkovich, A. J., Kuzniecky, R. I., Dobyns, W. B., Jackson, G. D., Becker, L. E. & Evrard, P. (1996). A classification scheme for malformations of cortical development. *Neuropediatrics*, **27**, 59–63.

Behar, T. N., Li, Y. X., Tran, H. T., Dunlap, V., Scott, V. & Barker, J. L. (1996). GABA stimulates chemotaxis and chemokinesis of embryonic cortical neurons via calcium-dependent mechanisms. *Journal of Neuroscience*, **16**, 1808–18.

Behar, T. N., Schaffner, A. E., Scott, C. A., O'Connell, C. & Barker, J. L. (1998). Differential response of cortical plate and ventricular zone cells to GABA as a migration stimulus. *Journal of Neuroscience*, **18**, 6378–87.

Behar, T. N., Scott, C. A., Greene, C. L. et al. (1999). Glutamate acting at NMDA receptors stimulates embryonic cortical neuronal migration. *Journal of Neuroscience*, **19**, 4449–61.

Bix, G. J. & Clarck, G. D. (1998). Platelet-activating factor receptor stimulation disrupts neuronal migration *in vitro*. *Journal of Neuroscience*, **18**, 307–18.

Brunstrom, J. E., Gray-Swain, M. R., Osborne, P. A. & Pearlman, A. L. (1997) Neuronal heterotopias in the developing cerebral cortex produced by neurotrophin-4. *Neuron*, **18**, 505–17.

Caviness, V. S., Misson, J. P. & Gadisseux, J. F. (1989). Abnormal neuronal migrational patterns and disorders of neocortical development. In *From Reading to Neuron*, ed. A. M. Galaburda, pp. 405–42. MIT Press, Cambridge.

Chae, T., Kwon, Y. T., Bronson, R., Dikkes, P., Li, E. & Tsai, L. H. (1997). Mice lacking p35, a neuronal specific activator of Cdk5, display cortical lamination defects, seizures, and adult lethality. *Neuron*, **18**, 29–42.

Changeux, J-P. & Danchin, A. (1976). Selective stabilization of developing synapses as a mechanism for the specification of neuronal network. *Nature*, **264**, 705–12.

Chevassus-Au-Louis, N., Congar, P., Represa, A., Ben-Ari, Y. & Gaïarsa, J. L. (1998). Neuronal migration disorders: heterotopic neocortical neurons in CA1 provide a bridge between the hippocampus and the neocortex. *Proceedings of the National Academy of Sciences, USA*, **95**, 10263–8.

Clarck, G. D., Mizuguchi, M., Antalffy, B., Barnes, J. & Armstrong, D. (1997). Predominant localization of the *LIS* family gene products to Cajal–Retzius cells and ventricular neuroepithelium in the developing human cortex. *Journal of Neuropathology and Experimental Neurology*, **56**, 1044–52.

Culican, S., Baumrind, N., Yammamoto, M. & Pearlman, A. (1990). Cortical radial glia: identification in tissue culture and evidence for their transformation to astrocytes. *Journal of Neuroscience*, **10**, 684–92.

Des Portes, V., Francis, F., Pinard, J. M. et al. (1998*a*). Doublecortin is the major gene causing X-linked subcortical laminar heterotopias. *Human Molecular Genetics*, **7**, 1063–70.

Des Portes, V., Pinard, J. M., Billuart, P. et al. (1998*b*). A novel CNS gene required for neuronal migration and involved in X-linked subcortical laminar heterotopia and lissencephaly syndrome. *Cell*, **92**, 51–61.

Edelman, G. M. (1981). Group selection as the basis for higher brain function. In *The Organization of the Cerebral Cortex*, ed. F. O. Schmitt, F. C. Worden, G. Adelman & S. G. Dennis, pp. 535–63. Cambridge: MIT Press.

Evrard, P., Kadhim, H. J., de St-Georges, P. & Gadisseux, J. F. (1989). Abnormal development and destructive processes of the human brain during the second half of gestation. In *Developmental Neurobiology*, ed. P. Evrard & A. Minkowski, pp. 21–42. New York: Raven Press.

Evrard, P., Miladi, N., Bonnier, C. & Gressens, P. (1992). Normal and abnormal development of the brain. In *Handbook of Neuropsychology*, vol. 6, *Child Neuropsychology*, ed. I. Rapin & S. Segalowitz, pp. 11–44. Amsterdam: Elsevier Science Publ.

Faust, P. L. & Hatten, M. E. (1997). Targeted deletion of the PEX2 peroxisome assembly gene in mice provides a model for Zellweger syndrome, a human neuronal migration disorder. *Journal of Cell Biology*, **139**, 1293–305.

Ferri, R. T. & Levitt, P. (1993). Cerebral cortical progenitors are fated to produce region-specific neuronal populations. *Cerebral Cortex*, **3**, 187–98.

Fishell, G., Mason, C. A. & Hatten, M. E. (1993). Dispersion of neural progenitors within the germinal zones of the forebrain. *Nature*, **362**, 636–8.

Fox, J. W., Lamperti, E. D., Eksioglu, Y. Z. et al. (1998) Mutations in filamin 1 prevent migration of cerebral cortical neurons in human periventricular heterotopia. *Neuron*, **21**, 1315–25.

Francis, F., Koulakoff, A., Boucher, D. et al. (1999). Doublecortin is a developmentally regulated, microtubule-associated protein expressed in migrating and differentiating neurons. *Neuron*, **23**, 247–56.

Friede, R. L. (1989). *Developmental Neuropathology*. 2nd edn. Berlin: Springer Publ.

Frotscher, M. (1997). Dual role of Cajal–Retzius cells and reelin in cortical development. *Cell Tissue Research*, **290**, 315–22.

Gadisseux, J. F. & Evrard, P. (1985). Glial–neuronal relationship in the developing central nervous system. *Developmental Neuroscience*, 7, 12–32.

Gilmore, E. C., Ohshima, T., Goffinet, A. M., Kulkarni, A. B. & Herrup K. (1998). Cyclin-dependent kinase 5-deficient mice demonstrate novel developmental arrest in cerebral cortex. *Journal of Neuroscience*, **18**, 6370–7.

Gleeson, J. G., Allen, K. M., Fox, J. W. et al. (1998). Doublecortin, a brain-specific gene mutated in human X-linked lissencephaly and double cortex syndrome, encodes a putative signaling protein. *Cell*, **92**, 63–72.

Gleeson, J. G., Lin, P. T., Flanagan, L. A. & Walsh, C. A. (1999). Doublecortin is a microtubule-associated protein and is widely expressed by migrating neurons. *Neuron*, **23**, 257–71.

Götz, M., Stoykova, A. & Gruss, P. (1998). *Pax6* controls radial glia differentiation in the cerebral cortex. *Neuron*, **21**, 1031–44.

Gressens, P. (1998). Mechanisms of cerebral dysgenesis. *Current Opinion in Pediatrics*, **10**, 556–60.

Gressens, P. & Evrard, P. (1993). The glial fascicle: a developmental unit guiding, supplying and organizing mammalian cortical neurons. *Developmental Brain Research*, **76**, 272–7.

Gressens, P., Baes, M., Leroux, P. et al. (2000). Neuronal migration in Zellweger mice is secondary to glutamate receptor dysfunction. *Annals of Neurology*, **48**, 336–43.

Gressens, P., Gofflot, F., Van Maele-Fabry, G. et al. (1992a). Early neurogenesis and teratogenesis in whole mouse embryo cultures. Histochemical, immunocytological and ultrastructural study of the premigratory neural-glial events in normal mouse embryo and in mouse embryos influenced by cocaine and retinoic acid. *Journal of Neuropathology and Experimental Neurology*, **51**, 206–19.

Gressens, P., Kosofsky, B. E. & Evrard, P. (1992b). Cocaine-induced disturbances of neurogenesis in the developing murine brain. *Neuroscience Letters*, **140**, 113–16.

Gressens, P., Lammens, M., Picard, J. J. & Evrard, P. (1992c). Ethanol-induced disturbances of gliogenesis and neurogenesis in the developing murine brain: an in vitro and in vivo immunohistochemical, morphological, and ultrastructural study. *Alcohol and Alcoholism*, **27**, 219–26.

Gressens, P., Richelme, C., Kadhim, H. J., Gadisseux, J. F. & Evrard, P. (1992d). The germinative zone produces most cortical astrocytes after neuronal migration in developing mammalian brain. *Biology of the Neonate*, **61**, 4–24.

Kadhim, H. J., Gadisseux, J. F. & Evrard, P. (1988). Topographical and cytological evolution of the glial phase during prenatal development of the human brain: histochemical and electron microscopic study. *Journal of Neuropathology and Experimental Neurology*, **47**, 166–88.

Kennedy, H. & Dehay, C. (1993). Cortical specification of mice and men. *Cerebral Cortex*, **3**, 171–86.

Komuro, H. & Rakic, P. (1992). Selective role of N-type calcium channels in neuronal migration. *Science*, **257**, 806–9.

Komuro, H. & Rakic, P. (1993). Modulation of neuronal migration by NMDA receptors. *Science*, **260**, 95–7.

Kostovic, I. & Rakic, P. (1990). Developmental history of the transient subplate zone in the visual and somatosensory cortex of the macaque monkey and human brain. *Journal of Comparative Neurology*, **297**, 441–70.

Kuban, K. C. K. & Gilles, F. H. (1985). Human telencephalic angiogenesis. *Annals of Neurology*, **17**, 539–48.

Lee, K. S., Schotter, F., Collins, J. L. et al. (1997). A genetic animal model of human neocortical heterotopia associated with seizures. *Journal of Neuroscience*, **17**, 6236–42.

Lee, K. S., Collins, J. L., Anzivino, M. J., Frankel, E. A. & Schottler, F. (1998). Heterotopic neurogenesis in a rat with cortical heterotopia. *Journal of Neuroscience*, **18**, 9365–75.

Lidow, M. S. (1995). Prenatal cocaine exposure adversely affects development of the primate cerebral cortex. *Synapse*, **21**, 332–41.

Lo Nigro, C., Chong, C. S., Smith, A. C., Dobyns, W. B., Carrozzo, R. & Ledbetter, D. H. (1997). Point mutations and an intragenic deletion of LIS1, the lissencephaly causative gene in isolated lissencephaly sequence and Miller–Dieker syndrome. *Human Molecular Genetics*, **6**, 157–64.

Lyon, G., Raymond, G., Mogami, K., Gadisseux, J. F. & Della Giustina, E. (1993). Disorder of cerebellar foliation in Walker's lissencephaly and Neu–Laxova syndrome. *Journal of Neuropathology and Experimental Neurology*, **52**, 633–9.

McConnell, S. K. & Kaznowski, C. E. (1991). Cell cycle dependence of laminar determination in developing neocortex. *Science*, **254**, 282–5.

Marin-Padilla, M. J. (1990). The pyramidal cell and its local-circuit interneurons: a hypothetical unit of the mammalian neocortex. *Cognitive Neuroscience*, **2**, 180–94.

Marin-Padilla, M. J. (1998). Cajal–Retzius cells and the development of the neocortex. *Trends in Neurosciences*, **21**, 64–71.

Marret, S., Gressens, P. & Evrard, P. (1996). Neuronal migration disorders induced by ibotenate in the neocortex. *Proceedings of the National Academy of Sciences, USA*, **93**, 15463–8.

Mountcastle, V. B. (1957). Modality and topographic properties of single neurons of cat's somatic sensory cortex. *Journal of Neurophysiology*, **20**, 408–34.

O'Rourke, N. A, Dailey, M. E., Smith, S. J. & McConnell, S. K. (1992). Diverse migratory pathways in the developing cerebral cortex. *Science*, **258**, 299–302.

Pilz, D. T., Matsumoto, N., Minnerath, S. et al. (1998). *LIS1* and *XLS* (*DCX*) mutations cause most classical lissencephaly, but different patterns of malformation. *Human Molecular Genetics*, **7**, 2029–37.

Purves, D., Riddle, D. R. & LaMantia, A-S. (1992). Iterated patterns of brain circuitry. *Trends in Neuroscience*, **15**, 362–8.

Rakic, P. (1971). Guidance of neurons migrating to the fetal monkey neocortex. *Brain Research*, **33**, 471–6.

Rakic, P. (1988). Specification of cerebral cortical areas. *Science*, **241**, 170–6.

Rakic, P., Knyihar-Csillik, E. & Csillik, B. (1996). Polarity of microtubule assemblies during neuronal cell migration. *Proceedings of the National Academy of Sciences, USA*, **17**, 9218–22.

Ringstedt, T., Linnarsson, S., Wagner, J. et al. (1998). BDNF regulates reelin expression and Cajal–Retzius cell development in the cerebral cortex. *Neuron*, **21**, 305–15.

Rio, C., Rieff, H. I., Qi, P. & Corfas, G. (1997). Neuregulin and erbB receptors play a critical role in neuronal migration. *Neuron*, **19**, 39–50.

Shatz, C. J., Chun, L. L. M. & Luskin, M. B. (1988). The role of the subplate in the development of the mammalian telencephalon. In *Development and Maturation of Cerebral Cortex*, vol. 7, *Cerebral Cortex*, ed. A. Peters & E. G. Jones, pp. 35–58. New York: Plenum.

Shibata, T., Yamada, K., Watanabe, M. et al. (1997). Glutamate transporter GLAST is expressed in the radial glia–astrocyte lineage of developing mouse spinal cord. *Journal of Neuroscience*, **17**, 9212–19.

Tamamaki, N., Fujimori, K. E. & Takauji, R. (1997). Origin and route of tangentially migrating neurons in the developing neocortical intermediate zone. *Journal of Neuroscience*, **17**, 8313–23.

Tan, S. S. & Breen, S. (1993). Radial mosaicism and tangential cell dispersion both contribute to mouse neocortical development. *Nature*, **362**, 638–40.

Voit, T. (1998). Congenital muscular dystrophies: 1997 update. *Brain and Development*, **20**, 65–74.

Walsh, C. & Cepko, C. L. (1992). Widespread dispersion of neuronal clones across functional regions of the cerebral cortex. *Science*, **255**, 434–40.

Walsh, C. & Cepko, C. L. (1993). Clonal dispersion in proliferative layers of developing cerebral cortex. *Nature*, **362**, 632–5.

Yuste, R., Peinado, A. & Katz, L. C. (1992). Neuronal domains in developing neocortex, *Science* **257**, 665–9.

Zhu, Y., Li, H. S., Zhou, L., Wu, J. Y. & Rao, Y. (1999). Cellular and molecular guidance of GABAergic neuronal migration from an extracortical origin to neocortex. *Neuron*, **23**, 473–85.

5

Synaptogenesis in the neocortex of the newborn: the ultimate frontier for individuation?

Jean-Pierre Bourgeois

Laboratoire de Neurobiologie Moléculaire, Institut Pasteur, Paris, France

Introduction

The development of the neocortex in mammals is a highly orchestrated cascade of histological events including, successively, the generation and differentiation of neurons (Rakic, 1995), the navigation and organization of the axonal projections between ensembles of neurons (Barone et al., 1995), then the formation and maturation of the synaptic contacts which constitute major final steps of corticogenesis (Bourgeois & Rakic, 1993; Bourgeois et al., 1994, 2000; Huttenlocher & Dabholkar, 1997; de Felipe et al., 1997). All these biological events ultimately lead to individuation, the process by which individual mammals become differentiated in their societies.

As reviewed by Zoli et al. (1998), intercellular communications in the neocortex can occur either via volume transmission or by wiring transmission. The present review describes the development of the wiring transmission via synaptic contacts.

The formation of synaptic contacts can be described at two distinct levels: on the one hand, one can describe the assembly of the numerous molecular components building up the pre- and postsynaptic domains of the neuron. On the other hand, one can describe the development of ensembles of synaptic contacts in the cortical neuropil. Putting in parallel these two aspects of synaptogenesis is not trivial since the synaptic contact constitutes a crucial point of articulation between the cellular properties of the single cortical neuron and the neurophysiological functions associated with large ensembles of these cortical neurons, which are under distinct categories of constraints.

(i) The constraints related to the multiple intracellular mechanisms control the type, amount and distribution of presynaptic active zones, and postsynaptic densities differentiated on the cell surface of a cortical neuron. Are these constrains all under strict genetic control?

(ii) The constraints related to intercellular mechanisms are linked to the neuro-physiological functions of large ensembles of these cortical neurons, and control the development of the topological distribution of the synaptic contacts in the neuropil. Are these constraints all under strict epigenetic control?

The interactions between genetically defined factors and experientially modifying factors are crucial in the development and the morphofunctional maturation of the neocortex, in which synaptogenesis is a key event. Knowing the exact timing of synaptogenesis in the cascade of histological events described above will provide a neuroanatomical base for the experimental identification of these interactions through the time course of development and maturation. The description of formation of ensembles of synaptic contacts is currently less explored than that of the mechanisms of assembling of synaptic macromolecules. We tried to redress this balance. The neocortex of the rhesus monkey provides an excellent animal model for the analysis of the developing synaptoarchitecture, plasticity and physiology of the human neocortex (Teller, 1997). Using quantitative electron microscopy, we first delineated the kinetics of synaptogenesis in several cortical areas of the macaque monkey from conception to death (Bourgeois & Rakic, 1993; Bourgeois et al., 1994, 2000).

Kinetics of synaptogenesis

In the primary visual cortex of the macaque, five different phases were identified (Fig. 5.1):

Phase 1

This is a very early synaptogenesis at a low density of synapses, first in the primordial plexiform layer (Marin-Padilla, 1988) then in the marginal zone (MZ, or prospective layer I) and in the subplate (SP), but not in the cortical plate (CP). These synapses are formed by axons of subcortical origin penetrating horizontally within the neuroepithelium (horizontal arrows in Fig. 5.1). This phase of synaptogenesis begins about 40 to 60 days after conception (DAC), and coincides with the onset of neurogenesis (Rakic, 1995).

Phase 2

This is an early synaptogenesis at a low density of synapses, now within the cortical plate itself, at mid-gestation between 70 and 100 days after conception, i.e. during the peak of neurogenesis and migration of neuroblasts. These synapses appear first in the infragranular layers and progressively in the more superficial cortical layers of the CP, following the vertical penetration of axonal projections (ver-

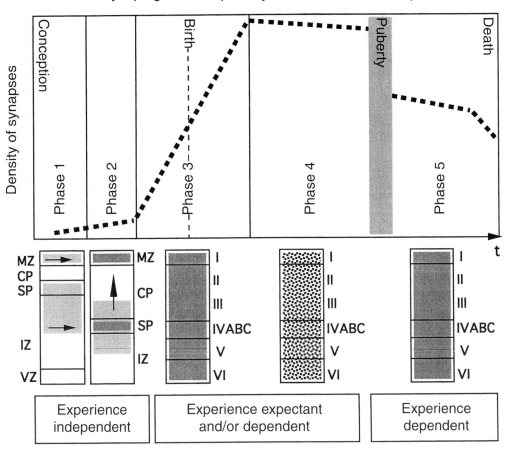

Fig. 5.1.   Changes in the relative density of synapses (discontinuous line in the upper frame) as a function of days after conception expressed on a log scale on the abscissa (t), in the primary visual cortex of the macaque monkey, during normal development. Five different phases of synaptogenesis are identified between conception and death, as described in the text. Each phase is superimposed above the density distribution of synapses in the cortical layers of the neocortex represented in vertical frames in the middle part of the figure. During phase 1, synapses appear first in the marginal zone (MZ), subplate (SP), and intermediate zone (IZ). During phase 2, synapses now appear also in the cortical plate (CP) with a gradient of density represented by a vertical arrow. Roman numbers indicate cortical layers. The proposed effects of experience on cortical development and maturation are represented in the lower part. (Reproduced from Bourgeois, 1997, with permission of Scandinavian University Press.)

tical arrow in Fig. 5.1) from cortical and subcortical origins (Bourgeois et al., 1994). All these 'early' synaptic contacts are formed on the dendritic shafts of the neurons (Fig. 5.2(*a*), (*b*)).

Phase 3

This is a phase of very rapid accumulation of synapses. This phase begins 2 months before birth (*ca.* 100 days after conception), and initially proceeds in the absence of patterned stimulation from the external world. The maximal density of synapses is reached about two months after birth. We have shown that the onset of phase 3 is not necessarily linked to the end of neurogenesis (Granger et al., 1995). The most rapid part of this phase 3 occurs around birth (in the macaque, delivery occurs 165 days after conception), when 40 000 new synapses are formed every second in each striate cortex of the macaque (Rakic et al., 1994), mainly on the dendritic spines (Fig. 5.2(*a*), (*b*)). This rapid accumulation of synapses coincides with the growth of the dendritic and axonal arbours. However, the onset of phase 3 of synaptogenesis may either precede, as in the primary visual cortex (Bourgeois & Rakic, 1993) or follow, as in the prefrontal cortex (Bourgeois et al., 1994), the segregation of the cortical columns.

Phase 4

This is a 'plateau' phase during which the mean density of synapses remains at a very high level, *ca.* 600–900 million synapses per mm³ of neuropil (Bourgeois & Rakic, 1993) throughout infancy and adolescence, until puberty (in macaque puberty occurs 3 years after birth).

Phase 5

This is a slow and steady decline in density of synapses from puberty throughout adulthood resulting mainly from the loss of synapses located on dendritic spines. This decline coincides with another crucial and lengthy phase in the late maturation of cortical functions. Finally, a drop in density of synapses is observed during senescence, before death (Fig. 5.1).

Our observations of these five distinct phases have been confirmed by studies done on the macaque using either brain imaging (Jacobs et al., 1995) or immunocytochemistry and histological techniques (Anderson et al., 1995). They have also recently been identified in the neocortices of mouse (de Felipe et al., 1998) and human brains (Huttenlocher & Dabholkar, 1997). These facts strongly suggest that the mechanisms of corticogenesis and synaptogenesis are highly conserved during the extensive evolution of the neocortex. In the human cortex, it is neither easy to obtain precise quantitative data on the time course of these phases, nor to establish time points equivalent to those described in the macaque. However, from the observations of Zecevic (1998) on the human occipital cortex, we tentatively propose that phase 1 might begin around 6–8 weeks of gestation. Phase 2 would begin near 12–17 weeks of gestation. The onset of phase 3 of rapid synaptogenesis would occur around mid-gestation (20–24 weeks). On the other hand, data from Huttenlocher and Dabholkar (1997) indicate that, in the primary visual cortex, phase 3 ends somewhere between 8 and 12 months after birth. For the phase 4 plateau of high density of synaptic contacts, differences appear between cortical areas. In the human primary visual cortex, the plateau phase has the same length as in the macaque: 2–3 years (Fig. 5.3), while in the prefrontal cortex it lasts for a decade, until puberty (Fig. 5.3; Huttenlocher & Dabholkar, 1997). Both in macaque and human neocortices, phase 5 begins after puberty and proceeds throughout adulthood with almost no decline in densities of synaptic contacts, and it is followed by a significant loss of synapses during senescence (Figs. 5.1 and 5.3).

Distinct waves of synaptogenesis

The curve presented here (Fig. 5.1) is actually an envelope covering many distinct waves of synaptogenesis differing in their location, timing, or tempo, as revealed by more detailed descriptions (Bourgeois & Rakic, 1993; Bourgeois et al., 1994). For location, we observed a wave of synaptogenesis outside the cortical plate during phase 1, and another one inside this plate later on, during phase 2 (Fig. 5.1). For timing, we observed sequential waves of synaptogenesis, first on dendritic shafts and later upon dendritic spines of the same neurons (Figs. 5.2(*a*) and (*b*)). For tempo, in the primary visual cortex, a protracted plateau was observed until puberty in supragranular layer III (Fig. 5.2(*a*)), while a short phase 4 of synaptogenesis on dendritic spines was observed postnatally in granular layer IVC (Fig. 5.2(*b*)). In layer III of the prefrontal cortex of the macaque, a protracted plateau of high density parvalbumin positive axon cartridges from chandelier cells was observed until puberty, while a short peak of density of dopaminergic varicosities was observed exactly during puberty (Anderson et al., 1995). These are the first examples of a long list of discrete synaptogenetic events we are just beginning to explore.

All these preliminary studies show that phase 3 is a period of rapid production of all categories of synaptic contacts, even if during the next phases different categories of synapses may display different kinetics in macaque (Anderson et al., 1995; Bourgeois & Rakic, 1993; Bourgeois et al., 1994; Zecevic et al., 1989; Zecevic & Rakic, 1991), mouse (de Felipe et al., 1997), and human (Fig. 5.3; Huttenlocher & Dabholkar, 1997) cerebral cortices.

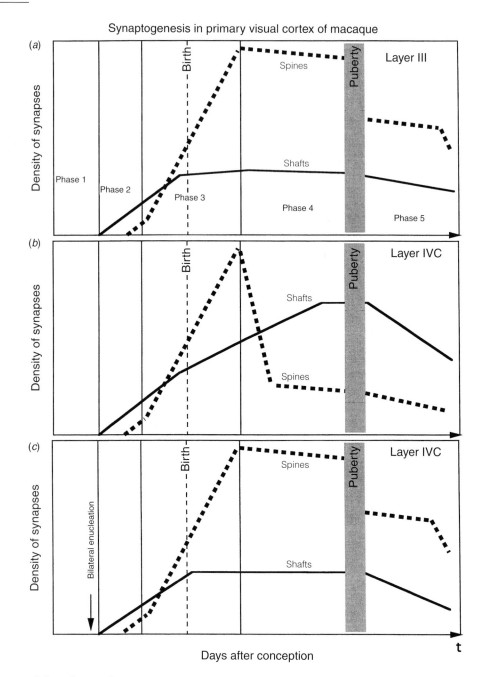

Synaptogenesis in primary visual cortex of macaque

Fig. 5.2.　Distinct classes of synapses appear in distinct waves of synaptogenesis in the primary visual cortex of the macaque monkey during normal development. As examples, changes in the relative densities of synaptic contacts located on dendritic shafts (black line) or on dendritic spines (discontinuous line), are represented here as a function of days after conception expressed on a log scale on the abscissae (t), in two cortical layers (layers III

Phase 3 of synaptogenesis in diverse cortical areas

In diverse cortical fields characterized by different cytoarchitecture, and subserving very different physiological functions, the same phases of synaptogenesis were found at the same developmental stage (Bourgeois & Rakic, 1993; Bourgeois et al., 1994, 2000; Granger et al., 1995; Zecevic et al., 1989; Zecevic & Rakic, 1991). The very same early developmental pattern of synaptogenesis, i.e. the ensembles of percentages of different classes of synapses at successive steps of development and maturation, is also observed in all cortical layers (see example in Figs. 5.2(*a*) (*b*) (*c*)), and all cortical areas examined.

Unexpectedly, during the perinatal period, we also observed that the rapid phase 3 of synaptogenesis occurs more concurrently than sequentially, in the sensory, motor and associational cortical areas (Bourgeois et al., 2000; Rakic et al., 1986, 1994). Excitatory and inhibitory synapses also accumulate concurrently during phase 3, in the prefrontal cortex of the macaque monkey (Anderson et al., 1995). These observations are corroborated by brain imaging studies on the cortical mantle of the macaque monkeys (Jacobs et al., 1995).

We have defined a 'time-window' of 41 days encompassing the midpoints of the rapid phase 3 of synaptogenesis in all the cortical areas described so far in the macaque (Granger et al., 1995). Using available data, we proposed that this is also the case in the human neocortex with a 'time-window' of about 3–5 months (Huttenlocher & Dabholkar, 997; Rakic et al., 1994; and see Fig. 5.3). Although the duration of this 'time-window' increases through evolution, it always remains short as compared to the long duration of the plateau phase 4 (a decade in the human cortex; see Fig. 5.3), which follows until puberty.

Caption to fig. 5.2 (*cont.*)

in (*a*) and IVC in (*b*)). The very same pattern of synaptogenesis is observed during the first three phases of synaptogenesis in all cortical layers (*a*) and (*b*), suggesting the existence of highly conserved mechanisms. During phase 2, a first wave of synaptogenesis occurs on dendritic shafts followed 2 weeks later by a second wave of synaptogenesis now on dendritic spines of the same neurons. During phase 3, before birth, the proportions of these classes of synapses are reversed. During phase 4 plateau, the kinetics of these waves of synaptogenesis differ. A protracted plateau of high density of synapses on dendritic spines is observed in supragranular layer III (*a*), while in granular layer IVC (*b*) we observed a very short wave of synaptogenesis on dendritic spines and a protracted wave of synaptogenesis on dendritic shafts. After an early bilateral enucleation was performed during phase 1 of synaptogenesis (arrow in *c*), the very same pattern of synaptogenesis unfolds normally during the first three phases, in granular layer IVC (compare (*a*), (*b*), (*c*)). However, during phase 4 plateau, the second reversal of densities of synapses on dendritic spines and shafts does not take place (*c*).

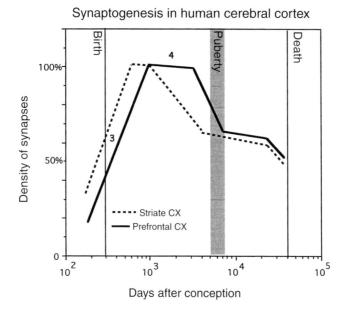

Fig. 5.3.   Changes in the relative densities of synapses in the primary visual cortex (discontinuous line) and prefrontal cortex (continuous line) of the human brain as a function of days after conception, expressed on a log scale on the abscissa. Phases 3 and 4 are indicated with numbers. This is a schematic representation of data published in Fig. 2 of Huttenlocher and Dabholkar (1997), with permission from the authors and John Wiley.

Recent observations reveal that the phases 2 and 3 of synaptogenesis also appear to occur concurrently in the prenatal human cerebral cortex as in the macaque (Zecevic, 1998). Similarly, corresponding analysis of the developmental patterns in several cytoarchitecturally distinct cortical areas also shows a concurrent morphological maturation of the whole cortical mantle in the human postnatal brain (Shankle et al., 1998).

Modifiability of phase 3 of synaptogenesis

The onset of synaptogenesis long before birth, its tempo, and the concurrent phase 3 in all cortical layers and in all cortical areas of the macaque, strongly suggested to us that these events might be determined by mechanisms intrinsic and common to the whole cortical mantle (Rakic et al., 1986; Goldman-Rakic et al., 1997; Rakic et al., 1994). We have tested this hypothesis in the following experiments:

First, with a mild intervention, using experimental preterm monkeys (Bourgeois et al., 1989), we found that a premature bilaterally equilibrated exposure to visual environment does not accelerate or delay the rate of synaptic accretion during the rapid phase 3 of synaptogenesis in the primary visual cortex. This phase of synaptogenesis proceeds in relation to the time of conception rather than to the time of delivery, i.e. the onset of visual stimulation.

Secondly, using a more drastic intervention, we found that an early bilateral enucleation (Bourgeois & Rakic, 1996) does not alter the final mean densities of synapses reached at the end of rapid phase 3, and maintained during the phase 4 plateau, in the striate cortex of blind monkeys. Our study also indicates that, a few weeks after birth, the proportions of synaptic contacts situated on dendritic spines (75%) and shafts (25%) were similar in all cortical layers of normal and enucleated animals. Four months after birth, the localization on dendritic spines or shafts in the thalamorecipient granular layers fails to mature properly in the absence of normal functional input from the periphery (Fig. 5.2(c)). The proportions indicated above, which normally become reversed during infancy in the sublayers IVAB and IVC, were not reversed in the enucleates. The proportion of symmetrical (20%) vs. asymmetrical (80%) synapses located on dendritic spines were within the normal range of variability in both groups of animals. As a result, the granular layers in the striate cortex of the early-blind macaque have more excitatory axodendrospines than normal animals.

This experimental model also provides an additional example showing that a perturbation at an early neurodevelopmental stage (before midgestation in the present case) may have a late (late infancy in the present case) and long-lasting effect of disorganization despite an apparently normal intermediate period (latency period for this aspect of synaptoarchitecture).

These experimental observations indicate that early synaptogenesis is a very robust neurodevelopmental process. They reinforce our hypothesis that the onset, time course, magnitude and rate of cortical synaptogenesis, during phase 3, in the primate striate cortex proceed without stimulation from the periphery. They are determined and coordinated by mechanisms intrinsic and common to the whole cortical mantle. The nature of these mechanisms and their interactions (metabolic, trophic, hormonal, genetic, etc.) are under investigation. However, final adjustments of some aspects of the synaptoarchitecture depend on normal functional input.

Effects of environment on diverse phases of synaptogenesis

The transition from intrinsic to extrinsic controls of synaptogenesis in the cerebral cortex most likely involves many steps. Experience, i.e. the presence of patterned evoked activities coming from the world external to the neocortex, has diverse effects on cortical maturation during the different phases of synaptogenesis described above. As sketched in Fig. 5.1, we tentatively propose the following interpretations:

(i) Phases 1 and 2 of very early synaptogenesis: the early events, such as neurogenesis, neuronal migration, neuritic navigation, individualization of cortical layers, neurochemical differentiation, and early synaptogenesis, are dominated by genetic and epigenetic mechanisms which are all intrinsic to the neocortex. These events can be severely disturbed by genetic mutations, viral infections, toxic agents, surgical interventions, etc. However, they are not yet influenced by experience coming from the world external to the neocortex. Using the terminology of Greenough (Greenough & Alcantara, 1993), these early events are said to be 'experience independent' (Fig. 5.1), and are possibly common to all mammals. Spontaneous activity most likely already occurs via synapses formed early and participates in the wiring of cortical neurons (Maffei & Galli-Resta, 1990; Mooney et al., 1996).

(ii) Rapid Phase 3 of synaptogenesis is dominated early on by 'experience-expectant' and later on by 'experience-dependent' mechanisms (Greenough & Alcantara, 1993; see Fig. 5.1). The intrinsic mechanisms become epigenetically modulated by 'experience' coming to the neocortex from the external world. 'Experience-expectant' means that the presence of some visual parameters in the external world (orientation, colour, movement, disparity, etc.) are necessary for the proper final adjustment of the cortical circuits being established for their specific processing. This phase 3 coincides with the beginning of critical periods. The mechanisms involved during this phase are assumed to be common to all individuals of a given mammalian species.

Huttenlocher and Dabholkar (1997) claimed that the onset of cortical functions occurs only at the end of the phase 3 of synaptogenesis, and at different ages in different cortical regions. This is in contradiction with much evidence for very early maturation of anatomical and physiological parameters in the neocortex of primates. In macaques, many sensory, motor, visceral and cognitive functions subserved by the neocortex are present very soon after birth, when the main aspects of synaptoarchitecture are still being laid down. The patterns of ocular dominance columns are already adult-like in the primary visual cortex of the newborn macaque (Horton & Hocking, 1996). Complex receptive field properties, such as face recognition, of inferotemporal neurons are already adult-like only a few weeks after birth in this species (Rodman, 1994). The possibility of a cortical circuitry prewired even for highly integrated functions has been raised (Rodman, 1994). The cardinal cognitive functions subserved by the dorsolateral prefrontal association cortex are present long before the end of the rapid phase 3 of synaptogenesis a few weeks after birth (Diamond & Goldman-Rakic, 1989; Bourgeois et al., 1994; Goldman-Rakic et al., 1997). Harlow and Harlow (1962) showed that critical periods for social skills of the macaque infant could also take place as early as 2 months after birth. Evoked activity in response to maternal voice seems to be present before birth in human fetuses (Lecanuet & Granier-Deferre, 1993), and the newborn human infant most certainly sees (Teller, 1997).

Our working hypothesis is that the very rapid and concurrent synaptogenesis in the whole cortical mantle during the phase 3 allows the early coordinated emergence of all these cortical functions (Rakic et al., 1986, 1994). This is essential for competitive and selective (Changeux & Danchin, 1976) interactions among the very heterogeneous cortical inputs at each point of the cortex. However, these cortical functions will also require up to three years to reach full maturity in the macaque (Goldman-Rakic et al., 1997) and more than a decade in human (Huttenlocher & Dabholkar, 1997; Rakic et al., 1994), i.e. until puberty.

(iii) Phase 4 plateau, is also dominated by 'experience-expectant' and 'experience-dependent' mechanisms (Greenough & Alcantara, 1993; see Fig. 5.1). This extended period of synaptic plasticity corresponds to a process of continuous reorganization of the intracortical axonal arborizations (Callaway & Katz, 1990; Lowel & Singer, 1992), allowing the fine tuning and maturation of the neuronal circuits, during the 3 years after birth, until puberty. This topological reorganization of synaptic contacts occurs with a constant density of synapses.

The phases 3 and 4 of synaptogenesis coincide with the diverse critical periods extending until puberty in cats (Daw et al., 1992), monkeys (LeVay et al., 1980) and humans (Johnson & Newport, 1989). Critical periods for different visual functions subserved by different cortical layers in the primary visual cortex have different timings. Neuronal plasticity lasts longer in the upper and lower cortical layers than in the granular layers. For example, the short postnatal peak of density observed in granular layer IVC in the striate cortex of the macaque (see pp. 97–98 and Fig. 5.2(b)) fits well with the short critical period for orientation selectivity subserved by this layer, while the long-lasting phase 4 plateau observed in supragranular layer III (see pp. 97–98 and Fig. 5.2(a)) coincides with the protracted critical periods described for contrast sensitivity, binocular selectivity and Vernier hyperacuity, subserved by this layer (Blakemore et al., 1981; Harwerth et al., 1986).

(iv) Phase 5, is dominated by 'experience-dependent' mechanisms (Greenough & Alcantara, 1993; see Fig. 5.1). It corresponds mainly to a very slow decrease in the density of synapses through adulthood. Over several decades of ageing, the efficacy and the local plastic reorganizations of synaptic contacts are now related only to the experience of each individual (Greenough & Alcantara,

1993), but the main aspects of synaptoarchitecture in the cortical networks remain unchanged.

We observed a true loss of synapses in the neocortex of the macaque monkey around puberty (Bourgeois & Rakic, 1993; Bourgeois et al., 1994). This observation is now confirmed by brain imaging in the macaque (Jacobs et al., 1995) and human cortices (Chugani et al., 1987). A similar loss of synapses near puberty was recently observed also in the cortices of the human brain (Huttenlocher & Dabholkar, 1997) and mouse brains (de Felipe et al., 1997), using quantitative synaptology. Although we arbitrarily included in phase 5 this period of rapid loss of synapses occurring during puberty, we do not exclude the possibility that it might be a single phase with its own mechanisms and tempo of synaptogenesis, distinct from the other phases.

One possibility is that the loss of synapses in the prefrontal cortex, during puberty, might correspond to a 'hormonal sanction' of neuronal plasticity. The deep hormonal 'reorganization' occurring in and near puberty would participate in the definitive elimination of labile synapses not stabilized during the preceding and long phase 4 plateau. In humans, central visual defects due to cataract are less curable near puberty (for review, see Mitchell & Timney, 1984). Twelve years of age corresponds to the point when people usually stop being able to learn non-maternal languages without effort and without accents (Johnson & Newport, 1989). As frequently stated in textbooks, the period around puberty corresponds to a 'freezing' of personality, and the end of several basic learning capacities and skills.

Selectionist vs. constructivist hypotheses for synaptogenesis

Studies addressing phases 3 and 4 of synaptogenesis are also the object of a confrontation between selectionist and constructivist hypotheses. Both classes of hypothesis relate the modifications of the synaptoarchitecture during development, maturation and learning in the neocortex to the activity evoked by individual experience. In both hypotheses, there is an early and rapid accumulation of synapses, with the most active ones being those which will ultimately be retained, but the sequence of events involved differs.

According to the selective stabilization hypothesis proposed by Changeux and Danchin (1976), the connectivity matures from a larger to a smaller number of connections and synapses. Intrinsic mechanisms control the initial formation of large pools of synaptic contacts, while the subsequent stabilization of the most active synapses, and the elimination of the less active ones, is regulated by evoked activity.

In the constructivist hypothesis proposed by Katz and Shatz (1996), Purves et al. (1996) and Quartz and Sejnowski (1997), the connectivity matures from a smaller to a larger number of connections and synapses. According to these instructionist models, the spontaneous activity and the patterns of evoked activities cause the formation of synapses, control the extent of their domains and orientate the elaboration of their synaptoarchitectural organization. Losses of neurons, axons and synapses, if any, are just epiphenomena.

In the primary visual system of the macaque or cat, the coincidence between the continuous increases in axono-dendritic branching, the segregation of ocular dominance columns (for reviews, see Katz & Shatz, 1996; Purves et al., 1996; Quartz & Sejnowski, 1997), and the rapid phase 3 of synaptogenesis (Bourgeois & Rakic, 1993) are taken as support for constructionist hypotheses. However, the fact that the onset of phase 3 of rapid synaptogenesis slightly precedes the loss of a few LGN axonal branches from contralateral ocular dominance columns, does not rule out a selective competition between these few axons subserving the two eyes. The massive growth and sprouting of axonal arbours which follow might as well just hide local selectionist competitions between diverse axons now subserving the same eye inside the same dominance column.

During the plateau phase of synaptogenesis, a selective stabilization of synapses might occur during reorganization of the tridimensional distribution of synapses in the neuropil, without any net loss of synapses, because different waves for different classes of synapses occur at different developmental stages (Fig. 5.2(*a*) (*b*); Bourgeois & Rakic, 1993). All these models include the existence of extensive production, remodelling and retraction of dendritic and axonal branches, and synapses, during development of the cortex. For example, synapses identified upon proximal axon collaterals at a juvenile stage relocate to distal axonal domains at the adult stage on local circuit neurons in cortex (Callaway & Katz, 1990).

The quantitative observations of Greenough and Alcantara (1993) suggest that learning induces formation of new synapses. However, if such an increase in density of synapses occurs everywhere, and permanently as primates learn, this density should increase constantly over whole life. This does not fit with the unambiguous losses of diverse classes of synapses, repeatedly observed at different times in phases 4 and 5, in different cortical layers and cortical areas of the macaque (Figs. 5.1 to 5.4; Anderson et al., 1995; Bourgeois & Rakic, 1993; Bourgeois et al., 1994; Zecevic & Rakic, 1991; Zecevic et al, 1989), mouse (de Felipe et al., 1997), or human (Huttenlocher & Dabholkar, 1997) cortices. Recently, Geinisman and colleagues (1999) showed that associative learning does not increase the number of synapses in the hippocampus. It is difficult to reconcile all these facts with a strict interpretation of the constructivist models.

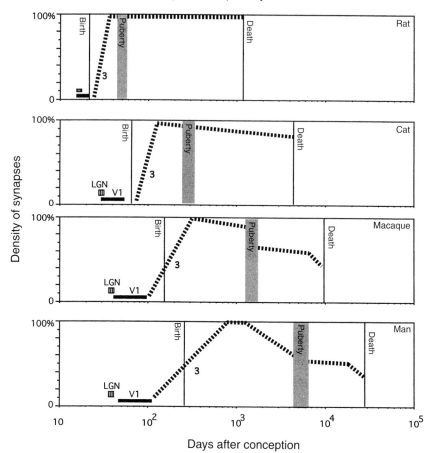

Fig. 5.4.   Changes in the relative density of synapses (discontinuous lines) in the primary visual cortices of four different mammalian species: rat, cat, macaque and man, as a function of days after conception, expressed on a log scale on the abscissa. Only phases 3, 4 and 5 of synaptogenesis are sketched here. Phase 3 is indicated with the number 3. The striped and the solid black horizontal bars represent the time of neurogenesis in the lateral geniculate nucleus (LGN) and primary visual cortex (V1). (Reproduced from Bourgeois, 1997, with permission of Scandinavian University Press.)

Evolution of phase 3 of synaptogenesis in the neocortex

Through evolution of the neocortex, there is a shift in the onset time of neurogenesis in the primary visual cortex (Fig. 5.4), which occurs respectively 14 days after conception (DAC) in the rat (Frantz et al., 1994), 30 DAC in the cat (Luskin &

Shatz, 1985), 40 DAC in the macaque and 43 DAC in the human neocortex (Rakic, 1995). For synaptogenesis, the comparison of the tempo of phase 3 in the primary visual cortices of these four mammalian species, also reveals two significant modifications, as indicated in Fig. 5.4.

First, the onset of the rapid phase 3 of synaptogenesis occurs progressively later after conception: from 23 DAC in the rat (Blue & Parnavelas, 1983) to 110 DAC in the human neocortex (Huttenlocher & Dabholkar, 1997; see data in Table 5.1 and Fig. 5.4). Through phylogeny of mammals, this shift is less pronounced than that of the time of delivery (Fig. 5.4). As a result, the onset of phase 3 of synaptogenesis, a postnatal event in rodents and carnivores, progressively becomes a precocious prenatal event in primates.

Secondly, more important for our present topic, the duration of the phase 3 in the primary visual cortex increases significantly from 14 days in the rat (Blue & Parnavelas, 1983) to 30 days in the cat (Cragg, 1975), 136 days in the macaque (Bourgeois & Rakic, 1993), and about 400 days in the human brain (Huttenlocher & Dabholkar, 1997; Table 5.1 and Fig. 5.4). Normalization of the duration of phase 3 of synaptogenesis to the onset time of puberty (Table 5.1) shows that it represents a constant proportion of 10–17% of this time in the four species studied, suggesting that phase 3 is a developmental process not apart from others. In an evolutionary perspective, this protracted phase 3 postpones the increase in volume of the primate brain well into the late postnatal period, a crucial parameter which, otherwise, could make delivery problematic.

These observations become even more interesting when one relates them to the evolution of synaptoarchitecture. The final mean density of synapses per unit volume of cortical neuropil in the mature striate cortex (column 5 in Table 5.1) is not higher in human than in rat, although it takes about 30 times longer to produce these synapses in each point of the cortex. Even the mean number of synapses per neuron in the striate cortex remains in the same range from rat to man (column 6 in Table 5.1).

Two working hypotheses, which are not mutually exclusive, are considered now as plausible mechanisms for this extension of phase 3 of synaptogenesis:

A genetic hypothesis

The time course of phase 3 is controlled by genetic mechanisms, and the number and/or the time needed by the developmental master genes to control phase 3 of synaptogenesis might increase during evolution. This hypothesis leads to one falsifiable experimental prediction: the mutation of these genes or the deregulation of their expression should result in a modification of the onset and/or time course of phase 3 of synaptogenesis.

Table 5.1. Parameters related to the development of the primary visual cortex of four distinct mammalian species

	Gestation	Puberty onset	Phase 3 duration (onset–end)	Density of synapses[a]	Synapses per neuron	Total number of cortical areas	Total number of 'visual areas'
Rat	21 DAC	82 DAC (2 months after birth)	14 days (P2–P16)	320–946	12 500–13 500	21	4–6
Cat	65 DAC	248 DAC (6 months after birth)	30 days (P9–P39)	276–406	5800–9300	30–50 ?	12–17
Macaque	165 DAC	1260 DAC (3 years after birth)	136 days (E90–P61)	276–620	2000–5600	72	25
Human	280 days	4660 DAC (12/13 years after birth)	470 days (E120–P310)	350	6800–10000	200 ?	50 ?

Notes:

[a] Density of synapses is expressed in millions per mm^3 of cortical tissue. DAC stands for Days After Conception, E for Embryonic day, and P for Post-natal day.

Source: The data are reproduced from Bourgeois (1997) with permission of Scandinavian University Press.

A morpho-functional hypothesis

Morphological and functional heterogeneities of the axonal inputs to the primary visual cortex increase with the addition of extrastriate cortical areas during mammalian evolution, and the increased diversity of synaptic inputs causes the extension of phase 3. During evolution of mammals, the neocortex grows more in surface than in the vertical dimension. From rat to human, the total surface area of the cortical mantle increases by three orders of magnitude. Cortical expansion in evolution is achieved largely by addition of radial units, and thus by increases in the number, not the size, of constituent columns (Rakic, 1995). Although the 2D shape of the primary visual cortex appears highly conserved across mammalian species (Duffy et al., 1998) its surface increases significantly. The total number of cortical areas also increases significantly (column 7 in Table 5.1). More relevant to our present purpose, the total number of visual areas increases from 4 in the rat (Coogan & Burkhalter, 1993) to about 25 in the macaque and probably many more in the human brain (Van Essen, 1985; column 8 in Table 5.1). Most of these visual areas are directly or indirectly connected to the primary visual cortex (Coogan & Burkhalter, 1993; Van Essen, 1985; Salin & Bullier, 1995), and their inputs are quite heterogeneous. This heterogeneity may be histologically related, for example, to the high diversity of cell adhesion molecules (Alcantara et al., 1992), and diffusible or signalling molecules (Edlund & Jessel, 1999). This heterogeneity may also be functional: in different cortical areas, neurons fire with different temporal patterns (Ferster & Spruston, 1995) and different conduction times (Salin & Bullier, 1995). In the morphofunctional hypothesis, all these heterogeneities increase the number and the complexity of cellular interactions between nerve endings during the formation of synapses, their selective stabilization, their elimination, or all these steps. This, along with an increased number of waves of synaptogenesis, might increase the duration of phases 3 and 4 of synaptogenesis.

This hypothesis leads to another falsifiable experimental prediction: the anatomical or functional suppression of a specified number of prestriate cortical areas should shorten the duration of phase 3 of synaptogenesis observed in the primary visual cortex. In contrast, the addition of cortical areas should prolong phase 3.

The two hypotheses considered above are not mutually exclusive: the two classes of mechanisms might be at work at different moments of phase 3 or/and for distinct ensembles of synapses. These mechanisms are expected to be identical in the whole cortical mantle.

New perspectives on genetics of synaptogenesis, evolution of epigenesis and individuation

In neocortices of non-human and human primates, neurogenesis and synaptogenesis are very precocious prenatal development events, while complete maturation of cortical functions is protracted until puberty. Although kinetics is not the whole story of synaptogenesis, our identification of distinct phases of synaptogenesis provides a new developmental frame for the description of the establishment and successive adjustment of synaptoarchitecture in the neocortex of primates. The density of synapses is the same at birth and after puberty. However, the developmental constraints on synaptogenesis are expected to be totally different. We observed that the onset and time course of phase 3 of synaptogenesis are very robust developmental events, while influences from environment increase thereafter. Among multiple mechanisms, this plasticity is related to the high variability in the density, localization, assembly and nature of many types of molecules in the pre- and postsynaptic domains of neurons. To cite only a few examples, one should refer to the large diversity and plasticity of the subunits of classical pharmacological receptors (Changeux et al., 1997; Craig, 1998; Vannier & Triller, 1997), as well as to new families of molecules such as class I MHC (Corriveau et al., 1998) and synaptic cadherins (Hagler & Goda, 1998), recently observed during formation of synaptic contacts. These numerous structural and signal-transducing molecules assemble and de-assemble in highly dynamic pre- and postsynaptic domains of morphologically permanent synaptic contacts.

We hypothesize that, upstream of all these molecular events, new families of genes control the onsets and durations of the different phases of synaptogenesis described above. Different groups of these genes may be activated, some transiently, some permanently, during distinct waves of synaptogenesis. The identification of the functional interactions between different groups of genes during critical periods of synaptogenesis will constitute an entirely new field of research. The regulatory genes controlling the onset of phase 3 of synaptogenesis will have to be identified first. The sequencing of the human genome will allow translation of the cascade of histological events observed during cortical development into a cascade of genetic events.

The aim of future projects is to explore the mechanisms of the transitions from strictly intrinsic (genes) to epigenetic environment control of the formation of synaptoarchitecture, during cortical normal or pathological development. Whether these transitions result from a changing overlap of independent mechanisms subserved by distinct ensembles of synaptic circuits, or whether it is a progressive epigenetic transformation from one mechanism to the next, is not yet known.

The existence of distinct and successive waves of synaptogenesis, along with these studies of genetic controls of synaptogenesis, will also provide new biological approaches to test diverse neurodevelopmental hypotheses for the origin of psychiatric disorders (Bloom, 1993; Feinberg, 1983, 1990; Stefan & Murray, 1997).

Synaptogenesis is a crucial part of the phylogenetic and ontogenetic histories of the neocortex. However, we do not yet know what is the sequence of causality, if any, between the extension of phases 3 and 4 of synaptogenesis, the appearance of many new local neuronal circuits, the functional refinement of the multiple receptive fields of the striate cortex, and the increased numbers and plasticity of the neuronal networks, all observed through phylogeny.

According to the heterochronic epigenesis hypothesis proposed recently (Bourgeois, 1997), the extension of the phase 3 of synaptogenesis increases significantly: (i) the scale and number of possible epigenetic combinations; (ii) the amplitude of the 'overshoot' of synapses; (iii) the extension of their plasticity well into adulthood, and (iv) the morphofunctional interindividual variabilities observed through mammalian phylogeny. This hypothesis also proposes that the extension of phases 3 and 4 of synaptogenesis during evolution of the neocortex significantly increases the process of maturation of cognitive and psychosocial competence, reaching its maximum in the human brain.

All these descriptions, including that of the development of the synaptoarchitecture in the cerebral cortex, participate in the identification of the mechanisms involved in the process of individuation.

Acknowledgements

I thank Professors Jean-Pierre Changeux, Patricia Goldman-Rakic and Pasko Rakic, for their constant support and numerous discussions about epigenesis. This work was supported at the origin by a Fogarty International Fellowship, and constantly by the Centre National de la Récherche Scientifique.

REFERENCES

Alcantara, A. A., Pfenninger, K. H. & Greenough, W. T. (1992). 5B4-CAM expression parallels neurite outgrowth and synaptogenesis in the developing rat brain. *Journal of Comparative Neurology*, **319**, 337–48.

Anderson, S. A., Classey, J. D., Condé, F., Lund, J. S. & Lewis, D. A. (1995). Synchronous development of pyramidal neuron dendritic spines and parvalbumin-immunoreactive chandelier neuron axon terminals in layer III of monkey prefrontal cortex. *Neuroscience*, **67**(1), 7–22.

Barone, P., Dehay, C., Berland, M., Bullier, J. & Kennedy, H. (1995). Developmental remodeling of primate visual cortical pathways. *Cerebral Cortex*, **5**, 22–38.

Blakemore, C., Vital-Durand, F. & Garey, L.J. (1981). Recovery from monocular deprivation in the monkey. I. Reversal of physiological effects in the visual cortex. *Proceedings of the Royal Society of London (B)*, **213**, 399–423.

Bloom, R. E. (1993). Advancing a neurodevelopmental origin of schizophrenia. *Archives in General Psychiatry*, **50**, 224–7.

Blue, M. E. & Parnavelas, J. G. (1983). The formation and maturation of synapses in the visual cortex of the rat. II. Quantitative analysis. *Journal of Neurocytology*, **12**, 697–712.

Bourgeois, J. P. (1997). Synaptogenesis, heterochrony and epigenesis in the mammalian neocortex. *Acta Paediatrica*, Suppl. **422**, 27–33.

Bourgeois, J. P. & Rakic, P. (1993). Changes of synaptic density in the primary visual cortex of the macaque monkey from fetal to adult stage. *Journal of Neuroscience*, **13**, 2801–20.

Bourgeois, J. P. & Rakic, P. (1996). Synaptogenesis in the occipital cortex of the macaque monkey devoid of retinal input from early embryonic stages. *European Journal of Neuroscience*, **8**, 942–50.

Bourgeois, J .P., Jastreboff, P .J. & Rakic, P. (1989). Synaptogenesis in the visual cortex of normal and preterm monkeys: evidence for intrinsic regulation of synaptic overproduction. *Proceedings of the National Academy of Sciences, USA*, **86**, 4297–4301.

Bourgeois, J. P., Goldman-Rakic, P. S. & Rakic, P. (1994). Synaptogenesis in the prefrontal cortex of the rhesus monkey. *Cerebral Cortex*, **4**, 78–96.

Bourgeois, J. P., Goldman-Rakic, P. S. & Rakic, P. (2000). Formation, elimination and stabilization of synapses in the primate cerebral cortex. *The Cognitive Neurosciences*, ed. M Gazzaniga, Cambridge, MA: MIT Press.

Callaway, E. M. & Katz, L. (1990). Emergence and refinement of clustered horizontal connections in cat striate cortex. *Journal of Neuroscience*, **10**, 1134–53.

Changeux, J-P. & Danchin, A. (1976). Selective stabilization of developing synapses as a mechanism for the specification of neural network. *Nature*, **264**, 705–12.

Changeux, J-P., Bessis, A., Bourgeois, J. P. et al. (1997). Nicotinic receptors and brain plasticity. Cold Spring Harbor Symposium on 'Function and Dysfunction in the Nervous system' Book Symposium No 61, 343–62.

Chugani, H. T., Phelps, M. E. & Mazziotta, J. C. (1987). Positron emission tomography study of human brain functional development. *Annals of Neurology*, **22**, 487–97.

Coogan, T. A. & Burkhalter, A. (1993). Hierarchical organization of areas in the rat visual cortex. *Journal of Neuroscience*, **13**(9), 3749–72.

Corriveau, R. A., Huh, G. S. & Shatz, C. J. (1998). Regulation of class I MHC gene expression in the developing and mature CNS by neural activity. *Neuron*, **21**, 505–20.

Cragg, B. G. (1975). The development of synapses in the visual system of the cat. *Journal of Comparative Neurology*, **160**, 147–166.

Craig, A. M. (1998). Activity and synaptic receptor targeting: the long view. *Neuron*, **21**, 459–462.

Daw, N. W., Fox, K., Sato, H. & Czepita, D. (1992). Critical period for monocular deprivation in the cat visual cortex. *Journal of Neurophysiology*, **67**, 197–202.

Diamond, A. & Goldman-Rakic, P. S. (1989). Comparison of human infants and rhesus monkeys on Piaget's AB task: evidence for dependence on dorsolateral prefrontal cortex. *Experimental Brain Research*, **74**, 24–40.

Duffy, K. R., Murphy, K. M. & Jones, D. R. (1998). Analysis of the postnatal growth of visual cortex. *Visual Neuroscience*, **15**, 831–9.

Edlund, T. & Jessel, T. M. (1999). Progression from extrinsic to intrinsic signalling in cell fate specification: a view from the nervous system. *Cell*, **96**, 211–24.

Feinberg, I. (1983). Schizophrenia: caused by a fault in programmed synaptic elimination during adolescence? *Journal of Psychiatric Research*, **17**, 319–34.

Feinberg, I. (1990). Cortical pruning and the development of schizophrenia. *Schizophrenia Bulletin*, **16**, 567–8.

de Felipe, J., Marco, P., Fairén, A. & Jones, E. G. (1997). Inhibitory synaptogenesis in mouse somatosensory cortex. *Cerebral Cortex*, **7**, 619–34.

Ferster, D. & Spruston, N. (1995). Cracking the neuronal code. *Science*, **270**, 756–7.

Frantz, G. D., Bohner, A. P., Akers, R. M. & McConnell, S. K. (1994). Regulation of the POU domain gene SCIP during cerebral cortical development. *Journal of Neuroscience*, **14**, 472–85.

Geinisman, Y., Disterhof, J. F., Gunderson, H. J. G., McEchorn, M., Persina, I. S. & Power, J. M. (2000). Structural substrate of hippocampus-dependent associative learning: remodelling of synapses. *Journal of Comparative Neurology*, **417**, 49–59.

Goldman-Rakic, P. S., Bourgeois, J. P. & Rakic, P. (1997). Synaptic development of the prefrontal cortex and the emergence of cognitive function. In *Development of the prefrontal Cortex: Evolution, Neurobiology and Behavior*, ed. N. A. Krasnegor, G. R Lyon & P. S. Goldman-Rakic, pp. 27–47, Baltimore: Paul Brookes Publishing Company.

Granger, B., Tekaia, F., LeSourd, A. M., Rakic, P. & Bourgeois, J. P. (1995). Tempo of neurogenesis and synaptogenesis in the primate cingulate mesocortex: comparison with the neocortex. *Journal of Comparative Neurology*, **360**, 363–76.

Greenough, W. T. & Alcantara, A. A. (1993). The roles of experience in different developmental information stage processes. In *Developmental Neurocognition*, ed. B. de Boysson-Bardies, S. de Schonen, P. Jusczyk, P. McNeilage & J. Morton, pp. 3–16. Dordrecht: Kluwer Academic Publishers.

Hagler, D. J. & Goda, Y. (1998). Synaptic adhesion: the building blocks of memory? *Neuron*, **20**, 1059–62.

Harlow, H. F. & Harlow, M. K. (1962). Social deprivation in monkeys. *Scientific American*, **207**, 136–46.

Harwerth, R. S., Smith III, E. L., Duncan, G. C., Crawford, M. L. J. & von Noorden, G. K. (1986). Multiple sensitive periods in the development of the primate visual system. *Science*, **232**, 235–8.

Horton, J. C. & Hocking, D. R. (1996). An adult-like pattern of ocular dominance columns in the striate cortex of newborn monkeys prior to visual experience. *Journal of Neuroscience*, **16**(5), 1791–807.

Huttenlocher, P. R. & Dabholkar, A. S. (1997). Regional differences in synaptogenesis in the human cerebral cortex. *Journal of Comparative Neurology*, **387**, 167–78.

Jacobs, B., Chugani, H. T., Allada, V. et al. (1995). Developmental changes in brain metabolism in sedated rhesus macaques and vervets monkeys revealed by positron emission tomography. *Cerebral Cortex*, **3**, 222–33.

Johnson, J. S. & Newport, E. L. (1989). Critical period effects in second language learning: the influence of maturational state on the acquisition of English as a second language. *Cognitive Psychology*, **21**, 60–99.

Katz, L. C. & Shatz, C. J. (1996). Synaptic activity and the construction of cortical circuits. *Science*, **274**, 1133–8.

Lecanuet, J. P. & Granier-Deferre, C. (1993). Speech stimuli in the fetal environment. In *Developmental Neurocognition*, ed. B. de Boysson-Bardies et al., pp. 237–48. Netherlands: Kluwer Academic Publishers.

LeVay, S., Wiesel, T. N. & Hubel, D. H. (1980). The development of ocular dominance columns in normal and visually deprived monkeys. *Journal of Comparative Neurology*, **191**, 1–51.

Lowel, S. & Singer, W. (1992). Selection of intrinsic horizontal connections in the visual cortex by correlated neuronal activity. *Science*, **255**, 209–212.

Luskin, M. B. & Shatz, C. J. (1985). Neurogenesis of the cat's primary visual cortex. *Journal of Comparative Neurology*, **242**, 611–31.

Maffei, L. & Galli-Resta, L. (1990). Correlation in the discharges of neighboring rat retinal ganglion cells during prenatal life. *Proceedings of the National Academy of Sciences, USA*, **87**, 2861–4.

Marin-Padilla, M. (1988). Early ontogenesis of the human cerebral cortex. In *Cerebral Cortex. Development and maturation of cerebral cortex*, **7**, ed. A. Peters & E. G. Jones, pp. 1–34. New York: Plenum Press.

Mitchell, D. E. & Timney, B. (1984). Postnatal development of function in the mammalian visual system. In *Handbook of Physiology*. Section I: *The Nervous System*, Vol. 3, Part 1. *Sensory Processes*, ed. I. Darian-Smith, pp. 507–55. Bethesda: American Physiological Society.

Mooney, R., Penn, A. A., Gallego, R. & Shatz, C. J. (1996). Thalamic relay of spontaneous retinal activity prior to vision. *Neuron*, **17**, 863–74.

Purves, D., White, L. E. & Riddle, D. R. (1996). Is neural development Darwinian? *Trends in Neuroscience*, **19**, 460–4.

Quartz, S. R. & Sejnowski, T. J. (1997). The neural basis of cognitive development: a constructionist manifesto. *Behavioral and Brain Sciences*, **20**(4), 1–60.

Rakic, P. (1995). A small step for the cell, a giant leap for mankind: a hypothesis of neocortical expansion during evolution. *Trends in Neuroscience*, **18**, 383–8.

Rakic, P., Bourgeois, J. P., Eckenhoff, M. F., Zecevic, N. & Goldman-Rakic, P. S. (1986). Concurrent overproduction of synapses in diverse regions of the primate cerebral cortex. *Science*, **232**, 232–5.

Rakic, P., Bourgeois, J. P. & Goldman-Rakic, P. S. (1994). Synaptic development of the cerebral cortex: implications for learning, memory, and mental illness. *Progress in Brain Research*, **102**, 227–43.

Rodman, H. R. (1994). Development of the inferior temporal cortex in the monkey. *Cerebral Cortex*, **5**, 484–98.

Salin, P. A. & Bullier, J. (1995). Corticocortical connections in the visual system: structure and function. *Physiological Reviews*, **75**, 107–54.

Shankle, W. R., Romney, A. K., Landing, B. H. & Hara, J. (1998). Developmental patterns in the cytoarchitecture of the human cerebral cortex from birth to 6 years examined by correspondence analysis. *Proceedings of the National Academy of Sciences, USA*, **95**, 4023–8.

Stefan, M. D. & Murray, R. M. (1997). Schizophrenia: developmental disturbance of brain and mind? *Acta Paediatrica* Suppl., **422**, 112–16.

Teller, D. Y. (1997). First glances: the vision of infants. *Investigative Ophthalmology and Visual Science*, **38**(11), 2183–203.

Van Essen, D. (1985). Functional organization of primate visual cortex. In *Cerebral Cortex, Vol. 3*, ed. A. Peters & E. G. Jones, pp. 259–329. New York: Plenum Press.

Vannier, C. & Triller, A. (1997). Biology of the postsynaptic glycin receptor. *International Review of Cytology*, **176**, 201–44.

Zecevic, N. (1998). Synaptogenesis in Layer I of the human cerebral cortex in the first half of gestation. *Cerebral Cortex*, **8**, 245–52.

Zecevic, N. & Rakic, P. (1991). Synaptogenesis in the monkey somatosensory cortex. *Cerebral Cortex*, **1**, 510–23.

Zecevic, N., Bourgeois, J. P. & Rakic, P. (1989). Synaptic density in the motor cortex of the rhesus monkey during fetal and postnatal life. *Developmental Brain Research*, **50**, 11–31.

Zoli, M., Torri, C., Ferrari, R. et al. (1998). The emergence of the volume transmission concept. *Brain Research Reviews*, **26**, 136–47.

6

Neurotrophic factors in brain development

Thomas Ringstedt

Department of Women and Child Health, Karolinska Institute, Neonatal Unit, Astrid Lindgren Children's Hospital, Stockholm, Sweden

The concept of neurotrophic factors

During nervous system development, neurons are generated in numbers exceeding those found in adults. The surplus neurons are eliminated by programmed cell death, a process which, in vertebrates and some invertebrates, is influenced by factors outside the cells themselves. Without understanding the molecular basis of programmed cell death, early investigators showed that many neurons in the peripheral nervous system are eliminated during a specific time window, referred to as 'the period of naturally occurring cell death'. Grafting experiments elegantly demonstrated that this naturally occurring cell death is regulated by the innervated target: when a target was removed, the rate of cell death in the innervating ganglion increased; when an extra target was added, it decreased. These effects were thought to be mediated by diffusible 'survival' or 'neurotrophic' factors generated by the targets. The first such factor was discovered in the 1950's, and since it increased neurite outgrowth from sympathetic ganglia, it was named nerve growth factor (NGF). Other proteins homologous to NGF were later discovered, and together these constitute a family of neurotrophic factors: the nerve growth factor family or the neurotrophins. To date, several families of proteins with neurotrophic actions have been described. Apart from the neurotrophins, this review will focus on the glial cell line-derived factor (GDNF) family.

Neurotrophic factors and their receptors are expressed during development and in adulthood. In addition to their neurotrophic role, several other functions for neurotrophins have been implicated. Their function in the CNS is less well understood, but appears to be distinctive from the PNS. What follows is a general introduction to the neurotrophin and GDNF families, and a summary of their functions during CNS development.

The neurotrophins

Structure

The neurotrophin family is comprised of nerve growth factor (NGF), brain derived neurotrophic factor (BDNF), neurotrophin-3 (NT-3) and neurotrophin-4 (NT-4). Additional neurotrophins are known in teleost fish, but it is most likely that these do not have any mammalian counterparts. Neurotrophins are diffusible peptide factors active in the form of homodimers. Heterodimers between different members of the family can be assembled in vitro, but there are as yet no indications that heterodimers are operational in the nervous system. The neurotrophin monomers are composed of about 120 amino acids, half of which are identical within the family. The monomer can be further subdivided in conserved and variable regions. Most of the variable regions have been implicated in receptor binding (for review, see Ibanez, 1998).

Receptors and signalling

The neurotrophins signals through two classes of receptors: the p75 neurotrophin receptor (p75NTR), and the trk (tropomyosin receptor kinase) receptors. Although discovered first, the functions and signalling pathways of the p75NTR are not as well characterized as those of the trk receptors.

Three different trk receptors are known in mammalians: trkA, trkB and trkC. They all exist in the form of transmembrane receptors with a tyrosine kinase activity in the intracellular region. In addition, there are various truncated forms of trkB and trkC that lack the intracellular domain. The different neurotrophins bind to and activate distinct trk receptors according to the following scheme: NGF binds to trkA, BDNF and NT-4 are both ligands of trkB, while NT-3, although considered mainly to be the ligand of trkC, can also activate trkA and trkB under certain conditions. The neurotrophin dimer binds two trk molecules, thereby bringing them together, a step necessary for intracellular signalling to occur. The ligand receptor complex is, in some instances, internalized and retrogradely transported to the neuron soma. Dimerization of the receptors induces autophosphorylation of intracellular tyrosine residues, whereby different effector molecules can bind to specific sites on the trk intracellular domain. There are indications that the truncated receptors can have some signalling activity as well, but the mechanisms are not known to date (for review, see Ibanez, 1998). (Fig 6.1.)

The p75 neurotrophin receptor (p75NTR) lacks an intracellular tyrosine kinase or other catalytic domain, but its intracellular domain shares a common motif with related receptors such as tumor necrosis factor receptor, (TNFR). This so called 'death domain' has been shown to induce apoptosis (programmed cell death), but the mechanisms by which it couples to intracellular signalling events is still largely unknown. p75NTR binds all the neurotrophins with similar affinity. Earlier hypotheses focused on p75NTR interaction with trk receptors. In some systems, the presence of p75NTR can enhance trkA signalling in response to NGF. This was thought to be a consequence of p75NTR binding to NGF and thereby concentrating it to the local environment where the trkA receptors could access it. Regardless

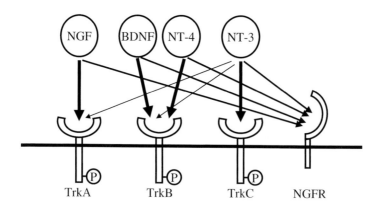

Fig. 6.1.   Schematic diagram of ligand–receptor interaction in the neurotrophin family. Large arrows indicate preferred neurotrophin–Trk receptor interactions, dotted arrows indicate alternate Trk receptor interactions. The importance of the alternate interactions are not fully understood, but the interaction between NT-3 and TrkB has been confirmed in vivo. Small arrows indicate neurotrophin–NGFR interaction. All neurotrophins bind to the NGFR with equal affinity.

of the validity of this model, it is now clear that p75NTR has a signalling activity of its own. Paradoxically for a neurotrophin receptor, the p75NTR seems to function as an apoptosis inducing receptor (for review, see Kaplan and Miller, 1997).

Expression

Most studies of the spatio-temporal localization of neurotrophins and their receptors during development are based on mRNA detecting technologies in rats and mice. Tissue levels of neurotrophin proteins are low, and specific antibodies (except for NGF) have, until recently, been unavailable. Recent studies with antibodies have partly confirmed the mRNA data, partly yielded different expression patterns. These differences have been interpreted to result from the neurotrophin being retrogradely transported in the areas in question. The following short survey, as well as the information in Table 6.1, is based on mRNA expression data obtained in rodents.

Somewhat surprisingly, the trk neurotrophin receptors are expressed earlier during development than their ligands. The earliest detected receptor mRNA is *trkC*, reported to be expressed in the mouse neuroectoderm already at embryonic day 7.5 (E7.5) (Tessarollo et al., 1993). Many tissues express more than on type of trk receptor. The dorsal root ganglia begins to express trk receptors at E9.5, the sympathetic ganglia slightly later (Martin-Zanca et al., 1990). The cranial sensory ganglia express trk receptors in distinct yet overlapping patterns from E10.5. The p75NGFR is expressed in the same ganglia as trkA, but expression begins later. Neurotrophins are quite often expressed in the peripheral target tissues during the period of naturally occurring cell death, but are, particularly in the case of BDNF and NT-3, also found within the ganglia themselves. TrkB and trkC are expressed in the brain throughout embryonic development, while expression of trkA and p75NGFR does not start until shortly before birth (Ernfors et al., 1992; Lu et al., 1989). During the first two postnatal weeks, expression of trkB and trkC decline, while that of trkA increases. NT-3 is probably the earliest expressed neurotrophin in the brain (Farinas et al., 1996). NT-4 and BDNF are expressed from at least E13 (probably earlier), but while BDNF expression is very low until birth and then rapidly increases, NT-4 is regulated in an opposite pattern (Timmusk et al., 1993). NGF is not detected in the brain until the first postnatal day, but thereafter the expression increases rapidly during postnatal development (Lu et al., 1989). Table 6.1.

Role of neurotrophins during PNS development

The concept of neurotrophic action is well established in the peripheral nervous system. As described in the previous section, the neurotrophic factors are expressed in several peripheral target areas, for example skin, while their receptors are found in the innervating ganglia. When the growing neuronal processes reach their targets, they compete for a specific growth factor, expressed by the target in limiting amounts. Excessive and incorrectly projecting neurons are eliminated by programmed cell death. By this mechanism, a correct wiring of the nervous system is ensured. In addition, it is possible that the excessive amount of neurons generated and subsequently eliminated is a necessary step in the pattern formation of the tissue in question.

The discovery that neurotrophins in many instances are expressed in the same parts of the nervous system as their receptors (see above and Table 6.1) led to the concept of local action, i.e. that neurotrophins also act in a para- or autocrine fashion. Local action of NT-3 has been demonstrated in the trigeminal and dorsal root ganglia. In the absence of NT-3, cell death occurs in these areas before target innervation. Furthermore, NT-3 does not act on mature neurons in this system, but on precursor cells (ElShamy et al., 1998; Farinas et al., 1996). Neurotrophins also affect cell differentiation. Primary cultures of neuronal stem cells (pluripotent cells capable of asymmetric division) from the brain or neuronal crest, differentiate in response to added neurotrophins (Sieber-Blum et al., 1993). Neuronal sprouting and fibre outgrowth is induced by neurotrophins. A limited number of studies have implicated the neurotrophins as having chemotropic (axon guiding) functions (Ming et al., 1997). Whether they have this function in vivo is still an open question, but in vivo studies have indicated them as important for the final stage in target innervation and the cessation of fibre outgrowth (Ringstedt et al., 1997). Many growth factors elicit mitogenic effects. Among the neurotrophins, NGF and NT-3 have been shown to promote proliferation in vitro (Memberg and Hall,

Table 6.1. Neurotrophin and neurotrophin receptor expression in rodents during embryonic and early postnatal development

Age	E7.5	E9.5	E10	E11	E13	E14	E16	E18	P0	P7
Neuroectoderm	*TrkC*									
Branchial arches		*NT-3[1]*								
Neural tube		*TrkC,*								
Dorsal root ganglia		*TrkC, TrkA,*	*NT-3[1,2]*	*NT-3, NGFR*	TrkB, BDNF,					
Sympathetic ganglia			*TrkB*		TrkC,	*BDNF, NGFR*	TrkA			
Sensory cranial ganglia			*TrkB*	NGFR	TrkC, TrkA	*BDNF*	BDNF			
Spiral ganglion							TrkC			
Enteric ganglia					*TrkC*					
Brain general		*TrkC, NT-3[1], TrkB*			TrkC, NT-4	*BDNF[a]*	NGFR[a]			BDNF
Neocortex					TrkC, TrkB			NT-3	*BDNF, NGF*	
Basal forebrain								TrkA		
Hippocampus					TrkC, TrkB		*NGF[2]*	NT-3, NGFR		
Basal ganglia					*(TrkB, TrkC)*		TrkC			
Cerebellum					TrkC, NT-3, TrkB		TrkC, NT-3			
Spinal cord					TrkC, NT-3, TrkB					
Eye			*NT-3[1]*		TrkA					
Ear			*NT-3[1]*		TrkB, TrkC, NT-3					

Tissue			
Skin	NGF	NT-3, NGF	
Heart		NT-3, NT-4, BDNF[a]	
Skeletal muscles	*NT-3*[1,3]	BDNF[a], NT-4	NT-3
Whisker/hair follicles		NGF	
Tongue		*NT3*	BDNF
Teeth			NGF, NT-3, NT-4
Lung		NT4, BDNF[a]	
Kidney			NT-4, BDNF
Liver		NT-4[a]	

Notes:

For each tissue, the earliest age at which mRNA expression has been been reported for a given factor is indicated. Normal letters denote data obtained in rats, letters in italics denote data obtained in mice. The sensitivity of the methods used in the original studies varies. In addition, several reports do not include early embryonic stages. Naturally, this biases the table.

Legends: E, embryonic day; 1, data obtained through the use of a knock in expression construct; 2, expression found in the surrounding mesenchyme only; [a], low levels detected by the sensitive RNase protection assay. The table is an overview, and not a complete list of the data available to date.

1995). However, when compared to other growth factors, the mitogenic effects of neurotrophins seem to be less pronounced.

Neurotrophins as survival factors in the CNS

The essential function as target derived survival (neurotrophic) factors demonstrated for the neurotrophins in the PNS has often been extrapolated to the CNS. Expression data can be used to support this view, but are also in accordance with a local action in many areas. Cell culture experiments have demonstrated that NGF and BDNF promote survival of cholinergic cells from the basal forebrain (Alderson et al., 1990), and that BDNF and NT-3 promote survival of motor neurons (Henderson et al., 1993). NT-4 promotes survival of striatal neurons in organotypic slice cultures (Ardelt et al., 1994). In an in vivo model, where the septo-hippocampal pathways of adult rats are transected, NGF and BDNF prevents degeneration of cholinergic neurons of the basal forebrain (Knusel et al., 1992). BDNF also acts on developing motor neurons after sciatic nerve transections during the prenatal period (Yan et al., 1992). NT-3 rescues noradrenergic cells from the locus coeruleus of adult rats from degeneration after chemically induced lesions (Arenas & Persson, 1994). More relevant for our understanding of CNS development, administration of BDNF to chick embryos prevents the extensive loss of motor neurons that normally occurs during the period of naturally occurring cell death (Oppenheim et al., 1992). As the above presented data indicate, neurotrophins can promote cell survival in the CNS. How prominent this role is during normal development remains less clear.

Life without neurotrophins

A landmark in the study of neurotrophins was the generation of mice with targeted gene deletions. Before this, several investigators using exogenously added neurotrophins or blocking antibodies had demonstrated the survival effects of neurotrophins in the PNS. When the PNS of the first neurotrophin ligand and receptor knockout animals was analysed, the results were in accordance with expression data and the known survival effects. Surprisingly, this turned out not to be true for the CNS. Despite the abundant and regulated expression of neurotrophins and neurotrophin receptors in the CNS during development, cell losses can unquestionably be detected in only a few cases. BDNF $-/-$ mice display a reduction in thickness of all cortical layers, but although the mechanism behind this is not clear yet (Jones et al., 1994), general malnourishment has been proposed. In the cerebellum of these mice, the granular cell layer is thinner, and the number of apoptotic granule cells is considerably increased (Schwartz et al., 1997). The number of apoptotic cells in the brains of trkB $-/-$ mice is also significantly increased. This is particularly evident in the dentate gyrus, but an increased apoptosis is also seen in other areas, including the basal ganglia, thalamus and cerebral cortex (Alcantara et al., 1997). While the number of motor neurons is reduced in the facial nucleus and the spinal cord of trkB $-/-$ animals (Klein et al., 1993), surprisingly no loss of motor neurons is described in neither the BDNF nor the BDNF/NT-4 double knockout animals (Liu et al., 1995). Interestingly, an enlarged basal forebrain structure is reported in the p75NGFR $-/-$ animals (Van der Zee et al., 1996). This phenotype is explained as an ablation of p75NGFR mediated apoptosis.

To summarize, the classical function of neurotrophins as target derived survival factors during development, as well as their later ascribed role as local survival factors, has not been fully corroborated in the CNS. Studies on neurotrophin ligand and receptor knockout animals have unexpectedly revealed largely intact cell populations in the CNS. These findings have been explained as a consequence of a high redundancy, with CNS cells supported by more than one neurotrophic factor. However, neither the BDNF/NT-4 (Liu et al., 1995) nor the trkB/trkC (Silos-Santiago et al., 1997) double knockouts display any additional cell loss. Naturally, this does not disprove the redundancy hypothesis, and it is possible that several other growth factors from different families are involved. Also, since all neurotrophin and neurotrophin receptor knockouts except NT4 $-/-$ die within the first postnatal weeks, it is possible that the CNS neurons are dependent on neurotrophins for their survival after the period of naturally occuring cell death, during later stages of development or adulthood. Still, the above data can be taken as an indication that the role of neurotrophins in the CNS is a different one from that in the PNS, and that their primary function should be sought in other areas of neuronal development than promotion of cell survival.

Neurotrophins affect neurotransmitter expression

Neurotrophin receptors are present in the brain throughout embryonic and postnatal development with distinct expression patterns, suggesting that their ligands have particular functions during development of the brain area in question. A picture is now emerging where the neurotrophins have various effects on differentiation of neurons in the developing CNS. In vitro and in vivo experiments have indicated that the basal forebrain cholinergic cells are dependent on NGF for their survival (a subpopulation depends on BDNF). However, there is no cell loss in this area in the brains of trkA $-/-$ or NGF $-/-$ mice. Instead, the cells have substantially reduced levels of acetylcholinesterase. This is particularly evident in the trkA $-/-$ animals. Cholineric cells in the striatum are not affected, although they also express trkA receptors in the wild-type animals (Crowley et al., 1994; Smeyne et al., 1994).

Similarly, neuropeptide Y (NPY) levels are reduced in the neocortex of BDNF $-/-$ mice (Jones et al., 1994). Conversely, injection of BDNF into the ventricles of newborn rats increases neuropeptide expression in the anterior neocortex, particularly of NPY and Substance P (SP). This increase is differentially restricted to specific cortical layers, probably reflecting the fact that the constituent cell's peptide phenotype has already been determined at birth (Nawa et al., 1994). BDNF levels in the brain increase during postnatal development, and it is possible that BDNF then acts to upregulate neuropeptide levels in the maturing neurons. BDNF also increases the levels of calcium binding proteins and microtubule associated protein 2 in the neocortex and hippocampal formation (Jones et al., 1994; Marty et al., 1996).

Neurotrophins affect cell migration

As shown in the previous section, interesting information can be obtained by adding exogenous neurotrophin to the brain. NT-4 added to organotypic slice cultures of embryonic mouse neocortex causes dramatic alterations. The number of cells in the marginal zone increases significantly 24 to 72 hours after addition of the neurotrophin. Intraventricular injection of NT-4 into rat fetuses in utero yields similar results (Brunstrom et al., 1997). The marginal zone houses a population of early pioneer neurons, the Cajal–Retzius cells, that are essential for the proper development and lamination of the neocortex. However, the additional cells, clustered together in heterotopic cell collections, are GABAergic and distinct from the Cajal–Retzius cells. It has been proposed that these cells are equivalent to the neurons of the subpial granule cell layer described in human fetuses. After the arrival of the Cajal–Retzius cells and the first cortical plate neurons, this layer builds up, presumably by lateral migration from the lateral ganglionic eminence (Brunstrom et al., 1997; Pearlman et al., 1998). NT-4 is expressed in the brain during embryonic development, and might be a regulator of this process.

Embryonic overexpression of BDNF in the brain of transgenic mice results in a striking and unexpected phenotype. In addition to a few heterotopic cell collections, the marginal zone of these animals contains clusters of Cajal–Retzius cells which are associated with sulci-like invaginations in the cortical plate. Some stretches of the marginal zone are completely missing or indiscernible, probably because they have been invaded by cells destined for the cortical plate. The Cajal–Retzius cells of these animals have a significantly reduced expression of reelin, an extracellular matrix protein which mediates the Cajal–Retzius cells' effect on neocortical lamination. As a consequence of this, the normal inside-out lamination of the neocortex is disturbed, with migration of neurons born later arrested in deeper layers of the cortical plate, or around their site of origin in the ventricular zone. BDNF expression in the embryonic mouse neocortex is all but absent before birth, but rises rapidly during the first two postnatal weeks. Reelin expression is, at the same time, downregulated at a pace inversely correlated to the rise in BNDF. This downregulation does not occur in mice with a targeted deletion of the

BDNF gene. It is therefore possible that BDNF acts as an intrinsic determinant of cortical maturation, terminating the mechanisms that regulate cortical lamination (Ringstedt et al., 1998). Although some of the effects described in the BDNF over-expressing mice undoubtedly are due to the reduced reelin expression of the Cajal–Retzius cells, a direct effect of BDNF cannot be excluded. In vitro studies have demonstrated that embryonic rat neurons migrate towards a BDNF or NT-4 gradient (Behar et al., 1997). The effect is most pronounced in cells from the ventricular zone of E18 brains. At this time in development, the cortical plate expresses weak levels of BDNF, which could act as an attractive force causing the later born neurons to leave the ventricular zone and enter the cortical plate.

Neurotrophins affect neurite outgrowth in the CNS

The neurotrophins are known to affect fibre outgrowth. NT-3 treatment of lesioned corticospinal tracts significantly increases regenerative sprouting in young adult rats. Interestingly, this increase is primarily in collateral branching, not in neurite elongation (Schnell et al., 1994).

Differentiated effects of neurotrophins on neurite outgrowth have been demonstrated in slice cultures of postnatal ferret visual cortex. The dendritic arborizations of neurons in layer 4 increase their length and complexity in response to exogenously added BDNF, while the other trkB ligand, NT-4, affects the neurons in layer 5 and 6 (McAllister et al., 1995). BDNF and NT-3 have opposing effects on neurons in layers 4 and 6. This has been shown by selectively blocking receptor binding of endogenous BDNF/NT-4 or NT-3 with trkB-, specifically, trkC receptor bodies (created by the fusion of the receptors ligand binding regions with the Fc region of an antibody). While blocking of BDNF decreases dendritic arborizations in layer 4, NT-3 blocking increases it. These effects are reversed in layer 6 (McAllister et al., 1997).

BDNF also affects dendritic arborization in cerebellar Purkinje cells. Normally the Purkinje cells send out one primary dendrite that subsequently branches. In the BDNF −/− mice however, this is replaced by multiple dendritic processes emanating at random angles from the cell body. The cerebellar foliation is also disturbed in these animals, perhaps due to the increased granule cell apoptosis, even though other mechanisms might be involved as well (Schwartz et al., 1997).

Neurotrophins affect cortical plasticity

Axons from the lateral geniculate nucleus entering layer IV of the visual cortex have their terminals segregated into eye-specific ocular dominance columns during postnatal development. Addition of either exogenous BDNF or NT-4 (Cabelli et al., 1995), or blockade of the endogenous trkB ligand (Cabelli et al., 1997) inhibits this process. It has been shown that cortical plasticity with respect to ocular dominance is possible only during a specific time window. A transgenic mouse line that over-expresses BDNF in the neocortex during postnatal development displays an early closure of this time window, as measured by electrophysiological methods. The innervation of pyramidal neurons by GABAergic interneurons is accelerated in the visual cortices of these mice. The precocious termination of cortical plasticity may therefore be due to a strengthening of postsynaptic inhibitory innervation. In accordance with this model BDNF is overexpressed primarily by the pyramidal neurons, which also express endogenous BDNF in wild type animals. The formation and maintenance of inhibitory synapses in the developing CNS are known to be activity regulated. This could be explained by a model were the firing activity of a pyramidal neuron determines its amount of BDNF, which then sets its level of GABAergic inhibitory innervation (Huang et al., 1999).

The GDNF family of neurotrophic factors

History and general introduction

Glial cell line derived neurotrophic factor (GDNF) was isolated in 1993 on the basis of its ability to promote dopamine uptake in cultures of rat embryonic midbrain cells (Lin et al., 1993). As the name indicates, it was first found as a factor secreted by a glioma derived cell line. Since it was shown to enhance survival of dopaminergic cells in cultures, it was regarded as a neurotrophic factor. Similar to members of the NGF family, GDNF was shown to adopt a cysteine knot fold, but possessed a conserved cysteine pattern most similar to the transforming growth factor β (TGFβ) superfamily. The fact that it shared less than 20% sequence homology with any known TGFβ subfamily, argued in favour of it constituting a new subfamily. This family, the GNDF family of neurotrophic factors, now includes three additional members: Neurturin, Persephin and Artemin. The members of this family are, like the neurotrophins, active in the form of homodimers. The monomer sizes are comparable to the neurotrophins (Baloh et al., 1998; Kotzbauer et al., 1996; Lin et al., 1993; Milbrandt et al., 1998).

Receptors and signalling

Neurturin and GDNF signal through the Ret tyrosine kinase receptor (Takahashi et al., 1988). However, they seem to be unable to bind to and activate Ret without the mediation of a second component, a GDNF receptor α (GFRα) coreceptor. There are four GFRαs known in mammals to date: GFRα1, GFRα2 GFRα3 and GFRα4. GFRα4 was until recently known only from the embryonic chick brain. Unlike Ret, the GFRαs are not transmembrane proteins, but linked to the cell membrane by glycosylphosphatidylinositol (GPI) bridges, (Buj-Bello et al., 1997; Jing et

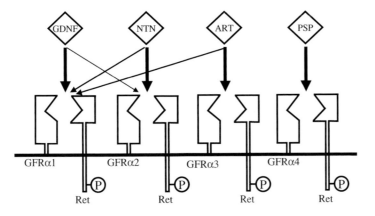

Fig. 6.2.   Schematic diagram of ligand–receptor interaction in the GDNF family of neurotrophic factors. Large arrows indicate preferred ligand-GFRα receptor interaction, whereas smaller arrows indicate alternative GFRα receptor interactions. In order for signalling to occur, the GDNF family ligands probably have to interact with Ret in addition to a GFRα receptor.

al., 1996; Thompson et al., 1998). The nature of the interaction between the ligand, Ret and the GFRα is not known, but it is likely that the GFRα receptor presents the ligand to Ret. Accordingly, ligand specificity seems to be determined by the GFRα component. Although there is some promiscuity in the receptor–ligand interaction, GFRα1 seems to be mainly the receptor for GDNF, GFRα2 the receptor for Neurturin, and GFRα3 the receptor for Artemin (Baloh et al., 1997, 1998; Klein et al., 1997). Mammalian Persephin binds and signals through chick (Enokido et al., 1998) and human (Lindahl et al., 2000a) GFRα4 coexpressed with Ret in mammalian cell lines. Rat GFRα4 has also been shown to bind Persephin, but no activation of Ret was demonstrated in this study (Masure et al., 2000). However, it seems clear that GFRα4 acts as the Persephin receptor in vivo.

Interestingly, the GFRα coreceptor does not have to be present in the same cell in order for signalling to occur. Soluble GFRα1 in combination with GDNF induces Ret autophosphorylation in vitro (Jing et al., 1996), and it is possible that the GFRα component can be supplied by cells adjacent to the responsive cell in vivo (Trupp et al., 1997) (Fig 6.2).

Since Ret, like the trk receptors, has a tyrosine kinase activity, intracellular signalling proceeds in a fashion similar to what has previously been described for the neurotrophin responsive cells.

Expression

The GDNF receptors are expressed by the cranial and dorsal root ganglia early during development. In the brain, a clear expression is detected from E12 or earlier.

While Ret expression increases until birth, and then starts to decline, GFRα1, GFRα2 and GFRα3 expression peaks before birth. In the case of GFRα1 and GFRα2, expression decreases to lower but still significant levels in the adult (Naveilhan et al., 1998; Nosrat et al., 1997; Widenfalk et al., 1997). Interestingly, GFRα3 expression is not detected in the brain after P3, indicating that this receptor might have a specific function in brain development (Naveilhan et al., 1998), even if the CNS levels are very low compared to the PNS. Ret, GFRα1, GFRα2 and GFRα3 are found in developing peripheral tissues, including kidney, lung and heart. Several splice variants of GFRα4 mRNA are expressed in the CNS as well as in peripheral tissues, including testis, thyroid and adrenals (Lindahl et al., 2000a, b) (Table 6.2).

GDNF, Neurturin and Artemin are expressed in various peripheral tissues during development. For example, GDNF and Neurturin are strongly expressed in the vibrissae and the gastrointestinal tract of rats. GDNF is also found in the kidney, where it has a morphogenetic function. Screening of human fetal tissue reveals that Artemin expression is highest in the kidneys and the lungs (Baloh et al., 1998). GDNF, but not NTN, is expressed by skeletal muscle. However, NTN is expressed by cardiac muscle. Expression of NTN and GDNF in the peripheral nervous system is weak or non-existent (Trupp et al., 1995; Widenfalk et al., 1997). Both factors are found in several areas of the CNS. While GDNF is expressed from E13 (Trupp et al., 1995), NTN expression is not detected until after birth. In addition, GDNF seems to be more widely expressed. Artemin is highly expressed in the DRG nerve roots during embryonic rat development, possibly by Schwann cell precursors. Low levels of *Artemin* mRNA can also be detected in human fetal brain (Baloh et al., 1998). *Persephin* mRNA levels are very low. The transcript is detected in several tissues including heart, kidney, liver and brain from E10. The levels remain constant throughout embryonic development, and then decline slightly to reach adult levels (Milbrandt et al., 1998) (Table 6.2).

The GDNF family as neurotrophic factors

While the neurotrophins were characterized early as survival factors for neurons in the peripheral nervous system, GDNF was isolated on the basis of it being a survival factor in vitro for embryonic midbrain dopaminergic neurons. This raised expectations not only as to its importance as a neurotrophic factor during brain development, but also concerning its potential therapeutic value in treating neurodegenerative diseases like Parkinson's disease (Lin et al., 1993). NTN, although first described as a survival factor for symphathetic neurons (Kotzbauer et al., 1996), was subsequently shown to promote survival of midbrain dopaminergic neurons as well (Klein et al., 1997). While GDNF, NTN and Artemin promote survival of both central and peripheral neurons in culture, Persephin promotes survival of central neurons exclusively (Baloh et al., 1998; Kotzbauer et al., 1996; Milbrandt et al., 1998).

In accordance with the in vitro findings, GDNF and NTN have been shown to prevent axotomy induced cell death in the brain. Physical transection of the projections from substantia nigra to striatum, as well as injection of retrogradely acting neurotoxins in this projection, results in an increased cell death in the substantia nigra which gives rise to a Parkinsonian state. Injections of GDNF or NTN in substantia nigra effectively reduces this cell death. Similar effects can be accomplished by injections into the striatum (Horger et al., 1998). An indication of GDNFs promising clinical potential has recently been published: aged and Parkinsonian monkeys injected in substantia nigra and striatum with *GDNF* mRNA expressing viral vectors displayed significantly reduced neurodegeneration, as well as functional improvement (Kordower et al., 2000)

Locus coeruleus is the most important noradrenergic nucleus in the brain. GDNF prevents the cell death that follows chemically induced lesions in this nucleus. In addition, it increases neuronal sprouting and the levels of tyrosine hydroxylase, the enzyme responsible for noradrenaline production (Arenas et al., 1995).

Motor neuron survival is significantly supported by GDNF, both in culture and after axotomy (Henderson et al., 1994). Further, addition of GDNF to developing chick embryos rescues 25% of the motor neurons that normally would undergo programmed cell death (Oppenheim et al., 1995). This points to a role for GDNF in motor neuron survival during normal development. Accordingly, P0 GDNF $-/-$ mice display a partial loss of motor neurons (Sanchez et al., 1996).

GDNF, Ret and GFRα1 knockouts

Several studies of mice with targeted gene deletions for *GDNF*, *ret* and *GFRα1* have been published to date. They all describe kidney agenesis, and aganglionosis of the intestinal enteric nervous system (Enomoto et al., 1998; Sanchez et al., 1996; Schuchardt et al., 1994). Greater phenotypical variances are found in other parts of the peripheral nervous system. While the superior cervical ganglion (SCG) is absent in Ret $-/-$ animals, it is only reduced by 35% in GDNF $-/-$ animals, and is fully intact in GFRα1 deficient animals. The GDNF $-/-$ mice also display reductions in sensory ganglia not observed in the GFRα1 $-/-$ animals.

Studies of mice with targeted gene deletions for Neurturin or GFRα2 have recently been published. Both studies describe reduced populations of parasympathetic neurons and of enteric neurons. The phenotypical similarities between GFRα2 $-/-$ and Neurturin $-/-$ mice, and the fact that these are distinct from the phenotype of GFRα1 /GDNF knockout mice, further strengthens the notion of GFRα2 being the receptor for Neurturin (Heuckeroth et al., 1999; Rossi et al., 1999).

A GFRα3 $-/-$ mouse has also been described. The only phenotypic aberrance

Table 6.2. Expression of members of the GDNF family and their receptors in rodents during embryonic and postnatal development

Age	E10	E12	E13	E14	E16	E17	PO	P7	Developing
Dorsal root ganglia			Ret	ARTM[1], GFRα3		GFRα2			
Sensory cranial ganglia				GFRα3	GDNF	GFRα2			Ret, GFRα1
Sympathetic ganglia			NTN, GFRα3						Ret
Parasympathetic ganglia									Ret, GFRα2
Brain general	GFRα3[a], PSP	GFRα1[a], GFRα2[a], NTN[a], GDNF[a], Ret[a]				GFRα2	NTN, GFRα4		
Neocortex								NTN	GDNF, NTN, GFRα1, GFRα2
Hippocampus						GFRα2		NTN	GDNF, GFRα1
Basal ganglia								GFRα2	GDNF, NTN, GFRα1
Cerebellum						GFRα2			GDNF, Ret, GFRα1
Spinal cord			Ret, GFRα1			GFRα2			
Eye									
Ear						GFRα2, NTN			
Intestine/stomach			GDNF, NTN, GFRα3, Ret				GFRα2		GFRα1
Skin									

Tissue			
Heart	PSP		NTN GFRα2
Whisker/hair follicles		*GFRα2, NTN*	
Lung		*GFRα2, NTN*	
Kidney	PSP	*GDNF, NTN,* *GFRα1,* *GFRα3, Ret*	
Liver	PSP	GDNF, NTN	GFRα2

Notes:

For each tissue, the earliest age at which mRNA expression has been reported for a given factor is indicated. The 'Developing' column contains data from reports that do not further specify age. Normal letters denote data obtained in rats, letters in italics denote data obtained in mice. The sensitivity of the methods used in the original studies varies. In addition, some reports do not include early embryonic stages.

Legends: E, embryonic day; 1, expression found in the nerve roots only; [a], detected by the sensitive RNase protection assay.

found by the authors is a severe defect in the superior cervical ganglion (SCG), and, as a consequence of this, drooping of the upper eyelid (ptosis). Interestingly, the SCG defect seems to be caused by a failure of the precursor cells to migrate in position and innervate their proper targets. A high proportion of them die later in development, probably since they lack necessary survival factors due to the incorrect target innervation. Since only a third of the cells express GFRα3 during the time of cell death, it is likely that survival factors other than the GFRα3 ligand (Artemin) are involved (Nishino et al., 1999).

In general, the reductions in the peripheral nervous system of the GDNF, Neurturin, GFRα1, GFRα2 and the Ret knockout animals give support to the notion that GDNF and Neurturin act as target derived survival factors. As in the case of the neurotrophins, this turns out not to hold true for the central nervous system. Even if GDNF's function as a major survival factor for motor neurons is partly corroborated by the loss of motor neurons reported in the GDNF deficient animals, the fact that this change amounts to not more than 20–30% of the cells indicates that GDNF is essential for only a subpopulation of the motor neuron pool. Quite contrary to the previously described effects on dopaminergic midbrain neurons, most investigators report no changes in the brains of GDNF, Neurturin, Ret, GFRα1 or GFRα2 knockout mice. However, a study describes a reduced packaging density of tyrosine hydroxylase (TH) positive cells in the locus coeruleus of GDNF −/− animals (Granholm et al., 1997). This is accompanied by lower TH levels in the individual cells, and the reduced number of TH positive cells probably reflects this general downregulation, rather than a loss of cells.

As in case of the neurotrophins, the GDNF family does not seem to have simple survival promoting functions in the CNS, although a high degree of redundancy in trophic dependence within the CNS might explain the observations that this conclusion is based on. The GDNF family members might be involved in cell differentiation and other essential processes in CNS development. They could also have a role in postnatal development, and it is possible that future studies will reveal subtle phenotypic defects in the brains of Neurturin and GFRα2 deficient mice. Unfortunately the GDNF, Ret and GFRα1 knockout mice die within the first days after birth. In a study designed to circumvent this problem, the authors transplanted fetal neural tissues from GDNF knockout mice into the brains of adult wild type mice. When compared to similar grafts from wild type mice, the GDNF −/− grafts displayed significantly reduced dopaminergic neuron numbers and fibre outgrowth. This effect was abolished when the grafts were soaked in a GDNF-containing solution prior to implantation (Granholm et al., 2000). There might also be still undiscovered phenotypic defects in the P0 animals. An indication of this is the observation that Ret deficient mice have a depressed ventilatory response to inhaled CO_2 (Burton et al., 1997).

Conclusions

Neurotrophic factors and their receptors are expressed in the central and the peripheral nervous system, as well as in peripheral tissues. The concept of neurotrophism (target derived survival promotion) is well established in the PNS, although local action, possibly on neuronal precursors, has also been described. Expression of neurotrophic factors in peripheral tissues can often be explained by the fact that these constitute targets for PNS projections, but it seems as if neurotrophic factors are also capable of influencing neuro- and organogenesis. In the central nervous system, neurotrophic factors have been shown to counter cell death induced by fibre transections or neurotoxins. Their role as target derived survival factors for neurons in the brain during the period of naturally occurring cell death is less clear. Apoptotic cell death increases in the brains of animals lacking in particular BDNF. However, this increased cell death is not of the magnitude one would derive from a model supporting a neurotrophic role for these factors in the brain, considering the abundance of neurotrophic factor ligands and receptors in the brains of wild-type animals. The possibility that neurotrophic factors have major functions as target derived or local survival factors still remains though. The developing CNS cells might be able to utilize several different factors for neurotrophic support. This notion is supported by the fact that the intracellular signalling pathways are highly similar for neurotrophic factors of different families. Regardless of their effects on cell survival it is however clear, particularly in the case of BDNF and NT-4, that neurotrophic factors have many other important functions in the developing central nervous system. These include the regulation of transmitter expression, axonal sprouting and cell migration. Neurotrophic factor and receptor expression during development suggests that more functions are yet to be elucidated, especially for NT-3 and the GDNF family.

Acknowledgements

I thank Miles Trupp, Joe Wagner and Rebecka Tuttle for valuable comments on the manuscript, and Carlos Ibáñez for good advice.

REFERENCES

Alcantara, S., Frisen, J., del Rio, J. A., Soriano, E., Barbacid, M. & Silos-Santiago, I. (1997). TrkB signaling is required for postnatal survival of CNS neurons and protects hippocampal and motor neurons from axotomy-induced cell death. *Journal of Neuroscience*, **17**, 3623–33.

Alderson, R. F., Alterman, A. L., Barde, Y. A. & Lindsay, R. M. (1990). Brain-derived neurotrophic factor increases survival and differentiated functions of rat septal cholinergic neurons in culture. *Neuron*, **5**, 297–306.

Ardelt, A. A., Flaris, N. A. & Roth, K. A. (1994). Neurotrophin-4 selectively promotes survival of striatal neurons in organotypic slice culture. *Brain Research*, **647**, 340–4.

Arenas, E. & Persson, H. (1994). Neurotrophin-3 prevents the death of adult central noradrenergic neurons in vivo. *Nature*, **367**, 368–71.

Arenas, E., Trupp, M., Akerud, P. & Ibanez, C. F. (1995). GDNF prevents degeneration and promotes the phenotype of brain noradrenergic neurons in vivo. *Neuron*, **15**, 1465–73.

Baloh, R. H., Tansey, M. G., Golden, J. P et al. (1997). TrnR2, a novel receptor that mediates neurturin and GDNF signaling through Ret. *Neuron*, **18**, 793–802.

Baloh, R. H., Tansey, M. G., Lampe, P. A. et al. (1998). Artemin, a novel member of the GDNF ligand family, supports peripheral and central neurons and signals through the GFRalpha3-RET receptor complex. *Neuron*, **21**, 1291–302.

Behar, T. N., Dugich-Djordjevic, M. M., Li, Y. X. et al. (1997). Neurotrophins stimulate chemotaxis of embryonic cortical neurons. *European Journal of Neuroscience*, **9**, 2561–70.

Brunstrom, J. E., Gray-Swain, M. R., Osborne, P. A. & Pearlman, A. L. (1997). Neuronal heterotopias in the developing cerebral cortex produced by neurotrophin-4. *Neuron*, **18**, 505–17.

Buj-Bello, A., Adu, J., Pinon, L. G. et al. (1997). Neurturin responsiveness requires a GPI-linked receptor and the Ret receptor tyrosine kinase. *Nature*, **387**, 721–4.

Burton, M. D., Kawashima, A., Brayer, J. A. et al. (1997). RET proto-oncogene is important for the development of respiratory CO_2 sensitivity. *Journal of the Autonomic Nervous System*, **63**, 137–43.

Cabelli, R. J., Hohn, A. & Shatz, C. J. (1995). Inhibition of ocular dominance column formation by infusion of NT-4/5 or BDNF. *Science*, **267**, 1662–6.

Cabelli, R. J., Shelton, D. L., Segal, R. A. & Shatz, C. J. (1997). Blockade of endogenous ligands of trkB inhibits formation of ocular dominance columns. *Neuron*, **19**, 63–76.

Crowley, C., Spencer, S. D., Nishimura, M. C. et al. (1994). Mice lacking nerve growth factor display perinatal loss of sensory and sympathetic neurons yet develop basal forebrain cholinergic neurons. *Cell*, **76**, 1001–11.

ElShamy, W. M., Fridvall, L. K. & Ernfors, P. (1998). Growth arrest failure, G1 restriction point override, and S phase death of sensory precursor cells in the absence of neurotrophin-3. *Neuron*, **21**, 1003–15.

Enokido, Y., de Sauvage, F., Hongo, J. A. et al. (1998). GFR alpha-4 and the tyrosine kinase Ret form a functional receptor complex for persephin. *Current Biology*, **8**, 1019–22.

Enomoto, H., Araki, T., Jackman, A. et al. (1998). GFR alpha1-deficient mice have deficits in the enteric nervous system and kidneys. *Neuron*, **21**, 317–24.

Ernfors, P., Merlio, J-P. & Persson, H. (1992). Cells expressing mRNA for neurotrophins and their receptors during embryonic rat development. *European Journal of Neuroscience*, **4**, 1140–58.

Farinas, I., Yoshida, C. K., Backus, C. & Reichardt, L. F. (1996). Lack of neurotrophin-3 results in death of spinal sensory neurons and premature differentiation of their precursors. *Neuron*, **17**, 1065–78.

Granholm, A. C., Srivastava, N., Mott, J. L. et al. (1997). Morphological alterations in the peripheral and central nervous systems of mice lacking glial cell line-derived neurotrophic factor (GDNF): immunohistochemical studies. *Journal of Neuroscience*, **17**, 1168–78.

Granholm, A. C., Reyland, M., Albeck, D. et al. (2000). Glial cell line-derived neurotrophic factor is essential for postnatal survival of midbrain dopamine neurons. *Journal of Neuroscience*, **20**, 3182–90.

Henderson, C. E., Camu, W., Mettling, C. et al. (1993). Neurotrophins promote motor neuron survival and are present in embryonic limb bud [see comments]. *Nature*, **363**, 266–70.

Henderson, C. E., Phillips, H. S., Pollock, R. A. et al. (1994). GDNF: a potent survival factor for motoneurons present in peripheral nerve and muscle [see comments] [published erratum appears in *Science*, 1995, Feb 10; **267**(5199): 777]. *Science*, **266**, 1062–4.

Heuckeroth, R. O., Enomoto, H., Grider, J. R. et al. (1999). Gene targeting reveals a critical role for neurturin in the development and maintenance of enteric, sensory, and parasympathetic neurons [In Process Citation]. *Neuron*, **22**, 253–63.

Horger, B. A., Nishimura, M. C., Armanini, M. P. et al. (1998). Neurturin exerts potent actions on survival and function of midbrain dopaminergic neurons. *Journal of Neuroscience*, **18**, 4929–37.

Huang, Z. J., Kirkwood, A., Pizzorusso, T. et al. (1999). BDNF regulates the maturation of inhibition and the critical period of plasticity in mouse visual cortex. *Cell*, **98**, 739–755.

Ibanez, C. F. (1998). Emerging themes in structural biology of neurotrophic factors. *Trends in Neuroscience*, **21**, 438–44.

Jing, S., Wen, D., Yu, Y. et al. (1996). GDNF-induced activation of the ret protein tyrosine kinase is mediated by GDNFR-alpha, a novel receptor for GDNF. *Cell*, **85**, 1113–24.

Jones, K. R., Farinas, I., Backus, C. & Reichardt, L. F. (1994). Targeted disruption of the BDNF gene perturbs brain and sensory neuron development but not motor neuron development. *Cell*, **76**, 989–99.

Kaplan, D. R. & Miller, F. D. (1997). Signal transduction by the neurotrophin receptors. *Current Opinion in Cell Biology*, **9**, 213–21.

Klein, R., Smeyne, R. J., Wurst, W. et al. (1993). Targeted disruption of the trkB neurotrophin receptor gene results in nervous system lesions and neonatal death. *Cell*, **75**, 113–22.

Klein, R. D., Sherman, D., Ho, W. H. et al. (1997). A GPI-linked protein that interacts with Ret to form a candidate neurturin receptor [published erratum appears in *Nature*, 1998 Mar 12; **392**(6672): 210]. *Nature*, **387**, 717–21.

Knusel, B., Beck, K. D., Winslow, J. W. et al. (1992). Brain-derived neurotrophic factor administration protects basal forebrain cholinergic but not nigral dopaminergic neurons from degenerative changes after axotomy in the adult rat brain. *Journal of Neuroscience*, **12**, 4391–402.

Kordower, J. H., Emborg, M. E., Bloch, J. et al. (2000). Neurodegeneration prevented by lentiviral vector delivery of GDNF in primate models of Parkinson's disease [In Process Citation]. *Science*, **290**, 767–73.

Kotzbauer, P. T., Lampe, P. A., Heuckeroth, R. O. et al. (1996). Neurturin, a relative of glial-cell-derived neurotrophic factor. *Nature*, **384**, 467–70.

Lin, L. F., Doherty, D. H., Lile, J. D., Bektesh, S. & Collins, F. (1993). GDNF: a glial cell-line-derived neurotrophic factor for midbrain dopaminergic neurons [see comments]. *Science*, **260**, 1130–2.

Lindahl, M., Poteryaev, D., Yu, L. et al. (2000a). Human GFR(alpha)4 is the receptor for perse-phin, and is predominantly expressed in normal and malignant thyroid medullary cells. *Journal of Biological Chemistry*, in press.

Lindahl, M., Timmusk, T., Rossi, J., Saarma, M. & Airaksinen, M. S. (2000b). Expression and alternative splicing of mouse Gfra4 suggest roles in endocrine cell development. *Molecular and Cellular Neuroscience*, **15**, 522–33.

Lindahl, M., Poteryaev, D., Yu, L. et al. (2001). Human glial cell line-derived neurotrophic factor receptor alpha 4 is the receptor for persephin and is predominantly expressed in normal and malignant thyroid medullary cells. *Journal of Biological Chemistry*, **276**, 9344–51.

Liu, X., Ernfors, P., Wu, H. & Jaenisch, R. (1995). Sensory but not motor neuron deficits in mice lacking NT4 and BDNF. *Nature*, **375**, 238–41.

Lu, B., Buck, C. R., Dreyfus, C. F. & Black, I. B. (1989). Expression of NGF and NGF receptor mRNAs in the developing brain: evidence for local delivery and action of NGF. *Experimental Neurology*, **104**, 191–9.

McAllister, A. K., Lo, D. C. & Katz, L. C. (1995). Neurotrophins regulate dendritic growth in developing visual cortex. *Neuron*, **15**, 791–803.

McAllister, A. K., Katz, L. C. & Lo, D. C. (1997). Opposing roles for endogenous BDNF and NT-3 in regulating cortical dendritic growth. *Neuron*, **18**, 767–78.

Martin-Zanca, D., Barbacid, M. & Parada, L. F. (1990). Expression of the trk proto-oncogene is restricted to the sensory cranial and spinal ganglia of neural crest origin in mouse develop-ment. *Genes and Development*, **4**, 683–94.

Marty, S., Carroll, P., Cellerino, A. et al. (1996). Brain-derived neurotrophic factor promotes the differentiation of various hippocampal nonpyramidal neurons, including Cajal–Retzius cells, in organotypic slice cultures. *Journal of Neuroscience*, **16**, 675–87.

Masure, S., Cik, M., Hoefnagel, E. et al. (2000). Mammalian GFRα-4, a divergent member of the GFRα family of coreceptors for glial cell line-derived neurotrophic factor family ligands, is a receptor for the neurotrophic factor Persephin. *Journal of Biological Chemistry*, **275**, 39427–34.

Memberg, S. P. & Hall, A. K. (1995). Proliferation, differentiation, and survival of rat sensory neuron precursors in vitro require specific trophic factors. *Molecular and Cellular Neuroscience*, **6**, 323–35.

Milbrandt, J., de Sauvage, F. J., Fahrner, T. J. et al. (1998). Persephin, a novel neurotrophic factor related to GDNF and neurturin. *Neuron*, **20**, 245–53.

Ming, G., Lohof, A. M. & Zheng, J. Q. (1997). Acute morphogenic and chemotropic effects of neurotrophins on cultured embryonic *Xenopus* spinal neurons. *Journal of Neuroscience*, **17**, 7860–71.

Nawa, H., Pelleymounter, M. A. & Carnahan, J. (1994). Intraventricular administration of BDNF increases neuropeptide expression in newborn rat brain. *Journal of Neuroscience*, **14**, 3751–65.

Naveilhan, P., Baudet, C., Mikaels, A., Shen, L., Westphal, H. & Ernfors, P. (1998). Expression and regulation of GFRalpha3, a glial cell line-derived neurotrophic factor family receptor. *Proceedings of the National Academy of Sciences, USA*, **95**, 1295–300.

Nishino, J., Mochida, K., Ohfuji, Y. et al. (1999). GFRα3, a component of the artemin receptor, is required for migration and survival of the superior cervical ganglion. *Neuron*, **23**, 725–36.

Nosrat, C. A., Tomac, A., Hoffer, B. J. & Olson, L. (1997). Cellular and developmental patterns of expression of Ret and glial cell line-derived neurotrophic factor receptor alpha mRNAs. *Experimental Brain Research*, **115**, 410–22.

Oppenheim, R. W., Yin, Q. W., Prevette, D. & Yan, Q. (1992). Brain-derived neurotrophic factor rescues developing avian motoneurons from cell death. *Nature*, **360**, 755–7.

Oppenheim, R. W., Houenou, L. J., Johnson, J. E. et al. (1995). Developing motor neurons rescued from programmed and axotomy-induced cell death by GDNF [see comments]. *Nature*, **373**, 344–6.

Pearlman, A. L., Faust, P. L., Hatten, M. E. & Brunstrom, J. E. (1998). New directions for neuronal migration. *Current Opinion in Neurobiology*, **8**, 45–54.

Ringstedt, T., Kucera, J., Lendahl, U., Ernfors, P. & Ibanez, C. F. (1997). Limb proprioceptive deficits without neuronal loss in transgenic mice overexpressing neurotrophin-3 in the developing nervous system. *Development*, **124**, 2603–13.

Ringstedt, T., Linnarsson, S., Wagner, J. et al. (1998). BDNF regulates reelin expression and Cajal–Retzius cell development in the cerebral cortex. *Neuron*, **21**, 305–15.

Rossi, J., Luukko, K., Poteryaev, D. et al. (1999). Retarded growth and deficits in the enteric and parasympathetic nervous system in mice lacking GFR alpha2, a functional neurturin receptor [In Process Citation]. *Neuron*, **22**, 243–52.

Sanchez, M. P., Silos-Santiago, I., Frisen, J., He, B., Lira, S. A. & Barbacid, M. (1996). Renal agenesis and the absence of enteric neurons in mice lacking GDNF. *Nature*, **382**, 70–3.

Schnell, L., Schneider, R., Kolbeck, R., Barde, Y. A. & Schwab, M. E. (1994). Neurotrophin-3 enhances sprouting of corticospinal tract during development and after adult spinal cord lesion [see comments]. *Nature*, **367**, 170–3.

Schuchardt, A., D'Agati, V., Larsson-Blomberg, L., Costantini, F. & Pachnis, V. (1994). Defects in the kidney and enteric nervous system of mice lacking the tyrosine kinase receptor Ret [see comments]. *Nature*, **367**, 380–3.

Schwartz, P. M., Borghesani, P. R., Levy, R. L., Pomeroy, S. L. & Segal, R. A. (1997). Abnormal cerebellar development and foliation in BDNF−/− mice reveals a role for neurotrophins in CNS patterning. *Neuron*, **19**, 269–81.

Sieber-Blum, M., Ito, K., Richardson, M. K., Langtimm, C. J. & Duff, R. S. (1993). Distribution of pluripotent neural crest cells in the embryo and the role of brain-derived neurotrophic factor in the commitment to the primary sensory neuron lineage. *Journal of Neurobiology*, **24**, 173–84.

Silos-Santiago, I., Fagan, A. M., Garber, M., Fritzsch, B. & Barbacid, M. (1997). Severe sensory deficits but normal CNS development in newborn mice lacking TrkB and TrkC tyrosine protein kinase receptors. *European Journal of Neuroscience*, **9**, 2045–56.

Smeyne, R. J., Klein, R., Schnapp, A. et al. (1994). Severe sensory and sympathetic neuropathies in mice carrying a disrupted Trk/NGF receptor gene [see comments]. *Nature*, **368**, 246–9.

Takahashi, M., Buma, Y., Iwamoto, T., Inaguma, Y., Ikeda, H. & Hiai, H. (1988). Cloning and expression of the ret proto-oncogene encoding a tyrosine kinase with two potential transmembrane domains. *Oncogene*, **3**, 571–8.

Tessarollo, L., Tsoulfas, P., Martin-Zanca, D. et al. (1993). trkC, a receptor for neurotrophin-3, is widely expressed in the developing nervous system and in non-neuronal tissues [published erratum appears in *Development*, 1993, August; **118**(4): following 1384]. *Development*, **118**, 463–75.

Thompson, J., Doxakis, E., Pinon, L. G. et al. (1998). GFRalpha-4, a new GDNF family receptor. *Molecular and Cellular Neuroscience*, **11**, 117–26.

Timmusk, T., Belluardo, N., Metsis, M. & Persson, H. (1993). Widespread and developmentally regulated expression of neurotrophin-4 mRNA in rat brain and peripheral tissues. *European Journal of Neuroscience*, **5**, 605–13.

Trupp, M., Ryden, M., Jornvall, H. et al. (1995). Peripheral expression and biological activities of GDNF, a new neurotrophic factor for avian and mammalian peripheral neurons. *Journal of Cell Biology*, **130**, 137–48.

Trupp, M., Belluardo, N., Funakoshi, H. & Ibanez, C. F. (1997). Complementary and overlapping expression of glial cell line-derived neurotrophic factor (GDNF), c-ret proto-oncogene, and GDNF receptor-alpha indicates multiple mechanisms of trophic actions in the adult rat CNS. *Journal of Neuroscience*, **17**, 3554–67.

Van der Zee, C. E., Ross, G. M., Riopelle, R. J. & Hagg, T. (1996). Survival of cholinergic forebrain neurons in developing p75NGFR-deficient mice [see comments]. *Science*, **274**, 1729–32.

Widenfalk, J., Nosrat, C., Tomac, A., Westphal, H., Hoffer, B. & Olson, L. (1997). Neurturin and glial cell line-derived neurotrophic factor receptor-beta (GDNF-beta), novel proteins related to GDNF and GDNFR-alpha with specific cellular patterns of expression suggesting roles in the developing and adult nervous system and in peripheral organs. *Journal of Neuroscience*, **7**, 8506–19.

Yan, Q., Elliott, J. & Snider, W. D. (1992). Brain-derived neurotrophic factor rescues spinal motor neurons from axotomy-induced cell death. *Nature*, **360**, 753–5.

The discovery of programmed neuronal death and nerve growth

It was well known at the beginning of the twentieth century that, by removing the target organ, some neurons innervating the organ disappear. Viktor Hamburger, who started as a student working with Hans Speeman (see p. 44) showed that, by removing the wing of the chick embryo the number of neurons disappeared. Hamburger gave his paper to an Italian neuro-anatomist, Guiseppi Levi, who together with a student, Rita Levi-Montalcini, challenged this finding and showed that the nerves first grow normally and then degenerate when the wing is removed. Thus the target organ seemed to keep the neurons alive.

These studies by Levi and Levi-Montalcini were performed under remarkable circumstances. These scientists were barred from working at the university in Mussolini's Italy, as they were Jewish. Therefore, Rita Levi-Montalcini set up a laboratory in her bedroom 'with a few indispensable pieces of equipment, such as an incubator, a light, a stereomicroscope and a microtome. The object of choice was the chick embryo, and the instruments consisted of sewing needles transformed with the help of a sharpening stone into microinstruments. My Bible and inspiration was an article by Viktor Hamburger . . .'. In July 1942 the heavy bombing of Turin forced Rita Levi-Montalcini to move to a small country house, where she continued her experiments. Due to food shortages, the eggs were scrambled for food after the experiments.

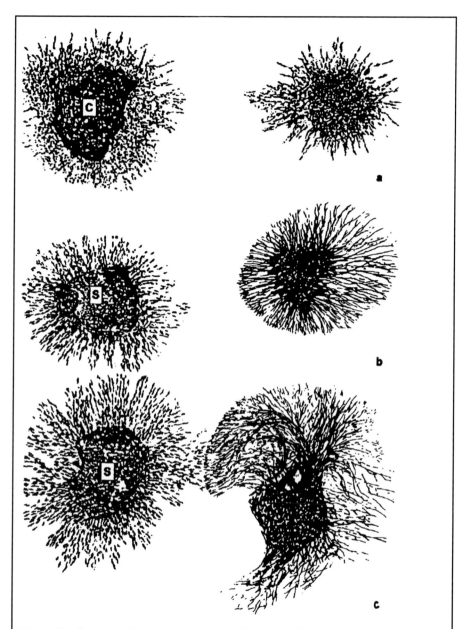

Fig. 1. The discovery of programmed neuronal death and nerve growth.

After the war Rita Levi-Montalcini was invited by Viktor Hamburger to St Louis in the United States to continue her research, where she stayed for several decades. A series of experiments was conducted, first with Hamburger and then with the biochemist Stanley Cohen, which led to the discovery of the nerve growth factor. A crude extract was first isolated from a mouse tumour and shown to produce the famous halo effect when incubating a naked ganglion cell. When trying to further purify NGF, a snake venom was used, but instead of degrading NGF it promoted the halo effect. In this way, the salivary glands were discovered to be a rich source of NGF. Rita Levi-Montalcini, together with Stanley Cohen, shared the Nobel Prize in physiology or medicine in 1986.

References

Levi-Montalcini, R. (1988). *In Praise of Imperfection.* NY: Basic Books.

Patterson P. H. & Purves, D. (1982). *Readings in Developmental Neurobiology.* Cold Spring Harbor Laboratory.

7

Neurotransmitters and neuromodulators

Hugo Lagercrantz and Eric Herlenius

Department of Women and Child Health, Karolinska Institute, Neonatal Unit, Astrid Lindgren Children's Hospital, Stockholm, Sweden

Although genes mainly determine the development of the scaffold of the CNS, the detailed wiring of the neuronal circuits is, to a large degree, self-generated dependent on the action of neurotransmitters and neuromodulators. They can promote, amplify, block, inhibit or attenuate the microelectric signals, which are passed on to neurones. Thereby, they give rise to the signalling patterns between myriads of neuronal networks providing the physical networks of cerebral neurones. Neurotransmitters such as the catecholamines appear in the embryos of vertebrate and invertebrate animals even before neurones are differentiated (Pendleton et al., 1998). Some of the cells in the neuronal crest contain noradrenaline from the outset, but become cholinergic due to environmental influences (Patterson & Chun, 1977).

Many neuroactive molecules change their functional role in the CNS during development. The same molecule may be crucial for differentiation, neuronal growth and establishment of neuronal networks in the immature CNS, while switching to a more modulatory role of the ongoing traffic in the mature CNS. Receptor subunits may exchange during development, i.e. the NMDA receptors, whose subunits allow longer open channel time during early development then switch to a shorter more stable adult subunit composition. This is of importance for the plasticity of the immature brain and subsequently for memory storage and preservation in the adult brain (Fox et al., 1999).

Noradrenaline and acetylcholine are regarded as classical neurotransmitters and dominate in the peripheral nervous system. They appear at an early stage during both phylogenesis and ontogenesis. Many of the neuropeptides were first identified in the gastrointestinal tract and probably appear early during CNS development. They act slowly since they have to be synthesized and packaged in the cell soma and carried to the terminals before they can be released. The recently evolved and more sophisticated mammalian brain requires more fast-switching neurotransmitters acting directly on ion-channels. Therefore, excitatory and inhibitory amino acids seem to dominate in the mature CNS, where the monoamines and neuropeptides may act more as neuromodulators (see Cooper et al., 1996).

The distinction between a transmitter and a modulator is far from clear, however, and several of the neuroactive agents described to date change their role during brain development or have different actions depending on brain region or innervated neurones. Furthermore, a given transmittor may have different effects depending on brain region, postsynaptic receptor configuration, G-protein coupling and second messenger system.

A neuroactive agent can be expressed in high amounts during certain stages of development, but then persists in only a few synapses (Cavanagh & Parnavelas, 1988). It is possible that this agent either has only a transitory role during a critical window during development or that it remains mainly as an evolutionary residue, with minor functions in, e.g. mammals. If the synthesis of some of these neurotransmitters/modulators is blocked pharmacologically or knocked-out by transgenic techniques, it does not seem to affect survival or even important physiological functions. This illustrates the plasticity of the brain during early development. Other neuroactive agents seem to be able to take over. Markers for neurotransmitters and neuromodulators during CNS development generally appear first in the caudal and phylogenetically older part of the brain probably due to earlier neurogenesis (see Semba, 1992).

Classification of the main neurotransmitters and modulators according to principal biochemical differences and tentative ontogenetic appearance is depicted in Table 7.1.

Receptors

The neurotransmitters or modulators can act on either metabotropic or ionotropic receptors (for reviews see, e.g. Bertrand & Changeux, 1995). The action of the metabotropic receptors is based on G- or N-proteins in the lipid bilayer of the membrane to affect their enzymes and channels. This effect is slower (tens of milliseconds) than for the ionotrophic receptors. Metabotropic receptors are probably expressed at an earlier stage during ontogeny and play a more modulatory role in the mature CNS.

The ionotropic receptors respond rapidly and are also termed class I receptors. They act on ion gates, which they can open or close in less than a millisecond. The ion channels consist of transmembrane proteins, which can be selective for cations (activatory receptors) or anions (inhibitory). The ionotropic nicotinic acetylcholine receptor (nAcR), the $GABA_AR$ and glycine receptor GlyR are members of the same evolutionary super family and have a similar structure. A fetal subunit of the acetylcholine receptor (gamma-AchR) is replaced by an adult type (epsilon-AchR) in the muscle end-plate to increase the conductance (Herlitz et al., 1996).

Small lipophilic or gaseous molecules that penetrate the cell membrane have,

Table 7.1. Major neurotransmitters and neuromodulators presented in presumed order of appearance during ontogeny

Purines
adenosine, ATP
Monoamines
serotonin (indoleamines)
dopamine, noradrenaline, adrenaline
Neuropeptides
opioids: enkephalins, endorphin, dynorphin
tachykinins: substance P, neurokinin
glucagon-related: vasoactive intestinal polypeptide (VIP), pituitary adenylate cyclase activating peptide (PACAP)
neuropeptide Y (NPY)
somatostatin
neurotensin, calcitonin gene-related peptide (CGRP)
Acetylcholine
Amino acids
glycine, GABA, glutamate, aspartate

since 1990 proved to be important neuroactive agents. These unconventional transmitters interact with nuclear receptors, i.e. retinoids, Vitamin D (Mangelsdorf et al., 1995) or enzymes in the cytosol (guanylyl cyclase), i.e. nitric oxide (NO) and carbon monoxide (CO). However, their roles during development of the CNS are still under investigation and they will not be included in the present review.

Ontogeny of neurotransmitter systems

The choice of neurotransmitter of a precursor neuron depends on the environment. In a series of remarkable experiments Nicole Le Douarin (1981) demonstrated that, when the sympathetic trunk crest from a quail was transplanted into the vagal region of a chick host, the nerves became cholinergic. Conversely, when vagal neurones were transplanted into the sympathetic trunk, the nerves became adrenergic. The expression of neurotransmitter type seemed to be dependent on a tissue factor. When sympathetic ganglia cells were cultivated in a medium from a heart cell culture, the adrenergic neurones became cholinergic (Patterson & Chun, 1977). The choice of transmitter could also be affected by corticosteroids. Thus, environmental factors are important for the differentiation and for which neuroactive agent will be used in communication with the surrounding cells.

Catecholamines

Catecholamines can be found in protozoa as well as in the very early embryo. The synthesizing enzyme tyrosine hydroxylase has been detected the first day of incubation of the chicken; dopamine the second day and noradrenaline and adrenaline the third day. High concentrations of catecholamines have been recorded in Hensen's node, corresponding to the notochord of the mammalian embryo (see Pendleton et al., 1998). Catecholaminergic neurones are generated at the time of telencephalic vesicle formation in rodents as well as in primates. The monoaminergic neurones reach the cerebral wall as cortical neurogenesis begins. Catecholamines play a crucial role in early development, which has been demonstrated by deleting the genes encoding for tyrosine hydroxylase (TH) (Zhou et al., 1995) and dopamine β-hydroxylase (DBH) (Thomas et al., 1995).

Noradrenaline

Noradrenaline is assumed to be involved in arousal and attention, fear and anxiety, and learning and memory. At one stage, about one out of four synapses contains noradrenaline. The cell bodies of the noradrenergic neurones are concentrated in the brain stem, particularly in the locus coeruleus (A6) within the caudal pons (Fig. 7.1). From this structure, five major noradrenergic tracts originate which innervate the whole brain. There are also clusters of noradrenergic cell bodies in, e.g. the nucleus tractus solitarius (A2), and in the lateral ventral tegmental field (A5). Fibres from these nuclei intermingle with those from the locus coeruleus. Noradrenergic neurones appear at an early stage in the CNS; 12–14th day in the rat (Olson & Seiger, 1972) (total gestational age 21 days) and 5–6 weeks in the human (Sundström et al., 1993), as detected by the formaldehyde reaction and immunofluorescence (see Fig. 7.2).

Adrenergic receptors seem to develop independently of the noradrenergic nerves. α_2-adrenergic receptors are expressed at a relatively early stage. They can either be presynaptic and inhibit noradrenaline release by negative feedback, or postsynaptic with mainly inhibitory effects (see Cooper et al, 1996).

Noradrenaline is essential for normal brain development. The noradrenergic system regulates the development of the Cajal–Retzius cells which are the first neurones to be born in the cortex and proposed to be instrumental in neuronal migration and laminar formation (Naqui et al., 1999). Administration of 6-OH-dopamine prevents the natural programmed cell death of these neurones and delays the formation of cortical layers. Lesioning the noradrenergic projections or blocking neurotransmission with receptor antagonist prevents astrogliosis and glial cell proliferation. Depleting noradrenaline during the perinatal period results in subtle dendritic changes and possibly also alterations in cortical differentiation (see Berger-Sweeny & Hohman, 1997)

Rat   Human

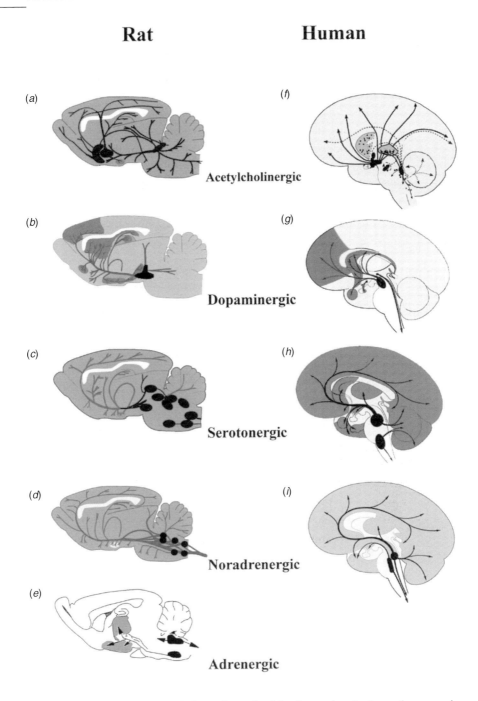

(a)   *(f)*

Acetylcholinergic

(b)   *(g)*

Dopaminergic

(c)   *(h)*

Serotonergic

(d)   *(i)*

Noradrenergic

(e)

Adrenergic

Fig. 7.1.   Figure shows schematic sagittal illustrations of cell bodies and projections of monoamine neurotransmittor systems. Acetylcholinergic pathways, dopaminergic pathways, serotoninergic pathways and noradrenergic pathways in the rat and human brain and adrenergic pathways in the rat. (Modified from Heimer, 1995, with permission.)

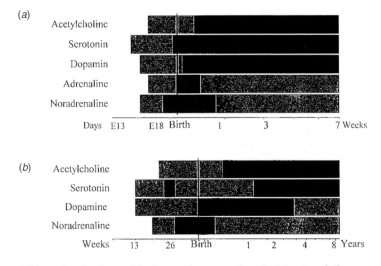

Fig. 7.2.   Arbitrary levels of acetylcholine and monoamines in (*a*) rat and (*b*) man vs. age (10-logarithmic scale). (Data from Olson & Seiger, 1972; Almqvist et al., 1996; Sundström et al., 1993; Herregodts et al., 1990; Naeff et al., 1992.)

The role of noradrenaline has been investigated by targeted disruption of the dopamine β-hydroxylase (DBH) gene. The DBH locus of the DBH proximal promoter and the first exon were replaced with a neomycin-resistance cassette (Thomas et al., 1995). This resulted in fetal death, probably due to cardiovascular failure. Only about 5% of the homozygotic mice survived until adulthood, presumably due to some placental transfer of noradrenaline. Most of the mice could be rescued to birth by providing them with dihydroxyphenylserine (DDPS), a precursor that can be converted to noradrenaline in the absence of DBH. These mice had a reduced ability of acquisition and retention for some tasks. Interestingly, female mice seemed to have deficient ability to take care of their offspring. Thus, there seems to be a critical window during early development when noradrenaline is involved in forming the pathways responsible for maternal behaviour (Thomas & Palmiter, 1997).

Dopamine

Dopamine plays a very important role in motor and cognitive programmes. The cell bodies of the dopaminergic neurones are concentrated in the substantia nigra, ventral tegmental area and retrorubral field and project to the basal ganglia, olfactory bulb, limbic regions, hippocampus and to the cortex (Fig. 7.1).

Dopaminergic neurones appear early during development at the gestational age of 10–15 days in the rat (Olson & Seiger, 1972) and 6–8 weeks in the human

(Sundström et al., 1993) (Fig. 7.2), earlier in females than in males. The dopamine turnover is relatively high during the perinatal period, compared to adults.

There are two main types of dopamine receptors: D_1 and D_2, but there are also D_3, D_4 and D_5 receptors. Stimulation of the D_1 receptors results in an increase in cAMP formation and phosphorylation of DARPP-32, while D_2 receptors mediate a decrease in cAMP formation. Extremely high levels of D_1 receptors have been reported in the pallidum during the perinatal period (Boyson & Adams, 1997). D_1 receptor stimulation regulates transcription of other genes, and it is possible that abnormal perinatal stimulation can result in long-term consequences (see below).

Disturbances of the development of the dopaminergic system may lead to dyskinesia, dystonia, tics, obsessive–compulsive disorders and abnormal eye movements. This has been observed in DA-depleted rats after 6-hydroxydopamine treatment but with preserved noradrenaline effect. Tyrosin-hydroxylase gene deleted mice were hypoactive and suffered from adipsia and aphagia which could be treated with l-dopa (Zhou et al., 1995).

Adrenaline

The existence of adrenaline in the brain was not accepted until the adrenaline synthesizing enzyme PNMT (phenylethanolamine-*N*-methyl transferase) was detected by immunohistochemical methods. This enzyme was localized in the lower brain-stem (Fig. 7.1) intermingled with noradrenergic neurones. Adrenaline in the brain is probably involved in neuroendocrine and blood pressure control. Adrenaline has inhibitory actions on locus coeruleus and brainstem respiratory rhythm. PNMT occurs predominantly before birth in the rat CNS, while there is a decline in PNMT-containing structures after birth (see Foster, 1992).

Serotonin

Serotonin (5HT) enhances motor neuron excitability. Serotoninergic tonic activity is highest during waking, arousal and absent during active or rapid-eye-movement sleep. If the gene encoding for 5HT1B receptors is knocked out the proportion of active sleep is increased (Boutrel et al.,1999).

Serotonin is localized in the midbrain, the pineal gland, substantia nigra, the hypothalamus and the raphe nuclei of the brain stem (Fig. 7.1).

Serotonin can already be detected in the fertilized egg and is involved in early morphogenesis of the heart, the craniofacial epithelia and other structures. If embryos are cultured in the presence of serotonin uptake inhibitors or receptor ligands, specific craniofacial malformations occur. Serotoninergic cells in the raphe are among the earliest to be generated in the brain (about E11 to E15 in the rat and between weeks 5 to 12 in the human fetus) (Fig. 7.2). These cells send axons to the forebrain and may be of importance in the differentiation of neuronal progenitors (Lauder et al., 1994). Excess of serotonin prevents the normal development of the somatosensory cortex, which has been demonstrated in monoamine oxidase knockout mice (Cases et al., 1998). At birth, serotonergic neurones penetrate all cortical layers, but then decline markedly after about 3 weeks. Depletion of serotonin after birth seems to have little effect on cortical development.

There is some indirect evidence that reduced serotoninergic innervation of the cortex results in impaired behaviour in juvenile rats. Autism has been suggested to be related to hyperserotonism.

Drugs affecting monoaminergic activity

Cocaine is probably the most well-known drug interacting with the catecholaminergic systems in the brain during development (Seidler et al., 1995). It inhibits the presynaptic transport mechanisms, removing and terminating the action of dopamine and noradrenaline. While cocaine potentiates the catecholamine effects in the adult, it inhibits the activity during the immediate postnatal period in most brain regions. Prenatal cocaine exposure results in disturbance of neuronal migration and consequently leads to severe neurobehavioural disturbances. Prenatal cocaine exposure in humans causes abnormal motor behaviour immediately after birth and abnormal behaviour is apparent at two and three years follow-up, probably mainly due to disturbance of the dopaminergic system. Neuroleptic drugs administered during pregnancy can block dopamine receptors and cause long-lasting effects (see Boyson & Adams, 1997).

Acetylcholine

Acetylcholine is one of the major neurotransmitters in the brain of importance for cortical activation, memory and learning. It has a major role in the control of motor tone and movement and probably counterbalances the effect of dopamine (see Johnston & Silverstein, 1998). It is involved in the control of autonomic functions. The cholinergic neurones in the brain are organized in local circuit cells, for example in the caudate–putamen nucleus and in longer projection neurones to the cortex, basal forebrain and mesopontine tegmentum (see Semba, 1992 and Fig. 7.1).

The development of cholinergic systems has been studied by analysing markers such as acetylcholine (ACh), the synthesizing enzyme choline acetyltransferase (ChAT) and acetylcholinesterase. The cholinergic innervation of the cortex occurs later than the monoaminergic, about E19 in the mouse and the rat and around week 20 in the human fetus. Mature levels in rodents are not reached until after 8 weeks postnatally (see Berger-Sweeney & Hohmann, 1997). The concentrations of ACh reach about 20% of the adult levels at E15 in the whole brain of the rat and about 40% at day P7 (Fig. 7.2). The levels of ChAT are much lower (1% and 8%) at the corresponding ages, indicating low firing rates of the cholinergic neurones. Conversely, the receptors reach adult levels earlier. The cholinergic markers appear sooner in the pons–medulla, probably due to earlier neurogenesis in the caudal and phylogenetically older part of the brain (see Semba, 1992).

The cholinergic afferents seem to have an important role in the differentiation of the cortex. After a considerable reduction of the cholinergic innervation a delay of cortical cytodifferentiation was revealed (see Berger-Sweeney & Hohmann, 1997). The cholinergic innervation has been found to be disturbed in Down's syndrome, lead and ethanol toxicity and asphyxia.

In conclusion, perinatal manipulations of the cholinergic system result in major changes of cortical structure. These changes can be correlated to cognitive deficits but do not affect motor behaviour.

Amino acid transmitters

The amino acids are involved in the main nervous process in the brain such as sensory input, encoding of memories and mediating movements. In the developing brain they seem to play an important role in the wiring of neuronal networks and building CNS cytoarchitecture (Ben-Ari et al., 1997) (Fig. 7.3).

Amino acid transmitters are the most abundant transmitters in the central nervous system. However, they were recognized as neurotransmitters in the mammalian brain much later than the monoamines and acetylcholine. This was probably due to the fact they are involved in intermediate metabolism and constitute important building blocks in the proteins.

Glutamate and aspartate

Glutamate and aspartate are the dominating excitatory amino acids (EAA) and the primary neurotransmitter in about half of all the synapses in the mammalian forebrain. They constitute the major transmitters of the pyramidal cells, the dominating neurones in the cortex. This has been demonstrated by injection of radioactively labelled D-(^{3}H) glutamate into the appropriate projection areas (see Cavanagh & Parnavelas, 1988). EAA pathways undergo striking developmental changes, involving transient overshoots, especially during critical periods as evident in visual cortex and hippocampus. EAA terminals are overproduced during the early postnatal period, for example, after 7–14 days in the rat cortex and after 1–2 years in the human cortex, which may be related to the high generation of synapses during those periods (see chapter by Bourgeois).

Glutamate acts on at least five types of receptors. The slower acting metabotropic receptors, of which eight subclasses are hitherto known, are expressed at a relatively

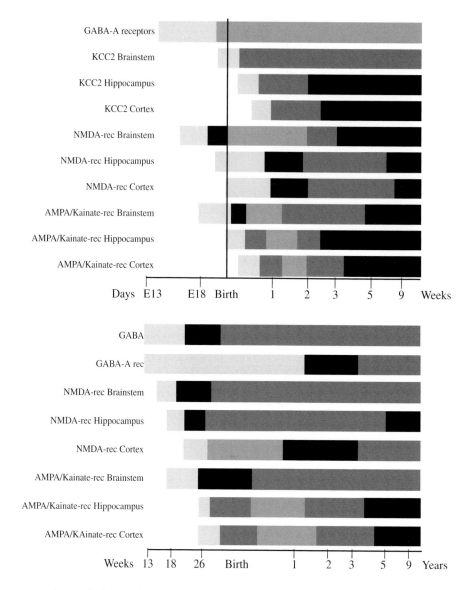

Fig. 7.3.   Expression and arbitrary levels of receptors of amino acid transmitter versus age in (*a*) rat and (*b*) man (10-logarithmic scale). (Data from Hagberg et al., 1997; Johnston & Silverstein, 1998; Herschkowitz et al., 1997; Rivera et al., 1999.) KCC2 is a neuron specific cotransporter of Cl^- ions and is responsible for the switch of GABA as an excitatory to an inhibitory neurotransmitter (see Fig. 7.9), NMDA receptors are expressed relatively earlier than the kainate and AMPA receptors. It is assumed that the NMDA receptors are more involved in the wiring of the brain, while the kainate and AMPA receptors are responsible for the fast traffic in the more mature brain.

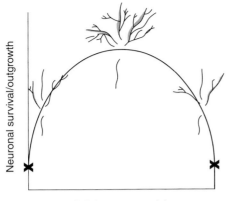

Neuronal survival/outgrowth

NMDA receptor activity

Fig. 7.4.   NMDA receptor activity vs. neuronal survival. Both too little and too much NMDA receptor activity may lead to neuronal death. Apoptosis can be induced in the developing CNS both by blocking the NMDA receptors or by overstimulation, for example after perinatal asphyxia. (Reproduced with permission from Lipton & Nakanishi (1999) in an article entitled 'Shakespeare in love – with NMDA receptors', Nature America Inc., since these receptors have potential for both tragic and comic (or at least therapeutic) consequences.

early stage. Of the ionotropic receptors the NMDA receptors dominate in the immature brain when synaptic transmission is weak and extremely plastic (Fig. 7.3). The NMDA receptors permit entry of Na^+ and Ca^{2+} when opened and may mediate neurotoxic effects during perinatal asphyxia (see Chapter 18). Furthermore, Ca^{2+} entry through NMDA channels seems to be crucially involved in the appearance of long-term potentiation (LTP) and memory storage. During maturation, the AMPA and kainic ionotropic receptors predominate and carry most of the fast neuronal traffic in the brain (Cooper et al., 1996).

Dark rearing or blocking the activity with tetrodotoxin results in preservation of the NMDA receptors in the visual cortex. Dark rearing also preserves the immature form of the NMDA receptors containing NR2B subunit and the expression of NR2A is delayed. This subunit switch is essential for development of rapid synaptic transmission (Fox et al., 1999).

Either too much or too little NMDA receptor activity can be life threatening to developing neurones. Fetal rats exposed to NMDA antagonists were found to have excessive apoptosis in the same way as the asphyxiated perinatal brain. NMDA receptor stimulation by excessive glutamate release leads to Ca^{2+} influx which may induce subsequent neuronal apoptosis. 'Thus either too much or too little NMDA receptor activity can be life-threatening to the developing neurones' (Lipton & Nakanishi, 1999) (Fig. 7.4).

Gamma-aminobutyric acid (GABA)

GABA is the dominating neurotransmitter in the non-pyramidal cells, as demonstrated by uptake of (^{3}H)-GABA and immunochemical labelling of the GABA-synthesizing enzyme glutamic acid (GAD). Perhaps 25–40 % of all nerve terminals contain GABA. GABA is regarded as the main inhibitory transmitter in the mature animal, but have a different role during early development.

There are two types of GABA receptors, $GABA_A$ and $GABA_B$. The $GABA_A$ receptor ($GABA_A$-R) is an ionotropic receptor that gates a chloride channel. It is a transmembrane protein built of several subunits where, for example benzodiazepines, barbiturates and ethanol can bind to specific sites and modulate the opening properties of the chloride channel. The $GABA_B$-R is coupled to a G-protein, is present in lower levels in the CNS than the $GABA_A$ receptor and starts to function late in CNS development (postnatal life in rodents).

During early development, the Cl^- concentration is high in the nerve cells. When GABA opens the Cl^- channels a depolarization, i.e. excitation, occurs. During maturation the Cl^- concentration decreases which results in an opposite effect of GABA, i.e. Cl^- ions are pumped out and the cell becomes hyperpolarized (Fig. 7.5). In this way GABA switches from an excitatory to an inhibitory neurotransmitter (Miles, 1999). This switch is due to the expression of the K^+/Cl^- cotransporter KCC2 that has recently been reported to be expressed around birth in the brainstem, one week after birth in the hippocampus and between 1 and 2 weeks in the cortex of the rat (Rivera et al., 1999; Miles, 1999) (Figs. 7.3 and 7.5).

Thus, GABA operates mainly as an excitatory transmitter on immature neurones. As described above, glutaminergic synapses initially lack functional AMPA receptors and the NMDA channels are blocked by Mg^{2+} at resting membrane potentials. GABA depolarizes immature neurones, which may result in Ca^{2+}-influx by removing the Mg^{2+} blockage of NMDA-channels. Thus, $GABA_A$ receptors play the role conferred to AMPA receptors in the more mature CNS (Ben-Ari et al., 1997; Onimaru et al., 1999). An increase in the intracellular Ca^{2+} concentration activates a wide range of intracellular cascades and is involved in neuronal growth and differentiation. Furthermore, GABA excitation and Ca^{2+} influx may act as triggers for plasticity of synaptic connections and for establishing and patterning of neural networks.

The $GABA_A$ receptors have a strong affinity for benzodiazepines. Several anxiolytic and anticonvulsant drugs increase the ability for GABA to open chloride channels. In neonatal neurones GABA currents are potentiated by barbiturates but are insensitive to benzodiazepines (Cherubini et al., 1991).

As GABA has a trophic role during early brain development, interference with the function of GABAergic transmission during this period may affect the develop-

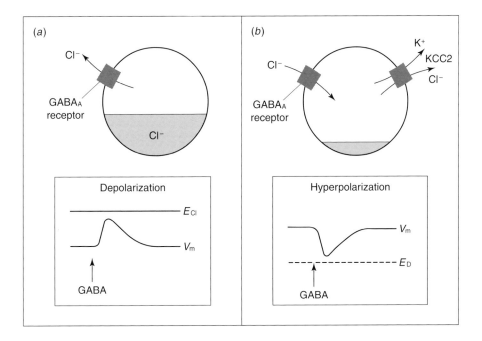

Fig. 7.5.   GABA switches from an excitatory to an inhibitory neurotransmitter (Miles, 1999) during neuronal maturation. Immature neurones start life as cells depolarized by GABA (*a*), and mature into cells in which GABA has a hyperpolarizing action (*b*). This switch is due to the expression of the K^+/Cl^- co-transporter KCC2 that recently has been reported to be expressed around birth in the brainstem, 1 week after birth in the hippocampus and between 1 and 2 weeks in the cortex of the mouse (Rivera et al., 1999; Miles, 1999). In immature neurones opening of Cl^- channels by activation of the GABA$_A$ receptor depolarizes the cell. (*b*) Expression of the KCC2 transporter (Rivera et al., 1999) maintains a low level of Cl^- E_{Cl} is negative relative to V_m and activation of the GABA$_A$ receptor inhibits the cell.

ment of neuronal wiring, plasticity of neuronal network and also have a profound influence on neural organization.

Ethanol abuse during pregnancy can interact with the GABA$_A$ receptor. The sensitive time window in rat cerebral cortex for ethanol exposure is situated between P3 and P10. It is worth noting that GABA during this same period seem to have mainly depolarizing and trophic effects on developing cortical neurones through effects on cell proliferation and migration (Belhage et al., 1998). In humans, the intellectual deficit produced by abnormalities of brain growth is the most important component of fetal alcohol syndrome (Kopecky & Koren, 1998). Craniofacial abnormalities in human fetuses related to first trimester alcohol exposure are similar to the facial defects seen in GABA$_A$ subunit receptor knockout mice (Condie et al., 1997).

Glycine

Glycine has both excitatory and inhibitory actions and can be regarded as the phylogenetically older inhibitory transmitter restricted to the brainstem and spinal cord in the adult. A similar switch as regarding the $GABA_A$ receptors from excitatory to inhibitory effects seems to occur with maturation (Miles, 1999).

The NMDA receptor has a modulatory site where glycine in submicromolar concentrations increases the frequency of NMDA receptor channel opening. Conditions that alter the extracellular concentration of glycine can dramatically alter NMDA receptor-mediated responses (see chapter by Edwards et al.).

Neuropeptides

More than 50 neuropeptides have been identified. In contrast to most of the other neurotransmitters/modulators, the neuropeptides are synthesized and packaged in large dense-cored vesicles in the cell soma and are carried to the nerve terminals by axonal transport at a rate of 1.5 mm/h. By this relatively slow process the neuropeptides cannot act as fast-switching neurotransmitters. Rather, they have a neuromodulatory role. They are often stored together with other neurotransmitters, i.e. monoamines or EAA, and it is possible that they play a role in setting of the sensitivity. Some of them are probably of less physiological importance and occur in the body mainly as evolutionary residues (Bowers, 1994). Still, they are of great neuropharmacological interest and their analogues or antagonists can be used as drugs. The most well-known examples are the opioids and naloxone.

Opioids

Endogenous opioids are involved in blood pressure and temperature regulation, feeding, sexual activity and memory storage besides pain perception.

Three major classes of opioid receptors: μ, δ, and κ have currently been identified, characterized and cloned, all with putative receptor subtypes. All are seven-transmembrane proteins and members of the G-protein-coupled receptor superfamily. Endogenous opioid peptides with distinctive selectivity profiles exist, namely the enkephalin (μ), endorphin (δ) and dynorphin (κ) groups.

β-endorphin-containing neurones have long projections and primarily occur in the pituitary, while proenkephalin- and prodynorphin-derived peptide-containing neurones are generally present in neurones with moderate to short projections (Morita, 1992). β-endorphin exists in two main forms with different production sites and effects on the brain. The non-acetylated form is found in the anterior pituitary, is involved in fetal growth and is expressed early during fetal brain development (E14 in the rat). The acetylated form is present in the intermediate lobe of the pituitary and is involved in postnatal development (Wang et al., 1992). μ-receptor binding sites are present during mid-gestation time and have a high

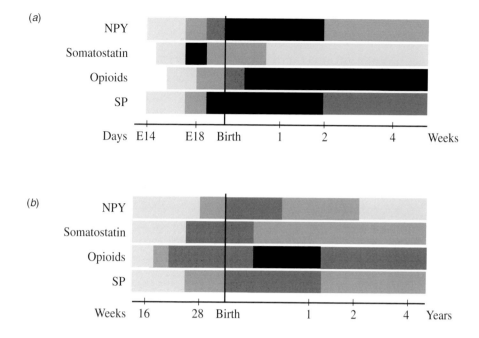

Fig. 7.6.   Expresssion and arbitrary levels of some major neuropeptides vs. age in rat (*a*) and man (*b*) (10-logarithmic scale). (Data on substance P from Sakanaka, 1992 and Bergström *et al.*, 1984, on somatostatin from Shiosaka, 1992; enkephalin Morita, 1992 and Foster, 1998; NPY Brana et al., 1995.)

density in cardiorespiratory-related brainstem nuclei, whereas the δ-opioid receptors primarily appear during the postnatal period in rats (Befort & Kiefer, 1997).

Although opioid binding sites progressively increase in the developing brain (Fig. 7.6), the effect of opioids appears to be dependent on the status of neuronal maturation. In addition, many neuronal populations exhibit transient expression of one or the other opioid genes but the physiological role of this is not clear. Opioid agonists inhibit mitosis and DNA synthesis in the developing brain, and endogenous opioids exert potent regulatory effects on brain development and morphogenesis, as demonstrated by the administration of exogenous opioid agonists and antagonists during the fetal period (Lichtensteiger, 1998). Human neonates who have been exposed in utero to opioids, such as heroin, have a smaller head circumference and reduced body weight due to a decrease in cell number (Kopecky & Koren, 1998).

Substance P and other tachykinins

Substance P is a primary sensory transmitter mediating pain sensations via the thin C-fibres. Substance P is also involved in the transmission of chemoreceptor and barometric input from the carotid and aortic chemo- and baroreceptors.

It is detected in the dorsal horn of the mammalian spinal cord and in a number of brain nuclei, especially in the substantia nigra and the nucleus tractus solitarius. The other mammalian tachykinins are neurokinin A and neurokinin B. Neurokinin A and substance P are encoded by the same gene, the preprotachykinin A gene. The neurokinin receptors for NK_1 have been cloned and found to belong to the G-protein coupled family; NK_2- and NK_3-receptors belong to the same superfamily.

Immunocytochemical studies have demonstrated that substance P appears in the rat brain stem at a gestational age of 14 days and reaches a maximum at a postnatal age of 21 days, and thereafter there is a successive decrease (Sakanaka, 1992). In humans there is an increase towards birth and then a levelling off during the first 6 months (Bergström et al., 1984) (Fig. 7.6).

Substance P may play a role in neurogenesis. It seems to counteract damage induced by neurotoxins and accelerates regeneration of cortical catecholamine fibres (see Sakanaka, 1992).

Increased expression of mRNA coding for preprotachykinin A, the substance P precursor, has been recorded in respiratory related nuclei in both the rabbit (see Lagercrantz, 1996) and the rat (Wickström et al., 1999). Increased expression of PPT-A mRNA has also been detected in patches in the caudale nucleus and putamen of the human newborn brain (Brana et al., 1995). Thus, there are suggestions that substance P is involved in the resetting and adaption of the organism to extrauterine life.

VIP-related peptides

Vasoactive intestitinal polypeptide (VIP) is structurally related to glucagon, secretin, GHRH and Pituitary adenylate cyclase-activating peptide (PACAP). Like these other neuropeptides, VIP was also first isolated from the intestine. However, VIP has subsequently been found to be an important neuropeptide in the autonomic nervous system and in the brain. It is co-stored and released together with acetylcholine (see Hökfelt, 1991). VIP appears to have important trophic effects on the development of the cerebral cortex. Radiolabelled VIP has been demonstrated to pass the placental barrier and stimulate growth of the brain in the mouse. VIP promotes astrocytogenesis in the germinative zone (see Chapter 4).

PACAP has a considerably higher potency in activating cAMP than its related peptide VIP. PACAP is upregulated at birth, particularly during perinatal asphyxia.

NPY-related peptides

Neuropeptide Y is probably the most important of the pancreatic polypeptide family in the brain. The peptides in the family are peptide YY (PYY), avian pancreatic polypeptide (APP) and human pancreatic polypeptide (HPP). NPY is released together with noradrenaline or adrenaline (see Hökfelt, 1991). It is a strong vasoconstrictor and increases the sensitivity of sympathetically innervated smooth muscle. In the brain NPY has been reported to be anxiolytic. It also has a role in the control of food intake. However, transgenic mice deficient in NPY seem to develop normally and exhibit normal food intake and body weight (Baraban et al., 1997).

CGRP

CGRP (calcitonin gene related peptide) is an example of a neuropeptide with trophic effects, which might be involved in synaptogenesis. It has been demonstrated to stimulate the synthesis of ACh receptors in cultured muscle cells from the chick. The expression of CGRP is most prominent from E11 to E19, when the motor end-plates are formed (Laufer et al., 1989, see also Hökfelt, 1991).

Somatostatin

Somatostatin is mainly an inhibitory neuromodulator coexisting with GABA. SRIF (somatostatin related immunofluorescence) neurones are transiently expressed to a high degree between E14 and E21 in the fetal rat. The peak is at E17 (Cavanagh & Parnavelas, 1988). Whether this high expression is crucial for the formation of the cortex or just reflects an evolutionary residue is not really known (Shiosaka, 1992).

Galanin

Galanin is involved in cognition, nociception, feeding and sexual behaviour (Bedecs et al., 1995). Eighty per cent of the noradrenaline neurones in the locus coerulos contain galanin. It hyperpolarizes these neurones and inhibits the release of noradrenaline, thus modulating the action of the noradrenaline. It can be detected at E19 in the rat fetus and is then upregulated at birth, while the galanin receptors seem to be downregulated (Wickström et al., 1999). It may possibly modulate the effects of the noradrenaline surge at birth. Furthermore, it may modulate/inhibit/depress excessive glutamate release during perinatal asphyxia (Ben-Ari, 1990).

Purines

Purines are fundamental components in the energy turnover of all cells, but also modulate neuronal activity through synaptic or non-synaptic release and interaction with specific receptors. The purinergic receptors are divided into type-1 receptors (P1) sensitive to adenosine and AMP, and type-2 (P2) sensitive for ATP and ADP. The action of purines is related as a rapid breakdown of ATP increases the levels of adenosine.

ATP

The purine nucleotide ATP is the main energy source of cells, but is also stored in synaptic vesicles and released together with classical transmitters such as noradrenaline and acetylcholine. The ratio between ATP and catecholamines in chromaffin granules has been found to be higher during early life than later suggesting that it is a phylogenetically and ontogenetically old signalling substance (O'Brien et al., 1972). During the last decade, evidence for ATP as a neural signalling substance has emerged from examining sites of storage, release and hydrolysis, as well as potential actions and targets. A variety of receptors for extracellular ATP have been identified. Some are involved in fast neuronal transmission and operate as ligand-gated ion channels ($P_{2T, X \text{ and } Z}$). Others are involved in the paracrine or autocrine modulation of cell function ($P_{2U \text{ and } Y}$). Many receptors of this type are coupled to phosphoinositide-specific phospholipase C (Fredholm, 1997). Intracellular ATP levels directly change the excitability of neurones by ATP-dependent potassium channels which may hyperpolarize cells, thus decreasing neuronal activity when energy resources are scarce.

Adenosine

Adenosine is a constituent of all body fluids, including the extracellular space of the central nervous system. It has multiple effects on organs and cells of the body. Thus, its levels are tightly regulated by a series of enzymatic steps (Fredholm, 1997). Adenosine can be regarded more as a neuromodulator in that it does not seem to be stored in vesicles with a regulated release from nerve terminals. Adenosine is produced by dephosphorylation of adenosine monophosphate (AMP) by 5'nucleotidase, an enzyme occurring in both membrane-bound and cytosolic forms. Degradation of intra- and extracellular ATP is the main source of extracellular adenosine. Specific bidirectional transporters maintain intra- and extracellular concentrations of adenosine at similar levels. During basal conditions, adenosine levels are 30–300 nM and can rise following stimuli that cause an imbalance between ATP synthesis and ATP breakdown. Thus, the levels during ischemia or hypoxia can rise 100-fold (Winn et al., 1981; Fredholm, 1997). The extracellular concentrations of adenosine might be higher in the fetal brain than postnatally, since fetal PaO_2 can decrease below the level (30 mm Hg) when a significant increase in extracellular adenosine can be expected (Winn et al., 1981). Overall, adenosine decreases oxygen consumption and has neuroprotective effects (Fredholm, 1997). However, hypoxia also induces a decrease in neonatal respiration. Theophylline and caffeine are adenosine antagonists that cause ventilation to increase and decrease the incidence of neonatal apnoeas when given systemically, mainly due to the antagonistic effect of theophylline on adenosine A_1-receptors in the medulla oblongata (see Herlenius, 1998).

Transition at birth

Before birth

The levels of most neurotransmitters and neuromodulators increase concomitantly with synapse formation. Some of them surge during the perinatal period (such as glutamate, catecholamines and some neuropeptides) and then level off. The interesting question is to what extent the expression of neuroactive agents is related to the functional state of the fetus and the newborn. On one hand, there is an intense firing and wiring in the fetal brain, particularly during active sleep. Therefore an inhibitory neurotransmitter such as GABA seems to be mainly excitatory in the fetal period (see above). Amino acid transmitters also act via NMDA receptors which are important for the wiring and plasticity of the immature brain, while the main excitatory fast-switching receptors (AMPA) are expressed later.

Activities such as respiratory movements are suppressed. The fetus seldom or never becomes aroused or wakes up. The sympathetic tonus is low. Furthermore, the fetus is adapted to the low oxygen level in the womb. If it is challenged by asphyxia, it is not excited as an adult responding with a flight or fight reaction, but rather becomes immobilized, stops breathing and becomes bradycardic (see Lagercrantz, 1996). This paralytic state of the foetus can be caused by inhibition of the chemical neurotransmission or lack of expression of excitatory neuroactive agents. Adenosine is such a neuromodulator which might be involved in this suppression of the fetal brain. It has a general sedatory effect. Its concentration increases during energy failure and hypoxia and it has been suggested that it can act as a modulator to cope with the hypoxic situation (Berne, 1986). Adenosine A_1-R activation depresses breathing substantially in the fetus and the neonate by inhibiting synaptic transmission and hyperpolarizing certain neurones (Herlenius & Lagercrantz 1999).

Neuropeptides which might be involved in the suppression of fetal activity are NPY, somatostatin and endogenous opioids. The levels of NPY are relatively high in the foetal brain and decline after birth. Plasma levels of endorphins and enkephalins are increased in the umbilical cord at birth. Blocking endogenous opioids with naloxone increases breathing in the newborn rabbit.

Birth

The healthy newborn baby is aroused and awake over the first 2 hours after birth and starts continuous breathing movements. Factors like squeezing and squashing of the fetus, increased sensory input and cooling are probably of importance. We can hypothesize that there is a surge of excitatory neurotransmitters and downregulation of inhibitory ones in the brain.

The increased neuronal activity is indicated by the increased expression of immediate early genes (Ringstedt et al., 1995). The arousal and vigilance of the newborn can probably partially be due to activation of the noradrenergic system in the brain, particularly locus coeruleus from where noradrenergic neurones are distributed in the whole brain (see above). The noradrenaline turnover as indicated by the ratio of the metabolite MHPG and NA was increased two- to threefold in the newborn rat (see Lagercrantz, 1996). There are indirect indications that there is also a noradrenaline surge in the human brain, by the finding of high levels of plasma catecholamines after birth.

The most important driving mechanism of respiration, coupling the ventilation to metabolic demand, is the CO_2-drive. This sensitivity seems to be mediated by a cholinergic mechanism (Nattie et al., 1989). The CO_2-drive seems to be strongly upregulated at birth. An increased expression of immediate early genes (c-fos) has been recorded at the ventral surface of the newborn rat (Wickström et al. 1999). Whether this could trigger an upregulation of the cholinergic neurotransmission is not yet known.

A neuropeptide involved in respiratory control at birth has been found to be substantially upregulated at birth. mRNA encoding for the Substance P precursor pre-protachykinin A is increased about fourfold in respiratory nuclei but not in others during the first day after birth in rabbit pups (see Lagercrantz, 1996).

A rapid decrease of the inhibitory neuromodulator adenosine in the brain occurs as partial pressure of oxygen in arterial blood rapidly increases after birth. In addition a decreased sensitivity for adenosine during the first postnatal days seems to contribute to the maintenance of continuous breathing (Herlenius, 1998; Herlenius & Lagercrantz, 1999).

Pre- and perinatal programming

The concept of fetal and neonatal programming first described by David Barker (Sayer et al., 1997) also applies to the ontogeny of neurotransmitters and neuro-modulators, i.e. an early stimulus or insult at a critical period can result in long-term changes in the structure and the function of the organism. For example, it can be postulated that prenatal or perinatal stress can disturb the timetable of the expression of neurotransmitters and neuromodulators and their receptors. Hydrocortisone given to neonatal rats has been found to enhance the maturation of the monoaminergic systems in the brain (Kurosawa et al., 1980). Administration of extra glucocorticosteroids to the rat fetus induces alterations of dopamine receptor responses, which affects spontanous motor control both short- and long-term (Diaz et al., 1997). Chronic prenatal hypoxia alters the monoamine turnover in the locus coeruleus and nucleus tractus solitarius in the adolescent rat (Peyronnet et al.,

2000). This was related to disturbed control of respiratory behaviour. Human handling of newborn rats for 15 min during the first weeks of life appeared to affect ascending serotonergic projections into the hippocampus and long-lasting increase in glucocorticoid receptors (see Sapolsky, 1999).

There are also clinical studies indicating that prenatal stress is associated with attention deficit disorders in children (Weinstock, 1997). Schizophrenic patients seem to have experienced more pregnancy and birth complications than their healthy siblings (Stefan & Murray, 1997). For example, mothers of schizophrenic patients suffered more often from severe infections during pregnancy, possibly affecting cytokines and indirectly the development of monoaminergic circuits in the fetal brain (Jarskog et al., 1997).

Conclusions

Monoamines are expressed in the very early embryo, at which stage the notochord already contains high noradrenaline levels. They may have an important role for neurotransmission in the fetus. Purines and neuropeptides are probably also expressed at an early stage, similar to how they occur early during phylogenesis. In the adult mammal the fast switching excitatory amino acids dominate. However, they also seem to be important for the wiring of the brain and the plasticity before birth. NMDA receptors that might mediate these effects dominate and are then substituted by AMPA-receptors. The main inhibitory amino acids GABA and glycine seem to be excitatory before birth, which could be of major importance for the wiring of neuronal circuits during development. Prenatal- or neonatal stress, for example hypoxia, can affect the programming of neurotransmitter and receptor expression, which can lead to long-term behavioural effects.

REFERENCES

Almqvist, P. M., Åkesson, E., Wahlberg, L. U., Pschera, H., Seiger, Å. & Sundström, E. (1996). First trimester development of the human nigrostriatal dopamine system. *Experimental Neurology*, **139**, 227–37.

Baraban, S. C., Hollopeter, G., Erickson, J. C., Schwartzkroin, P. A. & Palmiter, R. D. (1997). Knock-out mice reveal a critical antiepileptic role for neuropeptide Y. *Journal of Neuroscience*, **17**, 8927–36.

Bedecs, K., Berthold, M. & Bartfai, T. (1995). Galanin – 10 years with neuroendocrine peptide. *International Journal of Biochemistry and Cell Biology*, **27**, 337–49.

Belhage, B., Hansen, G. H., Elster, L. & Schousboe, A. (1998). Effects of gamma-aminobutyric acid (GABA) on synaptogenesis and synaptic function. *Perspectives on Developmental Neurobiology*, 5, 235–46.

Befort, K. & Kieffer, B. L. (1997). Structure–activity relationships in the delta opioid receptor. *Pain Reviews*, 4, 100–21.

Ben-Ari, Y. (1990). Galanin and glibenclamide modulate the anoxic release of glutamate in rat CA3 hippocampal neurons. *European Journal of Neuroscience*, 2, 62–8.

Ben-Ari, Y., Khazipov, R., Leinekugel, X., Caillard, O. & Gaiarsa, J-L. (1997). GABA-A, NMDA and AMPA receptors: a developmentally regulated 'ménage à trois'. *Trends in Neuroscience*, 20, 523–9.

Berger-Sweeney, J. & Hohmann, C. F. (1997). Behavioral consequences of abnormal cortical development: insights into developmental disabilities. *Behavioural Brain Research*, 86, 121–42.

Bergström, L., Lagercrantz, H. & Terenius, L. (1984). Post-mortem analyses of neuropeptides in brains from sudden infant death victims. *Brain Research*, 323, 279–85.

Bertrand, D. & Changeux, J-P. (1995). Nicotinic receptor: an allosteric protein specialized for intercellular communication. *Seminars in the Neurosciences*, 7, 75–90.

Boutrel, B., Franc, B., Hen, R., Hamon, M. & Adrien, J. (1999). Key role of 5-HT1B receptors in the regulation of paradoxical sleep as evidenced in 5-HT1B knock-out mice. *Journal of Neuroscience*, 19, 3204–12.

Bowers, C. W. (1994). Superfluous neurotransmitters? *Trends in Neuroscience*, 17, 315–20.

Boyson, S. J. & Adams, C. E. (1997). D_1 and D_2 dopamine receptors in perinatal and adult basal ganglia. *Pediatric Research*, 41, 822–31.

Brana, C., Charron, G., Aubert, I. et al. (1995). Ontogeny of the striatal neurons expressing neuropeptide genes in the human fetus and neonate. *The Journal of Comparative Neurology*, 360, 488–505.

Cases, O., Lebrand, C., Giros, B. et al. (1998). Plasma membrane transporters of serotonin, dopamine, and norepinephrine mediate serotonin accumulation in atypical locations in the developing brain of monoamine oxidase A knock-outs. *Journal of Neuroscience*, 18, 6914–27.

Cavanagh, M. E. & Parnavelas, J. G. (1988). Neurotransmitter differentiation in cortical neurons. In *The Making of the Nervous System*, ed. J. G. Parnavelas, C. D. Stern & R. V. Stirling, pp. 435–53. London: Oxford University Press.

Cherubini, E., Gaiarsa, J. L. & Ben-Ari, Y. (1991). GABA: an excitatory transmitter in early post-natal life. *Trends in Neuroscience*, 14, 515–19.

Condie, B. G., Bain, G., Gottlieb, D. I. & Capecci, M. R. (1997). Cleft palate in mice with a targeted mutation in the gamma-aminobutyric acid producing enzyme glutamic acid decarboxylase. *PNAS*, 94, 11451–5.

Cooper, J. R., Bloom, F. E. & Roth, R. H. (ed.) (1996). *The Biochemical Basis of Neuropharmacology*. Oxford: Oxford University Press.

Diaz, R., Fuxe, K. & Ögren, S. O. (1997). Prenatal corticosterone treatment induces long-term changes in spontaneous and apomorphine-mediated motor activity in male and female rats. *Neuroscience*, 81, 129–40.

Foster, G. A. (1992). Phenylethanolamine *N*-methyltransferase – the adrenaline-synthesizing enzyme. In *Ontogeny of Transmitters and Peptides in the CNS*, ed. A. Björklund, T. Hökfelt & M. Tohyama, pp. 133–56. Amsterdam: Elsevier.

Foster, G. A., (1998). *Chemical Neuroanatomy of the Prenatal Rat Brain; A Developmental Atlas*, p. 274. Oxford: Oxford University Press.

Fox, K., Henley, J. & Isaac, J. (1999). Experience-dependent development of NMDA receptor transmission. *Nature Neuroscience*, **2**, 297–9.

Fredholm, B. B. (1997). Adenosine and neuroprotection. *International Review of Neurobiology*, **40**, 259–89.

Hagberg, H., Bona, E., Gilland, E. & Puka-Sundvall, M. (1997). Hypoxia-ischaemia model in the 7-day-old-rat: possibilities and shortcomings. *Acta Paediatrica Suppl*, **422**, 85–8.

Heimer, L. (1995). *The Human Brain and Spinal Cord*. New York: Springer.

Herlenius, E. (1998). Respiratory activity in medulla oblongata and its modulation by adenosine and opioids. Dept of Woman and Child Health, Karolinska Institute, Stockholm. *Thesis*, pp. 1–152. http://diss.kib.ki.se/1998/91–628–3240–9.

Herlenius, E. & Lagercrantz, H. (1999). Adenosinergic modulation of respiratory neurones in the neonatal rat brainstem in vitro. *Journal of Physiology*, **518**, 159–72.

Herlitz, S., Villaroel, A., Witzemann, V., Koenen, M. & Sakmann, B. (1996). Structural determinants of channel conductance in fetal and adult rat muscle acetylcholine receptors. *Journal of Physiology*, **492**, 775–87.

Herregodts, P., Velkeniers, B., Ebinger, G., Michotte, Y., Vanhaelst, L. & Hooghe-Peters, E. (1990). Development of monoaminergic neurotransmitters in fetal and postnatal rat brain: Analysis by HPLC with electrochemical detection. *Journal of Neurochemistry*, **55**, 774–9.

Herschkowitz, N., Kagan, J. & Zilles, K. (1997). Neurobiological bases of behavioral development in the first year. *Neuropediatrics*, **28**, 296–306.

Hökfelt, T. (1991). Neuropeptides in perspective: the last ten years. *Neuron*, **7**, 867–79.

Jarskog, L. F., Xiao, H., Wilkie, M. B., Lauder, J. M. & Gilmore, J. H. (1997). Cytokine regulation of embryonic rat dopamine and serotonin neuronal survival in vitro. *International Journal of Developmental Neuroscience*, **15**, 711–16.

Johnston, M. V. & Silverstein, F. S. (1998). Development of neurotransmitters. In *Fetal and Neonatal Physiology*, ed. R. A. Polin & W. W. Fox, pp. 2116–17. Philadelphia: W. B. Saunders Company.

Kopecky, E. A. & Koren, G. (1998). Maternal drug abuse: effects on the fetus and neonate. In *Fetal and Neonatal Physiology*, ed. R. A. Polin & W. W. Fox, pp. 236–9. Philadelphia: W. B. Saunders Company.

Kurosawa, A., Kageyama H., John, T. M., Hirota, R. & Itoh, S. (1980). Effect of neonatal hydrocorticosterone treatment on brain monoamines in developing rats. *Japanese Journal of Pharmacology*, **30**, 213–20.

Lagercrantz, H. (1996). Stress, arousal and gene activation at birth. *News in Physiological Science*, **11**, 214–18.

Lauder, J. M., Moiseiwitsch, J., Liu, J. & Wilkie, M. B. (1994). Serotonin in development and pathophysiology. In *Brain Lesions in the Newborn*, Alfred Benzon Symposium 37, ed. H. C. Lou, G. Greisen & J. Falck Larsen, pp. 60–72. Copenhagen: Munksgaard.

Laufer, R., Fontaine, B., Klarsfeld, A., Cartaud, J. & Changeux, J-P. (1989). Regulation of acetyl-choline receptor biosyntheis during motor endplate morphogenesis. *News in Physiological Sciences*, **4**, 5–9.

Le Douarin, N. M. (1981). Plasticity in the development of the peripheral nervous system. *CIBA Symposium* 83, pp. 19–46.

Lichtensteiger, W. (1998). Developmental neuropharmacology. In *Fetal and Neonatal Physiology*, ed. R. A. Polin & W. W. Fox, pp. 226–39. Philadelphia: W. B. Saunders Company.

Lipton, S. A. & Nakanishi, N. (1999). Shakespeare in love – with NMDA receptors? *Nature Medicine*, **5**(3), 270–1.

Mangelsdorf, D. J., Thummel, C., Beato, M. et al. (1995). The nuclear receptor superfamily: the second decade, *Cell*, **83**, 835–9.

Miles, R. (1999). A homeostatic switch. *Nature*, **397**, 215–16.

Morita, Y. (1992). Ontogenic and differential expression of the preproenkephalin and predynor-phin genes in the rat brain. In *Ontogeny of Transmitters and Peptides in the CNS*. ed. A. Björklund, T. Hökfelt & M. Tohyama, pp. 257–95. Amsterdam: Elsevier.

Naeff, B., Schlumpf, M. & Lichtensteiger, W. (1992). Pre- and postnatal development of high-affinity [3H]nicotine binding sites in rat brain regions: an autoradiographic study. *Brain Research. Developmental Brain Research*, **68**, 163–74.

Naqui, S. Z. H., Harris, B. S., Thomaidou, D. & Parnavelas, J. G. (1999). The noradrenergic system influences in fate of Cajal–Retzius cells in the developing cerebral cortex. *Developmental Brain Research*, **113**, 75–82.

Nattie, E. E., Wood, J., Mega, A. & Goritski, W. (1989). Rostral ventrolateral medulla muscarinic receptor involvement in central ventilatory chemosensitivity. *Journal of Applied Physiology*, **66**(3), 1462–70.

O'Brien, R. A., Da Prada, M. & Pletscher, A. (1972). The ontogenesis of catecholamines and aden-osine 5'-triphosphate in the adrenal medulla. *Life Sciences*, **11**, 749–59.

Olson, L. & Seiger, Å. (1972). Early prenatal ontogeny of central monoamine neurons in the rat: fluorescence histochemical observations. *Z Anat. Entwickl. Gesch.*, **137**, 301–16.

Onimaru, H., Herlenius, E. & Homma, I. (1999). GABA-dependent responses of respiratory neurons in the fetal rat medulla. *Neuroscience Research*, Suppl. **23**, 77.

Patterson, P. H. & Chun, I. L. Y. (1977). The induction of acetylcholine synthesis in primary cul-tures of dissociated rat sympathetic neurons. I. Effects of conditioned medium. *Developmental Biology*, **56**, 263–80.

Pendleton, R. G., Rasheed, A., Roychowdhury, R. & Hillman, R. A. (1998). New role for catechol-amines: ontogenesis. *Trends in Pharmacological Sciences*, **19**, 248–51.

Peyronnet J., Roux, J. C., Géloën, A. et al. (2000). Prenatal hypoxia impairs the postnatal devel-opment of neural and functional chemoafferent pathway in rat. *Journal of Physiology (London)*, **524**(2), 525–37.

Ringstedt, T., Tang, L-Q., Persson, H., Lendahl, U. & Lagercrantz, H. (1995). Expression of c-fos, tyrosine hydroxylase, and neuropeptide mRNA in the rat brain around birth: effects of hypoxia and hypothermia. *Pediatric Research*, **37**, 15–20.

Rivera, C., Voipio, J., Payne, J. A. et al. (1999). The K+/Cl-cotransporter KCC2 renders GABA hyperpolarizing during neuronal maturation. *Nature*, **397**, 251–5.

Sakanaka, M. (1992). Development of neuronal elements with substance P-like immunoreactivity in the central nervous system. (1992). In *Ontogeny of Transmitters and Peptides in the CNS*, ed. A. Björklund, T. Hökfelt & M. Tohyama, pp. 197–250. Amsterdam: Elsevier.

Sapolsky, R. M. (1999). The importance of a well-groomed child. *Science*, 277, 1620–1.

Sayer, A. A., Cooper, C. & Barker, D. J. (1997). Is lifespan determined in utero? *Archives of Disease in Childhood*, 77, F161–4.

Seidler, F. J., Temple, S. W., McCook, E. C. & Slotkin, T. A. (1995). Cocaine inhibits central developmental period in which catecholamines influence cell development. *Developmental Brain Research*, 85, 48–53.

Semba, K. (1992). Development of central cholinergic neurons. In *Ontogeny of Transmitters and Peptides in the CNS*, ed. A. Björklund, T. Hökfelt & M. Tohyama, pp. 33–62. Amsterdam: Elsevier.

Shiosaka, S. (1992). Ontogeny of the central somatostatinergic system. In *Ontogeny of Transmitters and Peptides in the CNS*, ed. A. Björklund, T. Hökfelt & M. Tohyama, pp. 369–94. Amsterdam: Elsevier.

Stefan, M. D. & Murray, R. M. (1997). *Acta Paediatrica Suppl*, **422**, 112–16.

Stjärne, L., Hedqvist, P., Lagercrantz, H. & Wennmalm, Å. (ed.) (1981). *Chemical Neurotransmission. 75 years*. New York Academic Press.

Sundström, E., Kolare, S., Souverbie, F. et al. (1993). Neurochemical differentiation of human bulbospinal monoaminergic neurons during the first trimester. *Developmental Brain Research*, 75, 1–12.

Thomas, S. A. & Palmiter, R. D. (1997). Impaired maternal behavior in mice lacking norepinephrine and epinephrine. *Cell*, **91**, 583–92.

Thomas, S. A., Matsumoto, A. M. & Palmiter, R. D. (1995). Noradrenaline is essential for mouse fetal development. *Nature*, 374, 643–6.

Wang, Y-Q., Li, J-S., Li, H-M. & Tohyama, M. (1992). Ontogeny of pro-opiomelanocortin (POMC)-derived peptides in the brain and pituitary. In *Ontogeny of Transmitters and Peptides in the CNS*, ed. A. Björklund, T. Hökfelt and M. Tohyama, pp. 297–323. Amsterdam: Elsevier.

Weinstock, M. (1997). Does prenatal stress impair coping and regulation of hypothalamic–pituitary–adrenal axis? *Neuroscience Behavioral Reviews*, **21**, 1–10.

Wickström, H. R., Holgert, H., Hökfelt, T. & Lagercrantz, H. (1999). Birth-related expression of c-fos, c-jun and substance P mRNAs in the rat brainstem and pia mater: possible relationship to changes in central chemosensitivity. *Developmental Brain Research*, 112, 255–66.

Winn, H. R., Rubio, R. & Berne, R. M. (1981). Brain adenosine concentration during hypoxia in rats. *American Journal of Physiology*, 241, 235–42.

Zhou, Q-Y., Qualfe, C. J. & Palmiter, R. D. (1995). Targeted disruption of the tyrosine hydroxylase gene reveals that catecholamines are required for mouse fetal development. *Nature*, 374, 640–3.

Chemical neurotransmission

Chemical neurotransmission was first described in England by Elliot in 1905. Otto Loewi (1873–1961) in Austria demonstrated chemical transmission by transferring fluid of a stimulated heart preparation from the frog onto another isolated frog heart. He found that the second heart slowed down its rate when it was perfused with fluid from the first heart. This demonstrated that a chemical had been released from the nerve endings of the vagus 'vagusstoff', which was later determined to be identical with acetylcholine by Sir Henry Dale. However, it was a long time before neurophysiologists such as John Eccles accepted the idea of chemical transmission. For him and others it was so obvious that neurotransmission was electrical that he argued vigorously in stand-up discussions against Sir Henry Dale at the Physiological Society. It is said that Eccles changed his mind when one of his collaborators in Sydney cut his lawn with an electric lawn mower. Unfortunately, the young guest scientist (Bernard Katz) succeeded in cutting the electric wire to the lawn mower, which is why Dr Eccles decided to buy a lawn mower based on chemical transmission, i.e. a petrol-driven one.

Noradrenaline was described as a neurotransmitter by von Euler in 1946. For a long time it was believed that there were only two neurotransmitters: acetylcholine and noradrenaline. Dale claimed that there is only one type of neurotransmitter in one cell. However, since then

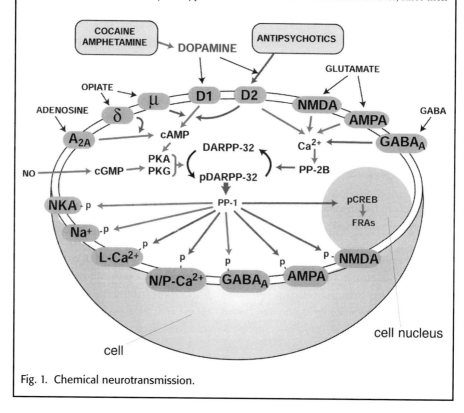

Fig. 1. Chemical neurotransmission.

a number of neuropeptides have been identified, which to some extent were co-stored and released in the same neurones as classical neurotransmitters (Hökfelt, 1991).

By studying end-plate potentials, Katz demonstrated that acetylcholine was released in discrete packages (quanta). Electron microscopical studies revealed the existence of clear vesicles with a diameter of about 40 nm, which were postulated to store and release acetylcholine. Small and large dense-cored vesicles were observed in the sympathetic nerve endings. Most neurotransmitters and modulators seem to be stored and released in quanta from vesicles (Stjärne et al., 1981).

The figure shows how DARPP-32 integrates the information from a variety of neurotransmitters. This explains the effects of some important drugs. This was discovered by Paul Greengard, who was awarded the Nobel Prize in physiology or medicine 2000, together with Arvid Carlsson and Eric Kandel. (Reproduced with permission from the Nobel Assembly.)

References

Hökfelt, T. (1991). Neuropeptides in perspective: the last ten years. *Neuron*, 7, 867–79.

Sjärne, L., Hedqvist, P., Lagercrantz, H. & Wennmalm, Å. (eds.) (1981). *Chemical Neurotransmission. 75 years.* New York: Academic Press.

8

Glial cell biology

Arne Schousboe and Helle S. Waagepetersen

NeuroScience PharmaBiotec Research, Royal Danish School of Pharmacy, Copenhagen, Denmark

Neuronal–glial interaction in nutrition and amino acid mediated neurotransmission.

Nutrition

The main substrate for brain energy metabolism is glucose and, in the adult human brain the glucose consumption, termed CMRgluc, is around $20\,\mu mol\,h^{-1}\,g^{-1}$ wet wt (Sokoloff, 1960). Alternative substrates may, however, be used and in this regard ketone bodies may play an important role particularly in the infant brain. The unique anatomical localization of astrocytes having their end feet closely apposed to capillaries (Fig. 8.1) has led to the proposal (Pellerin & Magistretti, 1994; Magistretti & Pellerin, 1996) that the astrocytes may be the major site for uptake of glucose in the brain. As glucose will be rapidly converted into glucose-6-phosphate, which is unable to cross the cell membrane, it is likely that metabolism of glucose proceeds to form lactate which may subsequently be transferred from the astrocytes to the neurons via the monocarboxylic acid transporters present in the membranes of both types of brain cells (Fig. 8.1) and possibly most prevalent in neurons (Pellerin et al., 1998). In this context, it is of interest that it has been shown that the distribution of lactate dehydrogenase isoenzymes in neurons favours metabolism of lactate to pyruvate (Bittar et al., 1996). Moreover, direct analysis of the metabolism of lactate in neurons and astrocytes using ^{13}C labelled lactate and NMR spectroscopy has shown that lactate is more actively metabolized to tricarboxylic acid (TCA) cycle intermediates and amino acids derived from TCA cycle intermediates in neurons compared to astrocytes (Waagepetersen et al., 1998a, b). The fact that neurons can utilize lactate as an energy substrate is important under conditions of short-lasting failures in the glucose supply, as this allows the use of astrocytic glycogen stores as an emergency fuel source in neurons. This is based on mobilization of glycogen by conversion to glucose-1-phosphate which, via glycolysis, is metabolized to lactate that is subsequently transferred to neurons. It has been demonstrated that stimulation of glycogen metabolism in astrocytes by activation

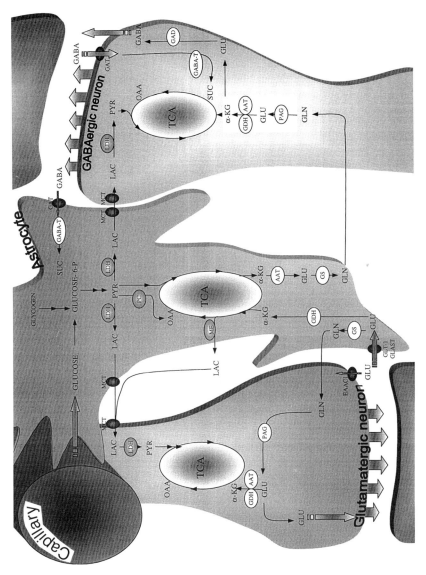

Fig. 8.1.   Schematic representation of a microenvironment in the brain consisting of a capillary, an astrocyte, and a GABAergic neuron. Release and uptake processes for the neurotransmitter amino acids glutamate (GLU) and GABA are indicated by bold arrows the size of which semiquantitatively reflects the corresponding activities. The membrane transporters for glutamate are named EAAC1 (neuronal) and GLT-1/GLAST (astrocytes) and those for GABA GAT. The lactate transporters are named MCT. Enzymes are abbreviated as follows: Glutamate dehydrogenase (GDH), phosphate activated glutaminase (PAG), aspartate aminotransferase (AAT), glutamine synthetase (GS), glutamate decarboxylase (GAD), GABA-transaminase (GABA-T), malic enzyme (ME), pyruvate carboxylase (PC) and lactate dehydrogenase (LDH). Metabolites are abbreviated as follows: lactate (LAC), pyruvate (PYR), oxaloacetate (OAA), α– ketoglutarate (α–KG), succinate (SUC) and glutamine (GLN). The tricarboxylic acid cycle is abbreviated TCA. It should be noted that succinate produced from GABA feeds into the TCA cycle.

of β-adrenergic receptors leads to production and release of lactate (Dringen et al., 1993). These aspects are illustrated in Fig. 8.1, which schematically shows the metabolic interactions between neurons and astrocytes with regard to exchange and transfer of metabolites.

Amino acid transmission

Neurotransmission mediated by the excitatory transmitter glutamate and the inhibitory neurotransmitter γ-aminobutyrate (GABA) obviously requires release of these amino acids from nerve endings (Fig. 8.1). The loss of glutamate and GABA from glutamatergic and GABAergic neurons, respectively is, to some extent, compensated for by reuptake of these amino acids (Schousboe, 1981; Hertz & Schousboe, 1987; Schousboe et al., 1988). However, for both amino acids there will be a net loss from the neurons, a loss which is most pronounced in the case of glutamate. This requires compensatory mechanisms allowing the neurons to perform a *de novo* synthesis of the amino acids. It was originally proposed that glutamine, which is synthesized exclusively in astrocytes by glutamine synthetase (Norenberg & Martinez-Hernandez, 1979), could function as a substrate for biosynthesis of the amino acids thus stoichiometrically compensating for the loss of glutamate and GABA (see Westergaard et al., 1995). Due to the subsequent demonstration that glutamate metabolism in astrocytes not only proceeds to glutamine but to a large extent involves oxidative metabolism to CO_2 or lactate (Yu et al., 1982; Sonnewald et al., 1993, 1997; McKenna et al., 1996), it is unlikely that the transfer of glutamine from astrocytes to neurons can occur in a stoichiometric manner as discussed in detail by Westergaard et al. (1995). The fact that neurons not only lack glutamine synthetase (see above) but also the main anaplerotic enzyme in the brain, pyruvate carboxylase (Yu et al., 1983; Shank et al., 1985; Cesar & Hamprecht, 1995) makes it essential that TCA cycle constituents can be replenished in neurons by transfer from astrocytes. As discussed by Westergaard et al. (1995), such compensatory transfer does occur to some extent. It thus appears that glutamine, together with TCA cycle constituents, represents the main source of precursors for biosynthesis of glutamate and GABA in neurons. It should be emphasized, however, that in quantitative terms, the flux of glutamine between astroglia and neurons is more important than transfer of TCA cycle constituents (Westergaard et al., 1995).

Developmental aspects of glial cell biochemistry

Enzymes

One of the important functions of astrocytes is to supply the metabolically handicapped neurons with energy substrates as well as precursors for synthesis of neuroactive amino acids (see Hertz et al., 1992). This means that astrocytes during the developmental period of the brain acquire high levels of activities of key enzymes such as lactate dehydrogenase, pyruvate carboxylase, malic enzyme, glutamate dehydrogenase, aspartate aminotransferase, glutamine synthetase and GABA-transaminase (Schousboe et al., 1977a,b; Hertz et al., 1978; Yu et al., 1983; Kurz et al., 1993), and the astrocyte-specific enzymes pyruvate carboxylase and glutamine synthetase exhibit almost identical developmental profiles in the brain in vivo in mice and in mouse neonatal astrocytes in culture (Hertz et al., 1978; Yu et al., 1983). It should, however, be noted that studies of the activity of glutamine synthetase in the intact tissue or neuronal–astrocytic cocultures indicate that the functional activity is influenced by neuronal factors (Wu et al., 1988).

One of the most important functions of astrocytes surrounding glutamatergic nerve terminals is to keep the concentration of glutamate in the synaptic cleft at a level below that which may induce excitotoxic damage to neurons (see Choi, 1988; Schousboe & Frandsen, 1995). It would therefore be expected that the enzymatic machinery for glutamate metabolism is present in astrocytes at a high expression level. As mentioned above, this is the case for glutamine synthetase which is only expressed in astrocytes. From studies of the activities in neurons and astrocytes of glutamate dehydrogenase (GDH) and from immunocytochemical labelling of the enzyme in brain slices (Schousboe et al., 1977b; Drejer et al., 1985; Larsson et al., 1985; Rothe et al., 1994), it is clear that this enzyme is expressed in astrocytes at a high level. Functional studies in intact astrocytes have shown that GDH primarily catalyses oxidative deamination of glutamate, a process which appears to be very important for metabolic degration of glutamate to α-ketoglutarate which can subsequently be oxidized in the tricarboxylic acid cycle (see Sonnewald et al., 1997). Alternatively, glutamate could be transaminated to α-ketoglutarate via aspartate aminotransferase which also has a high activity in astrocytes. It appears, however, that this enzyme preferentially catalyses production of glutamate from α-ketoglutarate (Westergaard et al., 1996). It should be noted that oxidation of glutamate in the TCA cycle leads to production of large amounts of lactate, a process that probably involves malic enzyme (Sonnewald et al., 1993). This lactate will subsequently be available for neurons which are able to utilize lactate in place of glucose (Magistretti & Pellerin, 1996; Waagepetersen et al., 1998a, b). In this context it should be kept in mind that lactate is also produced from glucose or glycogen in astrocytes and subsequently released to possibly serve as an energy substrate in neurons (Magistretti & Pellerin, 1996).

It has been shown by NMR analysis of [U-^{13}C]glutamate metabolism in astrocytes that its metabolism via GDH is particularly pronounced at high extracellular glutamate concentrations (McKenna et al., 1996; Sonnewald et al., 1997). This may be explained by the fact that GDH is allosterically activated by ADP (McCarthy &

Tipton, 1983), the concentration of which is likely to increase when glutamate uptake is intense since this is a process requiring energy in the form of ATP which is converted to ADP (see 'Glutamate transporters').

In addition to being able to metabolize glutamate, astrocytes are equipped to metabolize the inhibitory neurotransmitter GABA since the GABA metabolizing enzyme GABA-transaminase is present in astrocytes at high activity (Schousboe et al., 1977a). The carbon skeleton of GABA subsequently enters the TCA cycle in the form of succinate (Fig. 8.1). GABA which is metabolized in astrocytes or in neurons is lost from the neurotransmitter pool and this appears to be important for optimal function of inhibitory neurotransmission. Thus, drugs which block GABA metabolism, e.g. vigabatrin and valproate, act as anticonvulsants by increasing the availability of GABA in the neurotransmitter pool due to inhibition of metabolism (Schousboe, 1990; Waagepetersen et al., 1999).

Glutamate transporters

Glutamate is the major excitatory neurotransmitter in the CNS acting on a variety of receptors coupled to ion channels or G-proteins and second messenger systems (Schoep & Conn, 1993; Lodge, 1997). The extracellular concentration of glutamate is kept at a very low level by the highly efficient glutamate transporters in the membranes of neurons and glial cells (Nicholls & Attwell, 1990). From studies of glutamate transport in neural cellular and subcellular preparations, it has become clear that glutamate uptake into glial elements acts as the quantitatively most important mechanism for removal of glutamate from the extracellular space as indicated in Fig. 8.1 (Hertz, 1979; Schousboe, 1981; Lehre & Danbolt, 1998). The recent cloning of a series of glutamate transporters from CNS and subsequent studies of their cellular localization have confirmed this notion (Danbolt, 1994; Gegelashvili & Schousboe, 1997).

Uptake of glutamate increases as a function of postnatal development in the brain (Schousboe et al., 1976) and in astrocytes in culture the capacity for glutamate uptake is dependent upon the maturational and differentiational stage of the cells (Hertz et al., 1978; Gegelashvili & Schousboe, 1997). This is in all likelihood related to the fact that a variety of environmental cues such as factors released from neurons are known to enhance expression of glutamate transporters in astrocytes (Drejer et al., 1983; Gegelashvili et al., 1996, 1997; Gegelashvili & Schousboe, 1997). This probably explains the observation that destruction of glutamatergic neuronal pathways leads to a reduction of glutamate uptake in the brain areas in question (Levy et al., 1995).

Since glutamate uptake requires an intact sodium gradient and membrane potential in order to function optimally (Nicholls & Attwell, 1990), it is clear that conditions such as energy failure will affect the ability of cells to maintain the very high intra/extracellular glutamate gradient present under physiological conditions. This failure of glutamate uptake will reverse the direction of the carriers resulting in the dramatic increase in the extracellular glutamate concentration seen during ischemia (Benveniste et al., 1984; Levy et al., 1998). This is a major contributing factor in the neuronal degeneration associated with ischemia since glutamate acts as a very potent neurotoxin (Schousboe & Frandsen, 1995). In relation to this, it should be noted that other neurodegenerative disorders such as amyotrophic lateral sclerosis (ALS) have been associated with a reduction in the expression of GLT-1, the most important glial glutamate transporter (Rothstein et al., 1992, 1993). As pointed out above, failures in glutamate metabolism may also play important roles in this context (Plaitakis, 1990).

GABA transporters

GABA which is produced from glutamate by decarboxylation catalysed by glutamate decarboxylase (Schousboe, 1981; Waagepetersen et al., 1999) acts as the major inhibitory neurotransmitter in the CNS (Roberts, 1991). Its inactivation as a transmitter is mediated by high affinity transporters residing in GABAergic neurons and surrounding astrocytes (Schousboe, 1981). Contrary to glutamate, the highest capacity for GABA uptake appears to be associated with GABAergic nerve endings (Hertz & Schousboe, 1987). This may be compatible with the view that GABA neurotransmission to a large extent is based on reutilization of released transmitter GABA (Fig. 8.1). Thus, in GABAergic neurons, exogenously supplied GABA is accumulated into the vesicular neurotransmitter pool (Gram et al., 1988; Schousboe, 1990).

High affinity GABA transport is also expressed in astrocytes (Schousboe et al., 1977a) although, as mentioned above, the capacity for uptake seems lower than that present in GABAergic neurons (Hertz & Schousboe, 1987). Like GABA uptake in the brain, the astrocytic uptake process is developmentally regulated being increased in the course of postnatal development (Schousboe, 1981). As most other uptake systems for amino acids, GABA uptake is Na^+ dependent which makes the uptake electrogenic and thus dependent on the membrane potential (Martin, 1976; Schousboe, 1981). In this context, it is of functional importance that, in astrocytes, the coupling ratio between Na^+ and GABA (Na^+: GABA ratio) increases as a function of development (Larsson & Schousboe, 1981), a property which is shared by the neuronal GABA uptake (Larsson et al., 1983). As a consequence of this, the efficiency of GABA uptake increases in the brain during postnatal development. This may be of importance in the light of the fact that GABA appears to play an important role as a neurodifferentiating factor during early development (Meier et al., 1991). In order for GABA to fulfil this function, the extracellular concentration needs to be kept at a relatively high level compared to that seen in the adult brain, a condition which would be incompatible with a highly efficient uptake system since GABA synthesis and release is limited during the early developmental period (Waagepetersen et al., 1999).

It may also be of interest that astroglial GABA uptake may be influenced by neuronal stimuli. This was originally demonstrated in cultured cerebellar astrocytes where the expression of GABA transporters could be enhanced by conditioned media taken from cultured neurons (Drejer et al., 1983). It was subsequently shown that the active component in these media is a glycoprotein with a molecular weight of approximately 30 kD (Nissen et al., 1992). Although the mechanism of action of this protein termed GABACIP has not been fully characterized, it is clear that it acts via stimulation of the protein synthesis responsible for *de novo* synthesis of GABA carriers in astrocytes. In the light of the recent cloning of four different mouse brain GABA carriers (GAT 1–4) which exhibit different pharmacological and functional characteristics (Borden, 1996; Bolvig et al., 1999), it would be of interest to study the action of this neuronal factor on expression of these transporters in astrocytes.

Concluding remarks

Since 1980 the understanding of the functional significance of astrocytes in the brain has changed from that of a static role as a mechanical support for neurons to that of a highly dynamic one where a constant interplay between neurons and astrocytes exchanging metabolites and neurotransmitters appears to be a prerequisite for normal brain function. The present review has been concentrated on a discussion of nutritional and amino acid homeostatic functions of astrocytes. It should be emphasized, however, that astrocytes are involved in many other basic brain functions such as ion homeostasis, cell volume regulation and regulation of monoamine neurotransmission (Kettenmann & Ransom, 1995). Astrocytes therefore need to be considered as very active participants in essentially all brain functions and it should be noted that they express a large repertoire of neurotransmitter receptors thus allowing constant monitoring of neuronal activity (Kettenmann & Ransom, 1995). Proper development of astrocytes during embryogenesis and the neonatal period therefore is of utmost importance for proper function of the central nervous system in adulthood.

Acknowledgements

The expert secretarial assistance by Ms Hanne Danø is cordially acknowledged. The work has been supported by the Lundbeck Foundation and the Danish Medical Research Council (970671).

REFERENCES

Benveniste, H., Drejer, J., Schousboe, A. & Diemer, N. H. (1984). Elevation of the extracellular concentrations of glutamate and aspartate in rat hippocampus during transient cerebral ischemia monitored by intracerebral microdialysis. *Journal of Neurochemistry*, **43**, 1369–74.

Bittar, P. G., Charnay, U., Pellerin, L., Bouras, C. & Magistretti, P. J. (1996). Selective distribution of lactate dehydrogenase isoenzymes in neurons and astrocytes of human brain. *Journal of Cerebral Blood Flow Metabolism*, **16**, 1079–89.

Bolvig, T., Larsson, O. M., Pickering, D. S. et al. (1999). Action of bicyclic isoxazole GABA analogues on GABA transporters and its relation to anticonvulsant activity. *European Journal of Pharmacology*, **375**, 367–74.

Borden, L. A. (1996). GABA transporter heterogeneity: pharmacology and cellular localization. *Neurochemistry International*, **29**, 335–56.

Cesar, M. & Hamprecht, B. (1995). Immunocytochemical examination of neural rat and mouse primary cultures using monoclonal antibodies raised against pyruvate carboxylase. *Journal of Neurochemistry*, **64**, 2312–18.

Choi, D. W. (1988). Glutamate neurotoxicity and diseases of the nervous system. *Neuron*, **1**, 623–34.

Danbolt, N. C. (1994). The high-affinity uptake system for excitatory amino acids in the brain. *Progress in Neurobiology*, **44**, 377–96.

Drejer, J., Meier, E. & Schousboe, A. (1983). Novel neuron-related regulatory mechanisms for astrocytic glutamate and GABA high affinity uptake. *Neuroscience Letters*, **37**, 301–6.

Drejer, J., Larsson, O. M., Kvamme, E., Svenneby, G., Hertz, L. & Schousboe, A. (1985). Ontogenetic development of glutamate metabolizing enzymes in cultured cerebellar granule cells and in cerebellum in vivo. *Neurochemical Research*, **10**, 49–62.

Dringen, R., Gebhardt, R. & Hamprecht, B. (1993). Glycogen in astrocytes: possible function as lactate supply for neighboring cells. *Brain Research*, **623**, 208–14.

Gegelashvili, G. & Schousboe, A. (1997). High-affinity glutamate transporters: regulation of expression and activity. *Molecular Pharmacology*, **52**, 6–15.

Gegelashvili, G., Civenni, G., Racagni, G., Danbolt, N. C., Schousboe, I. & Schousboe, A. (1996). Glutamate receptor agonists up-regulate glutamate transporter glast in astrocytes. *NeuroReport*, **8**, 261–5.

Gegelashvili, G., Danbolt, N. C. & Schousboe, A. (1997). Neuronal soluble factors differentially regulate the expression of the GLT1 and GLAST glutamate transporters in cultured astroglia. *Journal of Neurochemistry*, **69**, 2612–15.

Gram, L., Larsson, O. M., Johnsen, A. H. & Schousboe, A. (1988). Effects of valproate, vigabatrin and aminooxyacetic acid on release of endogenous and exogenous GABA from cultured neurons. *Epilepsy Research*, **2**, 87–95.

Hertz, L. (1979). Functional interactions between neurons and astrocytes I. Turnover and metabolism of putative amino acid transmitters. *Progress in Neurobiology*, **13**, 277–323.

Hertz, L. & Schousboe, A. (1987). Primary cultures of GABAergic and glutamatergic neurons as model systems to study neurotransmitter functions. I. Differentiated cells. In *Model Systems of*

Development and Aging of the Nervous System, ed. A. Vernadakis, A. Privat, J. M. Lauder, P. S. Timiras & E. Giacobini, pp. 19–31. Boston: M. Nijhoff.

Hertz, L., Bock, E. & Schousboe, A. (1978). GFA content, glutamate uptake and activity of glutamate metabolizing enzymes in differentiating mouse astrocytes in primary cultures. *Developmental Neurosci*ence, **1**, 226–38.

Hertz, L., Peng, L., Westergaard, N., Yudkoff, M. & Schousboe, A. (1992). Neuronal-astrocytic interactions in metabolism of transmitter amino acids of the glutamate family. In *Alfred Benzon Symposium 32, Drug Research Related to Neuroactive Amino Acids*, ed. A. Schousboe, N. H. Diemer & H. Kofod, pp. 30–48. Copenhagen: Munksgaard.

Kettenmann, H. & Ransom, B. R. (eds.) (1995). *Neuroglia*. Oxford: Oxford University Press.

Larsson, O. M. & Schousboe, A. (1981). Comparison between (RS)-nipecotic acid and GABA transport in cultured astrocytes: Coupling with two sodium ions. *Neurochemical Research*, **6**, 257–66.

Larsson, O. M., Drejer, J., Hertz, L. & Schousboe, A. (1983). Ion dependency of uptake and release of GABA and (RS)-nipecotic acid studies in cultured mouse brain cortex neurons. *Journal of Neuroscience Research*, **9**, 291–303.

Larsson, O. M., Drejer, J., Kvamme, E., Svenneby, G., Hertz, L. & Schousboe, A. (1985). Ontogenetic development of glutamate and GABA metabolising enzymes in cultured cerebral cortex interneurons and in cerebral cortex in vivo. *International Journal of Developmental Neuroscience*, **3**, 177–85.

Lehre, K P. & Danbolt, N. C. (1998). The number of glutamate transporter subtype molecules at glutamatergic synapses: chemical and stereological quantification in young adult rat brain. *Journal of Neuroscience*, **18**, 8751–7.

Levy, L. M., Lehre, K.P., Walaas, S. I., Storm-Mathisen, J. & Danbolt, N. C. (1995). Down-regulation of glial glutamate transporters after glutamatergic denervation in the rat brain. *European Journal of Neuroscience*, **7**, 2036–41.

Levy, L. M., Warr, O. & Attwell, D. (1998). Stoichiometry of the glial glutamate transporter GLT-expressed inducibly in a Chinese hamster ovary cell line selected for low endogenous Na^+-dependent glutamate uptake. *Journal of Neuroscience*, **18**, 9620–8.

Lodge, D. (1997). Subtypes of glutamate receptors. In *The Ionotropic Glutamate Receptors*, ed. D. T. Monaghan & R. J. Wenthold, pp. 1–38. New Jersey: Humana Press.

McCarthy, A. D. & Tipton, K. F. (1983). Glutamate dehydrogenase. In *Glutamine, Glutamate and GABA in the Central Nervous System*, ed. L. Hertz, E. Kvamme, E. G. McGeer & A. Schousboe, pp. 19–32. New York: Alan R. Liss, Inc.

McKenna, M. C., Sonnewald, U., Huang, X., Stevenson, J. & Zielke, R. H. (1996). Exogenous glutamate concentration regulates the metabolic fate of glutamate in astrocytes. *Journal of Neurochemistry*, **66**, 386–93.

Magistretti, P. J. & Pellerin, L. (1996). The contribution of astrocytes to the ^{18}F-2-deoxyglucose signal in PET activation studies. *Molecular Psychiatry*, **1**, 445–52.

Martin, D. L. (1976). Carrier-mediated transport and removal of GABA from synaptic regions. In *GABA in Nervous System Function*, ed. E. Roberts, T. N. Chase & D. B. Tower, pp. 347–86. New York: Raven Press.

Meier, E., Hertz, L. & Schousboe, A. (1991). Neurotransmitters as developmental signals. *Neurochemistry International*, **19**, 1–15.

Nicholls, D. & Attwell, D. (1990). The release and uptake of excitatory amino acids. *TIPS*, **11**, 462–8.

Nissen, J., Schousboe, A., Halkier, T. & Schousboe, I. (1992). Purification and characterization of an astrocyte GABA-carrier inducing protein (GABA-CIP) released from cerebellar granule cells. *Glia*, **6**, 236–43.

Norenberg, M. D. & Martinez-Hernandez, A. (1979). Fine structural localization of glutamine synthetase in astrocytes of rat brain. *Brain Research*, **161**, 303–10.

Pellerin, L. & Magistretti, P. J. (1994). Glutamate uptake into astrocytes stimulates aerobic glycolysis: a mechanism coupling neuronal activity to glucose utilization. *Proceedings of the National Academy of Sciences, USA*, **15**, 10625–9.

Pellerin, L., Pellegri, G., Bittar, P. G. et al. (1998). Evidence supporting the existence of an activity-dependent astrocyte-neuron lactate shuttle. *Developmental Neuroscience*, **20**, 291–9.

Plaitakis, A. (1990). Glutamate dysfunction and selective motor neuron degeneration in amyotrophic lateral sclerosis: a hypothesis. *Annals of Neurology*, **28**, 3–8.

Roberts, E. (1991). Living systems are tonically inhibited, autonomous optimizers, and disinhibition coupled to variability generation is their major organizing principle: Inhibitory command-control at levels of membrane, genome, metabolism, brain, and society. *Neurochemical Research*, **16**, 409–21.

Rothe, F., Brosz, M. & Storm-Mathisen, J. (1994). Quantitative ultrastructural localization of glutamate dehydrogenase in the rat cerebellar cortex. *Neuroscience*, **62**, 1133–46.

Rothstein, J. D., Martin, L. J. & Kuncl, R. W. (1992). Decreased brain and spinal cord glutamate transport in amyotrophic lateral sclerosis. *New England Journal of Medicine*, **326**, 1464–8.

Rothstein, J. D., Jin, L., Dykes-Hoberg, M. & Kuncl, R.W. (1993). Chronic glutamate uptake inhibition produces a model of slow neurotoxicity. *Proceedings of the National Academy of Sciences, USA*, **90**, 6591–5.

Schoepp, D. D. & Conn, P. J. (1993). Metabotropic glutamate receptors in brain function and pathology. *Trends in Pharmacological Sciences*, **14**, 13–20.

Schousboe, A. (1981). Transport and metabolism of glutamate and GABA in neurons and glial cells. *International Review of Neurobiology*, **22**, 1–45.

Schousboe, A. (1990). Neurochemical alterations associated with epilepsy or seizure activity. In *Comprehensive Epileptology*, ed. M. Dam & L. Gram, pp. 1–16. New York: Raven Press.

Schousboe, A. & Frandsen, A. (1995). Glutamate receptors and neurotoxicity. In *CNS Neurotransmitters and Neuromodulators: Glutamate*, ed. T. W. Stone, pp. 239–51. Boca Raton, FL: CRC Press.

Schousboe, A., Lisy, V. & Hertz, L. (1976). Postnatal alterations in effects of potassium on uptake and release of glutamate and GABA in rat brain cortex slices. *Journal of Neurochemistry*, **26**, 1023–7.

Schousboe, A., Hertz, L. & Svenneby, G. (1977a). Uptake and metabolism of GABA in astrocytes cultured from dissociated mouse brain hemispheres. *Neurochemical Research*, **2**, 217–29.

Schousboe, A., Svenneby, G., & Hertz, L. (1977b). Uptake and metabolism of glutamate in astrocytes cultured from dissociated mouse brain hemispheres. *Journal of Neurochemistry*, **29**, 999–1005.

Schousboe, A., Drejer, J. & Hertz, L. (1988). Uptake and release of glutamate and glutamine in neurons and astrocytes in primary cultures. In *Glutamine and Glutamate in Mammals*, Vol. II, ed. E. Kvamme, pp. 21–38. Boca Raton, Fl.: CRC Press.

Shank, R. P., Bennett, G. S., Freytag, S. O. & Campbell, G. L. (1985). Pyruvate carboxylase: astrocyte-specific enzyme implicated in the replenishment of amino acid neurotransmitter pools. *Brain Research*, **329**, 364–7.

Sokoloff, L. (1960). The metabolism of the central nervous system *in vivo*. In *Handbook of Physiology-Neurophysiology*, Vol. 3, ed. H. W. Magoun & V. E. Hall, pp. 1843–64. Washington, DC: American Physiological Society.

Sonnewald, U., Westergaard, N., Petersen, S. B., Unsgård, G. & Schousboe, A. (1993). Metabolism of [U-^{13}C]glutamate in astrocytes studied by ^{13}C NMR spectroscopy: Incorporation of more label into lactate than into glutamine demonstrates the importance of the TCA cycle. *Journal of Neurochemistry*, **61**, 1179–82.

Sonnewald, U., Westergaard, N. & Schousboe, A. (1997). Glutamate transport and metabolism in astrocytes. *Glia*, **21**, 56–63.

Waagepetersen, H. S., Bakken, I. J., Larsson, O. M., Sonnewald, U. & Schousboe, A. (1998a). Metabolism of lactate in cultured GABAergic neurons studied by ^{13}C-NMR spectroscopy. *Journal of Cerebral Blood Flow Metabolism*, **18**, 109–17.

Waagepetersen, H. S., Bakken, I. J., Larsson, O. M., Sonnewald, U. & Schousboe, A. (1998b). Comparison of lactate and glucose metabolism in cultured neocortical neurons and astrocytes using ^{13}C NMR spectroscopy. *Developmental Neuroscience*, **20**, 310–20.

Waagepetersen, H. S., Sonnewald, U. & Schousboe, A. (1999). The GABA paradox: multiple roles as metabolite, neurotransmitter, and neurodifferentiative agent. *Journal of Neurochemistry*, **73**, 1335–42.

Westergaard, N., Sonnewald, U. & Schousboe, A. (1995). Metabolic trafficking between neurons and astrocytes: The glutamate/glutamine cycle revisited. *Developmental Neuroscience*, **17**, 203–11.

Westergaard, N., Drejer, J., Schousboe, A. & Sonnewald, U. (1996). Evaluation of the importance of transamination versus deamination in astrocytic metabolism of [U-^{13}C]glutamate. *Glia*, **17**, 160–8.

Wu, D. K., Scully, S. & de Vellis, J. (1988). Induction of glutamine synthetase in rat astrocytes by co-cultivation with embryonic chick neurons. *Journal of Neurochemistry*, **50**, 929–35.

Yu, A. C., Schousboe, A. & Hertz, L. (1982). Metabolic fate of [^{14}C]-labelled glutamate in astrocytes in primary cultures. *Journal of Neurochemistry*, **39**, 954–60.

Yu, A. C. H., Drejer, J., Hertz, L., & Schousboe, A. (1983). Pyruvate carboxylase activity in primary cultures of astrocytes and neurons. *Journal of Neurochemistry*, **41**, 1484–7.

9

Development of the somatosensory system

Sandra Rees and John Rawson

Department of Anatomy and Cell Biology, The University of Melbourne, Victoria, Australia

Introduction

The somatosensory system deals with information from a variety of sensory receptors that are located in the skin, muscles, joints and other deeper tissues. It enables us to feel touch, pain, warmth and cold and to sense the position and movements of our body. Understanding how this system develops structurally and functionally during fetal life provides an insight into how a fetus develops the capacity to receive and experience sensations delivered by noxious, tactile, thermal or mechanical stimuli. Although it will be difficult to determine, unequivocally, when the fetus is first aware of its surroundings and conscious of perceiving these stimuli, we can at least define when the minimum structural and functional apparatus necessary to do so is present. In this chapter we will first describe the structure of the main pathways that transmit nociceptive, tactile, thermal and proprioceptive information from the periphery to the cerebral cortex via synaptic connections in the spinal cord or brainstem. We will then describe the structural, neurochemical and functional development of the somatosensory system and the development of descending pathways from the brainstem which modify this activity. We will speculate on whether activity in the fetal somatosensory pathways is a necessary requirement for the appropriate development of these pathways as it is for the visual system (Goodman & Shatz, 1993). Very little experimentation can be performed on the human fetus, and laboratory animals are therefore used to answer these questions. We will draw on data from the fetal rat (gestation ~21.5 days) and from the fetal sheep (gestation 21 weeks). A considerable proportion of CNS development in sheep occurs in utero as it does in the human, making this animal a particularly useful animal model for the human fetus. Where available, data from humans will also be included.

Somatosensory receptors and pathways

Information from receptors in the body reaches the cerebral cortex via two main ascending systems: the dorsal column–medial lemniscal system and the

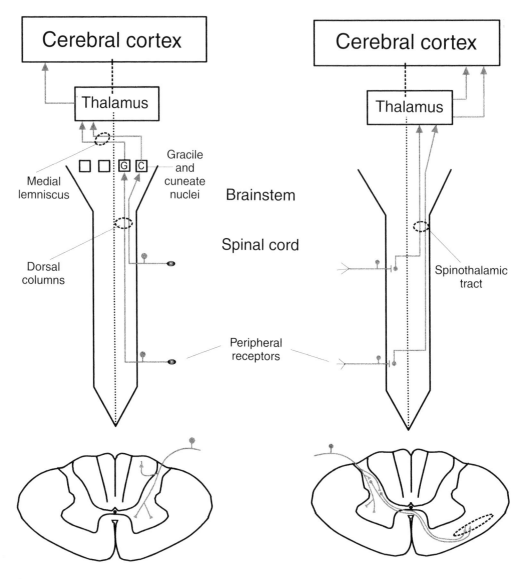

Fig. 9.1.   Diagrams of the main somatosensory pathways from the body. Dorsal column medial lemniscal systems (on left): Large diameter myelinated fibres connected with cutaneous mechanoreceptors, muscle spindle and tendon organ receptors provide collaterals or branches which ascend in the dorsal columns of the spinal cord and synapse in the dorsal column nuclei in the medulla. These are the gracile nucleus for the lower limbs and lower body and the cuneate nucleus for the upper limbs and upper body. From here, the input is transmitted via the medial lemniscus to the contralateral thalamus (ventral posterior lateral nucleus). This input system terminates in primary somatosensory cortex and is responsible for discriminative tactile sensation, kinesthesia and probably also for a sense of muscle tension. Although proprioceptive input from the upper limbs travels in the

spinothalamic or anterolateral system. The principal anatomical features of these systems are outlined diagrammatically in Fig. 9.1. The receptors that feed into the dorsal column–medial lemniscal system are encapsulated, low threshold, cutaneous mechanoreceptors and muscle spindle and tendon organ receptors. Low threshold mechanoreceptors (Meissner, Merkel, Ruffini and Paciniaw) in glabrous or smooth skin are innervated by large myelinated fibres of the Aβ group in the peripheral nerve. They respond to gentle mechanical stimulation of an area of skin that forms the receptive field. Afferents from Merkel and Ruffini endings have a static response; action potentials are elicited as long as deformation of the receptive field is maintained. Ruffini endings are particularly sensitive to lateral stretch of the skin. Fibres from Merkel endings are known as slowly adapting type 1; from Ruffini endings as type 2. Afferents from Meissner and Pacinian endings (which are encapsulated and have an alternating lamellar structure) have a dynamic response; action potentials are elicited only when deformation of the receptive field is changing. Meissner afferents (rapidly adapting type 1) respond preferentially to stimuli that are changing relatively slowly while Pacinian afferents (rapidly adapting type 2) are most sensitive to rapidly changing stimuli. In hairy skin, there are two further classes of afferents, both of which have large receptive fields and both of which are rapidly adapting; hair units are associated with hair follicles and field units are of unknown origin.

Muscle spindles provide precise signals about the lengths of muscles and the velocities of stretch and hence about the position and movement of attached

Caption for fig. 9.1 (*cont.*)

cuneate fasciculus to the cuneate nucleus, information from muscle spindles and Golgi tendon organs in hindlimb muscles follows a different route to the brainstem. Second-order fibres ascend in the dorsal spinocerebellar tract in the dorsolateral funiculus of the spinal cord. Tract fibres provide branches to nucleus Z in the medulla which then sends a projection to the contralateral medial lemniscus. This unusual route may help to explain why joint position sense from lower limb may be present after dorsal column lesions. Anterolateral or spinothalamic systems (on right): Unmyelinated and small diameter myelinated fibres connected with nociceptors, thermoreceptors and unencapsulated tactile receptors, project into the dorsal horn. The C fibre afferents terminate in lamina II (substantia gelatinosa) of the dorsal horn of the spinal cord (see Willis & Coggeshall, 1991), and Aβ fibres in laminae I and V (see Willis & Coggeshall, 1991). Large myelinated cutaneous afferents innervating low-threshold mechanoreceptors project to laminae III–V (see Willis & Coggeshall, 1991). From laminae I, II and V axons arise which project directly to the thalamus (ventral posterior, ventro-medial pars oralis, posterior and intralamina nuclei) via the contralateral spinothalamic tract. Recipient thalamic cells project to primary somatosensory cortex, limbic cortex and insula. A small number of touch and position sense fibres also travel in the spinothalamic system.

muscles. Spindles are composed of specialized muscle fibres, the intrafusal fibres, enclosed in a fluid-filled, fusiform, fibrous capsule. Motor nerve fibres (γ efferent fibres) innervate the intrafusal fibres and adjust their lengths according to the state of stretch of the muscle. This is detected by the primary ($A\alpha$) afferent fibres, which make spiral terminations around the intrafusal fibres. Golgi tendon organs which are encapsulated nerve endings are located at the musclo-tendinous junctions and signal tension in the muscles and hence forces in the limbs. There are receptors in joint capsules which signal joint angle, but they are relatively sparse and may respond only at extremes of joint angle.

The large diameter myelinated nerve fibres connected with these receptors provide collaterals or branches which ascend in the dorsal columns of the spinal cord and synapse in the dorsal column nuclei in the medulla. From these nuclei fibres project via the medial lemniscus to the contralateral thalamus and then to the somatosensory cortex (Fig. 9.1). The spinothalamic (or anterolateral) system mediates pain and thermal sensations and some light touch (Fig. 9.1). The receptor input originates from nociceptors, thermoreceptors and unencapsulated tactile receptors. There are two classes of thermoreceptors in the skin; cold receptors which are activated by a decrease in skin temperature and are innervated by small myelinated $A\delta$ axons. Warm receptors respond to an increase in temperature and are innervated by unmyelinated C fibres. Both fibres have a static and dynamic component to their response. There are three classes of nociceptors: mechanical nociceptors innervated by $A\delta$ fibres, mechanothermal nociceptors innervated by $A\delta$ and C fibres and polymodal nociceptors innervated by C fibres. The thermoreceptors and nociceptors are presumed to be free nerve endings.

The afferent nerve fibres of these receptors make synapses on neurons in the dorsal horn of the spinal cord. Axons arise from these neurons and project to the thalamus via the contralateral spinothalamic tract. Thalamic cells then project to the somatosensory cortex, limbic cortex and insular cortex (Fig. 9.1). The distinction between the two pathways is important clinically as they cross the nervous system at different levels (see Fig. 9.1). Sensation from the face is subserved by comparable trigeminal systems: fibres relaying discriminative touch and kinesthesia synapse in the trigeminal principal and mesancephalic nuclei, which then project to the thalamus via the medial lemniscus. Nociceptive and thermoreceptive afferents from the face connect with the spinal nucleus of the trigeminal, which sends crossed axons directly to the thalamus in the trigeminothalamic tract.

Development of cutaneous receptors and their afferent fibres

Functional receptor–afferent fibre units capable of transducing nociceptive, thermal and mechanical stimuli into propagated impulses represent an essential first stage for somatic sensation. In this section we will describe the structural, neurochemical and functional development of the receptors and their afferent projections to the spinal cord.

Structural development

Sensory neurons in the trigeminal and dorsal root ganglia (DRG) are largely derived from a distinct group of cells called the neural crest. The neural crest is a transient structure that arises from the dorsolateral edge of the neural plate just before neural tube closure. The neural tube gives rise to all the cells of the central nervous system. Neural crest cells migrate widely in the body to appropriate locations to form cranial and spinal ganglia. In the rat, DRG and trigeminal ganglion cells are born over the embryonic (E) period from day 11–14 and in humans by about the fourth week of gestational age. This data is not known for the sheep. Each DRG cell gives off one process, which bifurcates close to the soma and sends one process to the periphery, where it will innervate skin, muscle and visceral targets and the other centrally where it will grow into the spinal cord or brainstem.

An excessive number of neurons are produced; this number is reduced by a process of programmed cell death so that the final number of DRG cells is appropriate for the target fields. Factors which influence the regulation of neuronal number by cell loss are now being elucidated. The neurotrophins, nerve growth factor (NGF) and neurotrophin 3 and 4/5 are all thought to influence the survival of different subpopulations of neurons in the dorsal root ganglia (see Farinas et al., 1996). For example, in neonatal mice lacking NGF (Crowley et al., 1994) or its receptor trk A (Smeyne et al., 1994), all DRG nociceptive neurons are lost; NT-3/Trk C signalling is required for the survival of all proprioceptive neurons that convey information about the degree of muscle stretch and tension (Airaksinen et al., 1996); NT-3 also seems to be necessary for the survival of low threshold cutaneous mechanoreceptors innervating hair follicles and Merkel cells (Ernfors et al., 1994) and large diameter muscle spindle afferents (Oakley et al., 1995). It has been hypothesized that targets for developing neurons produce limiting amounts of these survival molecules such that, following target innervation, only those neurons successful in obtaining the factors survive (see Barde, 1989). Recent evidence suggests that neurotrophins (particularly NT-3) might also play a role in controlling events that occur prior to target innervation such as the genesis of sensory neurons (Ockel et al., 1996). As DRG cells mature, they lose their requirement for target-derived trophic support and appear to be sustained by autocrine or paracrine modes of delivery of growth factors, including brain-derived neurotrophic factor (BDNF) (Acheson et al., 1995).

Axons appear to grow directly to their targets in the periphery without sprouting and are possibly directed by chemotropic factors. Innervation of the skin of the

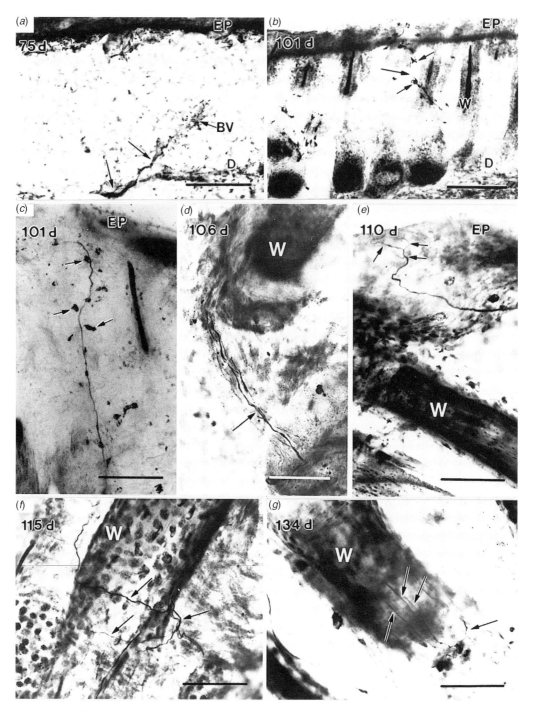

Fig. 9.2.   Photomicrographs of the skin of the hindlimb stained with a modification of the Winkelmann Schmitt technique. (*a*) 75 d, a bundle of nerve fibres at the border of the dermis and the subcutaneous tissue. Fibres (arrows) leave the bundle and traverse the

hind limb in sheep occurs by about mid-gestation (Rees et al., 1994a) (Fig. 9.2), coinciding with innervation of muscle fibres (Rees et al., 1994b). At this age, fibres have penetrated as far as the lower dermis and appear to be using blood vessels for axonal guidance (Fig. 9.2 (a)). Large macrophage-like granular cells are associated with developing axons in both sheep (Rees et al., 1994a) (Figs. 9.2(b) and (c)) and humans (Hogg, 1941). It has been shown that macrophages from embryonic rat brain release NGF in vitro when appropriately stimulated (Mallat et al., 1989). It is possible therefore, that these macrophages play a neurotropic role in skin innervation. Fibres can be seen penetrating the epidermis at 101 days (Fig. 9.2(b)) with more extensive branching at 100 days (Fig. 9.2(e)). In the rat, facial innervation begins on day E13 and hind limb innervation takes place over E15–E19. In the human, cutaneous innervation of the face, shoulder, axilla and thigh have begun at 8 weeks of gestation. In both rat and man, cutaneous nerve terminals initially form a dense plexus penetrating into the fetal epidermis. With time, fibres withdraw and reduce in density as receptors such as Meissner's corpuscles appear and become innervated some time after the initial innervation of the skin. Hair follicles are innervated later in gestation: at about 100–106 days in the sheep (Fig. 9.2(d)); postnatal day 7 in the rat and 22–24 weeks of gestation in the human fetus.

In fetal sheep, dorsal root afferent fibres have begun to penetrate the grey matter of the dorsal horn by 56 days of gestation (Fig. 9.3(a)) and by 67 days (Fig. 9.3(b)), innervation of the motoneuron pool is established; there is a marked increase in the number of fibres and in the extent of their arborization in the dorsal and ventral horns with increasing gestational age (Figs. 9.3(c) and (d)). From ultrastructural studies we were able to show that afferent fibres (immunoreactive for Substance P and CGRP, see below) form synaptic connections with dorsal horn cells within a few days of their arrival in lamina 1 of the dorsal horn (Rees et al., 1994b). In the rat, dorsal root fibres first reach the lumbar cord at E12, travel rostrocaudally in the

Caption for Fig. 9.2 (cont.)

dermis in association with blood vessels (BV) Bar = 100 μm. (b) 101 d, fibres traversing the dermis to innervate the epidermis. Note the presence of irregularly shaped densely stained cells (arrows) adjacent to the fibres. Bar = 80 μm. (c) 101 d, higher magnification to show the relationship of the cells (arrows) to a nerve fibre. Bar = 150 μm. (d) 106 d, simple innervation (arrow) of a wool/hair follicle, without any evidence of a terminal specialization. Bar = 50 μm. (e) 110 d, branched free nerve ending (arrows) penetrating to the edge of the epidermis. (f) 115 d, more complex innervation of the wool/hair follicle with first signs of circumferential wrapping by fibres (arrows). (g) 134 d, base of wool/hair follicle, innervated with a pallisade of parallel lanceolate endings. Bar = 60 μm for (e)–(g). EP, epidermis; D, dermis; W, wool/hair follicle. All sections 100 μm thick. (Taken with permission from Rees et al., 1994a.)

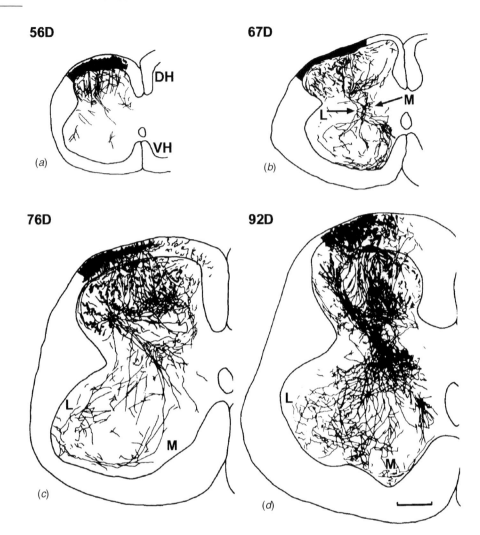

Fig. 9.3.   Drawings of the distribution of primary afferent fibres stained with the neural tracer
biocytin in the developing fetal sheep spinal cord. At each gestational age the section of
cord which contained the greatest number of stained fibres has been selected for
presentation. (*a*) At 56 days, fibres have entered the spinal cord and penetrated as far as
the intermediate zone with a few fibres projecting into the ventral horn. (*b*) By 67 days,
primary afferents converge in the intermediate zone (arrows) before they spread out and
extend into the medial (M) and lateral (L) motor neuron pools. With advancing
gestational age, at 76 d (*c*) and 92 d (*d*) the number of primary afferents entering the
spinal cord and following the trajectory described above increased. The density of
innervation of both the medial and ventral motor neuron pools increases concomitantly.
(*a*)–(d) Bar = 300 μm. DH: dorsal horn; VH: ventral horn. Taken with permission from Rees
et al., 1994b.)

bundle of His and begin to send collaterals into the dorsal grey matter at E15 (Fitzgerald et al., 1991; Mirnics & Koerber, 1995). The first sensory fibres to grow in are the large diameter myelinated afferents some of which are 1A muscle afferents projecting towards the motoneuron pool in the ventral horn and some are Aβ cutaneous afferents that remain in the dorsal horn (Smith, 1983; Fitzgerald, 1991). Some days later (E19–E20) smaller diameter unmyelinated C fibres grow into the substantia gelatinosa (Lamina II). The organized somatotopic projections and laminar location of C fibres is established early in development and requires little refinement to match that in the adult (Mirnics & Koerber, 1995). While somatotopy is also established early in gestation for A fibres, laminar location is not (Fitzgerald et al., 1994). A fibres are initially found throughout laminae 1 to V, including the substantia gelatinosa (Lamina II) which later becomes the major projection domain of C fibres. By postnatal day 22, A fibres have withdrawn to laminae III to V. It is not yet certain what causes this withdrawal, but it is possibly due to competitive interactions between the A fibres and the later arriving C fibres (Coggeshall et al., 1996), perhaps triggered by neurotrophic factors or a mismatch between activity levels in A fibres and neurons in the substantia gelatinosa. In a recent study of prenatal development of the central projections of primary afferents in the rat, Mirnics and Koerber (1995) concluded that: the initial penetration of the grey matter is a target-independent process; peripheral innervation is not invariably the stimulus for fibre ingrowth into the cord; the establishment of topography and modality in the cord is likely to be target dependent and that there is a postnatal component of development responsible for the subtle refinements of these projections probably requiring activity-dependent mechanisms. Our findings in the sheep concur with their observations in that central projections of afferent fibres grow into the dorsal horn prior to innervation of the distal hind limbs.

Neurochemical development

In addition to the development of the anatomical substrate for sensory perception, the development of neurochemicals in these pathways is also a prerequisite for a functional system. Neuropeptides, excitatory amino acids and monamines have all been implicated in sensory transmission mechanisms in the spinal cord as neurotransmitters or neuromodulators. Substance P is found in small diameter DRG cells and Aδ and C fibre sensory afferents and calcitonin gene-related peptide (CGRP) is found in small to large DRG cells and Aα, Aβ, Aδ and C fibres. The excitatory amino acid glutamate (GLU) has been implicated as a neurotransmitter for at least some of the primary afferent fibres (Jessell et al., 1986). In the sheep, afferent fibres immunoreactive (IR) for Substance P or CGRP (Fig. 9.4) were present in Lissaeur's tract and lamina I of the dorsal horn by 56–61 days of gestation (Fig. 9.4), that is,

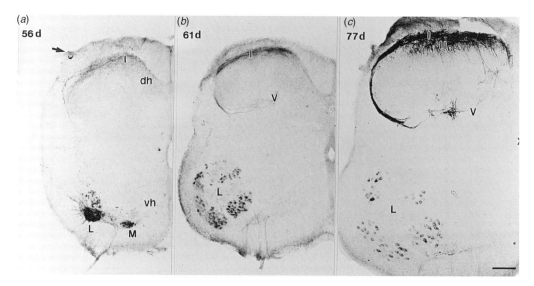

Fig. 9.4.   Photomicrographs of immunoreactivity for CGRP in the spinal cord of fetal and postnatal sheep. (*a*) At 56 d, CGRP-LI was seen in lamina I, the dorsolateral funiculus and in the tract of Lissauer (arrow). Medial (M) and lateral (L) motoneuron pools in the ventral horn were strongly immunoreactive. (*b*) By 61 d, fibres immunoreactive for CGRP were now present in the central region of lamina V. At this stage, intensely staining motoneurons were concentrated in the lateral motoneuron pool. (*c*) At 77 d, CGRP-LI fibres were found to extend into the central region of lamina II but this was predominantly in the outer layer of this lamina (II$_o$). A few fibres were also present in lamina X, the region surrounding the central canal. dh: dorsal horn; vh: ventral horn. Scale bar = 170 μm for (*a*)–(*c*).

within a few days of their arrival in the dorsal horn. The first appearance of peptides in the peripheral endings of primary afferent fibres in the skin of the fetal sheep is several weeks later at 85 days, at least 10 days after there is evidence of their presence with histological techniques. Similarly, in the rat, it has been reported that peptides were not present in the skin until some days after axons had innervated the dermis (Marti et al., 1987). In the human, a few CGRP-IR nerve fibres were first seen in the skin a few days after the time of skin innervation at 7 weeks. However, CGRP-IR was found more consistently at 17 weeks of gestation (Terenghi et al., 1993). CGRP is first detected in the dorsal horn at E17 in the rat and at week 10 in humans (Marti et al., 1987). Fibres immunoreactive for Substance P first appear in the dorsal horn at E16–E18 in the rat and at 11 weeks of gestation in the human. In terms of gestational period, the first appearance of these peptides is at 28% of gestation in humans, 38% in sheep and 79% in rats. In humans and sheep therefore, peptides are present for an extensive part of the intrauterine development of these pathways. It is possible that they play an important role in the normal growth and differentiation of the nervous system in addition to their role as neurotransmitters or neuromodulators. The reason for the delayed appearance of peptides in the periphery is not certain, but could be partly due to slower axonal transport in the peripheral branch of the developing sensory fibre or possibly to the peripheral release of peptides.

Functional development

In fetal sheep, the earliest age at which natural cutaneous stimulation could evoke activity in the DRG and dorsal horn was at 75 days gestation, that is at about mid-gestation (Rees et al., 1994a). These responses were low threshold with light stroking or indentation of the skin being an adequate stimulus to evoke brief discharge in DRG cells and in dorsal horn cells. Receptive fields were initially large, reducing in size with advancing gestational age. However, the overall impression we obtained from this study was that there was little change in the response patterns of the receptors with increasing gestational age. Although the action potentials of DRG cells tended to increase in size and decrease in duration and could be evoked at a higher frequency, there were no signs of an obvious shift in basic response types. It appears that very immature receptors are capable of responding to specific stimuli and further receptor development serves to enhance the fidelity of stimulus–response coding as indicated in Fig. 9.5. This impression was confirmed in the case of the wool/hair follicle receptors where it was possible to correlate functional and structural development. These afferents could be selectively stimulated by deflecting the wool/hair shaft and receptor units could be readily identified in microscopic analysis of the skin. The earliest response elicited from these afferents was phasic on/off and occurred at a stage when the follicle innervation was simple and just established (Fig. 9.2(*d*)). This pattern persisted throughout gestation even though there were major changes in the complexity and conformation of follicle innervation (Figs. 9.2(*f*), (*g*)). It is possible that the basic response properties of a receptor are already established at this stage of axon terminal formation and that further structural development refines the transduction process by shaping the sensitivity and firing sequence of the receptor–afferent unit.

Throughout gestation in the sheep, the majority of cells in the lumbar dorsal horn and DRGs responded to a low threshold cutaneous stimulus with cells responding to a high threshold mechanical stimulus being encountered less frequently. In the rat, primarily afferent fibres develop receptive fields to natural stimulation at E17 (Fitzgerald, 1987b) with dorsal horn cells developing receptive fields 2 days later at E19 (Fitzgerald, 1991): the delay possibly representing the maturation time of central synaptic connections. These results are consistent with behavioural studies in which stimulation of the plantar surface of the hind-limb produces a withdrawal reflex at E19 (Narayanan et al., 1971). In comparison to the sheep, the

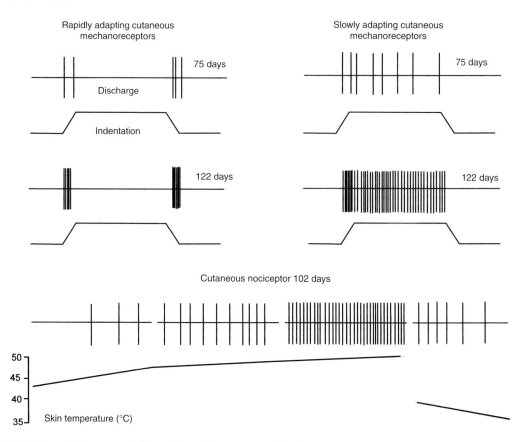

Fig. 9.5.   Diagrammatic illustrations of responses of developing cutaneous receptors in the sheep fetus. The top two traces show typical responses of receptor afferents to skin indentation at 75 days gestation (term ~147 days). The afferents signal the stimuli but do not respond with high frequency discharge. The traces underneath show responses of comparable receptor types in gestation where there is an improved ability to code both changing and steady pressure on the skin. The lowermost traces indicate the ability of a fetal cutaneous nociceptor to respond to noxious heat. This afferent was silent at normal skin temperature but started to discharge when the skin was heated to about 45 °C and fell silent again when heating was removed.

earliest responses in the rat from the skin of the hind paw were high threshold, requiring firm pressure to produce a few spikes (Fitzgerald, 1987b). The authors suggest that this might reflect an immaturity of synaptic connections rather than any preferential input from afferent nociceptors. In fact it has recently been shown that all direct cutaneous-evoked dorsal horn activity in the first postnatal week (and presumably before birth) results from activation of A fibres (Jennings & Fitzgerald, 1998). The formation of C fibre synaptic connections is almost entirely a postnatal event (Fitzgerald, 1987a) so C fibres do not become active until about P10 (Fitzgerald & Gibson, 1984).

As mentioned above, in the neonate, A fibres terminate in the dorsal horn in layers I–V withdrawing to layers III–V after about postnatal week 3; in the adult, layer II is the domain of C fibres. A fibre input in the neonate produces postsynaptic excitatory effects in dorsal horn cells, particularly sensitization, not seen in the adult; this might be important for normal sensory function in the developing mammalian system (Jennings & Fitzgerald, 1998). Large diameter primary afferent fibres in neonatal rats therefore, make synaptic contacts with presynaptic targets that presumably process nociceptive information (Coggeshall et al., 1996). Coggeshall et al. (1996) suggest that in ameliorating pain in neonates it might be more important to block low threshold sensory input whereas in adults it would be more important to block high threshold inputs. There is no direct evidence yet that a similar organizational change of A fibre input occurs in humans. If it does occur, we consider that it would most likely take place at some stage during fetal life in long gestational species such as sheep and humans where the spinal cord is far more developed at birth than it is in the rat. Clear lamination in the cord is not seen until E17 in the rat, while it is evident at week 13 in the fetus and at about day 61 in the sheep. It is known that cutaneous reflexes in the newborn human, as well as in the rat and kitten, are exaggerated compared to the adult. In neonatal humans, rats and kittens, flexor reflexes can be elicited by light touch rather than the noxious stimuli required in the adult (Ekholm, 1967; Fitzgerald & Gibson, 1984). This could be due to other aspects of developing spinal cord circuitry such as lack of descending inhibitory control and not necessarily to reorganization of input to lamina II.

There are further differences between the species in the functional development of cutaneous sensory input to the spinal cord. In the rat, spontaneous activity of cutaneous afferents in the DRG is present from E16, peaking at E18–19 (Fitzgerald, 1987b) and at E20–21 some dorsal horn cells displayed responses that outlasted the initial stimulus by 10–15s (Fitzgerald, 1991). Neither of these conditions was recorded in the sheep. These differences could relate to the different experimental conditions or could reflect species differences in the development of electrical properties of the sensory neurons or in the development of synaptic maturation.

In sheep we observed that the earliest responses of dorsal horn cells were sluggish and the action potential slow. It has been suggested that, during fetal development, there are significant changes in the ionic dependence of the inward current of the action potential in sensory neurons (Spitzer, 1994). This change frequently involves the gradual conversions of Ca^{2+}-dependent impulses of long duration into fast Na^+-mediated potentials. This conversion could explain the change in the shape of the action potential observed in sheep. It is not certain what role this alteration in ionic dependence might play in neural development, but it has been suggested that calcium transients might be important components in the pathway resulting in gene expression in differentiating cells (Spitzer, 1994).

Development of muscle afferents and their fibres

Structural development

The sequence of events involved in the innervation and structural development of mammalian muscle spindles has been well established in several species (Barker & Milburn, 1984), but much less is known about the functional development of muscle spindles in utero. Our work in the sheep (Rees et al., 1994b) has shown that the timing of the structural and functional development of muscle receptors and their afferent connections is closely associated with both the innervation of extrafusal muscle fibres and the appearance of early fetal movements. Immature afferent innervation of muscle spindles was evident at 67 days of gestation in the hind limb of fetal sheep (Fig. 9.6(a)). Innervation of extrafusal muscle fibres also occurs at about this time. At 67 days muscle spindle innervation was in the form of a fine network of fibres extending from two major branches; well formed annulospiral windings were not present and did not appear until approximately 83 days of gestation (Fig. 9.6(b)). With increasing gestational age (Fig. 9.6(c)–(e)) there was a progressive increase in the length of the spindle and in the complexity of its innervation, until ~127 days when it appears to have acquired the adult form. Fusimotor innervation of intrafusal fibres was evident from 83 days of gestation although specialized endings did not form until about 100 days. Muscle spindles in more rostral muscle groups such as the intercostal muscles develop earlier than the hind limbs at ~47 days.

Functional development

As with cutaneous receptors, the earliest age at which activity could be evoked in the DRG to muscle stretch was at 75 days of gestation (Rees et al., 1994b). It has been reported briefly that muscle afferents in the fetal rat discharge in response to a small change in limb position from E17 onwards, but there has not been an extensive developmental study in the fetal rat.

As mentioned above, muscle spindles in the sheep at 75 d are small and their afferent fibres are just beginning to form the annulospiral winding, characteristic of the mature spindle (Fig. 9.6(e)). Since it was possible to evoke activity in spindle afferents with an applied stretch at this age (Fig. 9.7), it appears that the annulospiral formation is not a necessary requirement for the generation of a response. The spindle at this age, however, does not appear to be capable of generating a consistent tonic response at resting muscle length, nor does it respond to stretch with a sustained train of discharges (Fig. 9.7). Within 2 weeks of the onset of activity (that is, by about 87 d) responses to stretch are easier to elicit. Receptors are beginning to

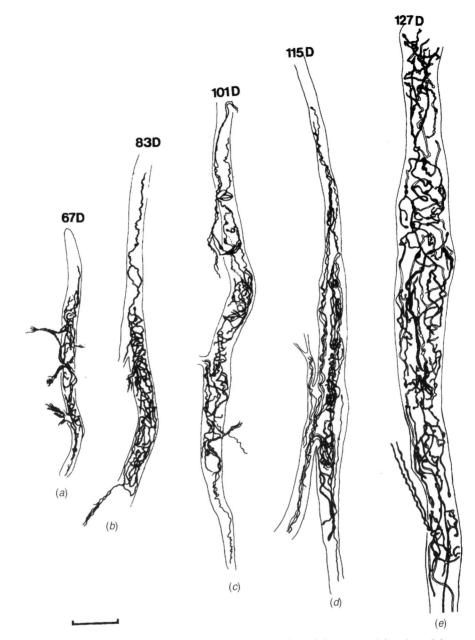

127 D

115 D

101 D

83D

67D

(a)

(b)

(c)

(d)

(e)

Fig. 9.6.   Camera lucida drawings of the entire sensory innervation of the equatorial region of the muscle spindles at 67(*a*), 83(*b*), 101(*c*), 115(*d*) and 127(*e*). These drawings were made to show the increase in the extent and complexity of the innervation with increasing gestational age. The solid lines represent the fibres on the upper surface of the intrafusal fibre and the unfilled lines, at the back of the fibres. The outlines of the individual intrafusal fibres have been omitted for clarity. Bar = 100 μm for all drawings. (Taken with permission from Rees et al., 1994b.)

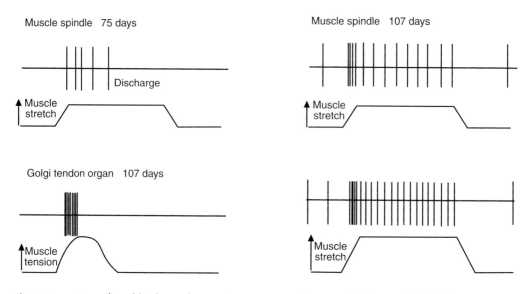

Fig. 9.7.   Examples of fetal muscle receptor responses. The upper left traces indicate the response
                of an immature muscle spindle afferent to a muscle stretch. The unit was responsive but
                only during the initial phase of the stretch and failed to signal the duration of the applied
                stretch. The sets of traces on the right show responses of a more mature muscle spindle
                at 107 days gestation. Here the afferent could signal a steady length change in the muscle
                and could also code muscle length by its discharge rate, as can be seen from the lower
                panel response where a greater stretch was applied to the muscle. Golgi tendon organs
                also develop functionally in utero as shown in the traces on the lower right which indicate
                an afferent responding to the rise of tension generated by a muscle twitch.

develop a tonic discharge at resting muscle length and the stretch-evoked response
displays clear static and dynamic sensitivities with the static component predomi-
nating. As indicated above, spindles are still relatively immature but annulospiral
windings are beginning to form and, in a few spindles, are well developed. These
results, in general, support the findings in the kitten (Patak et al., 1992), where
afferent responses demonstrating several features of the adult response are present
well before an annulospiral structure has developed.

   Spontaneous and evoked activity became more stable with increasing gestational
age (up to term). The frequency of the tonic discharge increased from 10 Hz at 87 d
to 35 Hz at 127 d and both static and dynamic sensitivities become more more pronounced. Parallel to this functional development was the progressive increase in the
complexity of the spindle innervation (Fig. 9.6). There were, however, no specific
structural changes which could be correlated with particular aspects of functional
development. Responses typical of Golgi tendon organs where the afferent responds
to the tension generated by a muscle twitch, were also evident in utero (Fig. 9.7).

Fusimotor innervation of intrafusal fibres was evident from 83 d although specialized endings did not form until about 101 d. Conduction velocity of all muscle receptor afferents increased markedly during the last four weeks of gestation. This is not unexpected in a precocious animal like the sheep which needs to have well developed motor control immediately after birth.

Experiments with the neural tracer biocytin revealed afferent projections to motoneuron pools by 67 d (Fig. 9.3(b)), that is just before muscle receptors had started to respond to stretch. The possibility therefore exists for even the earliest muscle receptor activity to influence motoneurons, and presumably other target neurons in the spinal cord. Furthermore, there was evidence of innervation of extrafusal muscle fibres by 67 d. Thus, the neural pathways required for reflex activity involving muscle spindles are present from early in gestation. In sheep, fetal movements can be observed with ultrasound by about 60 days.

Development of ascending pathways from spinal cord to brain

The most detailed information on the development of somatosensory projections to the thalamus and cerebral cortex has been obtained from the rat, and it appears that the first ascending projections reach their targets in synchrony and then undergo a phase of maturation in which the terminal arbors are fully developed. The cells of the central thalamus are born on E13 and have migrated and settled in position by E16–17 (Altman & Bayer, 1979). The first afferents from the trigeminal system (Leamey & Ho, 1998), and dorsal columns arrive in the thalamus at E17. After their arrival in the thalamus, the fibres continue to develop terminal arbors and at birth have formed a profuse innervation of the thalamus which continues to develop over several weeks postnatally (Asanuma et al., 1986). It appears that extensive maturation of the fibres is not required before they can transmit information, as they quickly establish functional synapses and are capable of activating thalamic cells at E7 (Leamey & Ho, 1998).

Fibres start to leave the thalamus at E16, arrive below the developing somatosensory cortex at E17 and then proceed to innervate the cortical tissue without any apparent delay (Catalano et al., 1991). The initial fibre arborizations in the cortex are rather simple and sparse but develop in size and complexity rather rapidly over a few days (Killackey et al., 1995). The growth of thalamic axons into the cortex and their maturation coincides with the establishment of structural and neurochemical patterns that are characteristic of cortical somatosensory representation of the body parts, which become clearly evident on the day of birth (Schlaggar & O'Leary, 1991).

The factors that guide and control the formation of the above connections are still poorly understood. The cortical subplate will be briefly mentioned, as it has been suggested that this structure may play an important role in the initial guidance of the thalamocortical axons up to and into the cortex. The subplate consists of a stratum of transient cells that are formed at E14, about a day before the cortex proper starts to develop above it (see Allendoerfer & Shatz, 1994). The thalamocortical fibres for some sensory systems such as the visual system in the cat (Ghosh & Shatz, 1992) pause for a time at the subplate as though waiting for a trigger signal which permits growth into the cortex. However, somatosensory thalamocortical fibres do not appear to wait at the subplate but grow directly through it to the developing cortex, and it has been suggested that the maturity of the cortex itself may be a factor in regulating the growth of thalamocortical projections (Catalano et al., 1991). For further discussion of the possible roles of the subplate in axon guidance see Allendoerfer and Shatz (1994) and Molnar and Blakemore (1995).

The overall picture which emerges from studies on the rat is that the substrates underlying discriminative sensation from the face and body start to develop just about halfway through gestation and progressively mature over several weeks of postnatal life with the refinement of afferent connections with the thalamus and cortex. In animals with a long gestation period, these stages of development are almost certainly attained in utero. For example, in humans cortical layer IV, which receives the thalamic afferents, begins to differentiate at about 18–20 weeks of gestation. Synapses begin to appear in the cortex shortly afterwards. Cortical evoked responses to somatosensory stimulation can be recorded at 25 weeks of gestation but are diffuse and largely undefined. By 29 weeks, a more mature response with a primary negative component has developed (Klimach & Cooke, 1988). In the sheep fetus, stimulation of the limbs evokes responses in somatosensory cortex at 120 days of gestation (Cook et al., 1987), indicating that the pathway to the cortex has already formed by this stage and is capable of transmitting somatosensory input. Very little is known about the development of the spinothalamic pathway which transmits information from nociceptors and thermal receptors. In the fetal sheep, fibre terminals from lumbar spinal cord cells appear in the thalamus between 120 and 130 days gestation (J. Rawson & S. Rees, unpublished observations), indicating that the spinothalamic projections are established before birth in this species.

Development of descending control systems

Transmission of all modalities of somatosensory input is potentially subject to control by descending systems that can 'gate' or modify the inflow of information to the thalamus or cerebral cortex according to functional requirements. Primary somatosensory cortex projects densely to the ventro–posterior thalamic complex where the medial lemniscus terminates (see Jones, 1984), and this projection presumably has an important role in finally regulating transmission of tactile and proprioceptive inputs to the cerebral cortex. In addition, the cortex also provides direct projections to the dorsal column nuclei, to the dorsal horn of the spinal cord (Coulter & Jones, 1977) and there is also a projection to Clarke's column which has been shown physiologically to control proprioceptive input from the hindlimb (McIntyre et al., 1989). Cortical input to the thalamus develops in utero, and a few projections from layer VI of somatosensory cortex to the thalamus are present in the rat as early as E16 (Catalano et al., 1991). However, it remains unclear when the cortex starts to influence transmission from the thalamus. Likewise, it is uncertain when the corticobulbar and corticospinal control systems first become operative, but this seems likely to happen postnatally.

Spinal transsection in rats has little influence on the reflex activity of the spinal cord before P12 (Weber & Stelzner, 1977) and in kittens before about 2–3 weeks of age (Ekholm, 1967). In humans, it seems that descending control from the cortex is also likely to develop after birth and mature over a prolonged period given that the corticospinal tract is poorly myelinated at birth and takes several years to develop fully. One of the first obvious signs of cortical modulation of sensory transmission in the spinal cord occurs at about 8–9 months of age when the plantar reflex changes from extensor to flexor.

The transmission of information from nociceptors can be potently inhibited by a descending anti-nociceptive pathway that projects to the spinal nucleus of the trigeminal and the dorsal horn of the spinal cord (for review, see Willis, 1988). A major component of this pathway originates in the raphe nuclei of the brainstem which provide serotonergic fibres that descend through the dorsolateral funinculus of the spinal cord and act via release of endogenous opioid peptides. Endogenous opioids and descending projections from the brainstem start to develop at an early intra-uterine stage in animals with a long gestation period. Encephalin-containing cells and fibres and opiate receptors are present in the human spinal cord at 4 weeks gestation (Charnay et al., 1984) and in the sheep fetus projections from the raphe nuclei are present in the lumbar spinal cord at 60 days gestation, which is less than halfway to term (J. Rawson & S. Rees, unpublished observations).

The most detailed information about development of this pathway has been obtained from the rat. Serotonergic fibres first appear in the spinal cord just before birth at E18 and continue to mature and establish connections in the dorsal horn, attaining an adult-like pattern at P21 (Bregman, 1987). Opioid peptides and receptors also start to appear just before birth, but the opioid system undergoes a prolonged phase of development and maturation that extends well into postnatal life and involves changes in the expression of different peptides and receptors (Rahman et al., 1998). This largely postnatal development of important components of the anti-nociceptive system in the rat correlates well with findings that stimulation of the dorsolateral funiculus of the spinal cord only starts to evoke inhibition in dorsal horn neurons after birth at P10 and inhibition becomes comparable with that seen in the adult by P22 (Fitzgerald & Koltzenburg, 1986). The sensitivity of C-fibre evoked responses to inhibition by morphine in the rat also develops postnatally and peaks at about P21.

Thus, in the rat, descending fibres and opiates are potentially capable of modulating nociceptive transmission by the first few weeks of postnatal life, but it is not yet clear for the rat or other species when the anti-nociceptive system begins to function under normal control.

Emergence of functional systems in utero

The onset of cutaneously evoked activity from the hind limb at E19 in the rat and 75 days of gestation in the sheep occurs at approximately similar stages of spinal cord development. In terms of gestational period, however, sensory pathways first become functional at 50% of gestation in the sheep but not until 87% of gestation in the rat. Muscle spindles in the hindlimb also respond to stretch at about 75 days of gestation in the sheep. As there is a rostro-caudal sequence of development, input from the face and snout in the sheep reach the spinal cord (and cortex) even earlier in gestation. As the sheep is a prenatal developer, required to exist independently at birth, it is not unexpected that these pathways begin to function earlier in the sheep than they do in an altricial species such as the rat.

The emergence of important features of somatosensory function in humans is summarized in Table 9.1. Observations of the human fetus with real-time ultrasound have shown that the first discernible movements are detectable at 7–8 weeks of postmenstrual age (de Vries et al., 1982). Movement of individual limbs occurs at about 9–10 weeks with more complex movements such as sucking and swallowing evident at 12–14 weeks. Recent ultrasound studies have suggested that handedness, the most prominent manifestation of behavioural lateralization in humans, develops from about 10 weeks of gestational age (Hepper et al., 1998). Fetuses showed a highly significant preference for arm movement with 85% exhibiting more right than left arm movement. In aborted fetuses it has been possible to evoke movements from light stimulation in the perioral region from 6–7 weeks (gestational age) (Hogg, 1941). This indicates that low threshold mechanoreceptors are operative at this age and have established functional connections with motoneurons. Structural connectivity has been confirmed in ultrastructural studies where synapses between sensory, interneurons and motoneurons have been demonstrated at 5.5 to 6 weeks of gestation (Okado, 1981). By 14 weeks, stimulation of most areas of the body surface can evoke reflex responses.

Why is it necessary for these pathways to become functional so early in gestation? In the developing mammalian visual system, it has been clearly demonstrated that

Table 9.1. Emergence of fetal behaviour in humans

Behaviour	Methods of assessment	Age of first appearance	Reference
Movement in response to peripheral stimulation	Cutaneous stimulation, ex utero fetus	6–7 weeks	(Hogg, 1941)
First discernible movement	Ultrasound	7–8 weeks	(de Vries et al., 1982)
Iolated arm movement	Ultrasound	9–10 weeks	(de Vries et al., 1982)
Jaw opening	Ultrasound	10–11 weeks	(de Vries et al., 1982)
Stretch	Ultrasound	10–11 weeks	(de Vries et al., 1982)
Evidence of handedness, right predominance	Ultrasound	10 weeks	(Hepper et al., 1998)
Marked increase in changes in fetal position	Ultrasound	10 weeks onwards, peaked 15 weeks	(de Vries et al., 1982)
Hand sensitive to touch	Cutaneous stimulation, ex utero fetus	10.5 weeks	(see Humphrey, 1978)
Sucking and swallowing movements	Ultrasound	12–14 weeks	(de Vries et al., 1982)
Reflex activity evoked by stimulation of most body areas	Cutaneous stimulation, ex utero fetus	14 weeks	(see Humphrey, 1978)
Cutaneous withdrawal reflex	Cutaneous stimulation, premature infant	26 weeks	(Andrews & Fitzgerald, 1994)
Cortical evoked responses to somatosensory stimulation	Cutaneous stimulation, premature infant	25–29 weeks	(Klimach & Cooke, 1988)
Coordinated facial actions indicative of pain	Heel prick, premature infant	26–31 weeks	(Craig et al., 1993)
Peak incidence of flexion and stretch during gestation	Ultrasound	28–31 weeks	(Kozuma et al., 1997)
Lateralized head position (mainly to right)	Ultrasound	38 weeks	(Ververs et al., 1994)

appropriate functional activity is a necessary requirement for normal development (Goodman & Shatz, 1993; Penn & Shatz, 1999). However, in relation to the somatosensory system it has been shown that, at least in some species, such as birds, patterned neuronal activity is not essential for the specification of pathways in the stretch reflex. Rather, it has been suggested that pre- and postsynaptic neurons have a distinctive molecular phenotype at the time of synaptogenesis and that this forms the basis for the formation of the correct patterning of synaptic connections. Whether this applies to mammals has yet to be determined. Currently, the only evidence of rearrangement of synaptic connections during development of the primary afferent innervation of the spinal cord is the withdrawal of A fibres from lamina II during the first 3 weeks postnatally in the rat. In any event, neural activity could play an important role in the reinforcement of pathways once they have formed. Certainly in the adult mammalian somatosensory system, activity in primary afferents plays an important role in shaping and maintaining receptive fields. This is well illustrated by findings that, after loss of input from a part of the body, the cortical receptive fields or representations of adjacent parts expand and occupy the area where the denervated part was present.

It must be pointed out, however, that input from somatosensory receptors is utilized by numerous functional systems and not just by those subserving conscious perception. The cerebellum receives a massive somatosensory input from several pathways originating in the spinal cord and brainstem. And, for example, there are somatosensory inputs to the hypothalamus, vestibular nuclei, inferior colliculus, parabrachial nuclei and respiratory control centres of the brainstem. In addition, the operations of the reflex circuitry of the spinal cord are dependent on input from receptors. Thus, there are potentially numerous circuits that might require somatosensory input during some stage of development.

Within the uterus, stimulation of low threshold cutaneous mechanoreceptors in the fetus could occur with movement of the amniotic fluid, contractions of the myometrium of the uterus or from self stimulation as limbs touch the body and fingers touch the face. This could then result in reflex contraction of muscles and activation of Golgi tendon organs and muscle spindles. Muscle spindles would also be activated by changes in limb position and these receptors also generate resting or background activity as they develop. Ultrasound studies have demonstrated that there is a marked increase in the rate of change in position of the fetus from about 10 weeks onwards peaking at 15 weeks, after which time there are spatial restrictions on fetal movement (de Vries et al., 1982).

Whether a fetus can 'feel' pain in utero is controversial. Some definitions of pain imply that the brain must achieve a certain level of neural functioning as well as having prior experience before pain can be understood (see Lloyd-Thomas &

Fitzgerald, 1996). Such a definition would exclude the fetus from 'feeling' pain. It is clear, however, that the fetal nervous system can respond to potentially damaging stimuli at the beginning of the last trimester. At about 26 weeks of gestation, premature infants show a measurable flexion withdrawal reflex to noxious stimulation suggesting that the nociceptive afferent input to the spinal cord is present and can function at this age (Andrews & Fitzgerald, 1994). It is reasonable to assume that such responses could also occur in utero, although it is difficult to envisage nociceptor activation occurring during fetal life except perhaps during fetal surgery. If the transient connections between A fibres (which originate from low threshold mechanoreceptors) and lamina II neurons described above for the rat also exist in humans, they might provide a means of generating input to nociceptive pathways during critical phases of development when none is likely to come from nociceptors themselves. In addition to spinal reflexes, infants delivered at 26–31 weeks show coordinated facial actions indicative of pain, such as brow bulging, eyes squeezed shut and open mouth in response to a heel prick (Craig et al., 1993).

It is still not certain whether nociceptor activation in the premature infant, or in the fetus, would be perceived as pain at this early age given the observations that sensory impulses do not evoke a mature cortical response until 29 weeks of gestational age (Klimach & Cooke, 1988). Any assessment of pain in the neonate must also take into account that the infant nervous system has a very low threshold for excitation. In the case of the cutaneous withdrawal reflex, features of the response evoked preferentially or specifically by noxious stimuli in the adult, can be evoked by non-noxious stimuli in the neonate. Apart from the question of pain perception, however, there is now increasing evidence that early exposure to noxious stimuli results in adverse effects on future neural development. That is to say, noxious stimulation might not need to reach consciousness to substantially alter the course of sensory development and postnatal outcome for the individual.

In summary, the essential anatomical substrates for transmitting somatosensory input to the cerebral cortex appear to be established prior to birth in man, in the sheep and presumably also in other species which undergo considerable development in utero during a long gestation period. This information still does not provide for an obvious answer to the question as to when stimulation of the body can first be perceived by a fetus or neonate. But, once essential projections are present and have matured in the cortex, there may be no obvious critical stage or defining point in development that results in a step from non-perception to perception of a stimulus. It seems more likely that these properties emerge gradually and mature over a long period of time in parallel with the maturation of cortical functions as a whole.

REFERENCES

Acheson, A., Conover, J. C., Fandl, J. P. et al. (1995). A BDNF autocrine loop in adult sensory neurons prevents cell death [see comments]. *Nature*, **374**, 450–3.

Airaksinen, M. S., Koltzenburg, M., Lewin, G. R. et al. (1996). Specific subtypes of cutaneous mechanoreceptors require neurotrophin-3 following peripheral target innervation. *Neuron*, **16**, 287–95.

Allendoerfer, K. L. & Shatz, C. J. (1994). The subplate, a transient neocortical structure: its role in the development of connections between the thalamus and cortex. *Annual Review in Neuroscience*, **17**, 185–218.

Altman, J. & Bayer, S. A. (1979). Development of the diencephalon in the rat. IV. Quantitative study of the time of origin of neurons and the internuclear chronological gradients in the thalamus. *Journal of Comparative Neurology*, **188**, 455–71.

Andrews, K. & Fitzgerald, M. (1994). The cutaneous withdrawal reflex in human neonates: sensitization, receptive fields, and the effects of contralateral stimulation. *Pain*, **56**, 95–101.

Asanuma, C., Ohkawa, R., Stanfield, B. B. & Cowan, W. M. (1986). Pre- and postnatal development of the medial lemniscus (ML), the branchium conjuctivum (BC) and the brachium of the inferior colliculus (BIC) in rats. *Society for Neuroscience*, **12**, 953 (Abstract).

Barde, Y. A. (1989) Trophic factors and neuronal survival. *Neuron*, **2**, 1525–34.

Barker, D. & Milburn, A. (1984). Development and regeneration of mammalian muscle spindles. *Science Progress*, **69**, 45–64.

Bregman, B. S. (1987). Development of serotonin immunoreactivity in the rat spinal cord and its plasticity after neonatal spinal cord lesions. *Brain Research*, **431**, 245–63.

Catalano, S. M., Robertson, R. T. & Killackey, H. P. (1991). Early ingrowth of thalamocortical afferents to the neocortex of the prenatal rat. *Proceedings of the National Academy of Sciences, USA*, **88**, 2999–3003.

Charnay, Y., Paulin, C., Dray, F. & Dubois, P. M. (1984). Distribution of enkephalin in human fetus and infant spinal cord: an immunofluorescence study. *Journal of Comparative Neurology*, **223**, 415–23.

Coggeshall, R. E., Jennings, E. A. & Fitzgerald, M. (1996). Evidence that large myelinated primary afferent fibers make synaptic contacts in lamina II of neonatal rats. *Brain Research. Brain Research Reviews*, **92**, 8–90.

Cook, C. J., Gluckman, P. D., Johnston, B. M. & Williams, C. (1987). The development of the somatosensory evoked potential in the unanaesthetized fetal sheep. *Journal of Developmental Physiology*, **9**, 441–55.

Coulter, J. D. & Jones, E. G. (1977). Differential distribution of corticospinal projections from individual cytoarchitectonic fields in the monkey. *Brain Research*, **129**, 335–40.

Craig, K. D., Whitfield, M. F., Grunau, R. V., Linton, J. & Hadjistavropoulos, H. D. (1993). Pain in the preterm neonate: behavioural and physiological indices [published erratum appears in *Pain*, **54**(1),111]. *Pain*, **52**, 287–99.

Crowley, C., Spencer, S. D., Nishimura, M. C. et al. (1994). Mice lacking nerve growth factor display perinatal loss of sensory and sympathetic neurons yet develop basal forebrain cholinergic neurons. *Cell*, **76**, 1001–11.

De Vries, J. I., Visser, G. H. & Prechtl, H. F. (1982). The emergence of fetal behaviour. I. Qualitative aspects. *Early Human Development*, **7**, 301–22.

Ekholm, J. (1967). Postnatal changes in cutaneous reflexes and in the discharge pattern of cutaneous and articular sense organs. A morphological and physiological study in the cat. *Acta Physiologica Scandinavica*, **297**, 1–130.

Ernfors, P., Lee, K. F., Kucera, J. & Jaenisch, R. (1994). Lack of neurotrophin-3 leads to deficiencies in the peripheral nervous system and loss of limb proprioceptive afferents. *Cell*, **77**, 503–12.

Farinas, I., Yoshida, C. K., Backus, C. & Reichardt, L. F. (1996). Lack of neurotrophin-3 results in death of spinal sensory neurons and premature differentiation of their precursors. *Neuron*, **17**, 1065–78.

Fitzgerald, M. (1987a). Prenatal growth of fine-diameter primary afferents into the rat spinal cord: a transganglionic tracer study. *Journal of Comparative Neurology*, **261**, 98–104.

Fitzgerald, M. (1987b). Spontaneous and evoked activity of fetal primary afferents in vivo. *Nature*, **326**, 603–5.

Fitzgerald, M. (1991). A physiological study of the prenatal development of cutaneous sensory inputs to dorsal horn cells in the rat. *Journal of Physiology (London)*, **432**, 473–82.

Fitzgerald, M. & Gibson, S. (1984). The postnatal physiological and neurochemical development of peripheral sensory C fibres. *Neuroscience*, **13**, 933–44.

Fitzgerald, M. & Koltzenburg, M. (1986). The functional development of descending inhibitory pathways in the dorsolateral funinculus of the newborn rat spinal cord. *Brain Research*, **389**, 261–70.

Fitzgerald, M., Butcher, T. & Shortland, P. (1994). Developmental changes in the laminar termination of A fibre cutaneous sensory afferents in the rat spinal cord dorsal horn. *Journal of Comparative Neurology*, **348**, 225–33.

Ghosh, A. & Shatz, C. J. (1992). Involvement of subplate neurons in the formation of ocular dominance columns. *Science*, **255**, 1441–3.

Goodman, C. S. & Shatz, C. J. (1993). Developmental mechanisms that generate precise patterns of neuronal connectivity. *Cell*, **72**, 77–98.

Hepper, P. G., McCartney, G. R. & Shannon, E. A. (1998). Lateralised behaviour in first trimester human fetuses. *Neuropsychologia*, **36**, 531–4.

Hogg, I. D. (1941). Sensory nerves and associated structures in the skin of human fetuses of 8 to 14 weeks of menstrual age correlated with functional capacity. *Journal of Comparative Neurology*, **75**, 371–410.

Humphrey, T. (1978). Function of the nervous system during prenatal life. In *Perinatal Physiology*, ed. U. Stave and A. A. Weech, pp. 651–83. New York: Plenum Press.

Jennings, E. & Fitzgerald, M. (1998). Postnatal changes in responses of rat dorsal horn cells to afferent stimulation: a fibre-induced sensitization. *Journal of Physiology (London)*, **509**, 859–68.

Jessell, T. M., Yoshioka, K. & Jahr, C. E. (1986). Amino acid receptor-mediated transmission at primary afferent synapses in rat spinal cord. *Journal of Experimental Biology*, **124**, 239–58.

Jones, E. C. (1984). *The Thalamus.* New York: Plenum Press.

Killackey, H. P., Rhoades, R. W. & Bennett, C. C. (1995). The formation of a cortical somatotopic map. *Trends in Neuroscience,* **18,** 402–7.

Klimach, V. J. & Cooke, R. W. (1988). Maturation of the neonatal somatosensory evoked response in preterm infants. *Developmental Medicine and Child Neurology,* **30,** 208–14.

Kozuma, S., Okai, T., Nemoto, A., Kagawa, H., Sakai, M., Nishina, H. & Taketani, Y. (1997). Developmental sequence of human fetal body movements in the second half of pregnancy. *American Journal of Perinatology,* **14,** 165–9.

Leamey, C. A. & Ho, S. M. (1998). Afferent arrival and onset of functional activity in the trigeminothalamic pathway of the rat. *Brain Research. Brain Research Reviews,* **105,** 195–207.

Lloyd-Thomas, A. R. & Fitzgerald, M. (1996). Do fetuses feel pain? Reflex responses do not necessarily signify pain. *British Medical Journal,* **313,** 797–8.

McIntyre, A. K., Proske, U. & Rawson, J. A. (1989). Corticofugal action on transmission of group I input from the hindlimb to the pericruciate cortex in the cat. *Journal of Physiology (London),* **416,** 19–30.

Mallat, M., Houlgatte, R., Brachet, P. & Prochiantz, A. (1989). Lipopolysaccharide-stimulated rat brain macrophages release NGF in vitro. *Developmental Biology,* **133,** 309–11.

Marti, E., Gibson, S. J., Polak, J. M. et al. (1987). Ontogeny of peptide- and amine-containing neurones in motor, sensory, and autonomic regions of rat and human spinal cord, dorsal root ganglia, and rat skin. *Journal of Comparative Neurology,* **266,** 332–59.

Mirnics, K. & Koerber, H. R. (1995). Prenatal development of rat primary afferent fibers: II. Central projections. *Journal of Comparative Neurology,* **355,** 601–14.

Molnar Z. & Blakemore, C. (1995). How do thalamic axons find their way to the cortex? *Trends in Neuroscience,* **18,** 389–97.

Narayanan, C. H., Fox, M. W. & Hamburger, V. (1971). Prenatal development of spontaneous and evoked activity in the rat (*Rattus norvegicus* albinus). *Behaviour,* **40,** 100–34.

Oakley, R. A., Garmer. A. S, Large, T. H. & Frank, E. (1995). Muscle sensory neurons require neurotrophin-3 from peripheral tissues during the period of normal cell death. *Development,* **121,** 1341–50.

Ockel, M., Lewin, G. R. & Barde, Y. A. (1996). In vivo effects of neurotrophin-3 during sensory neurogenesis. *Development,* **122,** 301–7.

Okado, N. (1981). Onset of synapse formation in the human spinal cord. *Journal of Comparative Neurology,* **201,** 211–19.

Patak, A., Proske, U., Turner, H. & Gregory, J. E. (1992). Development of the sensory innervation of muscle spindles in the kitten. *International Journal of Developmental Neuroscience,* **10,** 81–92.

Penn, A. A. & Shatz, C. J. (1999). Brain waves and brain wiring: the role of endogenous and sensory-driven neural activity in development. *Pediatric Research,* **45,** 447–58.

Rahman, W., Dashwood, M. R., Fitzgerald, M., Aynsley, G. A. & Dickenson, A. H. (1998). Postnatal development of multiple opioid receptors in the spinal cord and development of spinal morphine analgesia. *Brain Research. Brain Research Reviews.* **108,** 239–54.

Rees, S., Nitsos, I. & Rawson, J. (1994a). The development of cutaneous afferent pathways in fetal sheep: a structural and functional study. *Brain Research,* **661,** 207–22.

Rees, S., Rawson, J., Nitsos, I. & Brumley, C. (1994b). The structural and functional development of muscle spindles and their connections in fetal sheep. *Brain Research*, **642**, 185–198.

Schlaggar, B. L. & O'Leary, D. D. (1991). Potential of visual cortex to develop an array of functional units unique to somatosensory cortex. *Science*, **252**, 1556–60.

Smeyne, R. J., Klein, R., Schnapp, A. et al. (1994). Severe sensory and sympathetic neuropathies in mice carrying a disrupted Trk/NGF receptor gene. *Nature*, **368**, 246–9.

Smith, C. L. (1983). The development and postnatal organization of primary afferent projections to the rat thoracic spinal cord. *Journal of Comparative Neurology*, **220**, 29–43.

Spitzer, N. C. (1994). Spontaneous Ca2$^+$ spikes and waves in embryonic neurons: signaling systems for differentiation. *Trends in Neuroscience*, **17**, 115–18.

Terenghi, G., Sundaresan, M., Moscoso, G. & Polak, J. M. (1993). Neuropeptides and a neuronal marker in cutaneous innervation during human fetal development. *Journal of Comparative Neurology*, **328**, 595–603.

Ververs, I. A., de Vries, J. I., van Geijn, H. P. & Hopkins, B. (1994). Prenatal head position from 12–38 weeks. II. The effects of fetal orientation and placental localization. *Early Human Development*, **39**, 93–100.

Weber, E. D. & Stelzner, D. J. (1977). Behavioural effects of spinal cord transection in the developing rat. *Brain Research*, **125**, 241–55.

Willis, W. D. J. (1988). Anatomy and physiology of descending control of nociceptive responses of dorsal horn neurons: comprehensive review. *Progress in Brain Research*, **77**, 1–29.

Willis, W. D. & Coggeshall, R. E. (1991) Sensory mechanisms of the spinal cord. New York: Plenum Press.

10

Principles of endogenous and sensory activity-dependent brain development. The visual system

Anna A. Penn[1] and Carla J. Shatz[2]

[1]Department of Neonatology and Developmental Medicine, Lucille Salter Packard Children's Hospital at Stanford, CA, USA
[2]Department of Neurobiology, Harvard Medical School, Boston, MA, USA

Activity-dependent remodeling of early neural connections

Neural activity is critical for sculpting the intricate circuits of the nervous system from initially imprecise neuronal connections. Disruptions in early neural activity, and thus disruptions in the formation of precise circuits, may underlie many common neurodevelopmental disorders, ranging from subtle learning disorders to pervasive developmental delay. The necessity for sensory-driven activity has been widely recognized as crucial for infant brain development. Recent studies have revealed a similar requirement for endogenous neural activity generated by the nervous system itself, long before there is any sensory input. These patterns of sensory-driven and endogenously generated neural activity sculpt the precise circuits that are crucial to the many complex functions of the adult brain. In this chapter, the principles of activity-dependent development are illustrated by the mechanisms that form the precise connections of the mammalian visual system. Experiments that indicate that similar activity-dependent mechanisms are at work shaping many parts of the nervous system are also reviewed. Understanding the processes of activity-dependent development should contribute substantially to our future ability to identify, prevent, and treat many neurodevelopmental disorders that result from disruptions of neural activity during critical periods in brain development.

As the human brain develops, billions of neurons cause an average of 1000 synapses to become interconnected in precise neural circuits. How are these complex neural connections established? First, cells must be generated by successive cell divi-

This chapter is modified from a prior review entitled 'Brain waves and brain wiring: the role of endogenous and sensory-driven neural activity in development' *Pediatric Research* (1999) **45**, 447–58, by permission of the publishers.

sions and their identity must be determined – as neurons, and then as particular classes of neurons. Secondly, neurons from one region must extend axons along specific pathways to appropriate target regions to form the linked pieces of a functional system. However, the initial pattern of connections is often imprecise. The third step, focused on here, is the refinement of these connections to form the specific patterns of connectivity that characterize the mature brain.

The first two steps, cell type determination and pathway formation, are often referred to as 'activity-independent' processes because, in general, neuronal activity (i.e. transmission between presynaptic and postsynaptic partners via action potentials and neurotransmitter release) is not required for these processes to occur. Rather, signals for differentiation, cell type determination, and axonal guidance are given by genetically specified molecular cues that appear to provide for the reliable construction of a stereotyped framework (Goodman & Shatz, 1993). In contrast, the elaboration, retraction, and remodeling of neural connections within their targets is thought to be 'activity-dependent' because the ultimate patterns of connections can be disrupted by blockade of neuronal activity (Goodman & Shatz, 1993; Katz & Shatz, 1996).

Much laboratory and clinical work has focused on neurogenetics and the role of activity-independent factors in neurologic diseases of infants and children (for review, see Sarnat, 1992). Numerous 'activity-independent' neurologic diseases have been described: disorders of neural induction (anencephaly); disorders of neurogenesis (as seen in the 'minibrain' mutation); disorders of programmed cell death (spinal muscular atrophy); disorders of neural migration (focal dysplasias or heterotopias); and disorders of axonal pathfinding (agenesis of the corpus callosum). However, the list of 'activity-dependent' disorders is much shorter. It is not that these disorders do not exist, rather they are under recognized. Abnormal neuronal activity patterns have been implicated as the basis for widespread, diverse disorders including the progressive severity of some types of epilepsies (as in West syndrome in which hypsarrhythmia may promote the development of other epileptic circuits: Schwartzkroin, 1995; developmental delay: Huttenlocher, 1991; and autism: Bauman et al., 1997). Traditional histologic and radiologic studies in human subjects can visualize only the most profound disruptions in connectivity – those that result in major structural defects. Yet animal studies indicate that manipulations that disrupt normal neural activity can cause large changes in the detailed patterns of synaptic connections while leaving gross brain structure intact (Shatz & Stryker, 1988). Detailed histologic studies in pathology specimens from children who have epilepsy or metal retardation are rare, although they can show striking changes in dendritic patterning (Sarnat, 1992). In addition, the 'activity-independent' disorders mentioned above often result in abnormal neuronal circuitry making primary and secondary causes of neurologic diseases difficult to untangle. Non-invasive functional imaging techniques, such as positron emission tomography, functional magnetic resonance imaging, and spectroscopy, are beginning to allow the exploration of functional changes in neural circuitry during development. As the resolution of these techniques improves, there is likely to be an explosion in the number of developmental neurologic disorders identified as 'activity dependent'.

The developing visual pathway as a model system

The difficulties in studying the role of activity-dependent developmental processes in humans emphasizes the need for good animal models. The development of the mammalian visual pathway is a model system for illustrating the principles of activity-dependent synaptic refinement: the precise anatomy of this pathway is well-defined; the need for neural activity in the formation of visual connectivity has been documented; specific patterns of neural activity present in this pathway have been described; and the mechanisms of synaptic reorganization underlying the fine-tuning of these connections are being investigated intensively.

The anatomy of the system

In most adult mammalian visual systems, from mouse to human, RGC (retinal ganglion cell) axons from each eye project to the LGN (lateral geniculate nucleus) on both sides of the brain, with the axons from nasally placed ganglion cells projecting to the contralateral LGN, and axons from the temporally placed ganglion cells projecting to the ipsilateral LGN (see Fig. 10.1(a) in colour plate section). Within the LGN, the axons from the two eyes terminate in a set of separate, alternating layers in which LGN neurons receive purely monocular inputs. In addition to the ocular segregation pattern of the LGN, there is a topographic patterning to the connections such that the nearest neighbour relations of the RGC are preserved, projecting a retinotopic map of one hemisphere of the visual world onto the opposite LGN. In turn, LGN neurons project to layer IV of the primary visual cortex, where the axons are sorted into ODC (ocular dominance columns), in which alternating ½-mm wide columns of cortical neurons are driven only by input from one eye, and into orientation columns (or 'pinwheels'), and the retinotopic map is again preserved (Rodieck, 1979). RGC also project to the superior colliculus, and the axon terminals are again grouped in an eye-specific and cell class-specific manner (Stein, 1984).

In the initial development of the visual system, neither the layers in the LGN nor the cortical ODC are present, and the retinotopic map is crude (for review, see Chalupa & White, 1990). When RGC axons from each eye first innervate the LGN, they are intermingled in most of the nucleus (Fig. 10.1(b)) (Sretavan & Shatz, 1986). The LGN neurons receive binocular innervation during this period (Shatz

& Kirkwood, 1984), but, through a process of axon retraction and elaboration, connections are refined and the adult pattern emerges. Similarly, the LGN projections to layer IV are initially intermingled. LGN axons representing either the right or left eye then segregate to define ODC in the primary visual cortex (LeVay et al., 1978). In all mammals, the segregation of axons into eye-specific layers in the LGN precedes the formation of the cortical ODC.

General principles of activity-dependent development

Competition shapes the patterns of connections

Many experiments, beginning with those of Hubel and Wiesel (Hubel & Wiesel, 1965, 1970), have indicated that visual experience plays a key role in segregation of LGN axons to form ODC in layer IV of the primary visual cortex (Goodman & Shatz, 1993). Segregation is thought to be achieved by an activity-mediated competitive process involving the formation, and elimination, of specific synapses. The process is competitive in the sense that unequal levels of activity, or use, result in the dominance of connections from the more active eye at the expense of those from the less active eye. Segregation of LGN axons into ODC in the cortex is thought to occur from the initially intermixed state by a process in which interactions between LGN axons lead to the strengthening of those inputs that are simultaneously active, and activate the postsynaptic neuron, at the expense of those synapses that are not active synchronously and are consequently weakened and eliminated (Fig. 10.2(*a*)). These synapses are likely to have characteristics of Hebbian synapses – defined as synapses that are strengthened by the synchronous firing of both presynaptic and postsynaptic neurons (Hebb, 1949). In other words 'cells that fire together, wire together' and, as a corollary, 'those that don't, won't'. When this process is disrupted by unequal activity levels in the two sets of inputs, the active inputs have a competitive advantage and gain more connections.

As Hubel and Wiesel first observed in the 1960s (Hubel & Wiesel, 1965), closing one eye in a kitten during its early postnatal development profoundly disrupted the pattern of ODC; the eye that had visual input dominated the cortex, whereas the closed eye lost its connections. Cortical connections to the opened or closed eye as assessed both physiologically (Hubel & Wiesel, 1970; Blakemore & Van Sluyters, 1975) and anatomically (Antonini & Stryker, 1993) can be changed in less than a single week of deprivation. These experiments show that the balance of activity, not just vision itself, is crucial to the refinement of these connections. When both eyes are closed and consequently there is no imbalance in ocular activity, the ODC can still form, but much more slowly (Mower et. al., 1985). Even with binocular eye closure, columns can still form, most likely as a result of competition because ganglion cells are spontaneously active in the dark (Mastronarde, 1989). Visual deprivation does not abolish this spontaneous activity. Moreover, anatomic studies show

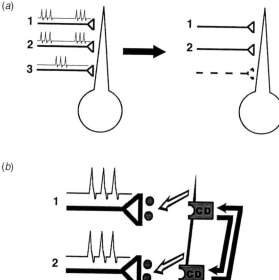

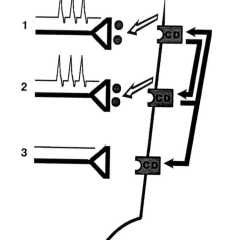

Fig. 10.2.   (a). Synaptic modifications based on patterns of activity. When coinnervating axons are synchronously active (axons 1 and 2; illustrated by the pattern of action potentials drawn schematically above each axon) with the postsynaptic neuron, they will both be maintained and strengthened. However, when a co-innervating axon is asynchronously active (axon 3), then this axonal connection will be lost. (b), Predicted signals for the activity-dependent refinement of connections. An enlargement of the schematic shown in (a) illustrates the basic mechanisms that are necessary for activity-dependent competition. When axons 1 and 2 fire action potentials synchronously and depolarize the postsynaptic neuron, the postsynaptic neuron must have a mechanism for detecting this coincident firing (a coincidence detector [CD], such as an NMDA receptor). When presynaptic axons are simultaneously active, a 'retraction' signal is produced (black arrows). The active axons (1 and 2) are protected from elimination, perhaps by a retrograde messenger that specifically stabilizes only active synapses (open arrows). When the inactive axon receives the retraction signal (axon 3), it is not protected and will therefore be eliminated. When all of the axons are inactive (not shown), no signals will be sent and the connection will remain (although they may be weaker than normal because of lack of support from retrograde messengers, such as neurotrophins; see text). Note that the messengers that govern protection and retraction may be presynaptically or postsynaptically generated (they are shown as postsynaptic here only for simplicity).

that in monkeys, the ODC are already segregating in utero (Horton & Hocking, 1996), and that in ferrets ODC start to form prior to eye opening (Crowley & Katz, 2000). There is current debate as to whether the initial segregation of ODC is therefore actually activity-dependent (Crowley & Katz, 2000), but it may depend on competitive interactions driven by spontaneous activity coming from the retina via the LGN (see below), or from the LGN itself.

ODC segregation can be blocked by eliminating all ascending activity in the visual pathway, achieved by silencing RGC activity intraocularly with the sodium-channel blocker TTX (tetrodotoxin) (Stryker & Harris, 1986). If the optic nerves are then stimulated electrically, the normal shift from initial binocular innervation of cortical neurons to the emergence of monocularly driven cells can be achieved (as assessed physiologically), indicating that neural activity drives this process (Stryker & Strickland, 1984). However, electrical stimulation only induces ocular segregation at the cortical level when it is applied to the two optic nerves in an alternating (asynchronous) manner. If the optic nerves are stimulated synchronously, cortical neurons remain binocularly innervated and segregation does not occur. This stimulation regimen does not alter the eye-specific LGN layers that have already formed. Additionally, recent experiments demonstrate that synchronous stimulation of RGC axons can disrupt the development of precise orientation tuning in the visual cortex (Weliky & Katz, 1997). Further support for the role of afferent activity in developing orientation tuning comes from studies in which visual axons are rerouted into auditory cortex, but still develop the connections necessary to create orientation tuned groups of neurons (Sharma et al., 2000). Because orientation tuning also depends on precisely patterned cortical connections, this experiment suggests a role for competitive, activity-dependent interactions in the development of yet another set of specific functional circuits.

Additional evidence for the role of neural competition in generating precise connections comes from studies of cold-blooded vertebrates (for review, see Cline, 1991). Neural activity is required for topographic map development in the tectum (the equivalent of the superior colliculus in mammals) and for the segregation of eye-specific stripes that can be experimentally induced in frog optic tectum. (The 'three-eyed' frog model is produced by grafting a third eye that sends its RGC axons to the tectum, normally monocular in frogs, such that the axons from the two eyes now innervating a single tectum segregate into eye-specific stripe.) Blockade of activity prevents refinement of the retinotectal map from an initially coarse projection and desegregates the eye-specific stripes in the tectum of the three-eyed frog, which require activity to be maintained even after they have formed because the frog tectum continues to grow throughout life. Again, experiments show that it is the temporal pattern of neural activity that is critical for the process of axonal refinement. Rearing goldfish or three-eyed frogs under strobe-lights, which synchronizes the activity of all ganglion cells, prevents topographic map refinement in the fish and eye-specific stripe formation in frogs. Taken together, these observations demonstrate that not just activity *per se,* but specific aspects of the timing of electrical activity, is necessary for this axonal segregation. Synapse formation on the basis of spatiotemporally correlated activity may be a general mechanism used throughout the vertebrate nervous system to establish precise connections (Goodman & Shatz, 1993; Katz & Shatz, 1996).

Critical periods for competition

The time when normal patterns of neural activity are necessary for the formation of the adult pattern of connections is called the 'critical period' for the development of those connections. In humans, one example of activity-driven rearrangements occurring during a critical period is the dramatic loss of functional vision (e.g. amblyopia) in one eye that occurs when a child younger than 18 mo with a cataract goes untreated for more than 1 to 2 wk (Daw, 1995). Even temporary disruption of appropriate sensory input can permanently affect cortical patterns of connections if it occurs during the appropriate critical period, as Hubel and Wiesel's studies of monocular visual deprivation in kittens demonstrated (Hubel & Wiesel, 1965). The plasticity of connections inherent in the critical period is followed by relative stability in the mature pattern of connections. This stability of adult neural connections is seen when a cataract forms in an adult. In contrast to the infant with a cataract, normal vision is restored in the adult who has the cataract removed, even if it has been present for many years, because the neural connections in the mature visual pathway do not change (Daw, 1995).

The synaptic plasticity present in the developing nervous system endows it with the ability to adapt to the many variations of the external world, as in language acquisition, or the ability to recover from early damage when one region of cortex subsumes the functions of a damaged area. However, this plasticity also leaves the developing nervous system uniquely vulnerable to injury from abnormal patterns of activity (see below). In the human, this period of neuronal vulnerability most likely extends from the end of the second trimester of gestation well into childhood (Huttenlocher & Dabholkar, 1997).

Neuronal activity: spontaneous and sensory driven

Requirement for spontaneously generated activity

How early in development is neural activity needed for the refinement of connections? As mentioned above, in the binocular eye-closure experiments, ODC still form, and the source of the activity that drives this process is presumed to be the retina, which is spontaneously active in the dark (Mastronarde, 1989). There is now strong evidence that even before the development of vision (before retinal photoreceptors develop), the RGC are spontaneously active (see below) and this activity may be transmitted through the entire developing visual pathway (Mooney et al., 1996). This observation can explain the fact that in primates, before visual experience, ODC and orientation columns are already forming in utero (Horton & Hocking, 1996; Wiesel & Hubel, 1974). The hypothesis that this spontaneous activity drives the initial establishment of ODC and orientation columns is currently being investigated intensively.

In addition, this spontaneous activity is required for the earlier formation of patterned visual system connections. Recall that before ODC form, RGC axons segregate to form the eye-specific layers in the LGN (Fig. 10.1(b)). This process occurs entirely during the period before photoreceptors mature, yet it depends on neural activity. Infusion of TTX into the LGN, which blocks both presynaptic and post-synaptic sodium action potentials, blocks this layer formation (Shatz & Stryker, 1988). Individual axons in TTX-treated LGN branch widely, rather than retracting inappropriate branches and growing selectively into their appropriate eye-specific layers (Sretavan et al., 1988). In recent experiments, we selectively blocked only the RGC activity (Penn et al., 1998). When activity was blocked binocularly, layers also failed to form, indicating a requirement for the presynaptic action potentials (Fig. 10.1(c)). But when the spontaneous retinal activity was blocked only in one eye, the projection from the active retina expanded greatly into territory normally belonging to the other eye, and the projection from the inactive retina was substantially reduced (Fig. 10.1(d)). Thus, as in the later occurring formation of the ODC, inter-ocular competition – this time driven exclusively by endogenous retinal activity – determines the pattern of connections. These experiments demonstrate that spontaneous activity can produce highly stereotyped patterns of connections long before the onset of visual experience. They also imply that disruptions in the competitive mechanisms of axonal segregation, either prenatally or postnatally, may result in profound disruptions in the appropriate patterning of neural connections and lead to neurologic dysfunction.

Patterns of spontaneous activity

The nervous system generates complex patterns of activity long before there is any patterned sensory input. Not only is neuronal activity required to drive the refinement of connections, but also the information contained in the patterns of this activity – the spatiotemporal correlations – that appears to be required for activity-dependent competition to occur (Goodman & Shatz, 1993).

For example, ex utero microelectrode recordings from fetal rat retinas indicated that cells in the ganglion cell layer are spontaneously active and fire together long before there is any visual input (Maffei & Galli-Resta, 1990). Simultaneous recordings from hundreds of neurons in developing retinas in vitro, using either a multielectrode array or optical recording techniques (Meister et al., 1991; Feller et al., 1996), reveal a particular spatiotemporal pattern of firing. Individual ganglion cells fire bursts of action potentials of 2–8 s in duration, separated by extended periods of quiescence 40–90 s long (Wong et al., 1993). Measurements from groups of cells show that neighbouring cells fire action potentials together and undergo increases in levels of intracellular calcium synchronously (Meister et al., 1991; Feller et al., 1996). On a larger spatial scale, the pattern of activity resembles a 'wave' that travels across local regions of the retina at about 100–300 μm/s, and involves cells situated within approximately 300 μm of each other (Wong et al., 1993). These waves 'tile' the retina with highly restricted domains of activity whose borders change over time (Feller et al., 1996). Significantly, the retinal waves are only present during the period of retinogeniculate axon terminal segregation and are gone by the time photoreceptors are present and visual input is available. After this early period, RGC are spontaneously active in the dark, but do not participate in waves of activity (Mastronarde, 1989; Wong et al., 1993). Similar spontaneous, correlated retinal activity is present in mammals (cat, ferret, and mouse; (Meister et al., 1991; Mooney et al., 1996), as well as in turtle and chick (Sernagor & Grzywacz, 1996; Catsicas et al., 1998), emphasizing that it may be a well-conserved mechanism for refining neural connectivity before vision.

The early pattern of spontaneous retinal activity is well suited to drive segregation not only because it is present during the appropriate period, but also because of these particular spatiotemporal characteristics. The short duration of the activity compared with the long intervening periods of silence makes it unlikely that presynaptic cells from the two eyes will be active simultaneously (Fig. 10.2(a)). Spurious correlations are unlikely because the location, timing, and direction of wave spread are highly variable within a single piece of retina (Meister et al., 1991; Wong et al., 1993; Feller et al., 1996). Within a retina, correlations in the timing of the bursts are stronger between neighbouring retinal neurons than for distant neurons. As mentioned earlier, lasting increases in synaptic strength are thought to require that presynaptic inputs be sufficiently correlated so that there is an overlap in postsynaptic response. For synaptic weakening, the inputs from the two eyes onto a single postsynaptic neuron should be significantly uncorrelated, resulting in the weakening of one of the two inputs (Fig. 10.2(a)). Thus, the correlations created by the retinal waves could underlie cooperative synaptic strengthening thought to be necessary to group monocularly driven cells into eye-specific layers in the LGN and, at slightly later ages, into ODC.

How are these correlated patterns of activity generated? In the retina, recent experiments point to a role for synaptic transmission (Feller et al., 1996). During the period when the waves are generated, the retina contains differentiated RGC and amacrine cells (a class of retinal interneurons). Both of these cell types participate in the waves (Feller et al., 1996; Wong et al., 1995). A synaptic circuit between RGC and the cholinergic amacrine cells is necessary for the generation and the propagation of the waves; blockade of cholinergic transmission blocks the waves (Feller et al., 1996; Penn et al., 1998). These results emphasize the extent to which even very immature circuits, in which few classic synaptic specializations are visible (Maslim & Stone, 1986), can produce sophisticated patterns of spontaneous activity.

The generation of spontaneous, correlated activity is not limited to the visual system. Spontaneously generated activity has been described in a variety of locations in the developing CNS, including cortex, hippocampus, cerebellum, thalamus, superior colliculus, locus coeruleus, spinal cord, and cochlea (for review, see Feller, 1999). It varies in pattern, but each pattern provides strong spatiotemporal correlations that may shape synaptogenesis. For example, in immature cortical slices, domains of neurons that tangentially span the thickness of the cortical layers and horizontally are within a 50 to 200 mm circular diameter undergo synchronous calcium increases (Katz & Shatz, 1996). Unlike the spontaneous activity in the retina, this pattern of activity appears to be coordinated not by synaptic connections, but rather by gap-junctional networks that transmit a chemical signal (inositol 1,4,5-trisphosphate), instead of creating classic electrotonic coupling between the neurons. It has been suggested that these cortical domains of activity help to shape the columnar structure of cortical connections (Katz & Shatz, 1996). The developing spinal cord is also endogenously active and appears to combine the use of synaptic and gap-junctional connections to generate patterned activity. Synaptic connections appear to underlie the spontaneous, oscillating bursts of activity that occur in dispersed groups of motoneurons that will innervate either flexor or extensor muscles. There also is extensive gap-junctional coupling in the spinal cord between motoneurons that innervate homonymous muscles (for review, see Feller, 1999). The spontaneous, coordinated oscillations of activity seen in developing motoneurons may drive the activity-dependent competition known to refine synaptic connections at the NMJ (neuromuscular junction) (Nguyen & Lichtman, 1996). The developing retina, cortex, and spinal cord illustrate the variety of neural circuitry – based on immature synapses, gap junctions, or a combination of the two – that can generate the correlated, spontaneous activity that may drive the activity-dependent refinement of connections throughout the developing nervous system.

Because spontaneous, highly patterned activity occurs in many areas of the nervous system, disruption of particular patterns of endogenous activity could result in abnormalities in neural circuitry. For example, damage could result from prepartum use of drugs that interfere with synaptic transmission (i.e. nicotine) or change gap-junctional connections (i.e. alcohols). Large-scale structural brain defects would not be expected to result from these exposures; rather, changes in the patterns of connections might result in subtle deficits, such as the mild cognitive impairments documented in prenatal nicotine or alcohol exposure (Levin et al., 1993; Olson et al., 1997). Although it is difficult to determine whether such deficits are simply the result of global insults from these agents (i.e. reduced oxygen delivery to the fetus or carbon monoxide poisoning), it is worth considering the specific changes in neural connections that may occur when the patterns of endogenous, correlated activity are disrupted.

Requirement for sensory-driven activity

Once sensory input becomes available, features of the external environment drive the activity that shapes connections. The shapes and forms present in our visual world provide multiple sources of correlated activity; just the edge of this page of paper can correlate the firing of many RGC across which the linear image falls simultaneously. Disruptions in these correlations, as discussed earlier, can lead to profound anatomic and functional changes in connectivity within the visual cortex during the appropriate critical periods. In addition, extreme manipulations of the visual environment, for example, raising kittens in an environment containing only vertical lines, preferentially selects for cortical neurons responding to vertical stimuli and leaves the rest of the cortex unresponsive (Stryker et al., 1978). In many other developing systems, neuronal receptive field properties and the underlying connections are also sensitive to alterations of sensory input (somatosensory system: Fox, 1994; auditory system: King, 1993). The ability of the developing brain to incorporate information from the external world into its precise circuitry allows it to adapt to a myriad of changing environments.

The use of these two sources of activity – endogenously produced and sensory-driven – should not be viewed as occurring in mutually exclusive periods. For example, studies of language acquisition demonstrate that infants are born with preferences for particular sounds present in their mother's language (Moon et al., 1993). This observation suggests that before birth (when spontaneous activity plays a dominant role in shaping connections) circuitry may also be modulated by auditory input that filters into the uterus. After birth, endogenous activity may still play a role in shaping connections. After the onset of vision, the local circuitry between the LGN and the surrounding reticular nucleus generates spontaneous, correlated waves of action potentials in the form of thalamic spindle oscillations that travel in waves of spike activity across the LGN (McCormick & Bal, 1997). These oscillations occur during sleep, and therefore do not normally disrupt the processing of sensory experience. In the normal brain, this activity could help shape thalamocortical connections because it creates highly synchronized inputs from neighboring LGN neurons. On the other hand, the mechanism that generates thalamic spindles during sleep also appears to underlie the classic 3 Hz spike-and-wave seizure discharges seen in children with absence epilepsy (McCormick & Bal, 1997). Because the mechanisms that shape the normal connectivity are tuned to be sensitive to highly correlated activity, it is possible that these highly synchronous epileptic discharges could generate abnormal neuronal connectivity by interrupting the normal pattern of sensory input. More generally, the highly synchronous activity of seizures may, in part, be responsible for the progressive nature of some epileptic syndromes (e.g. in Lennox–Gastaut syndrome: Oguni et al., 1996). The interplay between these two forms of activity – spontaneously generated and sensory-driven – is most likely the result of shared mechanisms underlying activity-dependent synaptic competition.

Mechanisms of activity-dependent competition

Physiologic and structural synaptic changes

What mechanisms operate so that correlated activity can drive the refinement of synaptic connections? The process is competitive in the sense that direct or indirect interactions between incoming axons for common postsynaptic targets drive the retraction of all but one (or one class of) axon and allow expansion and stabilization of the remaining axonal terminals. Ideas about how this process occurs on a cellular and molecular level in the developing CNS are drawn from primarily two sources: studies on synapse formation and elimination at the NMJ, and studies on long-term changes in synaptic strength in the hippocampus (Hall & Sanes, 1993; Malenka, 1994). Although the details of these systems differ, they share a common theme: synaptic refinement depends on a mechanism in which synapses that are synchronously active with the postsynaptic cell are reinforced ('Hebbian' synapses) whereas those synapses that are not synchronously active are eliminated (Fig. 10.2(*a*)).

The individual steps of synaptic refinement have been best studied at the NMJ (for review, see Nguyen & Lichtman, 1996). As in the visual system, axonal projections – in this case from motoneurons – are initially diffuse, with individual muscle fibres receiving innervation from multiple motoneurons before birth. These connections are then refined through an activity-dependent process so that each muscle fibre receives input from only one axon (possibly driven initially by the spontaneous patterns of activity generated by the developing spinal cord as mentioned above). The process of synaptic refinement at the NMJ has been monitored elegantly in vivo. Neurotransmitter receptor sites on the postsynaptic membrane (i.e. the muscle's acetylcholine receptors) first decrease, the presynaptic axon's terminals are eliminated from the muscle, and finally the nerve terminal resorbs into the main axonal trunk. Asynchronous receptor activation seems to be the signal that allows the muscle to destabilize particular synaptic sites: when focal postsynaptic blockade is produced by application of alpha-bungarotoxin (which blocks only the postsynaptic acetylcholine receptors, and not presynaptic transmitter release) then these blocked synapses are selectively eliminated. Elimination of the blocked synapse only occurs when there is activity at the rest of the junction, suggesting that active synaptic sites are stabilized and that this activity must somehow destabilize inactive sites. Studies of neurons and myocytes in tissue culture show similar results. Stimulation of one innervating neuron can suppress transmission from the synapse of a second, inactive neuron, whereas simultaneous stimulation of both neurons either results in strengthening of transmission at both synapses or no change (Dan & Poo, 1992). These results led to the proposal of the following scenario (Nguyen & Lichtman, 1996): when synapses are active they are somehow protected from elimination, but when they are inactive they receive a 'withdrawal' signal. When neither input is active, both remain stationary because no withdrawal signals are present; when both axons are simultaneously active, they are both protected from elimination (Fig. 10.2(*b*)). This dependence on the balance of activity, not on activity *per se*, is strikingly similar to the requirement for patterned activity discussed above for the developing visual system.

Cellular and molecular synaptic changes

Coincidence detection

Although the precise molecular mechanism that allows detection of coincident activity at the NMJ remains obscure, the cellular and molecular correlates of changes in synaptic strength have been studied in detail in the mature hippocampus. In area CA1 of the hippocampus, the application of high-frequency electrical stimulation leads to lasting increases in synaptic strength, known as LTP (long-term potentiation) (Malenka, 1994). In contrast, lower frequency stimulation can cause a lasting decrease in synaptic strength, LTD (long-term depression). LTP is also an appealing mechanism for synaptic modification during development because it requires cooperativity (a certain number of synapses must be active to induce LTP), associativity (the coincident firing of a weak synapse along with stronger synapses on a convergent input will potentiate both sets of synapses), and input specificity (only synchronously active inputs are potentiated), all of which are thought to operate at developing synapses. Additionally, LTP and LTD can occur homosynaptically (at the same synapse that is stimulated) and heterosynaptically (at other synapses on the same postsynaptic cell that is being depolarized by the active synapse; Abraham, 1996), allowing for the strengthening and weakening of multiple synapses, as is necessary in the refinement of developing connections (Fig. 10.2). These attributes have led to an exploration of the possible role of LTP and LTD as mechanisms underlying synaptic refinement during development.

In the developing visual system, both retinogeniculate and geniculocortical synapses demonstrate forms of synaptic enhancement similar to hippocampal LTP (Mooney et al., 1993; Kirkwood et al., 1995). Developing retinogeniculate synapses can undergo long-term increases in transmission with high-frequency stimulation or pairing of presynaptic and postsynaptic activity (Mooney et al., 1993). In the developing neocortex, LTP has been demonstrated directly at the geniculocortical synapse (Crair & Malenka, 1995). LTD has also been described in the neocortex (Dudek & Friedlander, 1996). Both LTP and LTD are easier to elicit at synapses during the period of synaptic refinement in the cortex (Crair & Malenka, 1995; Dudek & Friedlander, 1996).

The link between activity-dependent synaptic refinement and the mechanisms of LTP and LTD currently remains one of correlation rather than causation; however, the molecular mechanisms underlying LTP and LTD are presently the best-understood cellular correlates of activity-dependent synaptic changes. One molecular requirement that is necessary for LTP and LTD is a physiologic 'coincidence detector', a mechanism by which coincident activity of the presynaptic and postsynaptic neurons is sensed (Fig. 10.2(b)). The glutamatergic NMDA (N-methyl-D-aspartate) receptor is a molecular coincidence detector that has been studied in great detail in the CA1 region of the adult hippocampus (Malenka, 1994). This receptor can detect coincident activity because it fluxes Ca^{2+} ions only when glutamate, released by the active presynaptic neuron, binds to the receptor and the postsynaptic neuron is depolarized simultaneously, relieving a voltage-dependent Mg^{2+} gating of the channel pore. When NMDA receptors are blocked, LTP and LTD cannot be elicited at the CA1 synapse (Malenka, 1994). The level of Ca^{2+} influx into the postsynaptic neurons appears to determine whether LTP (high Ca^{2+}) or LTD (low Ca^{2+}) occurs (Bear, 1995).

Like the hippocampal synapse, the retinogeniculate and thalamocortical synapses use glutamate as their neurotransmitter, which has lead to an investigation of which glutamate receptors are critical for synaptic refinement during visual system development. At the retinogeniculate synapse, physiologic synaptic enhancement appears to depend on NMDA receptor activation, at least in some neurons (Mooney et al., 1993). In vivo infusion of NMDA receptor antagonists (such as MK801) into the ferret thalamus at appropriate ages can prevent retinogeniculate axons from segregating into the ON- and OFF-sublayers of the LGN (Hahm et al., 1991), although other NMDA receptor antagonists (such as 2-amino-5-phosphonovaleric acid) do not block the earlier occurring formation of eye-specific layers (Smetters et al., 1994). In the developing cortex, in vivo infusions of NMDA receptor antagonists block the physiologic shifts in ODC produced by monocular blockade (although the specificity of NMDA receptor blockade in the cortex has been called into question because these antagonists also block most activity in developing cortical neurons). The requirement for NMDA receptor-mediated plasticity is perhaps best defined for the optic tectum of lower vertebrates. In the three-eyed frog model, the eye-specific stripes in the tectum not only desegregate when all activity is blocked with TTX, as discussed earlier, they also desegregate when NMDA receptor antagonists are applied (reviewed in Cline, 1991). However, although NMDA receptor-mediated plasticity has been most thoroughly studied, there are many examples of plasticity mechanisms that do not require NMDA receptors, e.g. LTP in the hippocampal mossy fibres in CA3 and LTD in the cerebellum (Malenka, 1994; Ito, 1996). It has recently been found that some forms of AMPA (α-amino-3-hydroxy-5-methyl-4-isoazoleproprionic acid) receptors (the other major class of ion-fluxing glutamate receptors), can flux not only Na^+, but Ca^{2+} as well, which may allow them to participate in changing synaptic strength in some locations (Itazawa et al., 1997). There are not NMDA receptors in all brain regions that undergo activity-dependent refinement so additional mechanisms of coincidence detection will likely be critical for activity-dependent synaptic refinement.

The functioning of particular mechanisms for coincidence detection, such as a reliance on glutamate receptors, may increase the susceptibility of the developing brain to particular insults. In addition, recent experiments suggest that the earliest synapses that form during the development or rearrangement of glutamatergic circuits may contain solely NMDA receptors (optic tectum: Wu et al., 1996; hippocampus: Isaac et al., 1995). In the hippocampus, such synapses have been dubbed 'silent synapses' because they are undetectable at resting membrane potentials, but the NMDA receptor-dependent excitatory postsynaptic potentials are revealed when the postsynaptic cell is depolarized (Isaac et al., 1995). After LTP induction protocols, AMPA receptors appear at these synapses so that they are no longer functionally silent. It is possible that the severe disruption caused by glutamate or glycine toxicity in the developing brain is caused not only by acute cell death, but additionally by the disruption of this first step in the refinement of synaptic connections. Exacerbating this disruption may be the role that presynaptic activity can play in the regulation of postsynaptic ion receptor subtypes, which control ion flow and neuronal excitability (Spitzer et al., 1994). Changes in the properties of the glutamate receptor subunit composition during development also allow for increased calcium flux through these receptors. Neurons with glutamatergic synapses may be prone to death by toxicity because of excessive Ca^{2+} entry after the release of large amounts of glutamate during a hypoxic–ischemic episode, through activation of either NMDA receptors or AMPA receptors (Choi & Rothman, 1990). Similar damage can also follow the release of glycine (which at high levels can stimulate NMDA receptors) as seen in genetic disorders such as nonketotic hyperglycemia (McDonald & Johnston, 1990). The specific physiology of the developing circuitry is presumably intimately related to morphologic changes that are later seen in the brain, both in normal development and after injury.

Retrograde signals

Coincidence detection allows for anterograde information flow about correlated activity between the presynaptic and postsynaptic neuron (Fig. 10.2(*b*)). For this activity to result in a structural change in presynaptic connections during synaptic refinement, it seems there must also be a retrograde signal that allows communication back from the postsynaptic neuron to the active presynaptic terminals (Fig. 10.2(*b*)). Such a signal would need to be regulated by neuronal activity and cause selective stabilization and growth at synapses that are simultaneously active with the postsynaptic neuron. Again, studies of hippocampal LTP and NMJ synaptic refinement have provided possible candidates for retrograde messengers that could act in the activity-dependent refinement in the developing brain. At the NMJ, possible retrograde messengers that have been implicated in synaptic refinement include neurotrophins, particularly BDNF (brain-derived neurotrophic factor) and NT-3, NO (nitric oxide), ATP, and proteases (for review, see Nguyen & Lichtman, 1996). In the hippocampus, again both neurotrophins (BDNF and NT-3) and NO can potentiate CA1 synapses (Kantor et al., 1996; Kang & Schuman, 1995); antagonists of the neurotrophins and of NO can block LTP induction, and transgenic mice that lack BDNF or the ability to make NO have a diminished capacity for hippocampal LTP (Kantor et al., 1996; Korte et al., 1995). These experiments have lead to the investigation of the role of these compounds in activity-dependent development of the mammalian brain.

There is evidence accumulating that neurotrophins are good candidates for molecules that modulate activity-dependent developmental plasticity (Shatz, 1997). The receptors for BDNF and NT-4 (neurotrophin-4) (TrkB receptors) are expressed in mammalian LGN and cortex during the appropriate developmental period (TrkC receptors, which bind NT-3, are also expressed). Infusion of BDNF and NT-4 (but not other neurotrophins such as nerve growth factor or NT-3) into the visual cortex during the period of ODC development blocked ODC in the region of the infusion; blockade of the TrkB receptor also blocked ODC formation. Putting NT-4, but not BDNF or NT-3, into the visual cortex can also rescue LGN neurons from the shrinkage of their cell bodies that occurs with monocular deprivation. These experiments (for review, see Shatz, 1997) suggest that the competitive interactions that normally underlie synaptic remodeling are based on a limited supply of neurotrophins, and infusion of excess neurotrophins acted on the LGN axon terminals, removing this competition. When there is no activity, as in monocular deprivation, then the application of NT-4 can maintain the silenced LGN neurons, although it would be predicted that their terminals would still not have been able to segregate into ODC. Whether BDNF or NT-4 function endogenously during development has yet to be determined.

Although it seems likely that the neurotrophins may play a permissive role, allowing activity-dependent changes to occur, they are unlikely to function on the 10- to 100-ms scale on which coincidence detection must occur because the Trk receptor is likely to remain activated for a prolonged period once neurotrophin binds to it (Shatz, 1997). NO is a more rapidly acting candidate that could function rapidly to change synaptic strength during development. Experiments in chick tectum (Williams et al., 1994) and ferret LGN (Cramer et al., 1996) indicate that systemic blockade of NO synthesis can block refinement of some connections, but these effects are quite restricted.

It is likely that many molecular messengers play critical roles in activity-dependent development and are yet to be identified. In the future, it will be necessary to balance potential therapeutic effects of molecular messengers, such as the increased neuronal survival seen when BDNF is administered after an hypoxic–ischemic insult (Cheng et al., 1997), against the potential risk of creating abnormal neural circuitry.

Concluding remarks

Recent studies are beginning to forge a link between normally occurring activity-dependent synaptic modifications and specific neurologic disorders. Two examples are the reorganization of hippocampal connections after prolonged epilepsy (Parent & Lowenstein, 1997) and the activity-dependent translation of fragile X mental retardation protein at synapses (Weiler et al., 1997). In the hippocampus, rearrangement and sprouting of mossy fibre connections is a striking feature of temporal lobe epilepsy; current work is focusing on the similarity of the mechanisms that appear to underlie activity-dependent formation of hippocampal connections during development and the pathologic sprouting seen after seizures (Parent & Lowenstein, 1997). The link between the expression of the fragile X mental retardation protein and its role in normal development remains unknown, but its expression appears at least to be regulated by neural activity and could play a role in the initial formation of neural circuits that might in turn be disrupted when a pathologic form of the protein is produced. Information about the role of activity-dependent developmental changes in neurologic disease is just starting to emerge, but understanding normal activity-dependent developmental processes at the cellular and molecular levels should provide clues to human neurologic illness that may result from changes in the circuitry of the developing nervous system.

Activity-dependent development can be disrupted at many points. We have indicated a critical role for correlated activity, both spontaneous and sensory derived, in driving neuronal competition that shapes precise connectivity. Either subtle disruptions in the spatiotemporal patterns of activity or major disruptions in the overall balance of activity may result in abnormal connectivity. Such disruption of patterned neural activity may result from interference with synaptic transmission, with coincidence detection, or with retrograde signals, as might happen with prepartum use of drugs (such as nicotine, benzodiazepines, or narcotics) or postnatal exposure to a variety of medications. In addition, as different sensory systems become active at particular developmental stages in premature infants, it is worth considering what effect the sensory environment might have on neural activity patterns needed to drive synaptic remodeling. During critical periods, specific areas of the developing nervous system may be particularly susceptible to these types of disruption.

Disruptions of activity would affect the fine-tuning of neural circuits, a process that requires neural activity to shape the adult patterns of connectivity, not the large-scale wiring of the brain, which generally occurs independent of neural activity. It is all too common for a child to have neurologic deficits when no structural abnormalities can be identified. The current techniques in neuropathology and neuroradiology are just beginning to be able to detect the subtle, yet critical, changes that must be occurring. Consequently, the major challenge for the clinician and medical scientist is to develop techniques with high resolution that can monitor the normal or abnormal functioning of neural circuits on a fine-scale during development. Once disorders resulting from disruptions in activity-dependent development can be more accurately identified, therapies aimed at correcting the abnormal circuits (for example, by developing treatments to extend critical periods) or optimizing the use of the abnormal circuitry (as is being tried for specific language impairments: Tallal et al., 1996) can be further developed. Recognizing and understanding in detail the role of activity-dependent development in the formation of precise neural circuits should expand greatly the ability to identify, treat, and prevent many developmental brain disorders.

REFERENCES

Abraham, W. C. (1996). Induction of heterosynaptic and homosynaptic LTD in hippocampal sub-regions *in vivo*. *Journal of Physiology (Paris)*, **90**, 305–6.

Antonini, A. & Stryker, M. P. (1993). Rapid remodeling of axonal arbors in the visual cortex, *Science*, **260**, 1819–21.

Bauman, M. L., Filipek, P. A. & Kemper, T. L. (1997). Early infantile autism. *International Review of Neurobiology*, **41**, 367–86.

Bear, M. F. (1995). Mechanism for a sliding synaptic modification threshold. *Neuron*, 15, 1–4.

Blakemore, C. & Van Sluyters, R. C. (1975). Innate and environmental factors in the development of the kitten's visual cortex. *Journal of Physiology (London)*, 248, 663–716.

Catsicas, M., Bonness, V., Becker, D. & Mobbs, P. (1998). Spontaneous Ca^{2+} transients and their transmission in the developing chick retina. *Current Biology*, 8, 283–6.

Chalupa, L. M. & White, C. A. (1990). Prenatal development of visual system structures. In *Development of Sensory Systems in Mammals*, ed. J. R. Coleman, pp. 3–60. New York: John Wiley.

Cheng, Y., Gidday, J. M., Yan, Q., Shah, A. R. & Holtzman, D. M. (1997). Marked age-dependent neuroprotection by brain-derived neurotrophic factor against neonatal hypoxic–ischemic brain injury. *Annals of Neurology*, 41, 521–9.

Choi, D. W. & Rothman, S. M. (1990). The role of glutamate neurotoxicity in hypoxic–ischemic neuronal death. *Annual Review of Neuroscience*, 13, 171–82.

Cline, H. T. (1991). Activity-dependent plasticity in the visual systems of frogs and fish. *Trends in Neuroscience*, 14, 104–11.

Crair, M. C. & Malenka, R. C. (1995). A critical period for long-term potentiation at thalamo-cortical synapses. *Nature*, 375, 325–8.

Cramer, K. S., Angelucci, A., Hahm, J. O., Bogdanov, M. B. & Sur, M. (1996). A role for nitric oxide in the development of the ferret retinogeniculate projection. *Journal of Neuroscience*, 16, 7995–8004.

Crowley, J. C. & Katz, L. C. (2000). Early development of ocular dominance columns. *Science*, 290(5495), 1321–4.

Dan, Y. & Poo, M. M. (1992). Hebbian depression of isolated neuromuscular synapses *in vitro*. *Science*, 256, 1570–3.

Daw, N. W. (1995). *Visual Development*. New York: Plenum Press.

Dudek, S. M. & Friedlander, M. J. (1996). Developmental down-regulation of LTD in cortical layer IV and its independence of modulation by inhibition. *Neuron*, 16, 1097–1106.

Feller, M. B. (1999). Spontaneous correlated activity in developing neural circuits. *Neuron*, 22, 653–6.

Feller, M. B., Wellis, D. P., Stellwagen, D., Werblin, F. S. & Shatz, C. J. (1996). Requirement for cholinergic synaptic transmission in the propagation of spontaneous retinal waves. *Science*, 272, 1182–7.

Fox, K. (1994). The cortical component of experience-dependent synaptic plasticity in the rat barrel cortex. *Journal of Neuroscience*, 14, 7665–79.

Goodman, C. S. & Shatz, C. J. (1993). Developmental mechanisms that generate precise patterns of neuronal connectivity. *Cell*, 72 (Suppl.), 77–98.

Hahm, J. O., Langdon, R. B. & Sur, M. (1991). Disruption of retinogeniculate afferent segregation by antagonists to NMDA receptors, *Nature*, 351, 568–70.

Hall, Z. W. & Sanes, J. R. (1993). Synaptic structure and development: the neuromuscular junction. *Cell*, 72 (Suppl.), 99–121.

Hebb, D. O. (1949). *The Organization of Behavior*. New York: John Wiley.

Horton, J. C. & Hocking, D. R. (1996). An adult-like pattern of ocular dominance columns in striate cortex of newborn monkeys prior to visual experience. *Journal of Neuroscience*, **16**, 1791–807.

Hubel, D. H. & Wiesel, T. N. (1965). Binocular interaction in striate cortex of kittens reared with artificial squint. *Journal of Neurophysiology*, **28**, 1041–59.

Hubel, D. H. & Wiesel, T. N. (1970). The period of susceptibility to the physiological effects of unilateral eye closure in kittens. *Journal of Physiology (London)*, **28**, 1041–59.

Huttenlocher, P. R. (1991). Dendritic and synaptic pathology in mental retardation. *Pediatric Neurology*, **7**, 79–85.

Huttenlocher, P. R. & Dabholkar, A. S. (1997). Regional differences in synaptogenesis in human cerebral cortex. *Journal of Comparative Neurology*, **387**, 167–78.

Isaac, J. T., Nicoll, R. A. & Malenka, R. C. (1995). Evidence for silent synapses: implications for the expression of LTP. *Neuron*, **15**, 427–34.

Itazawa, S. I., Isa, T. & Ozawa, S. (1997). Inwardly rectifying and Ca^{2+}-permeable AMPA-type glutamate receptor channels in rat neocortical neurons. *Journal of Neurophysiology*, **78**, 2592–2601.

Ito, M. (1996). Cerebellar long-term depression [letter]. *Trends in Neuroscience*, **19**, 11–12.

Kang, H. & Schuman, E. M. (1995). Long-lasting neurotrophin-induced enhancement of synaptic transmission in the adult hippocampus. *Science*, **267**, 1658–62.

Kantor, D. B., Lanzrein, M., Stary, S. J. et al. (1996). A role for endothelial NO synthase in LTP revealed by adenovirus-mediated inhibition and rescue. *Science*, **274**, 1744–8.

Katz, L. C. & Shatz, C. J. (1996). Synaptic activity and the construction of cortical circuits. *Science*, **274**, 1133–8.

King, A. J. (1993). The Wellcome Prize Lecture. A map of auditory space in the mammalian brain: neural computation and development. *Experimental Physiology*, **78**, 559–90.

Kirkwood, A., Lee, H. K. & Bear, M. F. (1995). Co-regulation of long-term potentiation and experience-dependent synaptic plasticity in visual cortex by age and experience. *Nature*, **375**, 328–31.

Korte, M., Carroll, P., Wolf, E., Brem, G., Thoenen, H. & Bonhoeffer, T. (1995). Hippocampal long-term potentiation is impaired in mice lacking brain-derived neurotrophic factor *Proceedings of the National Academy of Sciences, USA*, **92**, 8856–60.

Levin, E. D., Briggs, S. J., Christopher, N. C. & Rose, J. E. (1993). Prenatal nicotine exposure and cognitive performance in rats. *Neurotoxicology and Teratology*, **15**, 251–60.

LeVay, S., Stryker, M. P. & Shatz, C. J. (1978). Ocular dominance columns and their development in layer IV of the cat's visual cortex. *Journal of Comparative Neurology*, **159**, 223–44.

McCormick, D. A. & Bal, T. (1997). Sleep and arousal: thalamocortical mechanisms. *Annual Review of Neuroscience*, **20**, 185–215.

McDonald, J. W. & Johnston, M. V. (1990). Nonketotic hyperglycinemia: pathophysiological role of NMDA-type excitatory amino acid receptors [letter]. *Annals of Neurology*, **27**, 449–50.

Maffei, L. & Galli-Resta, L. (1990). Correlation in the discharges of neighboring rat retinal ganglion cells during prenatal life. *Proceedings of the National Academy of Sciences, USA*, **87**, 2861–4.

Malenka, R. C. (1994). Synaptic plasticity in the hippocampus: LTP and LTD. *Cell*, **78**, 535–8.

Maslim, J. & Stone, J. (1986). Synaptogenesis in the retina of the cat. *Brain Research*, **373**, 35–48.

Mastronarde, D. N. (1989). Correlated firing of retinal ganglion cells. *Trends in Neuroscience*, **12**, 75–80.

Meister, M., Wong, R. O., Baylor, D. A. & Shatz, C. J. (1991). Synchronous bursts of action potentials in ganglion cells of the developing mammalian retina. *Science*, **252**, 939–43.

Moon, C., Cooper, R. P. & Fifer, W. P. (1993). Two-day-olds prefer their native language. *Infant Behaviour and Development*, **16**, 495–500.

Mooney, R., Madison, D. V. & Shatz, C. J. (1993). Enhancement of transmission at the developing retinogeniculate synapse. *Neuron*, **10**, 815–25.

Mooney, R., Penn, A. A., Gallego, R. & Shatz, C. J. (1996). Thalamic relay of spontaneous retinal activity prior to vision. *Neuron*, **17**, 863–74.

Mower, G. D., Caplan, C. J., Christen, W. G. & Duffy, F. H. (1985). Dark rearing prolongs physiological but not anatomical plasticity of the cat visual cortex. *Journal of Comparitive Neurology*, **235**, 448–66.

Nguyen, Q. T. & Lichtman, J. W. (1996). Mechanism of synapse disassembly at the developing neuromuscular junction. *Current Opinions in Neurobiology*, **6**, 104–112.

Oguni, H., Hayashi, K. & Osawa, M. (1996). Long-term prognosis of Lennox-Gastaut syndrome. *Epilepsia*, **37** (Suppl. 3), 44–7.

Olson, H. C., Streissguth, A. P., Sampson, P. D., Barr, H. M., Bookstein, F. L. & Thiede, K. (1997). Association of prenatal alcohol exposure with behavioral and learning problems in early adolescence. *Journal of the American Academy of Child and Adolescent Psychiatry*, **36**, 1187–94.

Parent, J. M. & Lowenstein, D. H. (1997). Mossy fiber reorganization in the epileptic hippocampus. *Current Opinions in Neurology*, **10**, 103–9.

Penn, A. A., Riquelme, P. A., Feller, M. B. & Shatz, C. J. (1998). Competition in retinogeniculate patterning driven by spontaneous activity. *Science*, **279**, 2108–12.

Rodieck, R. W. (1979). Visual pathways. *Annual Review of Neuroscience*, **2**, 193–255.

Sarnat, H. (1992). *Cerebral Dysgenesis: Embryology and Clinical Expression.* Oxford: Oxford University Press.

Schwartzkroin, P. A. (1995). Plasticity and repair in the immature central nervous system. In *Brain Development and Epilepsy*, ed. P. A. Schwartzkroin, S. L. Moshe, J. L. Noebels & J. W. Swann, pp. 234–67. Oxford: Oxford University Press.

Sernagor, E. & Grzywacz, N. M. (1996). Influence of spontaneous activity and visual experience on developing retinal receptive fields. *Current Biology*, **6**, 1503–8.

Sharma, J., Angelucci, A. & Sur, M. (2000). Induction of visual orientation modules in auditory cortex. *Nature*, **404**(6780), 841–7.

Shatz, C. J. (1997). Neurotrophins and visual system plasticity. In *Molecular and Cellular Approaches to Neural Development*, ed. W. M. Cowan, T. M. Jessell & L. Zipursky, pp. 509–24. Oxford: Oxford University Press.

Shatz, C. J. & Kirkwood, P. A. (1984). Prenatal development of functional connections in the cat's retinogeniculate pathway. *Journal of Neuroscience*, **4**, 1378–97.

Shatz, C. J. & Stryker, M. P. (1988). Prenatal tetrodotoxin infusion blocks segregation of retinogeniculate afferents. *Science*, **242**, 87–9.

Smetters, D. K., Hahm, J. & Sur, M. (1994). An *N*-methyl-D-aspartate receptor antagonist does not prevent eye-specific segregation in the ferret retinogeniculate pathway. *Brain Research*, **658**, 168–78.

Spitzer, N. C., Gu, G. X. & Olson, E. (1994). Action potentials, calcium transients and the control of differentiation of excitable cells. *Current Opinions in Neurobiology*, **4**, 70–77.

Sretavan, D. W. & Shatz, C. J. (1986). Prenatal development of retinal ganglion cell axons: segregation into eye-specific layers within the cat's lateral geniculate nucleus. *Journal of Neuroscience*, **6**, 234–51.

Sretavan, D. W., Shatz, C. J. & Stryker, M. P. (1988). Modification of retinal ganglion cell axon morphology by prenatal infusion of tetrodotoxin. *Nature*, **336**, 468–71.

Stein, B. E. (1984). Development of the superior colliculus. *Annual Review of Neuroscience*, **7**, 95–125.

Stryker, M. P. & Harris, W. A. (1986). Binocular impulse blockade prevents the formation of ocular dominance columns in cat visual cortex. *Journal of Neuroscience*, **6**, 2117–33.

Stryker, M. P. & Strickland, S. L. (1984). Physiological segregation of ocular dominance columns depends on the pattern of afferent electrical activity. *[Abstract] Investigative Ophthalmology and Visual Science*, **25** (Suppl.), 278.

Stryker, M. P., Sherk, H., Leventhal, A. G. & Hirsch, H. V. (1978). Physiological consequences for the cat's visual cortex of effectively restricting early visual experience with oriented contours. *Journal of Neurophysiology*, **41**, 896–909.

Tallal, P., Miller, S. L., Bedi, G. et al. (1996). Language comprehension in language-learning impaired children improved with acoustically modified speech. *Science*, **271**, 81–4.

Weiler, I. J., Irwin, S. A., Klintsova, A. Y. et al. (1997). Fragile X mental retardation protein is translated near synapses in response to neurotransmitter activation. *Proceedings of the National Academy of Sciences, USA*, **94**, 5395–400.

Weliky, M. & Katz, L. C. (1997). Disruption of orientation tuning in visual cortex by artificially correlated neuronal activity. *Nature*, **386**, 680–5.

Wiesel, T. N. & Hubel, D. H. (1974). Ordered arrangement of orientation columns in monkeys lacking visual experience. *Journal of Comparitive Neurology*, **158**, 307–18.

Williams, C. V., Nordquist, D. & McLoon, S. C. (1994). Correlation of nitric oxide synthase expression with changing patterns of axonal projections in the developing visual system. *Journal of Neuroscience*, **14**, 1746–55.

Wong, R. O., Meister, M. & Shatz, C. J. (1993). Transient period of correlated bursting activity during development of the mammalian retina. *Neuron*, **11**, 923–38.

Wong, R. O., Chernjavsky, A., Smith, S. J. & Shatz, C. J. (1995). Early functional neural networks in the developing retina. *Nature*, **374**, 716–18.

Wu, W. G., Malinow, R. & Cline, H. T. (1996). Maturation of a central glutamatergic synapse. *Science*, **274**, 972–6.

11

Fetal and neonatal development of the auditory system

S. Allen Counter

Neurology Department, The Biological Laboratories, Harvard Medical School, Cambridge, MA, USA

Introduction: traditional and modern biological approaches to embryology of the ear

The ear may be viewed as a doorway to the brain: an extension of the brain that reaches out to the periphery for input about the world of sound. The hearing apparatus provides the foundation for auditory interactions with the environment and serves as the essential component of two-way communication between organisms. In mammals, the mechanical vibrations of air particles that form the physical dimension of sound are collected by the external ear and channelled through a narrow canal within the skull to reach the sensitive eardrum or tympanic membrane. The external auditory canal and the tympanic membrane form the first portion of the superbly designed mammalian ear, which is an intricate sensory system that is composed of a series of complicated subsystems, linked in series, to perform vibro-mechanical conduction, hydrostatic pressure matching and mechano-electrical transformations (Fig. 11.1). Each of these unique subsystems must be intact for sound to reach the higher auditory tracts, nuclei and cortex of the brain and initiate perception. Auditory stimuli that are processed by the contiguous external, middle, and internal (cochlear) components of the ear system are conveyed as neuroelectric signals to the brain by the eighth cranial nerve. Sound frequency and feature analysis through tonotopic cellular organization take place from the cochlea and first order of neurons in the eighth nerve to higher auditory centres, including the inferior colliculus, medial geniculate and ultimately auditory cortex. During embryogenesis, each segment of the ear (from the most peripheral structures to the auditory cortex) is formed from specific cells, which follow predetermined genetic instructions, but different embryonic pathways. When these instructions are interrupted or go awry, a number of anomalies and diseases may ensue, resulting in abnormal development in one or more of the three components of the peripheral ear, the central nuclei, and ultimately leading to hearing impairment.

Approximately 4% of the world's population under 45 years of age suffer from

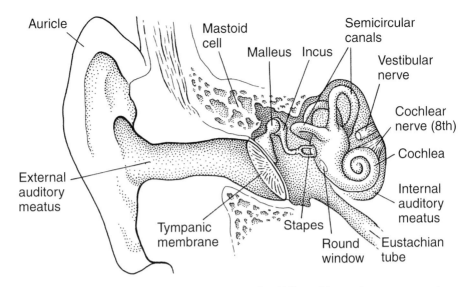

Fig. 11.1.   Drawing of the human ear illustrating the external, middle and internal ear components. The auricle or pinna, external auditory meatus, middle ear cavity, including ossicles, the inner ear, including the cochlea and semicircular canals, and the vestibular and auditory branches of the eighth cranial nerve are shown.

hearing impairment that is congenital or of early onset. One in 2000 children is born with significant hearing loss or deafness that is believed to be of genetic origin, with about 70% being non-syndromic, i.e. not associated with other clinical patterns. Some congenital hearing losses are conductive in nature, involving the blockage of the air conducting external and/or middle ear components, while others are of sensory–neural origin, involving the inner ear structures and retrocochlear neural elements. Autosomal recessive hearing impairment from defects in the inner ear is the most common form of genetic prelingual deafness in children. Some genes responsible for autosomal dominant, fully penetrant, non-syndromic inner ear hearing loss (about 15%) have been localized to specific chromosomes and their mutations identified (Lynch et al., 1997; Hardisty et al., 1998). Experimental manipulation of these identified genes has revealed specific effects on the morphogenesis of the ear, which have been beneficial to our understanding of the mechanisms of development and function of the entire auditory system.

The traditional approach to didactic discussions of the embryogenesis of the nervous system and the organogenesis of the vertebrate ear has involved mainly a description of the anatomical formation and cellular activities in the neural precursors, neural tube, neural crest and ectodermal placodes. Neural induction is the process of causing some ectodermal cells to become neural. Neurulation, which is the process of neural folding to form the neural tube, involves the specification of ectodermal cells into neural precursor cells. These processes are now known to be mediated by specific gene expressions. The differentiation of the ectodermal neural plate into the neural tube has been shown to follow a programmed pattern of specific cell fates, including the specification of dorsal vs. ventral. Earlier descriptions of the morphogenesis and histogenesis of the ear have focused on the structural integrity and detailed embryonic changes in anatomical structure of the developing ear (Deol, 1966; Anson & Davies, 1980; Sadler, 1990; Moore, 1988; Gulya, 1990). Recent findings, however, from a modern biological approach have added a new dimension to the discourse on fetal development and to our understanding of the molecular mechanisms underlying embryogenesis of the human ear.

Much of our present understanding of the neurogenetic factors involved in the embryogenesis of the human ear derives from studies of the morphogenesis in invertebrates such as in *Drosophila* (Lewis, 1978) and some lower vertebrates (for review, see Fritzsch, 1996a, b). The comparatively 'simpler' ears of certain amphibians, and avian species, for example, have served as useful models for a better understanding of the development and physiological mechanisms of the mammalian ear (Whitehead, 1986; Counter & Tsao, 1986; Borg & Counter, 1989; Fekete, 1996; Wu & Oh, 1996).

The embryonic and postnatal formation of the mammalian ear has been studied extensively in the mouse model (Deol, 1966, 1980; Sher, 1971). In mice, several molecules have been identified that are involved with cell fate and morphogenesis of the ear. These findings have been based on studies of gene mutations in knockout mice and the cloning of genes for deafness (Fekete, 1999). While some of the experimental gene deletions and mutations alter the formation of the outer and middle ear subsystems, others may inhibit neurogenesis and cellular formation of receptors in the cochlea (Bermingham et al., 1999). Hereditary deafness has become a major focus of research in the embryogenesis of the auditory system (Brown & Steel, 1994). More recent advances in molecular biology have revealed the contributions of a number of inductive factors and specific genes to the patterning of the cellular aggregates at each stage of the embryogenesis of the ear. Some 35 genes have been identified that are associated with ear abnormalities and deafness. These anatomical and physiological anomalies are seen in the outer, middle and inner ear components at various stages of embryogenesis (Deol, 1980; McPhee & Van De Water, 1988; Ruben et al., 1991; Ekker et al., 1992; Keynes & Krumlauf, 1994; Gallagher et al., 1996; Whitfield et al., 1996; Fritzsch, 1996a, b; Fekete, 1996, 1999; Holme & Steel, 1999).

The embryonic and fetal development of the human auditory system follows a precise extended timetable over the period of gestation in which the vital skeletal, muscular and neural structures are formed and mature to functional status. From the formation of the otic placode in the third week of gestation and the formation of the otocyst to the growth of the mesenchymal and endodermal tissues that form

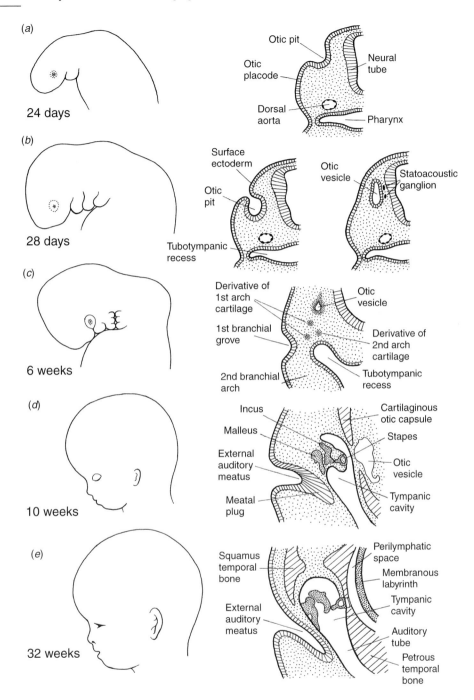

Fig. 11.2. Sequence of developmental changes in the fetus from day 24 involved in the formation of the outer and middle ear, showing the initial rhombencephalon invagination of the otic placode and otic pit and the appearance of the external auditory meatus and middle ear ossicles.

the outer and middle ear structures, the embryogenesis of the ear is guided predictably by intrinsic genetic inductive cues (Fig. 11.2). Each intricate subsystem must develop properly to form a seamless mechano-electric sense organ in order for the auditory system to function normally. A defect in any component of the outer, middle or inner ear may hinder the signal transmission capacity of the hearing organ and lead to deafness. Embryonic development of the ear may be disrupted by a variety of factors such as prenatal bacterial or viral infections, including bacterial meningitis, cytomegalovirus (CMV). For example, congenital CMV infection is believed to be a frequent cause of severe sensory–neural (inner ear or cochlear) hearing loss in neonates (Pappas, 1983). Also, human fetuses that are exposed to rubella in the first trimester of pregnancy may develop a significant bilateral sensorineural hearing loss or in some cases profound deafness.

The inner ear

Since the end organ of hearing, the cochlea, is the first of the subsystems to develop during embryogenesis of the ear, the development of the inner ear will be reviewed first. Table 11.1 (modified from Peck, 1995) shows a timetable for the development of each subsystem of the human ear.

The embryological development of the mammalian cochlea, like that of other sensory systems, proceeds in close association with the development of the central nervous system. The intricate inner ear consists of the organ of Corti, afferent and efferent neuronal endings of the auditory nerve and vestibular components: the otolith organs (the utricle and saccule), the endolymphatic duct and sac, and the three semicircular canals. Each of these structures is contained within a membranous labyrinth, which is housed in a surrounding bony labyrinth. The mechano-electric receptors of both the cochlea and vestibular organs are innervated by afferent fibres (otic placode) of the cochlear and vestibular ganglion cells. The receptors receive efferent neurons (from the brainstem basal plate) and autonomic nerve elements from the superior cervical ganglia (from the neural plate) (see Fritzsch et al., 1997). The vestibular portion of the inner ear is an integral but separate conglomerate of sensory organs that serve balance, spatial position, and acceleration, and as such will not be covered in this section on the ear and hearing.

The mammalian cochlea, which is embedded in the temporal bone, is a unit of coiled fluid-filled chambers or scalae (steps). The three chambers are the scala vestibuli, scala media and scala tympani (Fig. 11.3(a)). The fluid of the scala media, endolymph, is potassium rich and similar to cerebrospinal fluid in its protein composition, while the perilymph of the scala vestibuli and scala tympani has a substantially higher sodium and protein concentration. The scala media or cochlear duct contains the organ of Corti, which has a single row of differentiated epithelial

Table 11.1. Timetable of the embryological formation of the human ear from conception to term

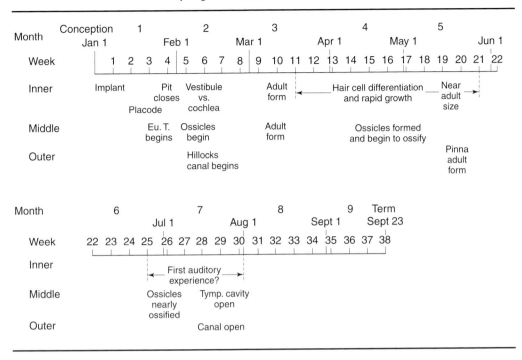

cells called the inner hair cells (around 3500), and three rows of approximately 20 000 outer hair cells (Fig. 11.3(*b*), (*c*)). The inner and outer hair cells interface with supportive cells and pillar cells which are separated by a tunnel (tunnel of Corti). On their apical surface, the hair cells contain contractile proteins, including an actin cuticular plate and about 100 stereocilia, which are graduated in their length, and which project to the overlying tectorial membrane. The stereocilia are composed of the active contractile proteins actin and myosin (Flock & Cheung, 1977; Flock, 1980). The stretching of the links of the tips of the stereocilia in relation to the tectorial membrane during sound-induced mechanical vibrations in the perilymphatic and endolymphatic fluids causes an opening in stereocilia transduction channels, an influx of endolymphatic K^+ at the hair cell, and ultimately, depolarization and release of neurotransmitter substance for synaptic communication with neurons at their base. The myosin, which is involved with hair cell adaptation and passive channel opening, works in conjunction with actin through ATP hydrolysis to provide a power force, and to readjust the tip links. The hair cells, their stereocilia and tectorial membrane contacts, convert through their motile actions the fluid disturbance caused by external sound waves to electrical activity in the contiguous synapses at their base (Hudspeth, 1989). The electromechanical

(a)

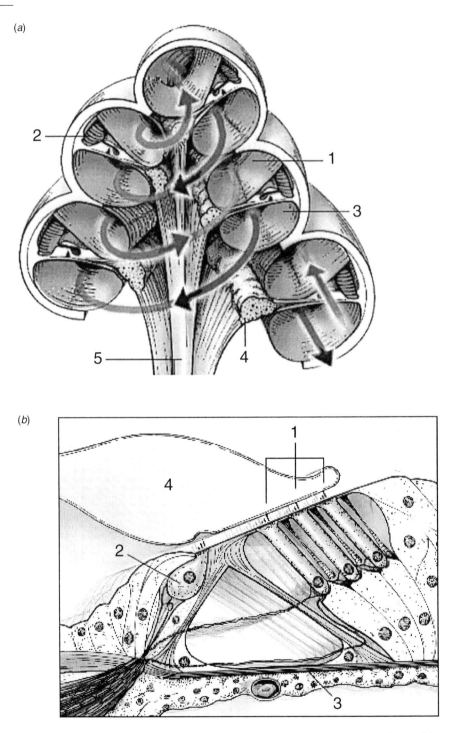

(b)

Fig. 11.3.   (a) Cross-section of the cochlea illustrating the scala vestibuli (1), scala media (cochlear duct (2)) and scala tympani (3), and the fluid spaces for perilymph and endolymph.

(c)

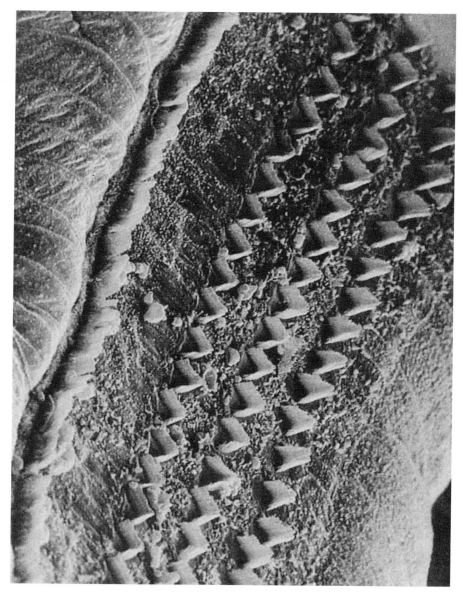

Caption for Fig. 11.3 (cont.)

Separating the scala vestibuli from the scala media is Reissner's membrane. The spiral
ganglion (4) and auditory nerve fibres (5) are also shown. (b) Schematic of the
organization of the organ of Corti illustrating the three rows of outer hair cells (1) and a
single row of inner hair cells (2), the basilar membrane (3) and tectorial membrane (4) in
the mammalian cochlea. (From S. Blatrix, M. Lavigne-Rebillard, L. Lenoir with permission:
Website 'The ear') (c) Scanning electron micrograph (SEM) of the three rows of outer hair
cells and a single row of inner hair cells in the mammalian cochlea. (Courtesy of Professor
Åke Flock.)

features of the outer hair cells, including their motility, are believed to underlie the frequency selectivity of the hair cells. The outer hair cells are an important physiological component of the cochlear amplifier, which is involved with the fine tuning of hearing.

The inner and outer hair cells of the cochlear duct are innervated at their base by afferent and efferent fibres from the eighth cranial nerve. Type I afferent auditory fibres (90%) are myelinated and innervate the inner hair cells. Type II fibres are unmyelinated and communicate with the outer hair cells. The efferent or centrifugal neurons, which inhibit mechano-electric transduction at the receptor level, originate in the brainstem superior olivary complex and innervate the inner and outer hair cells throughout the cochlea. The lateral olivo-cochlear bundle innervates the inner hair cells, and the medial olivo-cochlear bundle serves the outer hair cells. The hair cells convert sound-induced mechanical disturbances in the fluid and membranes of the scala media into neural impulses in the cochlear nerve. The inner and outer hair cells permit a broad range of sensitivity to sound, with the latter being more sensitive to a wide spectrum of sound intensities and frequencies. About 25 000 bipolar neurons in the cochlear nerve transmit the digital information of all sounds, including language, from the auditory periphery to the brain.

The embryogenesis of the inner ear initiates from interaction of inductive fields between the otocyst and the neural tube. The embryonic development of the mammalian inner ear begins at 25 days with a thickening of the surface ectoderm on the side of the head of the embryo called the otic placode, which emerges bilaterally on the caudal hindbrain (myelencephalon). The embryonic rhombencephalon and the chordamesoderm exert inductive influences on otic placode specification and invagination (Peck, 1994; Fekete, 1999). The otic placode invaginates to form the otic pit which when fused at the mouth becomes the otocyst or otic vesicle. The surface otic placode is formed at approximately 28 days when it begins to invaginate to form the otic pit, which is still open to the surface (Fig. 11.2). When the surface of the otic pit is fully closed, the otic vesicle (otocyst) is formed. The otic vesicle gives rise to the cochlea, its epithelial lining and the membranous labyrinth. The communication of inductive signals between the otocyst and the adjacent neural tube is necessary for the development of the membranous labyrinth. After several days, the otocyst divides into dorsal and ventral segments that will eventually become the vestibular apparatus (semi-circular canals, saccule and utricle) and auditory (cochlear) parts, respectively (Anniko & Wikström, 1984; Moore et al., 1988; Sadler, 1985; McPhee & Van de Water, 1988; Van de Water, 1988; Van de Water & Repressa, 1991; O'Rahilly & Müller, 1996; Peck, 1994; Fekete, 1996, 1999).

Development of the utricle, endolymphatic duct, saccule, cochlea and semicircular canals is associated with a localized distribution of apoptosis (Nishikori et al., 1999). At approximately 34 days morphogenesis begins: the endolymphatic

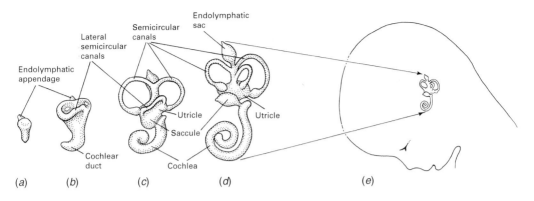

Fig. 11.4.   (*a*) Schematic summary of the development of the fetal cochlea and semicircular canals of the inner ear. (*a*) The otic vessel with an emerging endolymphatic appendage. (*b*) The lateral semicircular canals and cochlear duct appear. (*c*) The spiralling of the cochlear duct begins and the three semicircular canals and endolymphatic sac are clearly visible. (*d*) The developed embryonic inner ear shows the fully spiral cochlear duct, endolymphatic sac, utricle, saccule, and the anterior, posterior and lateral semicircular ducts (canals). (Modified from O'Rahilly and Müller, 1996.)

appendage appears dorsally and the cochlear duct elongates ventrally (see Fig. 11.4). The organ of Corti complex develops in the basal sections first, followed by the mid and apical regions. Afferent and efferent synaptogenesis begins during the late embryonic stages, and may not be complete until the postnatal period.

Development of the otic capsule begins with mesenchymal cells, and is induced by actions of the otic vesicle. The mesenchyme is remodelled by cavitation of the otic capsule to form the openings of the developing bony labyrinth. The cavitation results in the formation of the scala vestibuli and the scala tympani. The capsule is transformed from its cartilaginous state to an ossified form around the 16th week of development, from the base of the cochlea to the distal portions to the semicircular canals. The human inner ear reaches adult form at 10 weeks, and reaches adult size at around 20 weeks. During the embryological period of 9 to 20 weeks, the receptor cells undergo differentiation and grow to mature sizes. By the 26th week, the human inner ear is fully developed and believed to be functional (Kenna, 1990; Peck, 1995; Phippard et al., 1998). Congenital malformations of the inner ear may result in moderate to severe sensory–neural hearing loss or complete deafness (Jackler et al., 1987).

The outer ear

The outer (external) ear consists of the auricle or pinna, which collects airborne sound from the environment, the external auditory canal which channels the sound

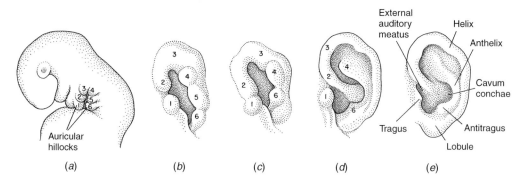

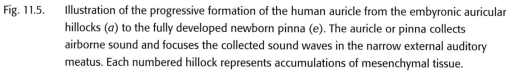

Fig. 11.5.   Illustration of the progressive formation of the human auricle from the embryonic auricular hillocks (*a*) to the fully developed newborn pinna (*e*). The auricle or pinna collects airborne sound and focuses the collected sound waves in the narrow external auditory meatus. Each numbered hillock represents accumulations of mesenchymal tissue.

waves toward the middle ear, and is bounded by the tympanic membrane or eardrum which converts the airborne vibrations to sympathetic mechanical vibrations (Fig. 11.1). The most visible part of the external ear is the auricle which first appears in the embryo as auricular hillocks (enlargements) around the pharyngeal (or branchial) arches 1 and 2. The mesenchymal auricular swellings appear at about 5 weeks in embryonic development and increase in size and number to six at about 6 weeks (Fig. 11.5(*a*)–(*e*)). The auricle derives from neural crest cells and mesenchyme, the embryonic connective tissue covered by cuboidal epithelium, in the first and second pharyngeal arches. The mesoderm in the first and second pharyngeal arches contributes the mesenchymal tissue in the hillocks.

The first three hillocks are the mandibular, and are believed to develop into the tragus and the crus of the helix. Auricular hillocks 4–6, the hyoid, form the helix and antitragus. Over the course of the embryonic period, as the mandible develops along with other craniofacial features, the auricles migrate from a ventrolateral position at the neck region to a dorsolateral position at the side of the head and the level of the eye with the lobule being the last part to develop (Anson & Davies, 1980; Moore, 1988; McPhee & Van De Water, 1988; O'Rahilly & Müller, 1996).

At approximately 8 weeks, the external auditory meatus develops from the dorsal aspect of the pharyngeal clefts, between the auricular hillocks. The ectodermal cells in the inferior aspect of the first pharyngeal groove multiply and invaginate to form an epithelial meatal plug (Fig. 11.6(*a*)–(*c*)). The fetal auricle and external auditory canal reach adult form at about 20 weeks, but continue to grow in size relative to the head into the puberty years (McPhee & Van De Water, 1988), with continued size modifications through life. The tympanic membrane forms at the point of contact between the ectodermal meatal plug and the endodermal tubotympanic recess, and is constructed in three layers: an outer ectodermal layer that is continuous with the tissue of the external auditory meatus, the intermediate layer of mesoderm, and the

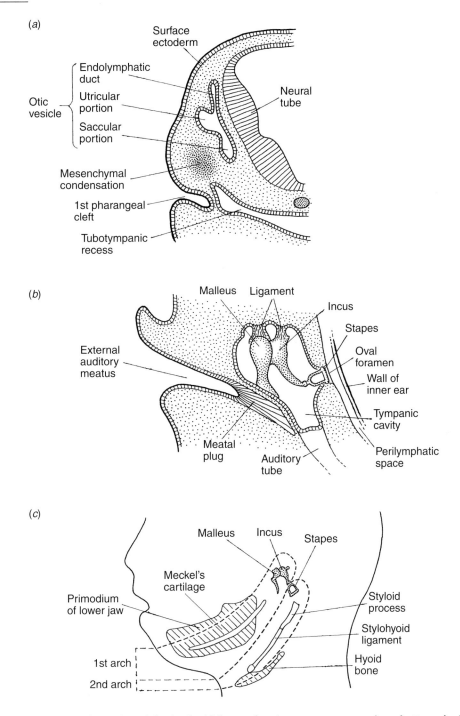

(a)

Surface ectoderm

Endolymphatic duct

Otic vesicle
- Utricular portion
- Saccular portion

Neural tube

Mesenchymal condensation

1st pharangeal cleft

Tubotympanic recess

(b)

Malleus   Ligament

Incus

Stapes

External auditory meatus

Oval foramen

Wall of inner ear

Tympanic cavity

Meatal plug

Auditory tube

Perilymphatic space

(c)

Malleus   Incus   Stapes

Meckel's cartilage

Primodium of lower jaw

Styloid process

Stylohyoid ligament

Hyoid bone

1st arch

2nd arch

Fig. 11.6.   Progressive formation of the fetal middle ear showing a transverse section of a 7-week-old embryo (a,b), and a schematic representation (c) of the middle ear and mandibulofacial structures derived from the first 3 branchial arches. The auditory malleus and incus derive from the first branchial arch and the stapes from the second. (Modified from Sadler, 1990.)

inner ectodermal layer that is continuous with the mucous membrane of the middle ear cavity (Anson & Davies, 1980).

Congenital defects of the human external ear include atresia of the external auditory meatus due to arrested development of the meatal plug or blockage by bone (Fig. 11.2). Atresia of the auditory canal causes a conductive hearing loss that is amenable to surgical correction. Malformation of the auricle is also seen in disruptions of the first branchial arch (first branchial arch syndrome). For example, Treacher–Collins syndrome is associated with congenital bilateral malformation of the auricles and external auditory meatus, mandibular and zygomatic hypoplasia, bilateral microtia and associated conductive hearing loss (Bergstrom, 1980). Common anomalies of the outer ear include microtia (abnormally small auricle) and macrotia (abnormally large auricle) ears that are often associated with syndromes.

It is now known that some forms of homeotic (Hox) genes guide the molecular differentiation of embryonic cells to form distinct auditory structures. In mice, for example, two defective copies of the Hoxa1 gene result in distortions in the embryonic development of the auricle and external auditory meatus. The congenital malformations seen in homozygous mutant mice probably result from a disruption of the critical inductive interactions between pharyngeal arches 1 and 2 mesenchyme and interactions between the arches, ear and hindbrain (Chisaka et al., 1992).

The middle ear

The middle ear is an air-filled cavity that serves as a hydrostatic pressure matching system and a mechanical sound transmission unit. The middle ear of mammals develops into a mucosal lined cavity that is defined by the tympanum, which forms the boundary with the external ear, the medial bony wall and the fenestrae (windows) of the cochlea. The middle ear arises near a portion of the developing skull that contains pneumatic (air-filled) mastoid cells that increase with growth of the petromastoid, stylus, squamous and tympanic components of the temporal bone. The middle ear subsystem consists of the auditory ossicles (malleus, incus and stapes), the ossicular muscles (tensor tympani and stapedius), the pharyngo-tympanic (eustachian) tube and the middle ear cavity. In the third and fourth weeks of development in the human embryo, the first pharyngeal pouch forms, giving rise to the mucosal layer of the tympanum, the tympanic cavity and eustachian tube (Figs. 11.2, 11.6). The mucosal layer of the tympanum, the eustachian tube and tympanic cavity originates from the endoderm, while the ossicles develop from the cephalic mesenchyme. The mesenchyme makes up a large proportion of the embryonic human temporal bone and is reorganized as the cavity expands (Piza et al., 1998). The tympanic cavity is lined with epithelial cells that are derived from the endoderm. The auditory ossicles, which derive from the first and second branchial (pharyngeal) arches, appear in the sixth week of human embryonic development and become fully formed in the area of the tubo-tympanic recess and external auditory meatus in the eighth week. After emerging from mesenchymal tissue, ossification of the auditory ossicles continues throughout the fetal development, reaching full adult size in 5 months.

The tiny middle ear muscles which attach the ossicles and the middle ear cavity wall, are also formed from mesenchymal tissue, and develop from the first and second branchial arches, respectively by the 16th week (McPhee & Van De Water, 1988). The m. tensor tympani, which inserts onto the handle of the malleus and tympanic membrane is innervated by a branch of the trigeminal (fifth cranial) nerve. The m. stapedius inserts onto the neck of the stapes and effectively abducts the stirrup-shaped ossicle from the oval window. The m. stapedius is innervated by the chorda tympani branch of the facial (seventh cranial) nerve. The smallest of the skeletal muscles, the stapedius, and the tensor tympani contract reflexively in response to loud sounds and during vocalization such as an infant's cry in order to attenuate and filter the sound reaching the cochlea (Borg & Counter, 1989).

The eustachian tube communicates with the nasopharyngeal cavity and adjusts middle ear air pressure relative to ambient pressure. This important pressure matching system maintains air equilibration and in so doing, protects the ear. For example, this automatic middle ear pressure adjustment action or the lack thereof is likely the reason for infant crying during dramatic ambient air pressure changes in the landing phase of aeroplane flight.

The middle ear is subject to a number of developmental abnormalities, including malformation of the ossicles and tympanic membrane. Perhaps the most common childhood middle ear disorder is otitis media, which may cause conductive hearing loss, discomfort, and in chronic cases permanent damage to middle ear structures as well as the inner ear. A second common middle ear disorder is otosclerosis, an autosomal dominant disorder that results in the production of excess osseous tissue in the tympanic cavity and fixation of the footplate of the stapes in the oval window. As with otitis media, otosclerosis causes a conductive hearing loss that is amenable to medical intervention. Congenital middle ear disorders are associated with other conditions and syndromes, such as Apert's acrocephalosyndactyly, Goldenhar's syndrome and Pierre Robin syndrome (Bergstrom, 1980).

Gene expression and neurotrophic factors in the embryonic development of the ear

During neurulation the hindbrain or rhombencephalon exhibits a series of transient bulges called rhombomeres that are critical for the subsequent development along different embryonic pathways of the inner, middle and external parts of the vertebrate ear, as well as the cranial nerve ganglia (Ruben et al., 1991; McPhee & Van

De Water, 1988; Moore, 1988; Sadler, 1990; Noden & Van de Water, 1992; O'Rahilly & Müller 1996). The inner ear, which develops first from the somatic ectoderm, can be observed adjacent to the developing rhombomere. The molecular mechanisms involved in the formation of bony labyrinth are not completely understood. However, the Brn4 gene has been strongly implicated in the formation of the bony labyrinth of the mammalian ear. Expression of this gene has been observed in the ventral portion of the otic capsule in the early embryonic stages (Phippard et al., 1998). The middle ear and external ear components develop later. Recent evidence suggests that inductive fields or signals in the ectoderm and mesoderm activate the formation of the otic disc or placode (Vendrell et al., 2000). These genetic inductive factors affect simultaneously the rhombencephalon, neural folds and otic disc. Interruptions in rhombomere development may cause congenital defects in the ear (Chisaka et al, 1992) that implicate specific gene transcription patterns in the embryological formation of the auditory outer, middle and inner ear components (Carpenter et al., 1993; Repressa et al., 2000; Pirvola et al., 1992, 2000).

Earlier studies of the genes from the *Drosophila* homeotic complex suggested that the homologous vertebrate homeotic Hox family of genes may specify segment identity in the anteroposterior axis of the mammalian embryo (Lewis, 1978; Redline et al., 1992). The Hox cluster of genes consists of 38 members, arranged in four linkage groups (HOXA-D) and on four distinct chromosomes in the genome (Chisaka et al., 1992). The genes can be experimentally manipulated or targeted for disruption by exogenous chemicals in order to study the mechanisms of expression. Using the mouse as a model for the human auditory system, Chisaka et al., 1992, for example, demonstrated that targeted disruption of the homeobox gene Hox-1.6 (Hoxa1) resulted in severe defects in the embryonic development of the outer, middle and inner ear, as well as the cranial nerves. Other genes such as fgf-3 (or int-2), a member of the fibroblast growth factor gene family, the Pax-3 gene and the Otx genes are believed to be involved in the formation of the inner ear (Torres & Giraldez, 1998).

Recent findings indicate that there are several groups of genes expressed during embryogenesis of the otic vesicle: genes encoding for transcription factors, such as dlx-3; dlx-4, GH6, SOHo-1, otx1, msx-D, Nkx-5.1, PAX-2; genes encoding secreted factors such as FGF-3, wnt-3, Xwnt-4, Bmp-4; genes encoding receptor tyrosine kinases: ret, sek-1; and Delta, a gene encoding membrane proteins of the Notch signalling system (Fekete, 1996; Fritzsch et al., 1995, 1997). Inductive signals expressed in the developing hindbrain at the level of rhombomeres 5 and 6, particularly int-2 (FGF-3), are required for the formation of the endolymphatic duct and sac (McKay et al., 1996). Lynch et al. (1997) identified DFNA1, a human homologue of diaphanous gene indrosphilla to be responsible for causing autosomal dominant, non-syndromic inner ear membranous defects and severe hearing loss.

An even more distinct effect is seen in the mouse atonal homologue (math) 1 gene, which has been reported to be responsible for the specification of the cochlear and vestibular hair cells (Bermingham et al., 1999). Two critical molecules have been identified in the induction of the otic placode. These signalling molecules, FGF-19, produced in the mesoderm and Wnt-8c from the neural plate, bring about the induction of the otic placode and inner ear organogenesis (Ladher et al., 2000).

It has been shown that a number of neurotrophins and their receptors are critical for the normal development of cochlear and vestibular neurons (Ernfors et al., 1995; Fritzsch et al., 1997; Phippard et al., 1998). Among the known molecules from the neurotrophin gene family that directly or indirectly modulate the afferent and efferent nerve fibres to the ear are nerve growth factor (NGF), brain-derived neurotrophic factor (BDNF), neurotrophin-3 (NT-3) (mice lacking NT-3 exhibit a reduction in cochlear neurons), and neurotrophin-4/5 (NT 4/5). These molecules bind selectively with receptor tyrosine kinases in the inner ear. NGF binds with the receptor TrkA, BDNF and NT-4/5 with TrkB and NT-3 with TrkC (Von Bartheld et al., 1991; Pirvola et al., 1992, 2000; Schecterson & Bothwell, 1994; Fritzsch et al., 1997). TrkB and TrkC receptors are expressed in early embryonic development of the cochlear and vestibular ganglia (Pirvola et al., 1992). The BDNF and NT-3 molecules and their receptors TrkB and TrkC are essential for survival of inner ear ganglion cells and ultimately the normal innervation of the inner ear (Fritzsch, et al., 1995).

Other recent findings on the molecular mechanisms involved with normal formation of the otic capsule have shown that the *Brn*4 gene is expressed in the otic capsule of mice in early otic embryogenesis. The *Brn*4 gene (human brain-4 orthologue, POU3F4) expression is believed to be regulated as the mesenchymal condensation forms the otic capsule (Phippard et al., 1998). Mutations in human *Brn*4 result in cochlear and middle ear hearing loss, defects in the bony labyrinth, partial hypoplasia of the cochlea, stapes fixation, dilated internal auditory meatus and blocked cochlear duct. The occurrence of this dysplastic phenotype in the cochlea (and internal auditory meatus) of patients with mutations in the human ortholog POU3F4 (around 27–47 days of gestation) appears to coincide with the timing of *Brn*4 gene expression in the developing otic capsule of the mouse (de Kok et al., 1995).

Mice that are homozygous for the int-2 gene have been found to have defective inner ears that are poorly developed and devoid of endolymphatic ducts and spiral ganglion cells (Mansour et al., 1993). The Otx genes (Otx1 and Otx2) play important roles in the morphogenesis of the mouse inner ear. Morsli et al. (1999), for example, observed a number of defects in the developing cochlea of Otx1 $-/-$ mutant mice (see Fig. 11.7 in colour plate section). Mutations in the Pax-3 gene in humans may lead to Waardenburg's syndrome, a condition characterized by disrupted melanocyte development and is associated with cochlear impairment and sensorineural hearing loss (Redline et al., 1992; Tassabehji et al., 1992). The cause of the lethal effects of these mutations is not fully understood. A mutant human myosin gene, myosin VIIA, which has been localized to a site on the long arm of chromosome 11, has been shown to cause both syndromic (in Usher's syndrome) and non-syndromic deafness (Steel & Brown, 1996; Petit, 1996). A human equivalent of the *Drosophila diaphanous* gene localized on chromosome 5 has been implicated in some cases of non-syndromic deafness (Lynch et al., 1997). The *diaphanous* gene is believed to be responsible for actions of the cytoskeletal protein actin in the inner ear hair cells and their stereocilia. The gene Connexin 26, which codes for a gap junctional protein that permits continuous electrical channels between neural elements, has been identified in the cochlea of rats (Lautermann et al., 1998). Mutations in Connexin 26 cause hearing loss and in some cases deafness, possibly by interfering with K^+ recycling in the sensory and non-sensory cells of the auditory epithelium (Zelante et al., 1997; Estivill et al., 1998). Identification of genes involved in the organogenesis of the mammalian ear is a significant advance in our understanding of fetal development, and will have major impact on our clinical approaches to hearing impairment and deafness.

Eighth nerve and brainstem auditory neuronal development

Both pre- and postnatal studies of auditory-evoked responses (ABR) indicate that the higher auditory tracts and nuclei develop rapidly and continue to develop during the first few years of life. Non-invasive, scalp surface recorded ABR measures represent summated electrophysiological activity from the eighth nerve through the ascending tracts and nuclei of the pons and lower midbrain (Chiappa, 1997). The ABR typically consists of six prominent surface positive wave peaks, with wave V being the earliest and most conspicuous in the newborn. Observations of ABR recordings show that wave peak amplitudes increased and neural conduction times (as indicated by the interpeak latencies of neural responses) shortened as the gestation period progressed to the last prenatal week (Salamy & McKean, 1976; Starr et al., 1977). Figure 11.8 shows ABR recordings in normal neonates during the first year of development which includes wave peaks I, II, III, IV, and V. The interpeak intervals (I–III, III–V, and I–V) indicate neural conduction times. The I–III interval reflects the neuronal transmission from the auditory nerve to the lower pons, while the III–V interval indicates the transmission time from the lower pons to the midbrain. The I–V ABR interval latency represents the neural conduction time throughout the ascending auditory tracts and nuclei from the eighth nerve to the lower midbrain, and is generally around 5 ms in full-term neonates (Levy, 1997). These ABR waves may be used to screen newborns for early detection of hearing loss and brain damage. The maturation of the central and peripheral

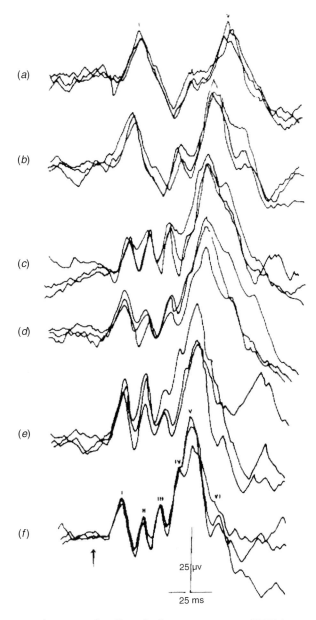

Fig. 11.8.   Development of auditory brainstem responses (ABR) in normal neonates during the first
year of development. The recordings show the absolute latencies of wave peaks I, II, III, IV,
and V. The inter-peak intervals (I–III, III–V, and I–V) indicate neural conduction times.
Ages: (*a*) newborn, (*b*) 6 weeks, (*c*) 3 months, (*d*) 6 months, (*e*) 12 months, (*f*) adult.
(From Salamy and McKean, 1976 with permission.)

auditory systems continues, albeit at different rates, for the first years of life (Salamy, 1984). Congenital hearing loss may impair development in the auditory tracts and nuclei of the developing brain (Hardie, 1998; Hardie et al., 1998).

The eighth cranial (auditory) nerve conveys the sensory cell information via 25 000 neurons from the cochlea to the brainstem. The eighth nerve ganglion develops from the otocyst at around the 28th day of embryonic development. The bipolar cells migrate to the basement membrane and the epithelium of the otic vesicle to form the eighth nerve ganglion. This ganglion divides into two portions: (i) the pars inferior that forms the cochlear nerve which innervates the hair cells of the organ of Corti, and the vestibular nerve which innervates the saccular macula of the posterior semicircular duct; (ii) the pars superior which develops into the vestibular nerve and which innervates the utricular macula and ampullae of the lateral semicircular ducts. The myelinated central processes of the eighth nerve ganglion (first-order neurons) travel through the internal auditory meatus to synapse at the cochlear nucleus. The cochlear nerve neurons bifurcate within the brainstem, sending an ascending tract to the anteroventral cochlear nucleus and a descending branch to the posteroventral cochlear nucleus. Second-order neurons of the higher auditory tract from the cochlear nucleus project to the ipsilateral lateral superior olive (near the midline of the ventral pons) and, through the trapezoid body to contralateral structures of the auditory tract. The ascending auditory tract includes the superior olivary bundle and the lateral lemniscus. The medial superior olive receives ascending auditory neurons from bilateral cochlear nuclei, the medial superior olive cells receive projections from the contralateral cochlear nucleus, and the lateral superior olive is innervated by auditory fibres from the ipsilateral cochlear nucleus. The third order of auditory neurons arises in the brachium of the inferior colliculus. The fourth order of ascending auditory neurons arise in the medial geniculate nucleus, which sends auditory radiations to the primary auditory cortex (A1 and A2) in the temporal lobe (Brodmann areas 31 and 32) (Kenna, 1990). Evidence suggests that early excitatory synaptic activity in the developing central auditory tracts and nuclei is necessary for normal function. Disruption of the development of structures in the auditory periphery or the central tracts and nuclei induces central hearing impairment (Moore, 1985, 1991; Kotak & Sanes, 1997).

Auditory function

Prenatal hearing

The functional development of the ear follows the maturation of the components of each of the three subsystems (outer, middle and inner ear). It has been shown that the ear is functionally active by the fifth month of gestation when the fetus is capable of responding to internal and external sounds at that stage of development (Johansson et al., 1964). At the 20th week of gestation, the human fetus shows an increase in heart rate in response to externally generated tones delivered to the abdomen of the mother (Johansson et al., 1964). During this period, the fetus has been bombarded with low frequency sounds at around 85 dB in the amniotic fluid, including the mother's heartbeat, muscular activities and possibly voice (Peck, 1995). Since sounds reaching the fetal ear in the amniotic sac are conducted by fluid (at a considerably higher velocity) rather than by air as in postnatal life, several acoustic features of the sound may differ. However, the fluid and bone-conducted sound still reaches the functional ear of the fetus and may evoke a measurable physiologic or motor reaction. Intrauterine startle responses to sound may be observed at week 28 of gestation. It is likely that the fetal ear is functionally capable of responding to a variety of biologically significant sounds by the 28th week of gestation.

Neonatal hearing

At birth, the human auditory system is sensitive to airborne as well as to bone-conducted sound. The neonate is bombarded with ambient noises as well as the voices of the mother, father, and caretakers. Auditory sensitivity in the neonate may be slightly less than that of older children with fully developed contiguous mechanical and neuro-electric subsystems. Acoustic reflex startle reactions in response to loud sounds may be evoked in the first postnatal days (Downs, 1967; Northern & Downs, 1991). Newborns may be calmed by low frequency sounds that accompany other stimulus-comforting modalities such as temperature and tactile. The neonate can also discriminate sounds on the basis of frequency, intensity and other acoustic features (Eisenberg, 1970). Downs (1967) found that sound could evoke the following behavioural responses in neonates: eyeblink or eyelid reflexes, Moro's response, cessation of activity, limb movement, head turning, grimacing, sucking, arousal, breathing changes, and widening of eyes. These acoustic reactions were further categorized by Eisenberg (1970) to include:

1. Overt reactions:
   (a) arousal
   (b) gross body movements
   (c) orienting behaviour
       (i) turning of head
       (ii) wide-eyed look
       (iii) pupillary dilation
   (d) motor reflexes
       (i) facial grimaces
       (ii) displacement of a single digit
       (iii) crying or cessation of crying
   (e) cardiac reactions
       (i) diphasic (deceleration–acceleration)
       (ii) latency changes with various acoustic signals

The normal infant is capable of sound localization in the environment at around 2 months after birth, and this skill becomes more refined over the next 4 months. At around 6 months, the infant can localize sound in the horizontal and vertical planes. Also, discrimination of ambient sound improves rapidly from birth, with the mother's voice probably being recognizable to the infant within the first month. At 4 weeks postnatal, the infant can discriminate phonemes, and at around 20 weeks is capable of 'learning' phonemic contrasts. At 12 weeks, the infant can attend to the mother's voice (Northern & Downs, 1991). Hearing acuity and speech sound discrimination continue to improve in the normal hearing infant through the first 3 years. Evidence of hearing impairment in the infant may be detected as early as the first month by objective auditory brainstem evoked response (ABR) tests and as early as 6 months by behavioural testing methods. With advances in physiological hearing testing technology, universal newborn hearing screening has become feasible using automated brainstem response (AABR) and otoacoustic emissions (OAE) techniques (Lutman, 2000). Otoacoustic emissions are essentially biological echoes of tonal stimuli that travel back from the cochlea through the middle ear to ear canal where they can be measured non-invasively by placing a small microphone at the entrance of the external auditory meatus. Otoacoustic emissions originate in the outer hair cells of the cochlea and reflect the integrity of the inner ear. Early identification of hearing loss in infants permits early intervention and possible corrective measures (Downs & Yoshinaga-Itano, 1999; Yoshinaga-Itano, 2000).

Higher auditory functions include the ability to localize sounds in space and speech discrimination. These abilities develop in early postnatal life in the normal neonate. Speech discrimination of phonemes and suprasegmentals (needed for normal speech and language development) is well developed around the tenth month of the postnatal period. Auditory experience and learning are important aspects of neonatal hearing development. Several features of experiential development are relevant to auditory development: (i) maturation or normal development of the auditory system, (ii) maintenance or the activation and normal use of the auditory system, (iii) facilitation or enabling perception and auditory experience, (iv) tuning or making the perceptual mechanisms more refined or sharper, and (v) induction or experientially based recognition and response (Werker, 1989; Peck, 1995).

Acknowledgements

The author thanks Dr Donna Fekete and Dr Göran Laurell for helpful suggestions and comments on the manuscript, and Dr Doris K. Wu for her kind permission to reproduce photomicrographs of the mutant ear.

REFERENCES AND RECOMMENDED READING

Anniko, M. & Wikström, S-O. (1984). Pattern formation of the otic placode and morphogenesis of the otocyst. *American Journal of Otolaryngology*, 5, 373–81.

Anson, B. J. and Davies, J. (1980). Embryology of the ear: developmental anatomy of the ear. In *Otolaryngology*, Vol. 1, ed. M. M. Paparella, D. A. Shumrick, W. L. Meyerhoff & A. B. Seil, Philadelphia: W. B. Saunders Co.

Bergstrom, L. (1980). Pathology of congenital deafness: present status and future priorities. *Annals of Otology, Rhinology and Laryngology*, 89, 31–2.

Bermingham, N. A., Hassan, B. A., Price, S. D. et al. (1999). Math 1: an essential gene for the generation of inner ear hair cells. *Science*, 284, 1837–41.

Borg, E. & Counter, S. A. (1989). The middle ear muscles. *Scientific American*, 260, 74–80.

Brown, S. D. & Steel, K. P. (1994). Genetic deafness – progress in mouse models. *Human Molecular Genetics*, 3, 1453–6.

Carpenter, E. M., Goddard, J. M., Chisaka, O., Manley, N. R. & Capecchi, M. R. (1993). Loss of Hox-A-1 (Hox-1.6) function results in the reorganization of the murine hindbrain. *Development*, 118, 1963–75.

Chiappa, K. H. (ed.) (1997). *Evoked Potentials in Clinical Medicine*. 3rd edn. Philadelphia: Lippincott-Raven.

Chisaka, O., Musci, T. S. & Capecchi, M. R. (1992). Developmental defects of the ear, cranial nerves and hindbrain resulting from targeted disruption of the mouse homeobox gene Hox-1.6. *Nature* , 355, 516–20.

Counter, S. A. and Tsao, P. (1986). Morphology of the seagull's inner ear. *Acta Otolaryngology (Stockholm)*, 101, 34–42.

de Kok, Y. J., van der Maarel, S. M., Bitner-Glindzicz, M. et al. (1995). Association between X-linked mixed deafness and mutations in the POU domain gene (POU3F4). *Science*, 267, 685–8.

Deol, M. S. (1966). Influence of the neural tube on the differentiation of the inner ear in the mammalian embryo. *Nature*, 209, 219–20.

Deol, M. S. (1980). Genetic malformations of the inner ear in the mouse and in the man. In *Morphogenesis and Malformation of the Ear*, ed. R. J. Gorlin, pp. 243–61.

Downs, M. P. (1967). A guide to newborn and infant hearing screening programs. *Archives of Otolaryngology*, 85, 15–22.

Downs, M. P. & Yoshinaga-Itano, C. (1999). The efficacy of early identification and intervention for children with hearing impairment. *Pediatric Clinics of North America*, 46, 79–87.

Eisenberg, R. (1970). *Auditory Competence in Early Life*. Baltimore: University Park Press.

Ekker, M., Akimenko, M. A., Bremiller, R. & Westerfield, M. (1992). Regional expression of three homeobox transcripts in the inner ear of zebrafish. *Neuron*, 9, 27–35.

Ernfors, P., Vandewater, T., Loring, J. & Jaenisch, R. (1995). Complementary roles of BDNF and NT-3 in vestibular and auditory development. *Neuron*, 14, 1153–64.

Estivill, X., Fortina, P., Surrey, S. et al. (1998). Connexin 26 mutations in sporadic and inherited deafness. *Lancet*, 351, 394–8.

Fekete, D. M. (1996). Cell fate specification in the inner ear. *Current Opinion in Neurobiology*, 6, 533–41.

Fekete, D. M. (1999). Development of the vertebrate ear: insights from knockouts and mutants. *Trends in Neuroscience*, **22**, 263–9.

Flock, Å. (1980). Contractile proteins in hair cells. *Hearing Research*, **2**, 411–12.

Flock, Å. & Cheung, H. C. (1977). Actin filaments in sensory hairs of inner ear receptor cells. *Journal of Cell Biology*, **75**, 339–43.

Fritzsch, B. (1996a). How does the urodele ear develop? *International Journal of Developmental Biology*, **40**, 763–71.

Fritzsch, B. (1996b). Development of the labyrinthine efferent system. *Annals of the New York Academy of Sciences*, **781**, 21–33.

Fritzsch, B., Silos-Santiago, I., Smeyene, A., Fagan, A. & Barbacid, M. (1995). Reduction and loss of inner ear innervation in trkB and trkC receptor knock out mice: a whole mount DiL and SEM analysis. *Aud Neuroscience*, **1**, 401–17.

Fritzsch, B., Silos-Santiago, I., Bianchi, L. M. & Farinas, I. (1997). The role of neurotrophic factors in regulating the development of inner ear innervation. *Trends of Neuroscience*, **20**, 159–64.

Gallagher, B. C., Henry, J. J. & Grainger, R. M. (1996). Inductive processes leading to inner ear formation during *Xenopus* development. *Developmental Biology*, **10**(175), 95–107.

Gulya, A. J. (1990). Developmental anatomy of the ear. In *Surgery of the Ear*, 4th edn., ed. M. E. Glasscock & G. E. Shambaugh, pp. 5–33. Philadelphia: W. B. Saunders Co.

Hardie, N. A. (1998). The consequences of deafness and chronic intracochlear electrical stimulation of the central auditory pathways. *Clinical Experimental Pharmacology and Physiology*, **25**, 303–9.

Hardie, N. A., Martsi-McClintock, A., Aitkin, L. M. & Shepherd, R. K. (1998). Neonatal sensorineural hearing loss affects synaptic density in the auditory midbrain. *NeuroReport*, **9**, 2019–22.

Hardisty, R. E., Fleming, J. & Steel, K. P. (1998). The molecular genetics of inherited deafness – current knowledge and recent advances. *Journal of Laryngology and Otology*, **112**, 432–7.

Holme, R. H. & Steel, K. P. (1999). Genes involved in deafness. *Current Opinion in Genetics and Development*, **9**, 309–314.

Hudspeth, A. J. (1989). How the ear's works work. *Nature*, **341**, 397–404.

Jackler, R. K., Luxford, W. M. & House, W. F. (1987). Congenital malformations of the inner ear: a classification based on embryogenesis. *Laryngoscope*, **97**, 2–14.

Johansson, B., Wedenberg, E. & Weston, B. (1964). Measurement of tone response by the human fetus. *Acta Otolaryngologica*, **57**, 188–92.

Kenna, M. A. (1990). The ear and related structures: embryology and developmental anatomy of the ear. In *Pediatric Otolaryngology*, 2nd edn, ed. C. D. Bluestone, S. E. Stool & M. D. Scheetz, pp. 77–87. Philadelphia: W. B. Saunders Co.

Keynes, R. & Krumlauf, R. (1994). Hox genes and regionalization of the nervous system. *American Review of Neuroscience*, **17**, 109–132.

Kotak, V. C. & Sanes, D. H. (1997). Deafferentation weakens excitatory synapses in the developing central auditory system. *European Journal of Neuroscience*, **9**, 2340–7.

Ladher, R. K., Anakwe, K. U., Gurney, A. L., Schoenwolf, G. C. & Francis-West, P. (2000). Identification of synergistic signals initiating inner ear development. *Science*, **290**, 1965–7.

Lautermann, J., ten Cate, W. J., Altenhoff, P. et al. (1998). Expression of the gap–junction connexins 26 and 30 in the rat cochlea. *Cell Tissue Research*, **294**, 415–20.

Lavigne-Rebillard, M. & Pujol, R. (1987). Hair cell innervation in the fetal human cochlea. *Acta Otolaryngologica*, **105**, 398–402.

Levy, S. R. (1997). Brainstem auditory evoked potentials in pediatrics. In *Evoked Potentials in Clinical Medicine*, 3rd edn, ed. K. H. Chiappa, Chapter 7. Philadelphia: Lippincott-Raven.

Lewis, A. B. (1978). A gene complex controling segmentation in *Drosophila*. *Nature*, **276**, 565–70.

Lutman, M. E. (2000). Techniques for neonatal hearing screening. *Seminars in Hearing*, **21**, 367–78.

Lynch, E. D., Lee, M. K., Morrow, J. E., Welsch, P. L., León, P. E. & King, M. C. (1997). Nonsyndromic deafness DFNA1 associated with mutation of a human homolog of the Drosophila gene diaphanous. *Science*, 1313–18.

McKay, I. J., Lewis, J. & Lumsden, A. (1996). The role of FGF-3 inner ear development: an analysis in normal and kreisler mutant mice. *Developmental Biology*, **174**, 370–8.

McPhee, J. R. & Van De Water, T. R. (1988). Structural and functional development of the ear. In *Physiology of the Ear*, ed. A. F. Jahn & J. Santos-Sacchi. New York: Raven Press.

Mansour, S. L., Goddard, J. M. & Capecchi, M. R. (1993). Mice homozygous for a targeted disruption of the proto-oncogene int-2 have developmental defects in the tail and inner ear. *Development*, **117**, 13–28.

Moore, D. R. (1985). Postnatal development of the mammalian central auditory system and the neural consequences of auditory deprivation. *Acta Otolaryngologica* (Stockholm) Suppl., **421**, 19–30.

Moore, D. R. (1991). Hearing loss and auditory brain stem development. In *The Fetal and Neonatal Brain Stem*, ed. M. A. Hanson. Cambridge: Cambridge University Press.

Moore, K. L. (1988). *Essentials of Human Embryology*. Toronto: B. C. Becker.

Morsli, H., Choo, D., Ryan, A., Johnson, R. & Wu, D. K. (1998). Development of the mouse inner ear and origin of its sensory organs. *Journal of Neuroscience*, **18**, 3327–35.

Morsli, H., Tuorto, F., Choo, D., Postiglione, M. P., Simeone, A. & Wu, D. K. (1999). Otx1 and Otx2 activities are required for the normal development of the mouse inner ear. *Development*, **126**, 2335–43.

Nishikori, T., Hatta, T., Kawauchi, H. & Otani, H. (1999). Apoptosis during inner ear development in human and mouse embryos: an analysis by computer-assisted three-dimensional reconstruction. *Anatomica Embryologica (Berlin)*, **200**, 19–26.

Noden, D. M. & Van de Water, T. R. (1992). Genetic analyses of mammalian ear development. *Trends in Neuroscience*, **15**, 235–7.

Northern, J. L. & Downs, M. P. (1991). *Hearing in Children*. 4th edn. Baltimore: Williams and Wilkins.

O'Rahilly, R. & Müller, F. (1996). *Human Embryology and Teratology*. 2nd edn. New York: John Wiley.

Pappas, D. G. (1983). Hearing impairments and vestibular abnormalities among children with subclinical cytomegalovirus. *Annals of Otology, Rhinology and Laryngology*, **92**, 552–7.

Peck, J. E. (1994). Development of hearing. Part II. Embryology. *Journal of the American Academy of Audiology*, **5**, 359–65.

Peck, J. E. (1995). Development of hearing. Part III. Postnatal development. *Journal of the American Academy of Audiology*, **6**, 113–23.

Petit, C. (1996). Genes responsible for human hereditary deafness: symphony of a thousand. *Nature Genetics*, **14**, 385–91.

Phippard, D., Heydemann, A., Lechner, M. et al. (1998). Changes in the subcellular localization of the Brn4 gene product precede mesenchymal remodeling of the otic capsule. *Hearing Research*, **120**, 77–85.

Pirvola, U., Ylikoski, J., Palgi, J., Lehtonen, E., Urumae, U. & Saarma, M. (1992). Brain-derived neurotrophic factor and neurotrophin 3 mRNAs in the peripheral target fields of developing inner ear ganglia. *Proceedings of the National Academy of Sciences, USA*, **89**, 9915–19.

Pirvola, U., Spencer-Dean, B., Xing-Qun, L. et al. (2000). FGF/FGFR-2 (IIIb) Signaling is essential for inner ear morphogenesis. *Journal of Neuroscience*, **16**, 6125–34.

Piza, J., Northrop, C. & Eavey, R. D. (1998). Embryonic middle ear mesenchyme disappears by redistribution. *The Laryngoscope*, **108**, 1378–82.

Redline, R., Neish, A., Holmes, L. & Collins, T. (1992). Biology of disease: homeobox genes and congenital malformations. *Laboratory Investigation*, **66**, 659–70.

Repressa, J., Frenz, D. A. & Van De Water, T. R. (2000). Genetic patterning of embryonic inner ear development. *Acta Otolaryngologica*, **120**, 5–10.

Ruben, R. J., Van De Water, T. R. & Steel, K. P. (1991).Genetics of hearing impairment. *Annals of the New York Academy of Sciences*, **630**, 329

Sadler, T. W. (1985). *Langman's Medical Embryology*, 5th edn, Chapter 17, *Ear*. Baltimore, London: Williams & Wilkins.

Sadler, T. W. (1990). *Langman's Medical Embryology*, 6th edn. Baltimore: Williams & Wilkins.

Salamy, A. (1984). Maturation of the auditory brainstem response from birth through early childhood. *Journal of Clinical Neurophysiology*, **1**, 293–329.

Salamy, A. & McKean, C. M. (1976). Postnatal development of human brainstem potentials during the first year of life. *Electroencephalography and Clinical Neurophysiology*, **40**, 418–26.

Schecterson, L. C. & Bothwell, M. (1994). Neurotrophin and neurotrophin receptor mRNA expression in developing inner ear. *Hearing Research*, **73**, 92–100.

Sher, A. E. (1971). The embryonic and postnatal development of the inner ear of the mouse. *Acta Otolaryngologica* (Suppl.), **285**, 1–20.

Starr, A., Amlie, R. N., Martin, W. H. & Sanders, S. (1977). Development of auditory function in newborn infants revealed by auditory brainstem potentials. *Pediatrics*, **60**, 831–9.

Steel, K. P. & Brown, S. D. (1996). Genetics of deafness. *Current Opinions in Neurobiology*, **6**, 520–5.

Tassabehji, M., Newton. V. E. & Read, A. P. (1992). Waardenberg syndrome type 2 caused by mutations in the human microphthalmia (MITF) gene. *Nature Genetics*, **8**, 251–5.

Torres, M. & Giraldez, F. (1998). The development of the vertebrate inner ear. *Mechanisms of Development*, **71**, 5–21.

Van de Water, T. R. (1988). Tissue interactions and cell differentiation: neurone–sensory cell interaction during otic development. *Development*, **103**(Suppl.), 185–93.

Van de Water, T. R. & Repressa, J. (1991). Tissue interactions and growth factors that control development of the inner ear. Neural tube-otic anlage interaction. *Annals of the New York Academy of Science*, **630**, 116–28.

Vendrell, V., Carnicero, E., Giraldez, F., Alonso, M. T. & Schimmang, T. (2000). Induction of inner ear fate by FGF3. *Development*, **127**, 2011–19

Von Bartheld, C. S., Patterson, S. L., Heuer, J. G., Wheeler, E. F. & Bothwell, M. (1991). Expression of nerve growth factor (NGF) receptors in the developing inner ear of the chick and rat. *Development*, **113**, 455–470.

Werker, J. F. (1989). Becoming a native listener. *American Scientist*, **77**, 54–9.

Whitehead, M. C. (1986). Development of the cochlea. In *Neurobiology of Hearing*, ed. R. A. Alschuler, D. W. Hoffman & R. P. Bobbin. New York: Raven Press.

Whitfield, T. T., Granato, M., van Eeden, F. J. et al. (1996). Mutations affecting development of the zebrafish inner ear and lateral line. *Development*, **123**, 241–54.

Wu, D. K. & Oh, S. H. (1996). Sensory organ generation in the chick inner ear. *Journal of Neuroscience*, **15**, 6454–62.

Yoshinaga-Itano, C. (2000). Successful outcomes for deaf and hard-of-hearing children. *Seminars in Hearing*, **21**, 309–26.

Zelante, L., Gasparini, P., Estivill, X. et al. (1997). Connexin 26 mutations associated with the most common form of non-syndromic neurosensory autosomal recessive deafness (DFNB1) in Mediterraneans. *Human Molecular Genetics*, **6**, 1605–9.

12

Cerebrovascular regulation in the neonate

William J. Pearce

Department of Physiology, Center for Perinatal Biology, Loma Linda University, CA, USA

In virtually all viviparous species, the end of gestation involves a diverse but well-coordinated acceleration of numerous developmental processes that prepare the fetus for birth and postnatal survival. From a cardiovascular perspective, this acceleration involves changes in blood vessel composition, reactivity, innervation, and reflex regulation, but most importantly these vascular changes parallel the parenchymal tissues' expanding metabolic demand. A key principle of cardiovascular homeostasis in the fetus, as well as the neonate and adult, is that tissue perfusion is matched to, and regulated by, tissue metabolic demand. Certainly, the developing brain is no exception to this general principle, even though many of the precise mechanisms responsible for flow-metabolism coupling in the immature brain remain unclear. The purpose of this chapter is to review recent advances in our understanding of cerebrovascular regulation in the immature brain, with an emphasis on findings made since 1995.

Neonatal cerebral metabolism

In the newborns of most species, including humans, cerebral metabolic rate is low at birth and rises steadily throughout early postnatal life. The rate of increase in metabolic demand varies in different brain areas, such that occipital demand rises early, followed by other brain areas including basal ganglia and primary cerebral cortex, with the frontal association cortex the last to demonstrate an increase to adult levels. In all these areas, respiratory quotient is often less than 1.0 during development, indicating the utilization of fuels other than glucose. Correspondingly, the abundances of the GLUT-1 and GLUT-3 glucose transporters are low in the neonate and increase as dependence on glucose increases. In terms of specific metabolic pathways, many exhibit high activity in the neonate including those involving the cytochrome P450 enzymes, the cyclooxygenases, the potentially excitotoxic glutaminergic pathways, and the ornithine decarboxylase pathways. Other key pathways, including those for free radical scavenging and nitric oxide synthesis, are depressed relative to adults in many brain regions. Altogether, the patterns of low cerebral metabolism unique to the term fetus enable it to survive the transient reductions in cerebral oxygenation that often accompany birth. At the same time, the marked regional heterogeneity in rates of cerebral metabolism render some areas more vulnerable than others during episodes of asphyxia or ischemia.

Cerebral vessel development and differentiation

Whereas the basic processes governing vasculogenesis apply to cerebral as well as systemic arteries, development of the cerebral vasculature exhibits several unique characteristics. First, cerebrovascular density correlates well with regional metabolic demand. Correspondingly, cerebrovascular conductance in the vertebrobasilar and carotid systems increases more slowly than brain weight, particularly during the postnatal period of rapid cerebral growth, myelination, and differentiation. In all brain regions, most cerebral arteries first arise as vertically oriented vascular trunks that later give rise to extensive radial branching. In general, the total number of cerebral arteries is at a maximum at birth, after which rarefaction begins to occur. Cerebral arteries typically make few arterio-venous connections, lack a vasovasorium, and exhibit an uneven medial distribution of elastic tissues that are more abundant in immature than in mature cerebrovascular networks. Compared to systemic arteries, cerebrovascular smooth muscle differentiation lags behind that observed in the aorta, umbilical, subclavian, and carotid arteries, even though cerebral arteries generally contain similar amounts of the intermediate filament proteins desmin and vimentin. Most immature human cerebral arteries appear to have, as part of normal development, regions of weakened media near vessel bifurcations. These weakened regions are reinforced during maturation via the deposition of additional smooth muscle, but can comprise areas of heightened vulnerability to rupture during early postnatal development.

Without doubt, the dramatic changes in cerebrovascular composition and phenotype characteristic of the perinatal period are strongly influenced by a variety of growth factor and hormonal influences, including vascular endothelial growth factor and basic fibroblast growth factor. Together with the gradual postnatal withdrawal of the effects of the steroids of pregnancy, these endocrine influences coordinate an overall decrease in extracellular water content, an increased synthesis and extracellular deposition of collagen, and ultimately a conversion to more Type III and less Type I collagen. The net result of these changes is an increase in mechanical stiffness that progresses with postnatal age (Pearce et al., 1991).

Cerebral perfusion during the perinatal period

Whereas our understanding of cerebral perfusion in the fetus and neonate in the late 1980s was dominated by relatively few measurements of animal cerebral blood flow using microspheres, inert gas clearance, and indicator dilution methods, the past decade has ushered in an abundance of new methods for the quantification of cerebral perfusion not only in immature animals but also in human neonates. Chief among these new methods is Doppler technology, which by virtue of its low cost and non-invasive nature, is now used widely in many different types of applications. For example, transcranial Doppler measurements of middle cerebral artery velocity are now routinely used to assess fetal status. Regional maps of cerebral perfusion patterns can be created using colour Doppler amplitude ultrasound, and transvaginal B-mode sonography combined with power Doppler flow mapping can provide serial images of fetal cerebrovascular development. Careful application of power flow Doppler measurements can even be used to construct three-dimensional images of cerebrovascular morphology. The rapid proliferation of Doppler-based technologies has had a dramatic impact on our ability to observe cerebral perfusion in the neonate, but often the interpretation of the data which these methods provide is not clear cut. Although blood flow velocities measured in the middle cerebral artery appear generally representative of overall cortical perfusion, the commonly measured and reported pulsatility index is affected by both mean arterial pressure and critical closing pressure as well as cerebral perfusion, and thus alone is a composite variable with no unique physiological relevance (Michel & Zernikow, 1998). In addition, the use of pulsed Doppler can deposit sufficient energy in cerebral tissues to raise brain temperature, and maternal plasma glucose levels, fetal hematocrit, and a patent ductus arteriosus can influence fetal Doppler velocity flow profiles in the fetal middle cerebral artery. Together, these findings demonstrate that Doppler measurements may be convenient and economical, but must be interpreted cautiously. With proper interpretation, these methods can provide valuable diagnostic information about many cerebrovascular complications, and can be particularly useful in evaluation of occlusive pathologies related to sickle cell disease, hydrocephalus, asphyxia, cerebral edema, and vasospasm.

Aside from Doppler-based methods, several other technologies have recently shown great utility for measurements of fetal cerebral perfusion. One of the most important of these is near-infrared spectroscopy (NIRS), which has proved to be a convenient bedside tool for assessment of cerebral oxygenation and perfusion in neonates. NIRS measurements are based on the spectral shifts related to the oxygenation and deoxygenation of hemoglobin and thus, unlike Doppler measurements, are generally independent of mean arterial pressure and hematocrit. NIRS-based methods can provide reliable measures of blood oxyhemoglobin, deoxyhemoglobin, total hemoglobin, and cerebral blood volume, and in combination with the use of the dye indocyanine green, can also be used to measure neonatal cerebral blood flow with reasonable accuracy. As for all methods that assess neonatal cerebral perfusion, NIRS measurements also have several limitations including sensitivity to probe position, hemoglobin concentration, and specificity for hemoglobin. Nonetheless, when properly implemented and interpreted, NIRS offers many important advantages (Barfield et al., 1999).

Another important methodology gaining popularity for assessments of cerebral perfusion in neonates is single photon emission computed tomography (SPECT). Although technologically more complex and costly than either Doppler or NIRS-based methods, SPECT is uniquely capable of providing information regarding regional cerebral perfusion, particularly in subcortical grey and cerebellar areas. SPECT radiotracers, such as technetium-99m hexamethylpropylene-amine-oxime, iodine-123 iodoamphetamine, and technetium-99m-ethylcysteinate dimer have demonstrated great utility for measurement of neonatal cerebral perfusion, particularly in patients afflicted with epilepsy, cerebral palsy, and other neurological disorders of the neonate. One particularly promising development along this line is our growing ability to synthesize receptor-specific radioligands that should, in the near future, enable non-invasive measurements to be made of various receptor densities and patterns of distribution in the neonatal brain (Gordon, 1998).

Perhaps the most expensive of all methods used to measure neonatal cerebral perfusion is positron emission tomography (PET). Although the ability to measure simultaneously regional cerebral perfusion, oxygen extraction fraction, oxygen consumption and blood volume with this method is unmatched by any other available method, the requirement for on-site synthesis of ^{15}O-containing compounds limits use of this method to a few centres. On the other hand, development of PET tracers using the more stable isotope ^{18}F is expanding rapidly and these tracers are beginning to find applications in studies of the neonatal brain in relation to both normal and pathological patterns of metabolism, oncology, epilepsy, and other cerebral pathologies.

Altogether, the various methods of neonatal cerebral blood flow measurement have enabled a relatively consistent view of cerebral perfusion as it changes during the perinatal period. From these studies it is clear that, with advancing gestation, the velocity of perfusion increases and overall cerebrovascular resistance decreases through term. However, cerebral perfusion in the fetus can be influenced by maternal emotional state, as shown in both experimental animals and humans (Sjostrom et al., 1997). During birth, cerebral perfusion can undergo dramatic fluctuations whose extent depends on the mode of delivery, as well as the size of the fetus. Following birth, human cerebral blood flow and oxygen consumption continue to increase through puberty, although the rates of increase vary significantly among different brain regions and individuals. Although occipital flow has been reported to be less than frontal or parietal flow in preterm neonates, the last brain region to exhibit adult levels of perfusion during postnatal development is typically the frontal association cortex (Takahashi et al., 1999). Consistent with functional asymmetry in the developing brain, human cerebral blood flow also often exhibits a right hemispheric predominance during the first few postnatal years.

Cellular mechanisms governing neonatal cerebrovascular reactivity

Coincident with the changing patterns of cerebral perfusion which characterize postnatal development, the contractile reactivity of individual cerebral arteries also undergoes dramatic alterations. In virtually all cerebral vessels, mechanical stiffness, wall thickness, smooth muscle cell size, and overall contractility increase with postnatal age (Pearce et al., 1991), but the extent of these changes is heterogeneously distributed between arteries and veins, between large and small arteries, between arteries of the brainstem and those of the cortex, and between pial and parenchymal arterioles. Amidst this complex variability, however, the basic principles of pharmacomechanical coupling still always apply. Most importantly, these principles dictate that reactivity to any agonist, whether physiological or pharmacological in origin, is determined mainly by the types of receptors present that are capable of binding the agonist in question. As is becoming increasingly clear, most agonists can bind multiple receptor types in any given tissue, and thus reactivity is largely governed by the receptor types present at the moment in time when the agonist appears. It is also important to recognize that the types and numbers of receptors present can be quite dynamic and subject to the processes of intracellular sequestration and/or downregulation, both of which reduce the numbers of receptors present. Thus, the density of each receptor type present is a critical determinant of overall reactivity to any agonist. Finally, the affinity of any receptor for its ligand largely determines the agonist concentrations necessary to activate the receptor. From a physiological perspective, this feature is particularly important because agonist affinity not only determines the magnitudes of the often measured ED50 values, but it is also physiologically up- and downregulated by a unique class of enzymes known as G-protein coupled receptor kinases (Pitcher et al., 1998). Although the effects of maturation on many of these determinants of pharmacomechanical coupling still await exploration in the developing cerebral circulation, certain features of this coupling are beginning to become clear.

In all tissues, the final effect of pharmacomechanical coupling is determined by the intracellular pathways that are activated by receptor occupation on the cell surface (see Fig. 12.1). In blood vessels, this coupling almost invariably influences the activity of the contractile proteins abundant in all smooth muscle cells. Typically, contractile agonists act to increase the cytosolic concentration of the key second messenger calcium, which in turn binds to calmodulin, activates myosin light chain kinase, increases the level of myosin light chain phosphorylation, and thereby stim-

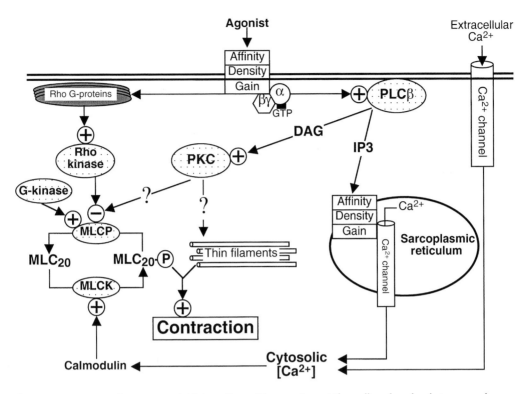

Fig. 12.1.   In most tissues, agonist interaction with receptors at the cell surface leads to second
messenger production as determined by receptor affinity, density, and gain (mass of
second messenger produced for each ligand–receptor interaction). Such agonist–receptor
binding may lead to activation of protein kinase C (PKC) via liberation of diacylglycerol
(DAG) which in turn can act on either thin filaments, or possibly on myosin light chain
phosphatase (MLCP). In some cells, receptor occupation can also stimulate activation of
the rho p21 via an unknown mechanism, that then activates Rho kinase which can
phosphorylate and inactivate MLCP, thereby leading to an apparent increase in Ca^{2+}
sensitivity. See text for details and references.

ulates development of contractile tone (Somlyo et al., 1999). Whereas the majority
of studies of contractile protein regulation since the 1970s have focused mainly on
the mechanisms whereby contractile and relaxant agonists influence cytosolic
calcium levels within smooth muscle cells, a broad range of more recent studies
clearly indicate that the sensitivity of the contractile proteins to calcium is also
physiologically regulated (Somlyo et al., 1999). By influencing contractile protein
calcium sensitivity, many agonists can dramatically influence contractile tone independent of their effects on cytosolic calcium concentration. A growing number of
studies now indicate that the ability of some agonists to influence contractile protein
calcium sensitivity varies with age, particularly in the cerebral circulation (Akopov

et al., 1997). In response to serotonin, for example, immature rabbit and lamb cerebral arteries exhibit a much more robust increase in contractile protein calcium sensitivity than observed in corresponding adult arteries (Akopov et al., 1997). The mechanism of this effect is apparently unrelated to age-related differences in protein kinase C activity, but in all likelihood involves the small G-protein rho, the specific kinase (rho-kinase) it activates, and the effects of this kinase on the extent of myosin light chain phosphorylation (Somlyo et al., 1999). This feature of immature cerebral arteries imparts to them an ability to regulate contractility with only modest effects on cytosolic calcium. In contrast, adult cerebral arteries exhibit more modest agonist-induced changes in calcium sensitivity, but more robust increases in cytosolic calcium concentration (Akopov et al., 1997, 1998). Overall, these data suggest that cerebrovascular responses to contractile agonists involve increases in both contractile protein calcium sensitivity and cytosolic calcium concentration, and that maturation decreases the importance of calcium sensitization, and increases the importance of calcium release in the cerebral circulation.

The relative inability of contractile agonists to increase cytosolic calcium in immature cerebral arteries is apparently not due to an absence of intracellular receptors for the second messenger inositol trisphosphate (IP3). For many contractile agonists, receptor occupation leads directly to the synthesis of IP3, which then diffuses to the surface of the sarcoplasmic reticulum where it activates specific receptors that mediate the release of sequestered calcium. Measurements of IP3 receptor density in fetal and adult cerebral arteries indicate that maturation has relatively little effect on the density of IP3 receptors present (Zhou et al., 1997). Similarly, maturation has relatively little effect on the ability of agonists to stimulate the synthesis of IP3 (Longo et al., 1996). Conversely, direct measurements of IP3-induced calcium release in permeabilized fetal and adult ovine cerebral arteries indicate that the size of the IP3 releasable calcium pool appears inadequate to support contraction in immature, but not mature, cerebral arteries. At the same time, immature cerebral arteries are highly dependent on the influx of extracellular calcium for activation (Akopov et al., 1998), much more so than are corresponding adult arteries. Together, these findings suggest that, in relation to cerebrovascular contractility, the physiological importance of calcium cycling between the cytosol and intracellular stores increases with advancing postnatal age. Correspondingly, the importance of calcium sensitization responses to agonist stimulation appear to diminish with maturation. From a dietary perspective this shift bears on the transition to extrauterine life where one of the first nutritional priorities is to increase the overall calcium mass of the neonate. This increasing calcium mass is apparently not only directed to the skeleton, but also appears to enhance the size, and physiological importance for contraction, of the releasable intracellular stores of calcium in developing cerebral arteries.

Maturation of cerebrovascular vasoconstrictor responses

A key developmental characteristic of the cerebral circulation is that overall cerebrovascular resistance generally parallels arterial pressure during maturation and thus is quite low in the fetus, increases dramatically with birth, and thereafter continues to increase toward adult levels during early postnatal life. The low cerebrovascular resistance typical of the fetal cerebrovascular circulation is not due to depressed vascular reactivity, because fetal cerebral arteries are highly sensitive to many contractile agonists. For some, such as norepinephrine and serotonin, sensitivity (as indicated by ED50 values) is significantly greater in fetal than in adult cerebral arteries, even though overall capacity for force generation is less in fetal than adult arteries. A key mechanism responsible for this difference appears to be agonist affinity for the receptor, which for both norepinephrine (Elliott & Pearce, 1994) and serotonin (Angeles et al., 2000) is greater in fetal than adult arteries. Receptor density also appears to play a role and is often greater in fetal than adult cerebral arteries, at least for norepinephrine (Longo et al., 1996). The coupling of norepinephrine to production of the contractile second messenger IP3 is apparently not different in fetal and adult cerebral arteries (Longo et al., 1996), which in turn suggests that much of the observed age-related difference in agonist sensitivity is probably attributable to corresponding differences in the agonist affinity and density of the receptors involved.

In contrast to norepinephrine and serotonin, prostaglandin F2α appears to promote vasodilatation at low concentrations in cerebral arteries from fetal baboons and newborn piglets, but marked vasoconstriction in corresponding adult arteries (Li et al., 1997). Although the effects of maturation on the agonist affinity of the PGF2α receptor have yet to be reported, several studies do suggest that receptor density for this agonist increases during development and maturation, and thereby imparts greater sensitivity to PGF2α with advancing postnatal age (Li et al., 1997). Correspondingly, PGF2α-induced IP3 synthesis closely follows age-related changes in receptor density (Li et al., 1997). Developmental regulation of PGF2α receptor density, in turn, appears to involve receptor downregulation in response to the circulating levels of PGF2α, synthesized mainly by cyclooxygenase-2, which are generally greater in the fetus and neonate than in the adult (Li et al., 1997).

Like prostaglandin F2α, sensitivity to angiotensin also appears to increase with age in cerebral arteries. Unlike prostaglandin F2α, however, responses to angiotensin appear to reflect developmental changes in the type of receptor mediating the response (Ardaillou, 1999). In many tissues, the AT1 family of angiotensin receptors is predominant in adult tissues, and stimulation of this subtype typically activates the phospholipase C cascade and thereby promotes cell activation and often vasoconstriction. Conversely, the AT2 receptor is predominant in many fetal tissues, and activation of this receptor appears to attenuate cell activation, particularly that induced by AT1 receptor activation, through unresolved mechanisms that may involve activation of protein tyrosine phosphatase (Ardaillou, 1999). In addition to the developmental shift in angiotensin receptor subtype, there is an important heterogeneity in tissue distribution that can be influenced by oestrogen levels. Administration of angiotensin II to immature animals generally produces cerebral vasodilatation mediated by activation of either AT2 receptors on the cerebrovascular smooth muscle, or by AT1 receptors located directly on the cerebrovascular endothelium. In isolated immature human cerebral arteries from the circle of Willis, however, angiotensin II is a vasoconstrictor (Bevan et al., 1998a,b) suggesting that the distribution of angiotensin receptor subtypes probably varies significantly among large and small arteries of the human cerebral circulation. In addition to developmental shifts in angiotensin receptor subtype, the distribution of these subtypes varies among different tissues and is strongly influenced by oestrogen.

Endothelin is another potent vasoconstrictor in fetal cerebral arteries (Yakubu et al., 1995). Circulating levels of endothelin are greater in neonates than adults, and the receptors mediating endothelin's effects are regulated in terms of both their density and their distribution, both as part of normal development and in response to disease states such as pulmonary hypertension and chronic hypoxia. Effects of endothelin receptor activation are mediated by increased influx of extracellular calcium, but the end-effects of endothelin are highly cell-type specific. Endothelin can depolarize neurones, modulate astrocyte growth and differentiation, and augment coagulation. In neonatal cerebral arteries, endothelin dilates at low concentrations and constricts at concentrations above 1 ng/ml and both of these effects involve increased prostanoid synthesis. The physiological stimuli that promote the release of endothelin from cerebral arteries during the perinatal period remain controversial but probably include hypoxia, flow-induced shear stress, and stretch of the cerebral arterial wall.

In addition to norepinephrine, serotonin, prostaglandin F2α, angiotensin, and endothelin, many other compounds typically stimulate vasoconstriction in immature cerebral arteries, including leukotrienes, thromboxanes, and neuropeptide Y. Multiple receptor types have been documented for several of these compounds, including endothelin and the leukotrienes, but studies have yet to be conducted to determine how maturation influences the expression and/or function of any of these receptors. The effect of maturation on responses to many of these agents remains largely unexplored. Thus the growing availability of specific ligands and antagonists for many of these receptors promises to provide numerous new opportunities to identify how the type, affinity, and density of these receptors contribute to maturation of cerebrovascular regulation.

Maturation of cerebrovascular vasodilator responses

As for many of the compounds that contract immature cerebral arteries, the effects of maturation on responses to most cerebral vasodilators remain largely unexplored. For the great majority of these compounds, very little is known about the subtype distributions, agonist binding affinities, and densities of the receptors that mediate these responses in the fetal cerebral circulation. Correspondingly, any discussion of the age-related changes in cerebral vasodilator responses is largely limited to consideration of the agents shown to be effective in the fetal cerebral circulation, their circulating levels, and the physiological responses to which they may contribute.

One of the most important vasodilators in the immature cerebral circulation is adenosine. Circulating adenosine levels are up to fourfold greater in the fetus than the adult and adenosine clearly exerts a strong tonic vasodilator influence in human infants, as indicated by vasoconstrictor responses to adenosine antagonists such as aminophylline and caffeine. Studies in fetal sheep further indicate that this tonic vasodilator influence may not become significant until sometime in the third trimester (Kurth & Wagerle, 1992). Given that adenosine potently vasodilates the fetal cerebral circulation, it is probable that the A2 family of receptors predominate in immature cerebral arteries (Kurth & Wagerle, 1992). Consistent with this (untested) view, is the observation that phenylisopropyl adenosine, which has greater affinity for the A1 than the A2 families of adenosine receptors, has little effect on medullary and pontine blood flows in the fetal sheep (Bissonnette et al., 1995). Adenosine contributes to cerebral vasodilator responses to hypoxia through mechanisms that appear sensitive to hypoglycemia, may also contribute to hypercapnic cerebral vasodilation in the neonate, and it probably plays a major role in cerebrovascular responses to systemic hypotension. Because responses to exogenous adenosine are generally inversely proportional to artery diameter (Gidday & Park, 1992), it is probable that the density, affinity, and/or coupling of adenosine receptors to the contractile proteins also changes with vessel size. Although this relation seems logical in light of the fact that the greatest adenosine concentrations are generated in the vicinity of the smallest arteries and arterioles, it remains an unexplored topic for future investigation.

Another important family of fetal cerebral vasodilators are the prostaglandins. In the fetus, high basal levels of prostaglandins, particularly PGE2 and PGI2, contribute to basal cerebral vasodilator tone. Correspondingly, administration of indomethacin generally decreases perfusion in the immature human cerebral circulation (Yanowitz et al., 1998). Whereas recent findings suggest that indomethacin can antagonize interactions between vasodilator prostaglandins and their receptors (Parfenova et al., 1995), the main effect of this drug is to inhibit prostaglandin synthesis. The major sources of vasodilator prostaglandins in the fetal cerebral circulation are probably the neurones and glia of the cortical cerebrum, although a significant portion of the basal production of vasodilator prostaglandins also resides within the cerebral arteries themselves because administration of indomethacin also constricts cerebral arteries isolated from human infants (Bevan et al., 1998a,b). The main enzyme responsible for prostaglandin synthesis in the neonate is cyclooxygenase-2, and the activity of this enzyme appears subject to regulation by tyrosine phosphorylation (Parfenova et al., 1999). The high fetal activity of this enzyme results not only in elevated levels of vasodilator prostanoids, but also in low levels of the receptors for these compounds due to receptor downregulation (Chemtob et al., 1996). Vasodilator prostaglandins participate in numerous physiological responses, including those to hypoxia, hypercapnia, and asphyxia. Prostanoids also participate in responses to hypotension and cerebral autoregulation, and are probably also involved in the altered patterns of cerebrovascular reactivity associated with intracranial haemorrhage in the neonate (Yakubu & Leffler, 1996). This broad involvement in multiple responses reflects the participation of vasodilator prostaglandins and their receptors not only in direct signal transduction pathways, but also in the potential permissive and modulatory actions of prostanoids in many cerebrovascular responses (Zucker & Leffler, 1998).

Opioid peptides are another class of compounds capable of vasodilating the immature cerebral circulation. This family includes methionine enkephalin, leucine enkephalin and dynorphin, which are endogenous agonists for mu, delta, and kappa opioid receptors, respectively. All three of these opioids can vasodilate immature piglet cerebral arteries, although their efficacies vary significantly with species. In the human preterm neonate, for example, continuous administration of morphine at $100\,\mu g/kg/h$ has little effect on cerebrovascular hemodynamics. Cerebral vasodilatation associated with opioids also often involves increased cyclic nucleotide levels in the cerebrospinal fluid and is attenuated by oxygen free radicals. The exact relation between opioid action and cyclic nucleotide levels remain unclear, as it has been proposed both that cyclic nucleotides elevate opioid levels (Armstead, 1997), and vice versa that elevated cyclic nucleotides facilitate opioid release (Wilderman & Armstead, 1997a). Under resting conditions in most species, opioids contribute little to basal cerebrovascular tone, but do appear to participate in neonatal cerebrovascular responses to hypoxia, hypercapnia, and possibly also hypotension. Despite evidence that opioids and their receptors are developmentally regulated and play key roles in the growth and differentiation of many tissues, the ontogeny of this signalling pathway in the cerebral circulation remains largely unexplored.

Receptor-dependent signal transduction pathways mediate the immature cerebral vasodilatory responses not only to adenosine, prostaglandins, and opioids, but also to many other agonists including NMDA, kainate, vasopressin, CGRP, and many other compounds whose vasoactivity and mechanisms of action in the neonatal cerebral circulation are just beginning to be explored. Aside from these receptor-dependent vasodilators, the fetal cerebral vasculature also dilates in response to several receptor-independent vasodilators, the most important of which is nitric oxide. In fetal as well as adult brains, nitric oxide is synthesized by endothelial, neuronal, and inducible isoforms of the enzyme nitric oxide synthase (Stuehr, 1999). The abundances of the endothelial and neuronal isoforms appear to increase with postnatal age, at least in rats and hamsters, but may change little with maturation in the human brain (Downen et al., 1999). The ontogeny of the inducible isoform has not been widely studied, but its abundance has been reported to transiently increase during fetal development and then in late term falls to very low levels typical of the adult (Galea et al., 1995). The human fetal cerebrovascular circulation is quite sensitive to nitric oxide, as indicated by ability of NO inhalation to increase fetal cerebral blood flow velocity (Polvi et al., 1996). In terms of physiological responses, nitric oxide is not only important for human brain development, but also appears to contribute to the vasodilatation associated with acute hypoxia and increased cerebral NMDA levels. Nitric oxide synthase activity exhibits a complex regulation that is isoform specific and modulated by phosphorylation not only of serine and threonine, but also possibly tyrosine, residues. Nitric oxide has multiple diverse targets of action within cerebrovascular smooth muscle, one of the most important of which is the enzyme soluble guanylate cyclase. Nitric oxide activates soluble guanylate cyclase and thereby increases vascular cGMP levels, which in turn promote vasodilatation. As for nitric oxide synthases, the expression of soluble guanylate cyclase is also developmentally regulated, and exhibits lower abundance in immature than in mature cerebral arteries (White et al., 2000).

Carbon monoxide, a molecule similar in structure and function to that of nitric oxide, is another possible mediator of receptor-independent cerebral vasodilatation in the neonate. The enzyme responsible for synthesis of endogenous carbon monoxide, heme oxygenase, is highly expressed in the piglet brain and in this model, application of exogenous carbon monoxide elicits cerebral vasodilatation (Leffler et al., 1999). The physiological roles and mechanisms of action of cerebral carbon monoxide, as well as the possible influence of this pathway in the human neonate, however, remain unclear.

For many cerebral vasodilators, both receptor dependent and receptor independent, the mechanism of action involves activation of potassium channels. For example, both opioids and prostacyclin have been reported to elicit cerebral vasodilatation, at least in part, via activation of ATP-sensitive and calcium-activated potassium channels. Because these channels appear to be developmentally regulated, and exhibit greater activity in adult than in neonatal cerebral arteries (Pearce

& Elliott, 1994), a significant component of the maturationally enhanced vasodilator activity of some stimuli may reflect the effects of advancing postnatal age on cerebrovascular potassium channel density, coupling and function.

From a more physiological perspective, a variety of other perturbations also increase fetal cerebral perfusion. Heat stress of several degrees centigrade increases fetal brain blood flow, as does hemodilution in human fetuses. Increased cerebrospinal fluid magnesium concentrations in the low millimolar range dilate fetal cerebral arteries (Kim et al., 1997), as do volatile anesthetics. Administration of dexamethasone (250 μg/kg/12h) also acutely increases cerebral perfusion in human neonates (Cabanas et al., 1997). Together, these observations strongly indicate that the fetal cerebral circulation should be regarded as a highly reactive vascular bed prone to vasodilatation. Regardless of the mechanisms involved, this heightened reactivity poses serious risks for the immature cerebral circulation, and may help explain the increased incidence of vascular rupture and intracranial hemorrhage observed in neonates, particularly those born prematurely.

Maturation of cerebrovascular endothelial function

One of the first functions recognized for the developing cerebral endothelium was that of the blood–brain barrier. In physical terms, this barrier is composed of endothelial cells interconnected with tight junctions that develop early in fetal life and continue to differentiate throughout fetal and early postnatal life. Early studies proposed that the fetal blood brain barrier was functionally immature due to its relatively greater permeability to small lipid-insoluble molecules and reduced capacity for amino acid and ion transport, but more recent work suggests that the fetal blood brain barrier is functionally specialized, utilizes mechanisms not found in adult cerebral endothelium, and is well adapted for fetal life (Saunders et al., 1999). Consistent with this view, the fetal blood brain barrier is largely impermeable to norepinephrine, angiotensin II and hydrogen ion, suggesting that the most important aspects of blood–brain barrier function are intact at birth. Nonetheless, maturation involves a complex pattern of environmentally sensitive changes that regulate the expression and function of the tight junction proteins throughout fetal and early postnatal life (Rubin & Staddon, 1999).

A second critical function of the cerebrovascular endothelium is its critical role in angiogenesis and regulation of the phenotype of the vascular smooth muscle of cerebral arteries. As in other vascular beds, cerebrovascular endothelium is influenced by a broad variety of circulating growth factors falling into at least five main classes including the heparin-binding growth factors, the non-heparin binding growth factors, the peptide inhibitory factors, the non-peptide inhibitory factors, and the angiogenic and metabolic stimulants (see Fig. 12.2). The endothelium

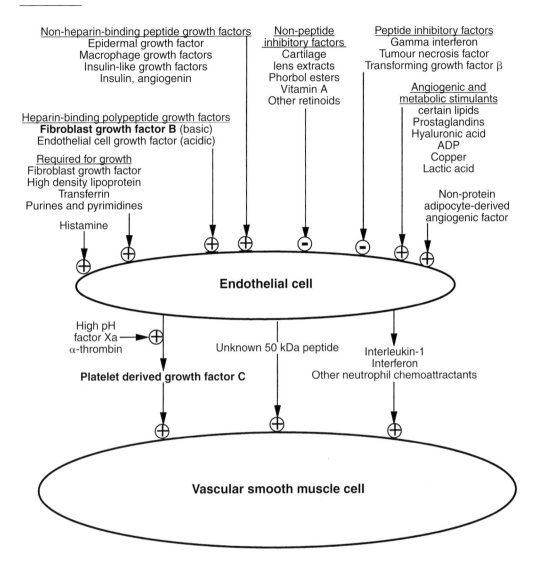

Fig. 12.2. Endothelial cells are responsive to, and also release, a broad variety of factors that both directly and indirectly influence smooth muscle growth and phenotype. Summarized here are a variety of factors, organized by class, that influence the growth of endothelial cells in culture. This summary is not meant to be exhaustive, but rather to indicate the complex nature of the mechanisms governing growth and proliferation of both endothelium and vascular smooth muscle. See text for details.

continuously integrates this cacophony of more the 30 growth-related signals and in response releases factors of its own that influence mitogenic activity within the adjacent vascular smooth muscle. Cerebrovascular smooth muscle phenotype is further influenced by multiple trophic factors released from the brain parenchyma, which together with the endothelial factors, assure maintenance of the unique vascular phenotypes characteristic of the cerebral circulation.

Another key role of the fetal cerebrovascular endothelium is the release of multiple vasoactive molecules. This aspect of endothelial function is heavily regulated during development, is influenced by oestrogen, and varies significantly among different vascular beds and species. In the fetal cerebral circulation, the vascular endothelium releases multiple vasodilator molecules, including nitric oxide, prostacyclin, and an as yet identified molecule known as endothelium derived hyperpolarizing factor (Faraci & Heistad, 1998). As in other vascular beds, maturation shifts the balance between prostacyclin and nitric oxide release, with greater relative release of prostacyclin in the neonate and greater nitric oxide release in the adult (Zuckerman et al., 1996). The nitric oxide released from fetal cerebrovascular endothelium is produced only by the endothelium isoform of nitric oxide synthase located exclusively in vascular endothelial cells. Endothelial prostacyclin release is dependent on endothelial cyclo-oxygenase, both forms of which are normally in low abundance in fetal arteries. Several influences, including ischemia and/or anoxia can upregulate endothelial cyclooxygenase-2 expression. Similarly, ischemia can also stimulate synthesis of endothelial nitric oxide synthase (Beasley et al., 1998). The cerebrovascular endothelium also releases vasoconstrictor molecules, the most important of which is endothelin for which endothelium is the main source. The physiological release of endothelial vasoactive molecules contributes significantly to cerebrovascular regulation in the fetus, particularly in response to changes in cerebral perfusion pressure, hypoxia, and pulsatile flow.

Postnatal development of cerebrovascular innervation

The perivascular innervation of cerebral arteries develops in three general phases. First, fibre bundles grow distally along the arteries, and then divide into a circumferentially distributed meshwork pattern. Next, transmitter synthesis and storage capacity develop, and finally the nerve varicosities expand and differentiate. Postsynaptic receptors generally develop earlier than do the mechanisms governing presynaptic transmitter release. The neurovascular system for which these processes are best understood is the sympathetic adrenergic innervation. In human fetal cerebral arteries, immature adrenergic nerves with few varicosities can be demonstrated at 19–23 weeks of gestation and their density is greatest in the most rostral vessels. In addition to well-documented trophic effects that influence

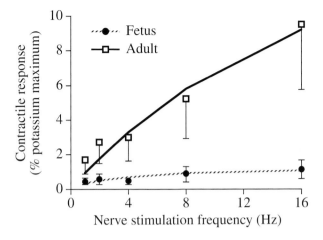

Fig. 12.3.   Transmural electric field stimulation at supramaximal current and 0.3 ms duration produced frequency-dependent increases in contractile tension in ovine middle cerebral artery segments. The resulting responses are expressed here relative to the maximum responses to 120 mM potassium Krebs. Electrical stimulation was administered in the presence of 10 μM capsaicin to inhibit release of vasoactive peptides, 1 μM atropine to inhibit activation of muscarinic receptor, and 10 μM L-NAME to prevent the local release of nitric oxide. Across all frequencies (ANOVA), responses to stimulation were significantly greater in the adult than in the fetus. All responses to stimulation were blocked by pretreatment with either 2 μM guanethidine or 0.3 μM tetrodotoxin. Vertical error bars indicate standard errors for artery segments from 10 fetuses and 6 adults. For details, see Pearce et al. (1999).

smooth muscle composition and reactivity, in vitro stimulation of the adrenergic perivascular innervation can constrict human infant cerebral arteries (Bevan et al., 1998a,b). In ovine cerebral arteries, the adrenergic response to transmural nerve stimulation increases dramatically with age (see Fig. 12.3). The mechanisms mediating this improved response do not involve postsynaptic sensitivity to norepinephrine, norepinephrine content, or norepinephrine uptake capacity, as all these variables have fetal values that are equivalent to or greater than those in adult ovine cerebral arteries (Pearce et al., 1999). Because stimulation-induced norepinephrine release is greater in fetal than adult cerebral arteries, these data suggest that adrenergic synaptic volume and/or cleft width may be greater in immature than mature cerebrovascular synapses (Pearce et al., 1999). Alternatively, corelease of other neurotransmitters may be greater in adult than in fetal arteries.

A probable candidate for corelease with norepinephrine is neuropeptide Y. Nerves containing this vasoconstrictor peptide can be demonstrated in immature cerebral arteries, and in some instances the peptide is colocated with norepinephrine (Sienkiewicz et al., 1995). Cerebral arteries are also innervated by nerves containing opioids, vasoactive intestinal polypeptide, CGRP, substance P, and galanin, but all these peptides are vasodilators and thus are unlikely to contribute to adrenergic cerebral vasoconstriction. Separate sensory nerves originating in the trigeminal ganglion also supply the major arteries of the Circle of Willis and the large pial arteries, and these nerves can contain substance-P, vasoactive intestinal polypeptide, cholecystokinin, somatostatin, and calcitonin gene-related peptide. Although the perivascular presence of these peptides in cerebral vasomotor neurones is generally well-documented, their effects on cerebral arteries, and the physiological stimuli which elicit their release during the perinatal period remain largely unexplored.

Despite the well-documented presence of serotonin receptors on cerebral arteries, there is now little evidence in favour of separate serotonergic cerebrovascular innervation. In contrast, nerves containing acetylcholine can be demonstrated in fetal human cerebral arteries between 19 and 23 weeks of gestational age and their development parallels that of the adrenergic system. Acetylcholine contracts fetal and newborn baboon cerebral arteries, but not corresponding arteries from adult baboons. Low concentrations of acetylcholine dilate newborn piglet pial arteries, whereas higher concentrations (100 μM) produce vasoconstriction. Indomethacin at 5 mg/kg can block pial artery contractile responses to 100 μM acetylcholine, suggesting that vasoconstrictor prostanoids, such as PGF2α or thromboxane A$_2$ may be involved in these responses.

Neonatal cerebrovascular autoregulation

A key general characteristic of cerebrovascular regulation is the ability to maintain a near constant cerebral blood flow despite changes in cerebral perfusion pressure (arterial pressure minus cerebrospinal fluid or cerebral venous pressure). This 'autoregulation' of cerebral blood flow can be observed in ovine fetuses as young as 0.6 gestation, but is less efficient or robust than in older fetuses. Neonatal piglets autoregulate quite efficiently to pressure changes and can maintain cerebral perfusion even when cerebral perfusion pressure is only one-third of its resting value. Preterm human infants (~33 weeks gestation) also autoregulate, often within a few seconds of transient changes in arterial pressure of as little as 5 mm Hg. The speed of autoregulatory responses is a good indicator of autoregulatory efficiency and can be used to identify human neonates with poor autoregulation (Panerai et al., 1998). For neonates of most species, the pressure range over which autoregulation can maintain cerebral perfusion is much narrower than in older individuals (see Fig. 12.4). In most neonates, including human infants, the autoregulatory range extends from perfusion pressures of 30–40 mm Hg to an upper limit of 70–100 mm Hg. With development and maturation throughout early childhood, auto-

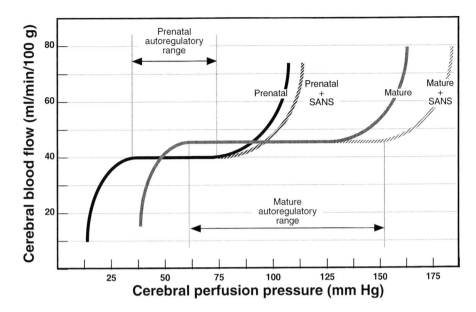

Fig. 12.4.   Summarized here are idealized age-specific responses of cerebral blood flow to changes in cerebral perfusion pressure. Note that in the fetus, the autoregulatory range extends from about 35 to 75 mm Hg, whereas it extends from about 60 to 125 mm Hg in adults. The general effect of perivascular sympathetic autonomic nerve stimulation (SANS) is to extend the upper limit of autoregulation, but note that the magnitude of this effect is much greater in mature than in immature brains.

regulatory capacity continues to develop and correspondingly, the autoregulatory range expands (Rodriguez et al., 1998). In adults, autoregulation extends from a lower limit of approximately 50 mm Hg to an upper limit of ~150 mm Hg of cerebral perfusion pressure.

In the fetus and neonate, arterial pressure is more labile and subject to fluctuations than in the adult. Correspondingly, autoregulation is essential to maintain cerebral perfusion during a wide variety of perturbations known to alter cerebral perfusion pressure, including fetal blood sampling, feeding in preterm infants, the presence of a patent ductus ateriosus, or complications due to maternal cardiomyopathy. Nonetheless, autoregulation of the immature cerebral circulation is a very fragile process that can be impaired by intraventricular haemorrhage (Menke et al., 1997), extracorporeal membrane oxygenation (Walker et al., 1996), and even by pancuronium in some preterm infants (Bohin et al., 1995).

The mechanisms mediating cerebral autoregulation have for many years been attributed largely to the myogenic properties of blood vessels that enable them to respond directly to increased stretch by increasing contractile tone (Davis & Hill, 1999). Whereas this view remains dominant in relation to cerebral autoregulation in the adult, very little is known of myogenic mechanisms in the neonate, particularly in the cerebral circulation. Alternatively, significant roles for adenosine, prostaglandins, and their receptors on cerebral arteries have been proposed. Mechanisms within the vascular smooth muscle of cerebral arteries also appear to be involved, given that isolated middle cerebral arteries from piglets exhibit autoregulatory responses to changes in stretch (Martinez-Orgado et al., 1998). Vasorelaxation responses to reduced stretch were antagonized by inhibitors of nitric oxide synthesis or calcium-sensitive potassium channels and vasoconstrictor responses to increased stretch were blocked by endothelin receptor antagonists or cyclooxygenase inhibitors. Together, these and other findings implicate a role for the vascular endothelium in cerebral autoregulation (Martinez-Orgado et al., 1998). Apart from potential endothelial mechanisms, sympathetic vasoconstriction limits increases in cerebral blood flow caused by elevated perfusion pressure and thus extends the upper limit of cerebral autoregulation in both fetuses and adults of most species. Multiple mechanisms are involved in autoregulation of fetal cerebral blood flow, but the relative importance of each of these, as well as their relevance to the human neonatal cerebral circulation, remains to be explored.

Reactivity to hypercapnia and hypoxia in the neonate

Elevated blood carbon dioxide tension is one of the best known and most widely studied vasodilators of the cerebral circulation. Reactivity to carbon dioxide appears well before birth in most species, but is depressed relative to that in adults and improves rapidly after birth. Carbon dioxide reactivity in the immature brain is heterogeneous throughout the brain and varies significantly between white matter, subcortical grey, and cortical grey matter. As for cerebral autoregulation, cerebral hypercapnic reactivity is fragile and can be easily damaged by a variety of insults, including brain trauma and asphyxia. Correspondingly, cerebral reactivity to carbon dioxide can be used to assess cerebral insult severity and to give a prognosis. Modern bedside methods based on Doppler and near infrared technologies are enabling more frequent and widespread assessments of carbon dioxide reactivity in hospitalized neonates, and these measurements reveal that a significant fraction of ill infants have altered CO_2 reactivity (Panerai et al., 1996). Whereas traditional strategies for management of the preterm infant focused on hyperventilation as a means to lower cerebral perfusion and attenuate the risk of intracranial artery rupture and hemorrhage, it is now recognized that the attenuated CO_2 reactivity typical of ill preterm infants, when combined with hypocapnia, actually increases the risk for periventricular leukomalacia and other types of white matter damage. Correspondingly, more modern management strategies aim to balance the concomitant risks of intracranial hemorrhage and white matter ischemia by maintaining normal to slightly elevated levels of arterial CO_2 and cerebral perfusion.

Despite the obvious importance of cerebral hypercapnic reactivity, the mechanisms that mediate this response remain unclear. In several species including newborn piglets, calves, and humans, indomethacin attenuates CO_2 reactivity, suggesting that a vasodilator prostaglandin is involved. The mechanisms responsible are not simple and straightforward, however, because only high dose (5 mg/kg) but not low dose (0.2 mg/kg) indomethacin can block the hyperemic response (Pourcyrous et al., 1999). In addition, ibuprofen (another inhibitor of cyclooxygenase) does not appear to alter hypercapnic reactivity in piglets, suggesting that some unique feature of indomethacin aside from its ability to inhibit cyclooxygenase may be involved. On the other hand, the finding that addition of prostacyclin receptor agonists to pial arteries pretreated with indomethacin restores their ability to respond to hypercapnia suggests that prostacyclin is not the final mediator of hypercapnic cerebral vasodilatation, but rather that it plays in intermediary or permissive role in the overall response in neonates (Mei & Gu, 1997). Because endothelial damage attenuates local responsiveness to hypercapnia, and hypercapnia promotes the release of prostacyclin from cultures of endothelial but not smooth muscle or glial cells, the source of the prostacyclin involved in hypercapnic cerebral vasodilatation appears to be the vascular endothelium. These effects of prostacyclin appear to require functional pertussis-toxin sensitive G-protein linked receptors and possibly also protein kinase C (Willis & Leffler, 1999). With advancing postnatal age, the indomethacin-sensitive component of hypercapnic reactivity diminishes in favour of increased involvement of the nitric oxide-dependent mechanisms that are predominant in adults. Apart from the roles played by prostaglandins and nitric oxide, extracellular pH also appears to play an important role and may be coupled to IP3 production within cerebrovascular smooth muscle and thereby contribute to hypocapnic cerebral vasoconstriction, as well as to hypercapnic vasodilatation (Albuquerque & Leffler, 1998).

Another important physiological stress that is coupled to cerebral vasodilatation is acute hypoxia. Typically, any perturbation that reduces either maternal oxygenation or uterine blood flow ultimately precipitates acute fetal hypoxia. Vasodilator responses to hypoxia appear in sheep fetuses by 0.75 gestation and these are adequate to maintain oxygen delivery throughout the brain, but are generally less than observed in near-term fetuses. Similarly, cerebral vasodilator responses to hypoxia are also evident in preterm fetal piglets (0.9 gestation), but the magnitude of these responses is less than observed in newborn piglets. Term human fetuses also appear responsive to hypoxia at an early age and exhibit 'fetal brain sparing', a response in which diastolic and mean blood flow velocities in the middle cerebral arteries increase in response to fetal hypoxia (Dubiel et al., 1997). Human fetuses also exhibit mild vasoconstrictor responses to hyperoxygenation and these responses are stronger at term than at mid-term (Almstrom & Sonesson, 1996). In general, this age-related pattern of responsiveness to hypoxia parallels the development of cerebral metabolic rate, suggesting that cerebral oxygen consumption is the main factor governing responses to hypoxia. Consistent with this view, the brainstem regions of both lambs and puppies, which are generally the most mature of any brain region at birth and have the highest metabolic rates, also exhibit greater responsiveness to hypoxia than other brain regions. In addition, hypoxia can also reduce fetal cerebral oxygen consumption (Shadid et al., 1999).

In many vascular beds, responses to acute hypoxia appear to be mediated by increased release of the metabolic vasodilator adenosine. Whereas this mechanism probably contributes to hypoxic cerebral vasodilatation in the immature brain, many other mechanisms are clearly involved. Calcium-sensitive potassium channels participate in neonatal cerebral responses to hypoxia, but unlike adult cerebral arteries, ATP-sensitive potassium channels do not play a consistent role. The cerebrovascular endothelium contributes to hypoxic cerebral vasodilatation, and the magnitude of this effect increases with postnatal maturation. Nitric oxide released from the endothelium participates in neonatal cerebrovascular responses to hypoxia. Nitric oxide synthesized by neuronal nitric oxide synthase also appears to contribute (Wilderman & Armstead, 1997a). Prostanoids, possibly from the endothelium, may also contribute to hypoxic cerebral vasodilatation although again their role is not clear. Hypoxic release of opioids also appears involved, and some of this effect appears secondary to hypoxic release of pituitary adenylate cyclase-activating peptide that, in turn, promotes the release of cerebral vasodilator opioids (Wilderman & Armstead, 1997b). A broad range of other factors also appear to participate in neonatal responses to hypoxia, as suggested by the varied findings that hypoxic vasodilatation can be attenuated by magnesium sulfate, chronic maternal ethanol exposure, NMDA receptor antagonists, or inhibitors of heme oxygenase. Finally, hypoxia influences not only the cells of the brain parenchyma and the vascular endothelium, but also the smooth muscle of the cerebral arteries directly (Pearce, 1995). Clearly, hypoxia is a complex stimulus which elicits multiple mechanisms of cerebrovascular response, and as for cerebral autoregulation and responses to hypercapnia, the relative contributions of many of these mechanisms change significantly with development and maturation.

Conclusions

The immediate perinatal period is a time of rapid change and adaptation for the immature brain. Not only must the brain adjust to a new hemodynamic environment in postnatal life, at the same time it must also accelerate a broad variety of synthetic processes to establish the neuronal processing essential for independent extrauterine survival. In turn, these processes require the increased delivery of fuels and substrates from the cerebral circulation in a manner that carefully matches metabolic supply and demand. The number and distribution of cerebral arteries is well established at birth, but their composition and reactivity changes dramatically in the first few days and weeks following birth. Extracellular matrix proteins are being synthesized at a rapid rate, smooth muscle membranes are becoming less leaky, membrane potential is shifting toward more negative potentials, the intracellular stores of calcium are growing, receptor numbers and coupling are shifting in an agonist specific manner, perivascular innervation is establishing more and more functional vasomotor synapses, and endothelial function is making a transition from predominant release of prostacyclin to release of nitric oxide. Despite this dramatic array of changes, cerebral autoregulation adapts to accommodate the increased perfusion pressures characteristic of postnatal life, hypercapnic reactivity improves, and responses to hypoxia remain fully functional. Certainly, it is no surprise that this period of rapid change is also a time of greatly increased vulnerability to cerebral insults such as asphyxia, hypoxia/ischemia, or brain trauma. Nonetheless, it is impressive that so many cerebrovascular changes can be so well coordinated and regulated in a manner that enables the great majority of neonates to survive birth without complication. Whereas our past efforts have revealed much about how the immature cerebral circulation changes in the perinatal period, our great challenge in the near future is to understand why these adaptations occur and what mechanisms govern this delicate transition to extrauterine life. Fortunately, a great many new technologies, such as magnetic resonance spectroscopy, PET, and NIRS are being used with increasing frequency and resolution to better understand the immature cerebral circulation. These new approaches, together with the unprecedented promise of new genetic approaches offered by the Human Genome Project, constitute good cause for excitement and high hopes that the next decade will substantially expand our understanding of fetal cerebrovascular regulation.

REFERENCES

Akopov, S. E., Zhang, L. & Pearce, W. J. (1997). Physiological variations in ovine cerebrovascular calcium sensitivity. *American Journal of Physiology*, **272**, H2271–81.

Akopov, S. E., Zhang, L. & Pearce, W. J. (1998). Maturation alters the contractile role of calcium in ovine basilar arteries. *Pediatric Research*, **44**, 154–60.

Albuquerque, M. L. & Leffler, C. W. (1998). pHo, pHi, and PCO_2 in stimulation of IP3 and $[Ca^{2+}]c$ in piglet cerebrovascular smooth muscle. *Proceedings of the Society for Experimental Biology and Medicine*, **219**, 226–34.

Almstrom, H. & Sonesson, S. E. (1996). Doppler echocardiographic assessment of fetal blood flow redistribution during maternal hyperoxygenation. *Ultrasound in Obstetrics and Gynecology*, **8**, 256–61.

Angeles, D. A., Williams, J. M., Zhang, L. & Pearce, W. J. (2000). Acute hypoxia selectively modulates 5HT receptor density and agonist affinity in fetal and adult ovine carotid arteries. *American Journal of Physiology*, **279**, H502–10.

Ardaillou, R. (1999). Angiotensin II receptors. *Journal of the American Society of Nephrology*, **10** (Suppl. 11), S30–9.

Armstead, W. M. (1997). Role of activation of calcium-sensitive K^+ channels and cAMP in opioid-induced pial artery dilation. *Brain Research*, **747**, 252–8.

Barfield, C. P., Yu, V. Y., Noma, O. et al. (1999). Cerebral blood volume measured using near-infrared spectroscopy and radiolabels in the immature lamb brain. *Pediatric Research*, **46**, 50–6.

Beasley, T. C., Bari, F., Thore, C., Thrikawala, N., Louis, T. & Busija, D. (1998). Cerebral ischemia/reperfusion increases endothelial nitric oxide synthase levels by an indomethacin-sensitive mechanism. *Journal of Cerebral Blood Flow and Metabolism*, **18**, 88–96.

Bevan, R., Dodge, J., Nichols, P. et al. (1998a). Responsiveness of human infant cerebral arteries to sympathetic nerve stimulation and vasoactive agents. *Pediatric Research*, **44**, 730–9, 1998.

Bevan, R. D., Vijayakumaran, E., Gentry, A., Wellman, T. & Bevan, J. A. (1998b). Intrinsic tone of cerebral artery segments of human infants between 23 weeks of gestation and term. *Pediatric Research*, **43**, 20–7.

Bissonnette, J. M., Hohimer, A. R. & Knopp, S. J. (1995). Effect of central adenosine on brainstem blood flow in fetal sheep. *Experimental Physiology*, **80**, 141–5.

Bohin, S., Fenton, A. C., Thompson, J. R., Evans, D. H. & Field, D. J. (1995). Circulatory effects of ventilator rate and end-expiratory pressure in unparalysed preterm infants. *Acta Paediatrica*, **84**, 1300–4.

Cabanas, F., Pellicer, A., Garcia-Alix, A., Quero, J. & Stiris, T. A. (1997). Effect of dexamethasone therapy on cerebral and ocular blood flow velocity in premature infants studied by colour Doppler flow imaging. *European Journal of Pediatrics*, **156**, 41–6.

Chemtob, S., Li, D. Y., Abran, D., Hardy, P., Peri, K. & Varma, D. R. (1996). The role of prostaglandin receptors in regulating cerebral blood flow in the perinatal period. *Acta Paediatrica*, **85**, 517–24.

Davis, M. J. & Hill, M. A. (1999). Signaling mechanisms underlying the vascular myogenic response. *Physiology Reviews*, **79**, 387–423.

Downen, M., Zhao, M. L., Lee, P., Weidenheim, K. M., Dickson, D. W. & Lee, S. C. (1999). Neuronal nitric oxide synthase expression in developing and adult human CNS. *Journal of Neuropathology and Experimental Neurology*, **58**, 12–21.

Dubiel, M., Gudmundsson, S., Gunnarsson, G. & Marsal, K. (1997). Middle cerebral artery velocimetry as a predictor of hypoxemia in fetuses with increased resistance to blood flow in the umbilical artery. *Early Human Development*, **47**, 177–84.

Elliott, S. R. & Pearce, W. J. (1994). Effects of maturation on alpha-adrenergic receptor affinity and occupancy in small cerebral arteries. *American Journal of Physiology*, **267**, H757–63.

Faraci, F. M. & Heistad, D. D. (1998). Regulation of the cerebral circulation: role of endothelium and potassium channels. *Physiological Reviews*, **78**, 53–97.

Galea, E., Reis, D. J., Xu, H. & Feinstein, D. L. (1995). Transient expression of calcium-independent nitric oxide synthase in blood vessels during brain development. *FASEB Journal*, **9**, 1632–7.

Gidday, J. M. & Park, T. S. (1992). Effect of 2-chloroadenosine on cerebrovascular reactivity to hypercapnia in newborn pig. *Journal of Cerebral Blood Flow and Metabolism*, **12**, 656–63.

Gordon, I. (1998). Cerebral imaging in paediatrics. *Quarterly Journal of Nuclear Medicine*, **42**, 126–32.

Kim, C. R., Oh, W. & Stonestreet, B. S. (1997). Magnesium is a cerebrovasodilator in newborn piglets. *American Journal of Physiology*, **272**, H511–16.

Kurth, C. D. & Wagerle, L. C. (1992). Cerebrovascular reactivity to adenosine analogues in 0.6–0.7 gestation and near-term fetal sheep. *American Journal of Physiology*, **262**, H1338–42.

Leffler, C. W., Nasjletti, A., Yu, C., Johnson, R. A., Fedinec, A. L. & Walker, N. (1999). Carbon monoxide and cerebral microvascular tone in newborn pigs. *American Journal of Physiology*, **276**, H1641–6.

Li, D. Y., Hardy, P., Abran, D. et al. (1997). Key role for cyclooxygenase-2 in PGE2 and PGF2alpha receptor regulation and cerebral blood flow of the newborn. *American Journal of Physiology*, **273**, R1283–90.

Longo, L. D., Ueno, N., Zhao, Y., Pearce, W. J. & Zhang, L. (1996). Developmental changes in alpha 1-adrenergic receptors, IP3 responses, and NE-induced contraction in cerebral arteries. *American Journal of Physiology*, **271**, H2313–19.

Martinez-Orgado, J., Gonzalez, R., Alonso, M. J., Rodriguez-Martinez, M. A., Sanchez-Ferrer, C. F. & Marin, J. (1998). Endothelial factors and autoregulation during pressure changes in isolated newborn piglet cerebral arteries. *Pediatric Research*, **44**, 161–7.

Mei, X. & Gu, Z. (1997). [Prostacyclin participates in regulation of hypoxic and high CO_2 cerebrovascular tension]. *Chung Kuo Ying Yung Sheng Li Hsueh Tsa Chih*, **13**, 29–31.

Menke, J., Michel, E., Hillebrand, S., von Twickel, J. & Jorch, G. (1997). Cross-spectral analysis of cerebral autoregulation dynamics in high risk preterm infants during the perinatal period. *Pediatric Research*, **42**, 690–9.

Michel, E. & Zernikow, B. (1998). Gosling's Doppler pulsatility index revisited. *Ultrasound in Medicine and Biology*, **24**, 597–9.

Panerai, R. B., Kelsall, A. W., Rennie, J. M. & Evans, D. H. (1996). Analysis of cerebral blood flow autoregulation in neonates. *IEEE Transactions on Biomedical Engineering*, **43**, 779–88.

Panerai, R. B., Rennie, J. M., Kelsall, A. W. & Evans, D. H. (1998). Frequency-domain analysis of cerebral autoregulation from spontaneous fluctuations in arterial blood pressure. *Medical and Biological Engineering and Computing*, **36**, 315–22.

Parfenova, H., Zuckerman, S. & Leffler, C. W. (1995). Inhibitory effect of indomethacin on prostacyclin receptor-mediated cerebral vascular responses. *American Journal of Physiology*, **268**, H1884–90.

Parfenova, H., Fedinec, A. & Leffler, C. W. (1999). Role of tyrosine phosphorylation in the regulation of cerebral vascular tone in newborn pig in vivo. *American Journal of Physiology*, **276**, H185–93.

Pearce, W. J. (1995). Mechanisms of hypoxic cerebral vasodilatation. *Pharmacology and Therapeutics*, **65**, 75–91.

Pearce, W. J. & Elliott, S. R. (1994). Maturation enhances the sensitivity of ovine cerebral arteries to the ATP-sensitive potassium channel activator lemakalim. *Pediatric Research*, **35**, 729–32.

Pearce, W. J., Hull, A. D., Long, D. M. & Longo, L. (1991). Developmental changes in ovine cerebral artery composition and reactivity. *American Journal of Physiology*, **261**, R458–465.

Pearce, W. J., Duckles, S. P. & Buchholz, J. (1999). Effects of maturation on adrenergic neurotransmission in ovine cerebral arteries [In Process Citation]. *American Journal of Physiology*, **277**, R931–7.

Pitcher, J. A., Freedman, N. J. & Lefkowitz, R. J. (1998). G protein-coupled receptor kinases. *Annual Review of Biochemistry*, **67**, 653–92.

Polvi, H. J., Pirhonen, J. P. & Erkkola, R. U. (1996). Nitrous oxide inhalation: effects on maternal and fetal circulations at term [see comments]. *Obstetrics and Gynecology*, **87**, 1045–8.

Pourcyrous, M., Busija, D. W., Shibata, M., Bada, H. S., Korones, S. B. & Leffler, C. W. (1999). Cerebrovascular responses to therapeutic dose of indomethacin in newborn pigs. *Pediatric Research*, **45**, 582–7.

Rodriguez, R. A., Weerasena, N., Cornel, G., Splinter, W. M. & Roberts, D. J. (1998). Cerebral effects of aortic clamping during coarctation repair in children: a transcranial Doppler study. *European Journal of Cardiothoracic Surgery*, **13**, 124–9.

Rubin, L. L. & Staddon, J. M. (1999). The cell biology of the blood–brain barrier. *Annual Review of Neuroscience*, **22**, 11–28.

Saunders, N. R., Habgood, M. D. & Dziegielewska, K. M. (1999). Barrier mechanisms in the brain, II. Immature brain. *Clinical and Experimental Pharmacology and Physiology*, **26**, 85–91.

Shadid, M., Hiltermann, L., Monteiro, L., Fontijn, J. & Van Bel, F. (1999). Near infrared spectroscopy-measured changes in cerebral blood volume and cytochrome aa3 in newborn lambs exposed to hypoxia and hypercapnia, and ischemia: a comparison with changes in brain perfusion and O_2 metabolism. *Early Human Development*, **55**, 169–82.

Sienkiewicz, W., Majewski, M., Kaleczyc, J. & Lakomy, M. (1995). Immunohistochemical study of the existence and coexistence of catecholamine synthesizing enzymes and some neuropeptides in perivascular nerve fibres of the main thoraco-cranial arteries in the pig. *Folia Histochemica et Cytobiologica*, **33**, 59–67.

Sjostrom, K., Valentin, L., Thelin, T. & Marsal, K. (1997). Maternal anxiety in late pregnancy and fetal hemodynamics. *European Journal of Obstetrics, Gynecology and Reproductive Biology*, **74**, 149–55.

Somlyo, A. P., Wu, X., Walker, L. A. & Somlyo, A. V. (1999). Pharmacomechanical coupling: the role of calcium, G-proteins, kinases and phosphatases. *Reviews of Physiology Biochemistry and Pharmacology*, **134**, 201–34.

Stuehr, D. J. (1999). Mammalian nitric oxide synthases. *Biochimica et Biophysica Acta*, **1411**, 217–30.

Takahashi, T., Shirane, R., Sato, S. & Yoshimoto, T. (1999). Developmental changes of cerebral blood flow and oxygen metabolism in children. *American Journal of Neuroradiology*, **20**, 917–22.

Walker, L. K., Short, B. L. & Traystman, R. J. (1996). Impairment of cerebral autoregulation during venovenous extracorporeal membrane oxygenation in the newborn lamb [see comments]. *Critical Care Medicine*, **24**, 2001–6.

White, C. R., Hao, X. & Pearce, W. J. (2000). Maturational differences in soluble guanylate cyclase activity in ovine carotid and cerebral arteries. *Pediatric Research*, **47**, 369–75.

Wilderman, M. J. & Armstead, W. M. (1997a). Role of PACAP in the relationship between cAMP and opioids in hypoxia-induced pial artery vasodilation. *American Journal of Physiology*, **272**, H1350–8.

Wilderman, M. J. & Armstead, W. M. (1997b). Role of neuronal NO synthase in relationship between NO and opioids in hypoxia-induced pial artery dilation. *American Journal of Physiology*, **273**, H1807–15.

Willis, A. P. & Leffler, C. W. (1999). NO and prostanoids: age dependence of hypercapnia and histamine-induced dilations of pig pial arterioles [In Process Citation]. *American Journal of Physiology*, **277**, H299–307.

Yakubu, M. A. & Leffler, C. W. (1996). Role of endothelin-1 in cerebral hematoma-induced modification of cerebral vascular reactivity in piglets. *Brain Research*, **734**, 149–56.

Yakubu, M. A., Shibata, M. & Leffler, C. W. (1995). Hematoma-induced enhanced cerebral vasoconstrictions to leukotriene C4 and endothelin-1 in piglets: role of prostanoids. *Pediatric Research*, **38**, 119–23.

Yanowitz, T. D., Yao, A. C., Werner, J. C., Pettigrew, K. D., Oh, W. & Stonestreet, B. S. (1998). Effects of prophylactic low-dose indomethacin on hemodynamics in very low birth weight infants. *Journal of Pediatrics*, **132**, 28–34.

Zhou, L., Zhao, Y., Nijland, R., Zhang, L. & Longo, L. D. (1997). Ins(1,4,5)P3 receptors in cerebral arteries: changes with development and high-altitude hypoxia. *American Journal of Physiology*, **272**, R1954–9.

Zucker, B. & Leffler, C. W. (1998). PTX-sensitive G proteins and permissive action of prostacyclin in newborn pig cerebral circulation. *American Journal of Physiology*, **275**, H259–63.

Zuckerman, S. L., Armstead, W. M., Hsu, P., Shibata, M. & Leffler, C. W. (1996). Age dependence of cerebrovascular response mechanisms in domestic pigs. *American Journal of Physiology*, **271**, H535–40.

13

The description of the early development of the human central nervous system using two-dimensional and three-dimensional ultrasound

Harm-Gerd K. Blaas and Sturla H. Eik-Nes

National Center for Fetal Medicine, Women's Hospital RiT, Trondheim, Norway

Ultrasound in the early pregnancy

With the technical development of ultrasound equipment, major advances in the imaging of early pregnancy have been made. Transabdominal ultrasonography has been used to describe embryonic cerebral ventricles such as the rhombencephalic cavity (Cyr et al., 1988) and the lateral ventricles (Cullen et al., 1990). The use of the transvaginal route has improved the image quality to such an extent that a detailed anatomical description of the living embryo and early fetus has become possible; the large hypoechogenic cavities of the embryonic brain have, naturally, attracted the attention of ultrasound examiners (Cullen et al., 1990; Timor-Tritsch et al., 1988, 1990, 1991; Warren et al., 1989; Bree & Marn, 1990; Achiron & Achiron, 1991; Takeuchi, 1992). The first detailed transvaginal sonographic imaging of embryonic development with descriptions of the brain at different gestational age was published in 1988 (Timor-Tritsch et al., 1988). Two-dimensional measurements of the embryonic brain have been made to describe the normal development and dimensions of the cavities of the hemispheres, the diencephalon, the mesencephalon (Blaas et al., 1994, 1995a) and of the rhombencephalon (Blaas et al., 1995a; Zalen-Sprock et al., 1996). Linking real-time ultrasonography with computer technology has made three-dimensional ultrasound feasible, allowing us to analyse the recorded ultrasound volume off-line in any plane. This has made it possible to measure the diameters and volumes of interest more precisely as well as make more precise diagnoses (Blaas et al., 1995b, 1998, 2000).

Embryology

(All times are based on the last menstrual period, expressed in complete weeks and completed days, assuming a regular cycle with ovulation at 2 weeks 0 days.)

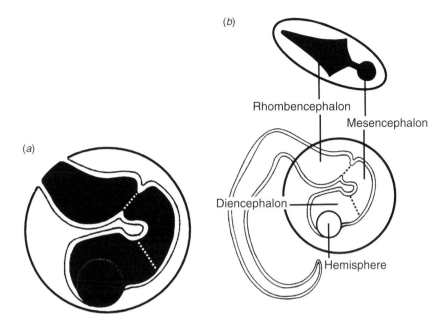

Fig. 13.1.   Sketch of the sagittal section of the embryonic central nervous system at 7 weeks gestation (Carnegie stage 16). (*a*) = horizontal section superior through the embryonic head showing the rhomboid shape of the rhombencephalon; anteriorly the section shows the mesencephalic cavity. (*b*) = sagittal section through the cavities of the rhombencephalon, mesencephalon, diencephalon, and a hemisphere.

The human embryo develops from the fertilized ovum, through the bilaminar and three-laminar disc, into a cylindrical body, and only at the end of the embryonic period does it acquire the unique structural proportions of an immature human being. The first visible indication of the central nervous system is the appearance of the neural groove during Carnegie stage 8 (O'Rahilly & Müller, 1987) at the gestational age of about 4 weeks and 4 days. During the 2 weeks that follow, the neuroectoderm is transformed into the neural tube and further into the ventricular system, with its five brain regions on its rostral pole, before the end of week 6: the telencephalon (future hemispheres) and the diencephalon (future midbrain) derive from the prosencephalon (forebrain); the mesencephalon (midbrain) remains undivided, and the metencephalon (future cerebellum and pons) and the myelencephalon (medulla oblongata) derive from the rhombencephalon (hindbrain). The future lateral ventricles develop at Carnegie stage 14, which is about 6 weeks and 4 days (based on LMP), and appear as bilateral evaginations of the telencephalon (Streeter, 1948; O'Rahilly & Gardner, 1971; O'Rahilly & Müller, 1990; O'Rahilly et al., 1982). At the same time, the fourth ventricle becomes apparent as a large rhomboid shallow cavity in the head of the embryo, while the brain is bent

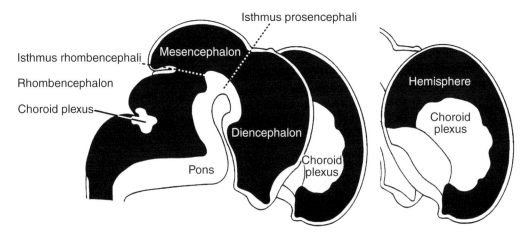

Fig. 13.2.   Sketch of the sagittal and parasagittal section through the embryonic brain at 10 weeks, Carnegie stage 23.

forward by the mesencephalic and cervical flexures. During the following weeks, the brain compartments enlarge and alter both in shape and in their relation to each other (O'Rahilly & Müller, 1990; Jenkins, 1921).

Description of the sonoanatomic development of the brain

This chapter describes the development of the central nervous system of embryos and fetuses as seen with ultrasound from about 7 weeks of gestation to 12 weeks of gestation (Blaas et al., 1994, 1995a, b, 1998). Table 13.1 shows the estimated volumes of embryonic brain compartments from three-dimensional ultrasound reconstructions of 34 embryos and fetuses with crown–rump length (CRL) from 9.3 mm to 39 mm (Blaas et al., 1998).

7 weeks 0–6 days, CRL 8–14 mm

Sonographically, the embryonic body appears as a triangle in the sagittal section. The sides consist of (i) the back, (ii) the roof of the rhombencephalon and (iii) the frontal part of the head, the basis of the umbilical cord, and the embryonic tail. The embryonic head is slender when viewed in the coronal plane.

The hypoechogenic brain cavities, including the separated cerebral hemispheres, can be identified. The lateral ventricles appear as small, rounded vesicles located lateral and rostral to the cavity of the diencephalon. The cavity of the diencephalon (future third ventricle) runs posteriorly and continues directly into that of the mesencephalon. The medial telencephalon forms a continuous cavity between the lateral ventricles. The future foramina of Monro are wide during week 7. In the

Table 13.1. Mean (±2 SD) volumes of embryonic body and cavities of the brain

CRL (mm)	Body (mm³)	Total brain (mm³)	Hemispheres (mm³)	Diencephalon (mm³)	Mesencephalon (mm³)	Rhombencephalon (mm³)
10	96 (209;26)	5.2 (18.2; 0.1)	0.5 (2.7; 0.0)	1.7 (4.8; 0.2)	1.1 (3.3; 0.1)	7.3 (15.9; 2.0)
15	402 (611; 237)	25.6 (49.4; 9.5)	6.7 (15.1; 2.2)	4.4 (9.0; 1.5)	3.6 (7.1; 1.3)	13.4 (24.4; 5.7)
20	918 (1222; 657)	61.3 (96.1; 34.3)	25.9 (44.6; 13.4)	6.7 (12.1; 2.8)	6.6 (11.2; 3.2)	18.8 (31.6; 9.4)
25	1644 (2044; 1288)	112.4 (158.1; 74.4)	65.7 (98.7; 41.0)	7.5 (13.3; 3.4)	9.4 (14.7; 5.3)	22.6 (36.4; 12.0)
30	2581 (3076; 2129)	178.8 (235.3; 129.9)	133.4 (184.8; 92.6)	6.7 (12.1; 2.9)	11.5 (17.3; 6.9)	23.9 (38.1; 13.0)
35	3727 (4318; 3180)	260.5 (328.0; 200.7)	236.6 (310.4; 175.5)	4.5 (9.1; 1.5)	12.5 (18.6; 7.7)	22.7 (36.5; 12.1)

Notes:

CRL = crown–rump length.

CRL 10 mm ≅ 7 weeks 2 days gestational age based on the last menstrual period.

CRL 15 mm ≅ 8 weeks 0 days.

CRL 20 mm ≅ 8 weeks 5 days.

CRL 25 mm ≅ 9 weeks 2 days.

CRL 30 mm ≅ 9 weeks 6 days.

CRL 35 mm ≅ 10 weeks 2 days.

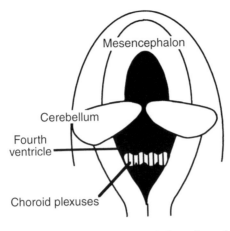

Fig. 13.3.   Sketch of the posterior coronal plane through the embryonic/early fetal brain.

sagittal plane, the height of the cavity of the diencephalon (future third ventricle) is slightly greater than that of the mesencephalon (future Sylvian aqueduct). Thus, the wide division between the cavities of the diencephalon and the mesencephalon is indicated. The curved tube-like mesencephalic cavity (future Sylvian aqueduct) lies anteriorly, its rostral part pointing caudally. The mesencephalon straightens considerably during the weeks that follow. By week eight it is regularly identified. The isthmus rhombencephali represents the connection to the rhombencephalic cavity and future fourth ventricle. The rather broad and shallow rhombencephalic cavity, which is located superiorly in the head, represents the largest brain cavity. It then has a well-defined rhombic shape in the cranial pole of the embryo. The future spine appears as two parallel lines.

8 weeks 0–6 days, CRL 15–22 mm

The brain cavities are easily seen as large 'holes' in the embryonic head. The shape of the lateral ventricles gradually changes, from small round vesicles (CRL ≥ 14 mm) via thick round slices originating antero-caudally from the third ventricle (CRL 15–19 mm), into the crescent shape of the larger embryos (CRL ≥ 20 mm). The choroid plexuses in the lateral ventricles become visible as tiny echogenic areas. The future foramina of Monro become more accentuated during week 8. The third ventricle is still rather wide, as is the mesencephalic cavity. Now, the mesencephalon lies at the top of the head. The increased growth of the rostral brain structures and the deepening of the pontine flexure lead to the deflection of the brain. The rhombencephalic cavity (future fourth ventricle) has a pyramid-like shape with the central deepening of the pontine flexure as the peak of the pyramid. It deepens gradually with the growth of the embryo, at the same time decreasing in length. The

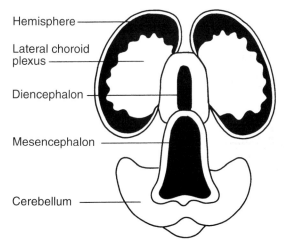

Hemisphere

Lateral choroid plexus

Diencephalon

Mesencephalon

Cerebellum

Fig. 13.4.   Sketch of the horizontal plane through the embryonic/early fetal brain. The mesencephalon actually lies higher than the diencephalon and the cerebellum.

first signs of the bilateral choroid plexuses are lateral echogenic areas originating near the branches of the medulla oblongata caudal to the lateral recesses. Within a short time, the choroid plexuses traverse the roof of the fourth ventricle, meeting in the midline and dividing the roof into two portions, about two-thirds located rostrally and one-third caudally. In the sagittal section, the choroid plexuses can be identified as an echogenic fold of the roof.

9 weeks 0–6 days, CRL 23–31 mm

The lateral ventricles are always visible. They are best seen in the parasagittal plane, where the C-shape becomes apparent. The cortex is smooth and hypoechogenic. The bright choroid plexuses of the lateral ventricles are regularly detectable at 9 weeks 4 days. They show rapid growth, similar to the hemispheres, and soon fill most of the ventricular cavities. The width of the diencephalic cavity narrows gradually, while the width of the mesencephalon remains wide. A distinct border (isthmus prosencephali) has developed between the cavity of the mesencephalon and the third ventricle. The wall of the diencephalon, initially very thin, thickens considerably starting from week eight to nine. The isthmus rhombencephali is always distinct. The cavity of the mesencephalon remains relatively large, especially the posterior part. The height and width are about the same. The choroid plexuses of the fourth ventricle are bright landmarks dividing the ventricle into a rostral and a caudal compartment. The cerebellar hemispheres are easily detectable. The primordia of cerebellar hemispheres are clearly separated in the midline during the embryonic period.

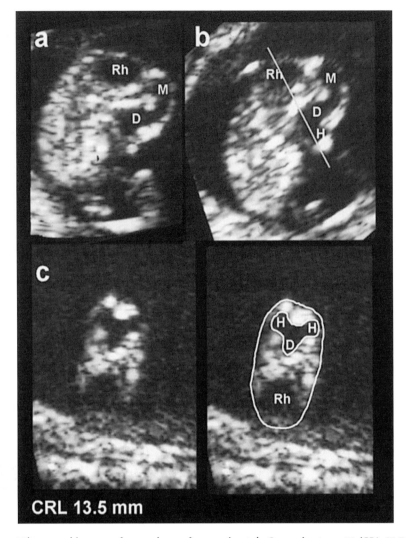

CRL 13.5 mm

Fig. 13.5.   Ulltrasound images of an embryo of approximately Carnegie stage 17 (CRL 13.5mm); compare also with Fig. 13.1.(*a*) Midsagittal section through the cavities of the rhombencephalon (Rh), mesencephalon (M) and diencephalon (D). (*b*) The ultrasound plane is slightly moved parasagittally, showing the future foramen of Monro leading from the third ventricle (D = diencephalon) into the small lateral ventricle (H = hemisphere). Rh = rhombencephalon. The line indicates the ultrasound section as shown in (*c*) and (*d*). (*c*) Section through the rhombencephalon and the forebrain with outlining of the head, the cavity of the diencephalon (D) and of the hemispheres (H).

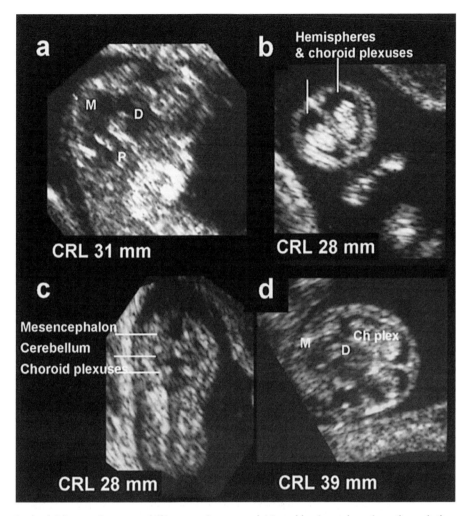

Fig. 13.6.   Sagittal (*a*), anterior coronal (*b*), posterior coronal (*c*) and horizontal sections through the brain of embryos/fetuses. (*a*) Sagittal view of the diencephalon (D), mesencephalon (M) and rhombencephalon of a 10-week-0-day-old embryo, CRL 31 mm. P = pons; the echogenic structure to the left of the pons is the choroid plexus of the fourth ventricle. Compare also with Fig. 13.2. (*b*) Coronal section through the hemispheres of a 9-week-6-day-old embryo, CRL 28 mm; the bright choroid plexuses fill the dark lateral ventricles. The wall of the hemispheres is still thin. Compare also with Fig. 13.2. (*c*) Coronal section through the mesencephalon, the cerebellum and the choroid plexuses of a 9-week-6-day-old embryo, CRL 28 mm; the dark area in the mesencephalon represents the wide Sylvian aqueduct. The cerebellar hemispheres can be identified. The bright echogenic choroid plexuses have not yet met in the midline. Compare also with Fig. 13.3. (*d*) Horizontal section through the head of a 10-week-5-day-old fetus, CRL 39 mm; the bright choroid plexuses fill the lateral ventricles. The diencephalon (D) lies central in the head, its dark cavity is clearly narrower than the cavity of the midbrain (M). Compare also with Fig. 13.4.

10 weeks 0–6 days, CRL 32–42 mm, and 11 weeks 0–6 days, CRL 43–54 mm

Early postembryonic period

The head is relatively large with a prominent forehead and a flat occiput. The future skull can be distinguished; at about 11 weeks ossification starts with the occipital bone (Zalen-Sprock et al., 1997). The thickness of the cortex is about 1 mm at the end of the first trimester. Three-dimensional reconstructions show that the thick crescent lateral ventricles fill the anterior part of the head and conceal the diencephalic cavity, which becomes smaller. After an initial increase, the width of the third ventricle becomes narrow towards the end of the first trimester. The mesencephalon gradually moves towards the centre of the head. The cerebellar hemispheres seem to meet in the midline during weeks 11 to 12. After 10 weeks 3 days, the image of the choroid plexuses of the fourth ventricle can always be seen. The distance between the choroid plexuses and the cerebellum becomes shorter during weeks 9 to 11. At the end of the first trimester, the choroid plexuses are found close to the caudal border of the cerebellum.

Summary and future aspects

The introduction of transvaginal ultrasound has opened new possibilities for describing and measuring organs of the growing conceptus in vivo. Longitudinal 2D ultrasound descriptions of the human embryonic brain gave insight into the brain development, which takes place during the first trimester (Blaas et al., 1994, 1995a), and show agreement with the developmental time schedule of human embryos described by the Carnegie staging system (O'Rahilly & Müller, 1987, 1994). The extension of the ultrasound techniques to 3D has made it possible to reconstruct the shape of the brain cavities and even to measure their volumes (Blaas et al., 1995b, 1998, 2000). Being able to achieve these measurements is a significant innovation.

There is no reason to believe that the development of ultrasound technology and its integration with computer technology has reached its end-point. We can expect to see ultrasound devices with even higher frequencies and improved resolution in the near future. Three-dimensional ultrasound has made its entry into the first trimester, making it possible to analyse the recorded ultrasound volume off-line in any plane for a more precise measurement of diameters and volumes of any structure of interest. Thus, 2D and 3D ultrasound have become major tools for the clinical evaluation of early human central nervous system development.

Our previous knowledge about the development of brain malformations was limited. The classical embryologists were dependent on the accidental cases of aborted embryos and fetuses to study eventual brain anomalies. Now, we are able to study the human embryo longitudinally, and to describe step by step the development, and possible maldevelopment, of organs. In the field of human embryology, this implies a major development which 'puts life' into descriptive human embryology.

REFERENCES

Achiron, R. & Achiron, A. (1991). Transvaginal ultrasonic assessment of the early fetal brain. *Ultrasound in Obstetrics and Gynecology*, **1**, 336–44.

Blaas, H-G., Eik-Nes, S. H., Kiserud, T. & Hellevik, L. R. (1994). Early development of the forebrain and midbrain: a longitudinal ultrasound study from 7 to 12 weeks of gestation. *Ultrasound in Obstetrics and Gynecology*, **4**, 183–92.

Blaas, H-G., Eik-Nes, S. H., Kiserud, T., Berg, S., Angelsen, B. & Olstad, B. (1995a). Three-dimensional imaging of the brain cavities in human embryos. *Ultrasound in Obstetrics and Gynecology*, **5**, 228–32.

Blaas, H-G., Eik-Nes, S. H., Kiserud, T. & Hellevik, L. R. (1995b). Early development of the hindbrain: a longitudinal ultrasound study from 7 to 12 weeks of gestation. *Ultrasound in Obstetrics and Gynecology*, **5**, 151–60.

Blaas, H-G., Eik-Nes, S. H., Berg, S. & Torp, H. (1998). In-vivo three-dimensional ultrasound reconstructions of embryos and early fetuses. *Lancet*, **352**(9135), 1182–6.

Blaas, H-G., Eik-Nes, S. H., Vainio, T., & Vogt Isaksen, C. (2000). Alobar holoprosencephaly at 9 weeks gestational age visualized by two- and three-dimensional ultrasound. *Ultrasound Obstetrics and Gynecology*, **15**, 62–5.

Bree, R. L. & Marn, C. S. (1990). Transvaginal sonography in the first trimester: embryology, anatomy, and hCG correlation. *Seminars in Ultrasound, CT and MR*, **11**,12–21.

Cullen, M. T., Green, J., Whetham, J., Salafia, C., Gabrielli, S. & Hobbins, J. (1990). Transvaginal ultrasonographic detection of congenital anomalies in the first trimester. *American Journal of Obstetrics and Gynecology*, **163**(2), 466–76.

Cyr, D. R., Mack, L. A., Nyberg, D. A., Shepard, T. H., & Shuman W. P. (1988). Fetal rhombencephalon: normal US findings. *Radiology*, **166**, 691–2.

Jenkins, G. B. (1921). Relative weight and volume of the component parts of the brain of the human embryo at different stages of development. *Contributions in Embryology Carnegie Institution*, **13**, 41–60.

O'Rahilly, R. & Gardner, E. (1971). The timing and sequence of events in the development of the human nervous system during the embryonic period proper. *Zeitschrift Anatomie Entwicklung-Gesellschaft*, **134**, 1–12.

O'Rahilly, R. & Müller, F. (1987). *Developmental Stages in Human Embryos*. Washington, DC: Carnegie Institution Publication, vol 637.

O'Rahilly, R. & Müller, F. (1990). Ventricular system and choroid plexuses of the human brain during the embryonic period proper. *American Journal of Anatomy*, **189**, 285–302.

O'Rahilly, R. & Müller, F. (1994). *The Embryonic Human Brain. An Atlas of Developmental Stages.* New York: Wiley-Liss.

O'Rahilly, R., Müller, F. & Bossy, J. (1982). Atlas des stades du développment du système nerveux chez l'embryon humain intact. *Archives d'Anatomie, d'Histologie et d'Embryologie*, **65**, 57–76.

Streeter, G. L. (1948). Developmental horizons in human embryos, *Contributions in Embryology Carnegie Institute*, **211**(32), 133–203.

Takeuchi, H. (1992). Transvaginal ultrasound in the first trimester of pregnancy. *Early Human Development*, **29**, 381–4.

Timor-Tritsch, I. E., Farine, D. & Rosen, M. G. (1988). A close look at the embryonic development with the high frequency transvaginal transducer. *American Journal of Obstetrics and Gynecology*, **159**, 678–81.

Timor-Tritsch, I. E., Peisner, D. B. & Raju, S. (1990). Sonoembryology: an organ-oriented approach using a high-frequency vaginal probe. *Journal of Clinical Ultrasound*, **18**, 286–98.

Timor-Tritsch, I. E., Monteagudo, A. & Warren, W. B. (1991). Transvaginal ultrasonographic definition of the central nervous system in the first and early second trimesters. *American Journal of Obstetrics and Gynecology*, **164**, 497–503.

Warren, W. B., Timor-Tritsch, I. E., Peisner, D. B., Raju, S. & Rosen, M. G. (1989). Dating the pregnancy by sequential appearance of embryonic structures. *American Journal of Obstetrics and Gynecology*, **161**, 747–53.

Zalen-Sprock, R. Mv., Vugt, J. M. Gv. & Geign, H. Pv. (1996). First-trimester sonographic detection of neurodevelopmental abnormalities in some single-gene disorders. *Prenatal Diagnosis*, **16**, 199–202.

Zalen-Sprock, R. Mv., Brons, J. T. J., Vugt, J. M. Gv., Harten, H. Jvd. & Geijn, H. Pv. (1997). Ultrasonic and radiologic visualization of the developing embryonic skeleton. *Ultrasound in Obstetrics and Gynaecology*, **9**, 392–7.

14

Imaging of the infant brain

Olof Flodmark[1] and A. James Barkovich[2]

[1]Department of Pediatric Neuroradiology Research, Karolinska Institute Stockholm, Sweden
[2]Department of Radiology, University of California, San Francisco, USA

Brain maturation

Many techniques are currently available for assessing the brain of the fetus, neonate and infant. These include ultrasound and magnetic resonance imaging (MR) of the fetus and transfontanelle sonography, X-ray computed tomography (CT), and MR of the neonate and infant. In general, the choice of imaging modality depends upon which features of brain development must be evaluated. In the infant with a large anterior fontanelle, ultrasound can assess development of the gyri and sulci nearly as well as CT and MR, but does not give information about brain myelination. CT allows fairly good assessment of sulcal development and gives some information about myelination. MR allows excellent assessment of myelination, sulcation and biochemical status (via magnetic resonance spectroscopy, MRS). Fetal MR imaging is being successfully utilized in some centres (Girard et al., 1995; Levine & Barnes, 1999.). The studies from these centres indicate that sulcation may develop slightly earlier in utero than in prematurely born infants. However, precise differences between in utero and ex utero sulcal development have not been fully defined.

Preterm infants

The following comments on sulcal development apply to all imaging modalities, while those on signal intensity and myelination apply only to MR. Prior to 24 weeks of gestation, the brain is essentially agyric with the exception of the wide, vertically oriented Sylvian fissures. At this stage of maturity, the cerebral cortex is very hyperintense with respect to the underlying white matter on T_1-weighted images and very hypointense compared to white matter on T_2-weighted images. The germinal matrix is isointense to the cortex on T_1- and T_2-weighted images. MR also shows a layer of migrating cells in the cerebral white matter, separate from the more peripheral cerebral cortex and more central germinal matrix; this layer is believed to represent migrating glial cells. No myelination is seen at this age, and little will be detected until after 35 weeks. Between 24 and 28 weeks, the cerebral cortex shows development of shallow Rolandic (central), calcarine, pericallosal/callosomarginal, interparietal, and superior temporal sulci, and sometimes the precentral, postcentral, superior frontal and middle temporal sulci may be visualized. By 31–32 weeks, an increased number of gyri and shallow sulci become visible. The Sylvian fissures retain an immature appearance, although some development of the opercula can be detected. The germinal matrix has involuted to some degree, but some grey matter signal remains present along the lateral walls of the lateral ventricles, most prominently seen in the region of the caudate heads and around the tips of the frontal horns (Van Wezel-Meijler et al., 1998). The thalami and globi palladi are contrasted by the unmyelinated internal capsule, which is relatively hypointense on T_1-weighted images and hyperintense on T_2-weighted images. The signal intensity of the entire cerebral cortex is uniform at this age on both T_1- and T_2-weighted images. The superior and inferior cerebellar peduncles are bright on T_1-weighted images. T_2-weighted images show hypointensity in the dorsal brainstem, superior and inferior cerebellar peduncles, far lateral putamen, and ventrolateral thalamic nucleus (Sie et al., 1997). The cerebral white matter still appears completely unmyelinated. At 34 to 36 weeks, the cerebral cortex has further thickened and more sulci have developed. Little change occurs in the signal intensity of the white matter between 32 and 36 postconceptional weeks (Sie et al., 1997). Considerable variation in brain maturity can be seen at this age, some infants having a gyral pattern that resembles a term infant and others still appearing quite immature (Barkovich, 1995).

Term neonates and infants

By 38 to 40 weeks, the brain has a nearly normal adult sulcal pattern. The sulci are formed, but are not as deep as they will become in the next several weeks. The medial lemniscus, lateral lemniscus, median longitudinal fasciculus, brachium of the interior colliculus, and the inferior and superior cerebellar peduncles are bright on T_1-weighted images (Barkovich, 1998). Above the tentorium, the decussation of the superior cerebellar peduncles, the ventral lateral region of the thalamus, the globus pallidus, and the posterior portion of the posterior limb of the internal capsule exhibit high signal intensity. In addition, small foci of grey matter intensity are seen just anterior to the tips of the frontal horns of the lateral ventricles in term neonates and premature infants. These persistent foci of germinal matrix disappear by about 44 postconceptional weeks (Childs et al., 1998; Van Wezel-Meijler et al., 1998). The development of high signal intensity proceeds rostrally from the pons along the corticospinal tracts into the cerebral peduncles, posterior limb of the internal capsule and the central portion of the centrum semiovale. Subsequently, the visual cortex, the corpus callosum, the more anterior frontal regions, the parietal lobes and the temporal lobes become hyperintense, with the final changes complete by 8–11 months in the frontal and temporal white matter (Barkovich et al., 1988).

T_2-weighted images are probably superior to T_1-weighted images for assessment of maturation of the cerebellum and brainstem (Barkovich, 1998; van der Knaap et al., 1991; Martin et al., 1991). At birth, low signal intensity is present in the inferior and superior cerebellar peduncles, cerebellar vermis, flocculi, and the cranial nerve nuclei (particularly cranial nerves VI, VII and VIII). Small foci of grey matter intensity are seen just anterior to the tips of the frontal horns in premature and term neonates, probably representing persistent germinal matrix (Van Wezel-Meijler et al., 1998; Childs et al., 1998). The ventral brainstem becomes of similar low intensity to the dorsal brainstem at about the fifth postnatal month. The middle cerebellar peduncles begin to decrease in signal intensity during the second month of life and are of uniform low intensity by age 3 months (Hittmair et al., 1996). Above the tentorium, low signal is present at birth in many mesencephalic and deep cerebral nuclei; a small patch of the posterior portion of the posterior limbs of the internal capsules, and a small linear region in the lateral putamina (Barkovich, 1998). By less than 1 month of age, the perirolandic cerebral cortex has low intensity; this disappears as the surrounding cortex diminishes in intensity. Most deep white matter tracts of the cerebrum decrease in signal intensity between 6 and 12 months of age. The corpus callosum is entirely hypointense by 11 months. The subcortical white matter (other than the calcarine and rolandic areas) matures last, proceeding from the occipital region anteriorly to the frontal and temporal lobes. This process begins at 9 to 12 months of age in the occipital lobe and at 11 to 14 months frontally. Peripheral extension of the low signal intensity into the subcortical white matter begins at about 1 year and is essentially complete by 22 to 24 months (Barkovich et al., 1988; Barkovich, 1998).

MR spectroscopy can be used to assess biochemical neonatal brain development (Kreis et al., 1993), although the consequences of delayed biochemical development have not been determined.

Infections

Both congenital and acquired infections can cause neurological signs and symptoms in the neonate. This chapter discusses the imaging appearance of congenital cytomegalovirus, toxoplasmosis, and rubella infection. Congenital syphilis and congenital AIDS, which do not generally cause symptoms in neonates, will not be considered. We will also discuss the use of neuroimaging in neonatal herpes meningoencephalitis and neonatal meningitis.

Congenital cytomegalovirus

Congenital cytomegalovirus (CMV) disease is the most common serious viral infection among newborns in the USA (Alford et al., 1990). Congenital CMV infection occurs in approximately 40 000 newborns each year, or approximately 1% of all births. Of these, 10% have the various hematological, neurological, and developmental symptoms and signs that define the disease; these include hepatosplenomegaly, microencephaly, impaired hearing, and small head size. An additional 10–15% of infected infants subsequently develop neurological or developmental abnormalities in the first year of life (Yow, 1989). Severe, permanent neurological conditions were found in 55%, including intracranial calcification (43%), microcephaly (27%), chorioretinitis (15%) and seizures (10%) (Dobbins et al., 1992). 'Less severe neurological abnormalities' (not specified) were found in 31% and hearing loss of variable degree was noted in 27% (Dobbins et al., 1992).

Findings on cross-sectional imaging examinations are variable, depending upon the degree of brain destruction and the timing of the injury. Transfontanelle ultrasound shows branching curvilinear hyperechogenicity in the basal ganglia. This appearance is called 'lenticulostriate vasculopathy' (Teele et al., 1988; Hughes et al., 1991). It is seen in patients with congenital infections of many types and is also described in patients with trisomy 13, trisomy 21 and a variety of anoxic and toxic injuries to the developing brain. Postmortem studies have shown evidence of a mineralizing vasculopathy as the cause (Teele et al., 1988; Hughes et al., 1991). Ultrasound may also show ventriculomegaly and foci of hyperechogenicity and shadowing from calcification. On CT and MR, some patients, presumably infected during the first half of the second trimester, have complete lissencephaly with a thin cortex, hypoplastic cerebellum, delayed myelination, marked ventriculomegaly and significant periventricular calcification. Those injured later, presumably in the middle of the second trimester, have more typical polymicrogyria (cortical dysplasia), less ventricular dilatation, and less consistent cerebellar hypoplasia. Patients infected near the end of gestation have normal gyral patterns, mild ventricular and sulcal prominence, and scattered periventricular calcification or hemorrhage (Barkovich & Linden, 1994). Calcifications can be seen on CT as foci of high attenuation (Barkovich, 2000). Although in young infants and neonates, calcifications can be detected on MR as foci of short T_1 and T_2 relaxation times, they are much more easily and reliably detected on CT than on MR, particularly in older infants and children. Differentiation of calcification from hemorrhage may be difficult by either modality (Barkovich & Linden, 1994). It is important to recognize that calcification is not specific by itself, as any injury to the brain, including that caused by ischemia and metabolic disorders, can cause dystrophic calcification. MR can often be helpful in the detection of cortical dysplasia, which is far more common in CMV than in other causes of cerebral calcification, myelination delay and cerebellar hypoplasia (Barkovich & Linden, 1994). When these four findings are present in a child with developmental delay or seizures, a diagnosis of congenital CMV is likely.

Congenital toxoplasmosis

Toxoplasmosis is caused by the protozoan *Toxoplasma gondii*. Pregnant women usually acquire the infection by ingestion of oocysts in uncooked meat (Robertson, 1962; Desmonts & Couvreur, 1974). The infection may be generalized or primarily concentrated in the developing nervous system. The principal CNS findings are chorioretinitis (bilateral in 85% of affected patients), abnormal cerebrospinal fluid, hydrocephalus and seizures (Eichenwald, 1956).

A diffuse inflammatory infiltration of the meninges is found on pathological examination, with large and small granulomatous lesions or a diffuse inflammation of the brain. Hydrocephalus is frequent, most often caused by ependymitis causing occlusion of the aqueduct (Friede, 1989). Porencephaly or hydranencephaly may occur if the disease is severe and occurs in the second trimester (Altschuler, 1973). It is important to note that, in contrast to congenital CMV, malformations of cortical development, such as polymicrogyria, are not a common feature of congenital toxoplasmosis.

The findings of cross-sectional imaging studies reflect the pathological findings of meningeal infiltration, small and large granulomata and diffuse brain inflammation (Friede, 1989). Calcifications are common; they usually involve the basal ganglia, periventricular region and cerebral cortex. Large ventricles are common and may be the result of hydrocephalus, brain destruction, or both. As with cytomegalovirus, a spectrum is seen from relatively mild disease, with a few periventricular calcifications and mild atrophy, to severe disease with near total destruction of the cortex and brain accompanied by marked, diffuse cerebral calcification. Diebler et al. (1985) have related the severity of the brain involvement to the date of maternal infection. They found that early infection (before 20 weeks) results in ventricular dilatation, areas of porencephaly and extensive calcifications, particularly in the basal ganglia. Ultrasound shows lenticulostriate vasculopathy (Teele et al., 1988; Hughes et al., 1991) and hyperechogenicity/shadowing from the calcifications. Infection between 20 and 30 weeks leads to a more variable outcome. On CT scan, multiple periventricular calcifications and ventricular dilatation are present. Infection after the 30th week is generally associated with small periventricular and intracerebral calcifications that are only rarely accompanied by ventricular dilatation (Diebler et al., 1985). An important differentiating feature is the absence of cortical dysplasia, which is a common finding in congenital CMV infection; cortical dysplasia is rare in congenital toxoplasmosis.

Congenital rubella

Congenital rubella is now extremely rare in western countries because of screening techniques now performed on pregnant women. In the USA, the incidence is now less than 1 per 1 000 000 live births (Preblud & Alford, 1990). This virus affects the fetus more commonly during the first and second trimester; ocular, cardiac and neurological defects are most common when infection occurs in the first and second postconceptional months. Rubella infection is nearly benign when occurring during the third trimester (Miller et al., 1982).

The appearance of the brain on imaging studies varies depending upon the time of the in utero infection. Early infection will result in congenital anomalies whereas late infection will result in a non-specific generalized edema or loss of brain tissue. Ultrasound shows lenticulostriate vasculopathy, identical to that in congenital toxoplasmosis and congenital CMV (Teele et al., 1988; Hughes et al., 1991). CT typically shows multifocal regions of hypodensity throughout the cerebral white matter, often in association with calcification (Ishikawa et al., 1982). In addition, calcification may be seen in the basal ganglia and cortex. In severe cases, nearly total brain destruction and microcephaly are present (Barkovich, 2000). MR imaging shows multifocal regions of prolonged T_2 relaxation and myelination delay (Yamashita et al., 1991).

Neonatal herpes simplex encephalitis

Infection of the fetus with herpes simplex virus may result in a fatal generalized disease. Most cases of HSV infection result from exposure of the fetus to maternal type II herpetic genital lesions as he/she passes through the birth canal. The incidence of neonatal herpes simplex infections is estimated to be 1 per 2000–5000 deliveries per year (Whitley & Hutto, 1985). The brain is involved in approximately 30% of infected infants.

Imaging studies of patients with neonatal herpes encephalitis show patchy, widespread areas of abnormal signal (hyperechogenicity on ultrasound, low attenuation on CT, prolonged T_1 and T_2 on MR) in the grey and white matter, which rapidly progress in prominence and area of involvement during the course of the disease. Some contrast enhancement occurs in a meningeal pattern, presumably reflecting meningeal involvement. As the disease progresses, the cortical grey matter undergoes a change in signal (increase in attenuation on CT, shortening of T_1 and T_2 on MR) that persists for weeks to months (Noorbehesht et al., 1987; Barkovich, 2000). Loss of brain substance occurs rapidly, often as early as the second week. Eventually, severe diffuse cerebral atrophy evolves, with profound cortical thinning, leukomalacia (often multicystic in nature) and punctate or gyriform calcification. The cerebellum is involved in about half of affected infants (Noorbehesht et al., 1987). The combination of a meningeal pattern of enhancement and the increased attenuation/short T_1/T_2 of cortical grey matter that may persist for weeks to months should lead to a suggestion of the diagnosis of neonatal herpes simplex encephalitis.

Neonatal meningitis

Bacterial meningitis can cause severe brain damage to the neonatal brain as a result of accompanying vasculitis and ventriculitis (Friede, 1989; Volpe, 1995a). Imaging studies are not performed routinely in neonates and infants with meningitis; they are indicated if the clinical diagnosis is unclear, if neurological deterioration occurs secondary to increased intracranial pressure, if the meningitis is associated with persistent seizures or focal neurological deficits, or if patient recovery from the disease is slow (Dunn et al., 1982; Snyder, 1992; Volpe, 1995a).

CT and MR studies in uncomplicated cases of purulent meningitis are usually normal. Occasionally, some enhancement of the meninges will be seen on post-contrast scans (Barkovich, 2000). Contrast-enhanced MR is more sensitive than contrast-enhanced CT in detecting inflammatory changes in the meninges (Mathews et al., 1988); however, enhancement of the meninges is only occasionally seen, even with MR. Hydrocephalus is a common sequel of meningitis that is well evaluated by all imaging modalities; MR is the most effective at localizing the level of the obstruction. Deep vein, cortical vein and sinus thrombosis are uncommon complications of meningitis; they are more likely in the presence of dehydration. Sinus thrombosis can be recognized by Doppler ultrasound by the absence of flow in the superior sagittal sinus or straight sinus. On CT, acute sinus thrombosis is diagnosed by increased density in the affected sinus on a noncontrast scan. When the clot is subacute, it is seen as a low density filling defect in the sinus on a contrast-enhanced scan. This filling defect is only visible after the clot becomes less dense than the contrast enhanced blood flowing within it (Rao et al., 1981; Virapongse et al., 1987). Acute or subacute dural sinus thrombosis is easily diagnosed by MR when the sinus is hyperintense on T_1-weighted images. When the thrombus is hyperacute, it is isointense to brain on T_1-weighted images and hypointense on T_2-weighted images. This appearance can be mistaken for slow flow of pseudogating (in which the sinus is always imaged during diastole). To establish a lack of blood flow, MR venography using a phase contrast technique with gradient timing set to detect a phase change of 180° at 20 cm/s (Venc = 20 cm/s) or two-dimensional time of flight MR venography (with images acquired in the coronal plane) is necessary to make the diagnosis. Venous infarcts have characteristic location and appearance. Typically, infarcts from sagittal sinus thrombosis are parasagittal, infarcts from straight sinus/vein of Galen thrombosis involve the thalami, and infarcts from vein of Labbé, transverse sinus, or sigmoid sinus thrombosis involve the temporal lobe. Sonography shows venous infarcts as hyperechogenic regions with mass effect, often with heterogeneity resulting from hemorrhage. On CT, venous infarcts are usually poorly delimited, hypodense or mixed attenuation areas involving the subcortical white matter and producing a slight mass effect on ventricular structures. The low attenuation is probably due to localized cerebral edema, whereas high attenuation areas usually represent hemorrhage. Following contrast administration, linear or round gyral enhancement frequently overlies the hypodensity (Chiras et al., 1985). On MR, the oedematous areas have prolonged T_1 and T_2 relaxation times; T_2 shortening from hemorrhage is common (Barkovich, 2000). Twenty-five per cent of venous infarcts are hemorrhagic and have an imaging appearance that varies from large subcortical hematomas to petechial hemorrhages within edematous brain parenchyma (Rao et al., 1981; Chiras et al., 1985; Raybaud et al., 1996). The hemorrhages are generally subcortical and often multifocal with irregular margins. They are occasionally linear in nature indicating hematoma in and around the vein; this appearance is quite specific. Arteritis accompanying meningitis can be reliably diagnosed by CT or MR because of the resulting infarcts, which tend to be sharply marginated and confined to a specific arterial vascular territory. Large or small vessels can be affected. When major vessels, such as the middle or anterior cerebral arteries are involved, large, usually cortical infarctions result. Frequently, multiple lacunar-type infarcts are seen in the distribution of perforating vessels in the brain stem and basal ganglia, presumably resulting from involvement of the basilar cisterns and vessels contained therein (Barkovich, 2000). Cerebritis and abscesses develop when the infectious process travels through thrombosed venules into the cerebral parenchyma. The only differences between cerebritis/abscess in neonates and in older children are the speed at which brain destruction occurs and the amount of reactive astrogliosis that occurs. Because of the reduced immune response of the neonate, brain destruction is rapid, resulting in macrocystic encephalomalacia with relatively minimal atroglial response. When ventriculitis is present, the ependyma manifests hyperechogenicity (ultrasound) and intense enhancement following contrast administration (CT and MR). MR has, perhaps, a greater sensitivity to the inflammatory process. The ventricles are nearly always dilated as a result of the obstruction of CSF flow that is typically present in meningitis. Loculations of CSF within and external to the ventricles often result from obstruction of ventricular outlets, the formation of septations across the ventricles, or necrosis of periventricular brain tissue (Schultz & Leeds, 1973; Naidich et al., 1983). Septations are better identified by ultrasound or MR than by CT.

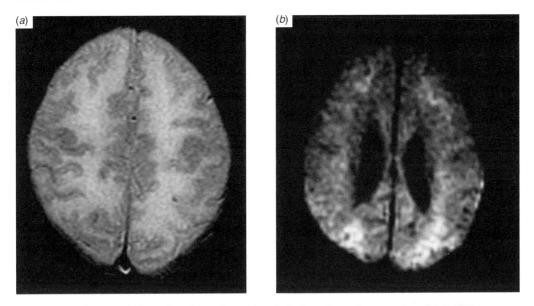

Fig. 14.1.   This term baby suffered a prolonged period of moderate hypotension. (*a*) Axial T$_2$-
weighted (SE 3000/60) image shows blurring of the interface between cortical and
subcortical structures in the anterior and posterior watershed regions. (*b*) Axial isotropic
diffusion image shows increased signal indicating reduced diffusion in the same regions.

Hypoxic–ischemic injury in the term neonate

Factors determining patterns of injury

Many different patterns of brain injury can result from hypoxic–ischemic episodes
in neonates (Barkovich & Hallam, 1997). These patterns can be best interpreted as
resulting from three primary factors: (i) severity of hypotension; (ii) maturity of
the brain at the time of the injury; and (iii) duration of the event.

Severity of hypotension

When blood flow to the brain is mildly or moderately reduced in the setting of
impaired autoregulation, blood flow is shunted from the anterior to the posterior
circulation in order to maintain adequate perfusion to the brainstem, cerebellum
and basal ganglia (Ashwal et al., 1981). As a result, damage is limited to the cerebral cortex, with the most severe damage in the intervascular boundary zones
(Barkovich & Hallam, 1997) (Fig. 14.1(*a*), (*b*).) When reduction of cerebral blood
flow is severe, resulting in complete or nearly complete cessation of cerebral blood
flow, shunting of blood is no longer adequate to save the deep structures from

damage. In this situation, the deep cerebral nuclei (thalami and basal ganglia), peri-rolandic cortex and dorsal brain stem are initially damaged; these are the areas with highest metabolic activity in the neonate (Chugani et al., 1987; Tokumaru et al., 1999). Damage to the remainder of the cortex and white matter occurs only later in the course of the hypotensive episode (Roland et al., 1988, 1998; Pasternak et al., 1991; Barkovich, 1992; Rutherford et al., 1994; Barkovich et al., 1995; Pasternak & Gorey, 1998).

Maturity of the brain

The patterns of injury secondary to mild to moderate hypotension and those secondary to profound hypotension both change with the postconceptional age of the child.

Premature infants who suffer mild to moderate hypotension typically sustain injury to the periventricular white matter with sparing of the subcortical white matter and cerebral cortex (Barkovich & Truwit, 1990; Volpe, 1995b) (see Chapter 12). In contrast, term infants who suffer similar degrees of hypotension sustain injury in the watershed portions of the cerebral cortex and in the underlying subcortical and periventricular white matter (Barkovich & Truwit, 1990; Volpe, 1995b).

Differences in pattern of injury from profound hypotension are also seen as the brain matures (Barkovich & Sargent, 1995). Certain regions of the brain mature sooner than others; these changes in maturity are reflected in relative blood flow (Tokumura et al., 1999), glucose uptake (Chugani et al., 1987) and myelination (Azzarelli et al., 1996). The thalami and brainstem have the highest blood flow and metabolic activity in the early third trimester; from the middle of the third trimester through 40 postconceptional weeks, the brainstem, thalami, basal ganglia and perirolandic region have the highest activity (Chugani et al., 1987; Kinnala et al., 1996; Tokumaru et al., 1999). By the end of the first postnatal month (44 postconceptional weeks), the visual cortex becomes more active (Chugani et al., 1987; Kinnala et al., 1996; Tokumaru et al., 1999). By the third or fourth postnatal month, the remainder of the cerebral cortex and the basal ganglia become increasingly metabolically active and the regions more likely to be damaged shift from the thalami and perirolandic cortex to the basal ganglia and the entire cerebral cortex (Chugani et al., 1987; Kinnala et al., 1996; Barkovich & Hallam, 1997; Tokumaru et al., 1999).

Duration of the injury

Although the precise duration of an arrest is not usually known, particularly in a neonate, it is our experience that the longer the duration of an episode of profound hypotension, the greater the region of brain involved. The least injured patients (those with short episodes of hypotension) have damage only to the ventrolateral thalami and posterior putamen. Longer duration of profound hypotension results in progressively more damage to the basal nuclei and in damage (in progressive order) to the perirolandic cortex, superior cerebellar vermis, visual cortex and ultimately the entirety of the cerebral cortex.

The duration of cerebral ischemia necessary to cause injury to the watershed zones and periventricular white matter is probably similar to that needed to cause damage from circulatory arrest. However, because the region suffering hypoperfusion is limited, the region that is damaged does not extend as the duration of the hypotension progresses unless the hypotension becomes more severe. Therefore, in our experience, patients who suffer mild to moderate ischemia for many hours, or even days, have watershed patterns of injury similar to those who suffer injuries of shorter duration.

Imaging appearances

Watershed injury in the neonate is very similar to watershed injury at other ages and from any cause. When injury is primarily cortical, as in the watershed zones, ultrasound is usually normal; it is difficult to see watershed injury by this method. CT will show low density of the cortex in the watershed zones in the acute phase. MR shows reduced diffusion in the watershed zones in the acute phase. By 24 hours, T_2 prolongation will be seen in the affected cortex on the first echo of T_2-weighted sequences. On either CT or MR, volume loss starts to be seen about 10–14 days after the injury. By 2 months after injury, the cortex and underlying white matter is shrunken and atrophic in both anterior and posterior watershed zones (Barkovich & Truwit, 1990).

When the neonate has suffered severe injury to the brain secondary to profound hypotension, ultrasound may show diffuse hyperechogenicity and blurring of normal landmarks within the first few days after injury (Babcock & Ball, 1983; Siegel et al., 1984). If injury is less severe, hyperechogenicity will be limited to the thalami, globi palladi, putamina and periventricular white matter and will appear by the second or third day after injury. This hyperechogenicity can easily be overlooked if the sonographer is not actively searching for it (Phillips et al., 1993); the finding of thalamic hyperechogenicity portends a poor neurological outcome (Connolly et al., 1994; Rutherford et al., 1994). Transcranial Doppler seems to show a decreased resistive index in the first days after injury, probably because of impaired autoregulation (Stark & Seibert, 1994; Siebert et al., 1998). CT shows hypoattenuation of the thalami and basal ganglia, which can be easily overlooked, as these grey matter structures become isodense with surrounding white matter (Barkovich, 1992; Roland et al., 1998). It is therefore, essential to specifically assess the thalami and basal ganglia to be sure that their attentuation values are similar to other grey matter structures. The presence of low attenuation in the thalami on postnatal days 2–4 is highly predictive of poor neurological outcome (Roland et al., 1998). Standard MR imaging will typically be normal if performed on the day of birth. Diffusion imaging, however, will show loss of the normally restricted diffusion in the lateral thalami (Cowan et al., 1994). T_1- and T_2-weighted images will become positive on the second or third day, but findings are subtle (Barkovich et al., 1995; Barkovich & Hallam, 1997). By day 2, the first echo of the T_2-weighted sequence will show that the basal nuclei, particularly the posterior thalami, are isointense with white matter. By day 2 or 3, T_1-weighted images will be abnormal, showing diffuse high signal in the lateral thalami, globi palladi and posterior putamina and in deep areas of the cerebral cortex, particularly in the perirolandic area. Extensive cortical injury portends a very poor neurological outcome (Kuenzle et al., 1994). When severely injured, the basal ganglia will become isointense with white matter on T_2-weighted images and the normal dot of T_1 and T_2 shortening (Barkovich, 1998) will not be seen in the posterior limb of the internal capsule.

By 7 to 10 days after the injury, ultrasound shows better definition of the hyperechogenic areas and some increase in ventricular size as the edema resolves. CT scans also show resolution of edema and may begin to show high signal, probably representing hemorrhage, in the affected grey matter nuclei (Pasternak et al., 1991; Barkovich, 1992). On MR, the high signal seen in the deep grey matter on T_1-weighted images becomes heterogeneous, with small areas of marked focal hyperintensity near the junction of the anterior commissure and the globi palladi. Heterogeneous high and low signal is seen in the basal nuclei on the T_2-weighted images (Barkovich & Hallam, 1997). The extent of injury is variable, being limited to the hippocampi, lateral thalami, posterior putamina and perirolandic cortex in the least severely injured patients, involving all of the deep cerebral nuclei and central mesencephalon in more severely injured patients, and involving much of the cerebral cortex, all the deep cerebral nuclei and many brainstem nuclei in the most severely injured patients (Steinlen et al., 1991; Kuenzle et al., 1994; Barkovich et al, 1995; Barkovich & Hallam, 1997). The short T_1 and T_2 relaxation times slowly fade as atrophy of the injured tissues develops over the subsequent 6 to 10 weeks (Figs. 14.2(*a*)–(*c*), 14.3(*a*), (*b*).)

Diseases of the premature brain

Neuroradiological investigation of the brain in the premature neonate has been practised since 1975 and all available modalities have been used: first computed tomography (CT) scanning and neurosonography and later positron emission tomography (PET) and magnetic resonance imaging (MRI). The delicate physiology of the preterm neonate and the risks associated with any manipulation, have

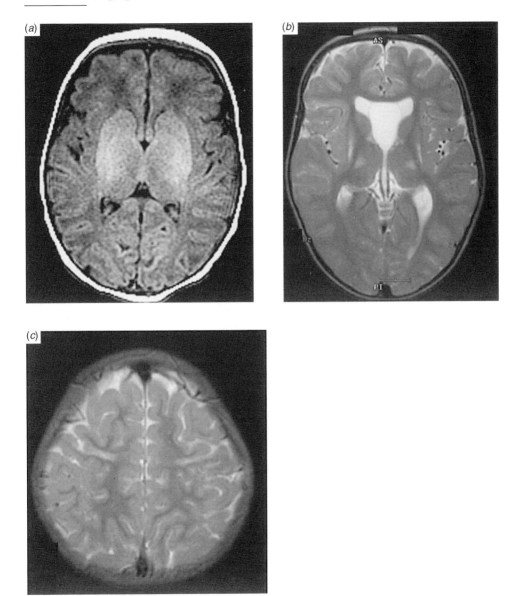

Fig. 14.2.   (*a*) A term baby who suffered profound hypotension (Apgars 0 and 1 at 1 and 5 minutes). Axial T$_1$-weighted image shows abnormally low signal in the posterior limbs of the internal capsules and abnormally high signal intensity in the lateral thalami and putamina. (*b*) A different infant born at term who also suffered profound asphyxia. Axial T$_2$-weighted image at 2 years of age shows permanent damage with abnormally increased signal bilaterally in lateral thalamus and posterior putamen. (*c*) Same infant as in (*b*) in whom an axial T$_2$-weighted image of the parietal lobes shows symmetrically increased signal adjacent to the central sulcus.

(a)

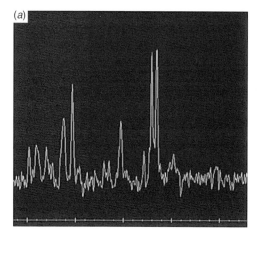

(b)

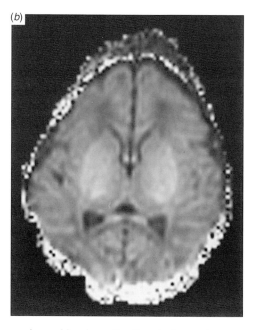

Fig. 14.3.   A baby born at term, who suffered severe prolonged bradycardia after uterine rupture. (*a*) MR spectroscopy of tissue in the basal ganglia/thalamic region shows reduced NAA, reduced choline and markedly elevated lactate. A spectrum with similar appearance was also obtained in the centrum semiovale. (*b*) Isotropic diffusion image shows reduced diffusion throughout the brain, indicating severe, diffuse injury.

had the consequence that cribside neurosonography has remained the imaging modality of choice in most neonatal intensive care units. While CT scanning has lost its role for the preterm neonate during the neonatal period almost altogether, MR imaging may provide so much additional value that it may be well indicated, provided that the environment around the neonate can be controlled.

Neurosonography is a technically simple procedure requiring equipment available in most paediatric hospitals. However, great care must be used in selecting the proper probe for the desired investigation. Thus different probes are used to investigate superficial cortical structures than deeper structures such as the posterior fossa. However, most cerebral pathology found in the preterm neonate is located centrally in the brain and therefore in an ideal location to be visualized by neurosonography. Investigation of more difficult areas can be improved by using other acoustic windows, such as the posterior and posterio-lateral fontanelles (Merrill et al., 1998) in addition to the usual anterior fontanelle. Despite meticulous technique, neurosonography has important limitations that must be known to the investigator. The diagnostic quality of the procedure is very much dependent on the skill and knowledge of the operator. The very nature of the procedure, as a clinical examination, provides great freedom in interpreting the images, thus giving clinical bias an opportunity to play a major role in the final interpretation. However good or experienced the sonographer, neither the sensitivity nor specificity of neurosonography is even close to 100%. Thus both false-positive (Grant et al., 1983) and false-negative results (DiPietro et al., 1986, Baarsma et al., 1987) may result from the search for both periventricular leukomalacia (PVL), the most important diagnosis in preterm neonates, and other diagnoses (Merrill et al., 1998). Thus neonatal neurosonography cannot be used prospectively to select, for instance, a group of high-risk neonates to be followed for future development of PVL.

Germinal matrix and intraventricular hemorrhage

Germinal matrix hemorrhage and secondary intraventricular hemorrhage are readily identified using neurosonography. The origin of this hemorrhage is found in the germinal zone, the part of the brain in which the cells that compose the brain are generated (Hambleton & Wigglesworth, 1976; Wigglesworth & Pope, 1978). The germinal zones show most activity during the period from 8 to 28 weeks of gestation. The germinal matrix diminishes in activity toward the end of the second trimester and begins to involute. The last part of the germinal zone to involute, known as the ganglionic eminence, is adjacent to the head of the caudate nucleus. The frequency of hemorrhage decreases with increasing maturity and germinal matrix hemorrhage is unusual after 34 weeks of gestation (Greisen, 1992).

Germinal matrix hemorrhage is usually described in four grades with some significant but not absolute relationship to severity (Papile et al., 1978): Grade I is defined as hemorrhage confined to the germinal zone and without intraventricular extension. Grade II is diagnosed when the hemorrhage has extended into the lateral ventricle but the ventricle remains normal in size. Grade III hemorrhage is when the bleed has extended into the ventricle, which is dilated due to hydrocephalus. Grade IV hemorrhage describes a combination of hemorrhages in the germinal matrix, lateral ventricle and adjacent cerebral parenchyma. This grade usually needs further qualification, as the amount of hemorrhage in the cerebral hemisphere may be anywhere from minimal to massive. The presence of massive parenchymal hemorrhage and ventricular dilatation is an excellent prognosticator of very poor short- and long-term neurologic outcome of the neonate (Van de Bor et al., 1993; Pikus et al., 1997). Neurosonography as well as CT scanning are imaging modalities capable of showing the hemorrhagic components of hypoxic/ischemic injury to the preterm neonate.

Neurosonography is the method of choice to follow the evolution of ventricular dilatation in posthemorrhagic hydrocephalus of the preterm neonate. In most cases this hydrocephalus is resolved without further treatment, without negative prognostic value. However, in some neonates, the ventriculomegaly may develop into secondary hydrocephalus a poorly understood etiology (Fukumizu et al., 1995). Such secondary hydrocephalus carries a less favourable prognosis.

The parenchymal hemorrhage in Grade IV bleed represents secondary hemorrhage into an area of venous infarction and is sometimes referred to as periventricular hemorrhagic infarction (Volpe, 1995c). Obstruction of the terminal veins by the germinal matrix hemorrhage may play an important role in the pathogenesis of the periventricular hemorrhage, a hypothesis that can be studied with the help of Doppler ultrasound (Taylor, 1995). In the acute phase, the hemorrhage is seen on ultrasound as areas of mixed hyper- and hypodensities. The damaged part of the brain will, with time, undergo liquefaction and a large parenchymal cyst develops. This cyst is separated from the ventricle by a thin membrane representing the ependyma. This membrane is usually incomplete and will eventually disappear; the cyst becomes part of the ventricle and lined with ependyma. This process is well seen on serial neurosonography studies.

Periventricular leukomalacia – PVL

Periventricular leukomalacia is an ischemic brain injury that is more or less symmetrical in distribution and involves the periventricular white matter most often adjacent to the trigone or foramina of Monro of the lateral ventricles. PVL has been demonstrated pathologically in as many as 85% of infants with birthweight between 900 and 2200 g who survived more than 6 days (Shuman & Selednik, 1980). The true incidence of PVL in all preterm children is not known but recent studies of an entire population in northern Finland has revealed that about one-third (32%) of all prematurely born children had MR evidence of end-stage PVL at 8 years of age (Olsén et al., 1998). This is far more frequent than suggested by studies in which neonatal neurosonography was used in the diagnosis of PVL (Claris et al., 1996).

Neuroradiological diagnosis of PVL is not easy. CT and MRI do not play a major role in early diagnosis of PVL, owing to difficulties in transporting the very fragile neonate to the scanner. Thus neurosonography, despite its shortcomings, remains the modality of choice in the neonatal period. Very early diagnosis of PVL, during the first week of life, is exceedingly difficult. The first sign of pathology is increased echogenicity in the periventricular regions. However, edema in brain tissue will also show increased echogenicity and edema may resolve without being associated with subsequent brain damage (Vannucci et al., 1993). To complicate the picture further, increased echogenicity can be seen without either edema or PVL (Grant et al., 1983). Even severe forms of PVL have been shown to develop in children known to have had normal ultrasound studies during the neonatal period (Di Pietro et al., 1986; Baarsma et al., 1987). Thus early ultrasound diagnosis of PVL can only be confirmed when periventricular cavities and subsequent cyst formation in the periventricular regions are demonstrated. These cysts develop 2–6 weeks after the initial brain injury (Sudakoff et al., 1991). A recently suggested grading scheme classifies PVL into three categories. Grade I represent periventricular areas of increased echogenicity present for 7 days or more. Grade II PVL is said to be present when the areas of increased echogenicity evolve into small, localized fronto-parietal cysts. Grade III PVL is diagnosed when the periventricular echodense areas develop into extensive periventricular cystic lesions involving the occipital as well as fronto-parietal white matter (deVries et al., 1992).

The finding on neurosonography of increased periventricular echogenicity without subsequent cavitation has generated great interest as it is often discussed as an imaging finding in neonatal clinical studies of preterm neonates. Lack of a standard nomenclature increases the difficulties of comparing results from the different studies published on this subject. The grading indicated above does not take into account what some authors describe as a 'flare', an area of increased echogenicity that may resolve early or late without any subsequent ultrasound abnormality (Appleton et al., 1990). Other descriptions are used to define the same phenomenon (Ringelberg & Van de Bor, 1993; Aziz et al., 1995). An addition to previous grading of PVL has been suggested in which a 'flare' is 'restricted to any hyperechoic image that resolves completely without leaving any abnormality in its place'. The 'flare' should be termed 'brief' if it resolves within 6 days of its appearance, 'intermediate' if it disappears between 7 and 13 days after onset, and 'prolonged' if it disappears on day 14 or later (Dammann & Leviton, 1997) (Fig. 14.4(a)–(c).)

Although MR does not play a major role in early diagnosis of PVL, it is occasionally used early in life on premature neonates. It has been shown that small periventricular areas of short T_1 and T_2 can be seen for several weeks in the periventricular white matter (Battin et al., 1998). Later stages show development of cysts which will eventually become incorporated in the lateral ventricles and show the typical features of end stage PVL. These characteristic features in mild cases include abnormal signal (short T_1 and T_2) in the periventricular white matter, which may also be slightly reduced in volume. The lateral ventricles remain normal in size and shape in mild cases, but become dilated in more severe cases in which the periventricular white matter may be locally absent and grey matter abuts directly the ventricular wall. The lateral ventricles become irregular in shape with cortical structures at the deepest reaches of the sulci, particularly the posterior sylvian fissures, indenting the walls of the lateral ventricles. The deep portions of the sylvian fissures often show focal dilatation; when present this provides a quite specific proof that PVL is indeed the cause of reduced amounts of periventricular white matter. The corpus callosum is thinner than usual (Flodmark et al., 1987, 1989).

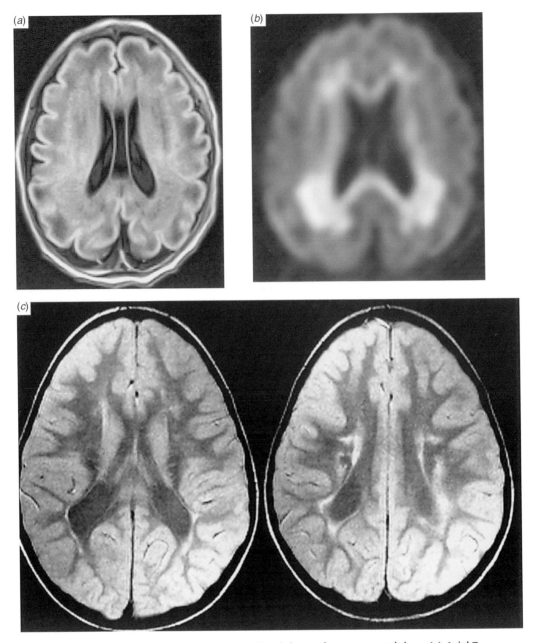

Fig. 14.4.   This baby born at 32 weeks of gestation is imaged at 6 postnatal days. (a) Axial T_1-weighted image shows some T_1 shortening in the white matter surrounding the frontal horns and some possible microcavitations in the white matter around the trigones of the lateral ventricles. (b) Axial isotropic diffusion weighted image shows markedly reduced diffusion (manifest as hyperintensity) in the white matter around the frontal horns and trigones. (c) This 8-year-old girl has periventricular leukomalacia. Note the widened lateral ventricles with grey matter directly abutting the ventricular wall. The white matter more anteriorly has abnormally increased signal on these proton dense images.

Profound hypotension or circulatory arrest in the premature infant

It is well recognized that partial hypoxia and profound asphyxia cause damage of different patterns in the term neonate (Barkovich, 1992). A similar situation appears to be applicable also in the prematurely born neonate. A study of four prematurely born neonates showed decreased amount of hemispheric white matter and shrunken basal ganglia, thalami, brain stem structures and cerebelli. The pattern differed considerably from that of partial hypoxia causing periventricular leukomalacia in the immature brain, but showed similarities to those described in term neonates following profound asphyxia (Barkovich & Sargent, 1995). Although similar, the difference from the term neonate is the perirolandic cortex that was spared and the basal ganglia being less involved in the preterm neonate. Although imaging support for these observations is sparse, pathological studies seem to concur in their description of damage following profound asphyxia before 32 weeks gestational age (Parisi et al., 1983; Cohen & Roessmann, 1994). As in the term neonate, the pattern of injury appears to relate to the progress of myelination in the developing brain. There is an almost exact correlation between the highest glucose uptake and the location of most advanced myelination (Chugani et al., 1987; Hasegawa et al., 1992). Thus thalami myelinate at 23–25 weeks gestation while the basal ganglia myelinate at 33–35 weeks of gestation. This may explain why the basal ganglia are less involved with profound asphyxic damage in the preterm neonate less mature than 32 weeks than in the mature neonate (Fig. 14.5(*a*), (*b*).)

An important concept is that hypoxia/ischemia and asphyxia/arrest can occur in utero. The imaging pattern of brain injury seen in those infants who have suffered in utero damage is identical to that found in neonates who have been damaged postnatally during the same stage of development (Barkovich & Truwit, 1990). Thus periventricular leukomalacia found in an infant born at term should be considered a sequel to a prenatal insult (Krägeloh-Mann et al., 1995).

Hypoglycemia

Although hypoglycemia is common in neonates, isolated hypoglycemia uncommonly causes brain damage (Volpe, 1995d). The less mature brain can withstand lower glucose levels than the more mature; thus, the definition of hypoglycemia depends on the maturity of the neonate. In preterm neonates, hypoglycemia is defined as glucose levels below 20 mg/dl, in term neonates as below 30 mg/dl and in adults as below 45 mg/dl. Hypoglycemia has many causes, providing different pathophysiological mechanisms that may lead to more or less severe clinical symptoms (Cornblath & Schwartz, 1991). Although hypoglycemia may be underdiagnosed, its damaging effects on the brain may be even less recognized. Hypoglycemia has only minor effects on the cardiovascular system in the newborn (Vannucci et al.,

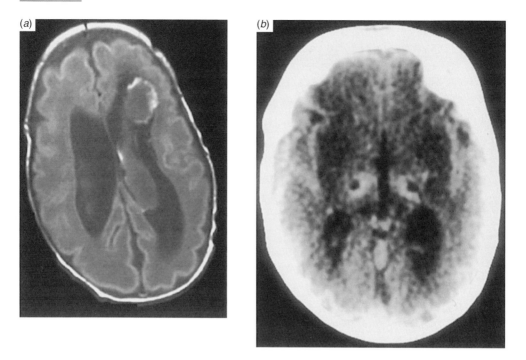

Fig. 14.5.   (a) Periventricular hemorrhagic infarction. Axial T_1-weighted image of a neonate born at 24 weeks postconceptional age and studied at 6 weeks of age. Note the resolving parenchymal hemorrhage in the left frontal region. (b) Axial CT image in a child who suffered cardiac arrest at postconceptional age of 28 weeks. Bassal ganglia are very hypodense. Thalami show a central hole with surrounding calcification.

1981); thus cerebral perfusion and cerebral oxygen delivery are maintained during neonatal hypoglycemia. The ability of the neonatal brain to utilize energy sources other than glucose and the maintenance of cerebral perfusion during hypoglycemia probably account for the different patterns of brain damage seen in neonatal hypoglycemia and hypoxic–ischemic injury (Flodmark et al., 1989; Keeney et al., 1991; Barkovich, 1992; Barkovich & Sargent, 1995; Barkovich et al., 1998). Hypoxic–ischemic brain injury is often superimposed upon hypoglycemic damage, as ischemia will secondarily cause lack of glucose transportation to the brain. As hypoglycemia appears to potentiate the effect of hypoxic–ischemic injury, the combined effect may be devastating (Volpe, 1995b). The brain damage due to hypoxia/ischemia alone is therefore identical to that of a combination of hypoxia/ischemia and hypoglycemia (Griffiths & Laurence, 1974).

The pattern of brain injury, as seen on neuroimaging, has recently been described (Spar et al., 1994; Barkovich et al., 1998). In all neonates reported, there has been predominant involvement of cortical and subcortical structures in the

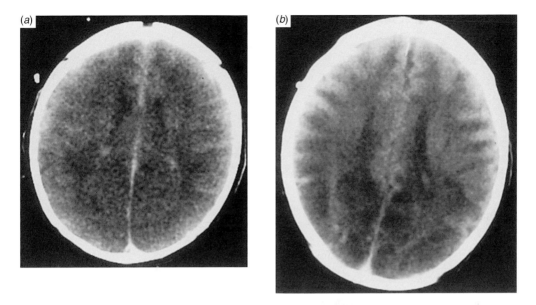

Fig. 14.6.   This child born at term suffered profound hypoglycemia for several days during the first week of life. (*a*) Axial CT at age 8 days shows edema involving the parietal and occipital lobes. (*b*) Axial CT at age 6 months shows severe encephalomalacia in the same areas as in (*a*).

parietal and occipital lobes of the cerebral hemispheres. In more severe cases, damage has also been detected in the frontal lobe and in the globus pallidus. CT scans have been reported to show edema in the parietal and occipital locations during the first days of life, while knowledge about the findings on MR imaging are limited to a later subacute stage when T_1 and T_2 prolongation is detected in the parietal and occipital white matter. The signal in cortical structures is more mixed. Short-term follow-up of these patients shows atrophy with cystic encephalomalacia developing in the damaged areas (Barkovich et al., 1998).

Although the causes of hypoglycemia have been different in the neonates described in the literature, the imaging features have been consistent. It is therefore reasonable to assume that the pattern of damage detected by neuroimaging reflect the injury caused by hypoglycemia and not the underlying disorder (Barkovich et al., 1998) (Fig. 14.6(*b*).)

The pattern of brain damage in neonatal hypoglycemia is distinctly different from that of hypoxic–ischemic injury (Barkovich & Hallam, 1997). Damage caused by hypoxic–ischemic injury does not cause the pattern described here and can therefore be separated from that of neonatal hypoglycemia on the basis of the imaging appearance of the injuries (Barkovich et al., 1998) (Fig. 14.7.)

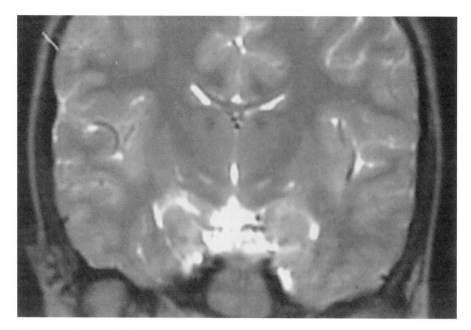

Fig. 14.7.   This coronal T$_2$-weighted image of a 10-year-old child with clinical symptoms of kernicterus shows symmetrically located areas of increased signal in the medial aspects of glubus pallidus.

Hyperbilirubinemia

The ability of bilirubin to injure the neonatal brain has been well known for a long time. The relationship between serum levels of unconjugated bilirubin and toxic effect on the brain is complicated. The role of neuroimaging is limited, as no abnormal findings have been reported in the acute phase of hyperbilirubinemia. However, children with bilirubin encephalopathy have been shown to have abnormal findings on MRI with bilaterally marked increased signal in the medial portions of the globus pallidus. This is a location known from pathological descriptions of kernicterus (Volpe, 1995e).

REFERENCES

Alford, C. A., Stagno, S., Pass, R. F. & Britt, W. J. (1990). Congenital and perinatal cytomegalovirus infections. *Review of Infectious Diseases* (Suppl. 7), S745–53.

Altschuler, G. (1973). Toxoplasmosis as a cause of hydranencephaly. *American Journal of Disease in Childhood*, **125**, 251–2.

Appleton, R. E., Lee, R. E. J. & Hey, E. N. (1990). Neurodevelopmental outcome of transient neo-natal intracerebral echodensities. *Archives of Disease in Childhood*, **65**, 27–9.

Ashwal, S., Majcher, J. S. & Longo, L. (1981). Patterns of fetal lamb regional cerebral blood flow during and after prolonged hypoxia: studies during the post-hypoxic recovery period. *American Journal of Obstetrics and Gynecology*, **139**, 365–72.

Aziz, K., Vickar, D. B., Sauve, R. S., Etches, P. C., Pain, K. S. & Robertson, C. M. T. (1995). Province-based study of neurologic disability of children weighing 500 through 1249 grams at birth in relation to neonatal cerebral ultrasound findings. *Pediatrics*, **95**, 837–44.

Azzarelli, B., Caldemeyer, K. S., Phillips, J. P. & DeMyer, W. E. (1996). Hypoxic–ischemic enceph-alopathy in areas of primary myelination: a neuroimaging and PET study. *Pediatric Neurology*, **14**, 108–16.

Baarsma, R., Laurini, R. N., Aerts, W. & Okken, A. (1987). Reliability of sonography in non-hemorrhagic periventricular leukomalacia. *Pediatric Radiology*, **17**, 189–91.

Babcock, D. S. & Ball, W. S. J. (1983). Postasphyxial encephalopathy in full term infants: ultra-sound diagnosis. *Radiology*, **148**, 417–23.

Barkovich, A. J. (1992). MR and CT evaluation of profound neonatal and infantile asphyxia. *American Journal of Neuroradiology*, **13**, 959–72.

Barkovich, A. J. (1995). Normal development of the neonatal and infant brain, skull and spine. In *Pediatric Neuroimaging*, 2nd edn, ed. A. J. Barkovich, pp. 9–54. New York: Raven Press.

Barkovich, A. J. (1998). MR of the normal neonatal brain: assessment of deep structures. *American Journal of Neuroradiology*, **19**, 1397–403.

Barkovich, A.J. (2000). Infections of the nervous system. In *Pediatric Neuroimaging*, 3rd edn, ed. A. J. Barkovitch, pp. 715–70. Philadelphia: Lippincott Williams & Wilkins.

Barkovich, A. J. & Hallam, D. (1997). Neuroimaging in perinatal hypoxic–ischemic injury. *MRDD Research Reviews*, **3**, 28–41.

Barkovich, A. J. & Linden, C. L. (1994). Congenital cytomegalovirus infection of the brain: imaging analysis and embryologic considerations. *American Journal of Neuroradiology*, **15**, 703–15.

Barkovich, A. J. & Truwit, C. L. (1990). *American Journal of Neuroradiology*, **11**, 1087–96.

Barkovich, A. J. & Sargent, S. K. (1995). Profound asphyxia in the preterm infant: imaging find-ings. *American Journal of Neuroradiology*, **16**, 1837–46.

Barkovich, A. J., Kjos, B. O., Jackson, D. E. Jr. & Norman, D. (1988). Normal maturation of the neonatal and infant brain: MR imaging at 1.5T. *Radiology*, **166**, 173–80.

Barkovich, A. J., Westmark, K. D., Ferriero, D. M., Sola, A. & Partridge, J. C. (1995). Perinatal asphyxia: MR findings in the first 10 days. *American Journal of Neuroradiology*, **16**, 427–38.

Barkovich, A. J., Al Ali, F., Rowley, H. A. & Bass, N. (1998). Imaging patterns of neonatal hypo-glycemia. *American Journal of Neuroradiology*, **19**, 1397–403.

Battin, M. R., Maalouf, E. F., Counsell, S. J. et al. (1998). Magnetic resonance imaging of the brain in very preterm infants: visualization of the germina matrix, early myelination and cortical folding. *Pediatrics*, **101**, 957–62.

Childs, A. M., Ramenghi, L. A., Evans, D. J. et al. (1998). MR features of developing periventric-ular white matter in preterm infants: evidence of glial cell migration. *American Journal of Neuroradiology*, **19**, 971–6.

Chiras, J., Dubs, M. & Bories, J. (1985). Venous infarctions. *Neuroradiology*, **27**, 593–600.

Chugani, H. T., Phelps, M. E. & Mazziotta, J. C. (1987). Positron emission tomography study of human brain functional development. *Annals of Neurology*, **22**, 487–97.

Claris, O., Besnier, S., Lapillonne, A., Picaud, J. C. & Salle, B. L. (1996). Incidence of ischemic–hemorrhagic cerebral lesions in premature infants of gestational age ≤28 weeks: a prospective ultrasound study. *Biology of the Neonate*, **70**, 29–34.

Cohen, M. & Roessmann, U. (1994). In utero brain damage: relationship of gestational age to pathological consequences. *Developmental Medicine and Child Neurology*, **36**, 263–71.

Connolly, B., Kelehan, P., O'Brien, N. et al. (1994). The echogenic thalamus in hypoxic ischaemic encephalopathy. *Pediatric Radiology*, **24**, 268–71.

Cornblath, M. & Schwartz, P. (1991). *Disorders of Carbohydrate Metabolism in Infancy*, 3rd edn. Boston, MA: Blackwell Scientific.

Cowan, F. M., Pennock, J. M., Hanrahan, J. D., Manji, K. P. & Edwards, E. D. (1994). Early detection of cerebral infarction and hypoxic ischemic encephalopathy in neonates using diffusion weighted magnetic resonance imaging. *Neuropediatrics*, **25**, 172–5.

Dammann, O. & Leviton, A. (1997). Duration of transient hyperechoic images of white matter in very-low-birthweight infants: a proposed classification. *Developmental Medicine and Child Neurology*, **39**, 2–5.

Desmonts, G. & Couvreur, J. (1974). Congenital toxoplasmosis. *New England Journal of Medicine*, **290**, 1110–12.

De Vries, L. S., Eken, P. & Dubowitz, L. M. S. (1992). The spectrum of leukomalacia using cranial ultrasound. *Behavioral Brain Research*, **49**, 1–6.

Diebler, C., Dusser, A. & Dulac, O. (1985). Congenital toxoplasmosis: clinical and neuroradiological evaluation of the cerebral lesions. *Neuroradiology*, **27**, 125–30.

Di Pietro, M. A., Brody, B. A. & Teele, R. L. (1986). Periventricular echogenic 'blush' on cranial sonography: pathologic correlates. *American Journal of Neuroradiology*, **7**, 305–10.

Dobbins, J. G., Stewart, J. A. & Demmier, G. J. (1992). Surveillance of congenital cytomegalovirus disease, 1990–91. *Collaborating Registry Group. MMWR CDC Surveillance Summaries*, **41**(2), 35–9.

Dunn, D. W., Daum, R. S., Weisberg, L. & Vargas, R. (1982). Ischemic cerebrovascular complications of haemophilus influenza meningitis. *Archives of Neurology*, **39**, 650–2.

Eichenwald, H.F. (1956). *Human Toxoplasmosis.* Baltimore: Williams & Wilkins, pp. 226.

Flodmark, O., Roland, E. H., Hill, A. & Whitfield, W. F. (1987). Perventricular leukomalacia: radiologic diagnosis. *Radiology*, **162**, 119–24.

Flodmark, O., Lupton, B., Li, D., Stimac, G. K., Roland, E. H., Hill, A., Whitfield, M. F. & Norman, M. G. (1989). Magnetic resonance imaging of periventricular leukomalacia (PVL) in childhood. *American Journal of Neuroradiology*, **10**, 111–8.

Friede, R. L. (1989). *Developmental Neuropathology*, 2nd edn. Berlin: Springer-Verlag.

Fukumizu, M., Takashima, S. & Becker, L. E. (1995). Neonatal posthemorrhagic hydrocephalus: neuropathologic and immunohistochemical studies. *Pediatric Neurology*, **13**, 230–4.

Girard, N., Raybaud, C. & Poncet, M. (1995). In vivo MR study of brain maturation in normal fetuses. *American Journal of Neuroradiology*, **16**, 407–13.

Grant, E. G., Schellinger, D., Richardson, J. D., Coffey, M. L. & Smirniotopoulous, J. G. (1983).

Echogenic periventricular halo: normal sonographic finding in neonatal cerebral hemorrhage? *American Journal of Neuroradiology*, **4**, 43–6.

Greisen, G. (1992). Ischemia of the preterm brain. *Biology of the Neonate*, **62**, 243–7.

Griffiths, A. & Laurence, K. (1974). The effect of hypoxia and hypoglycaemia of the brain in the newborn human infant. *Developmental Medicine and Child Neurology*, **16**, 308–19.

Hambleton, G. & Wigglesworth, J. S. (1976). Origin of intraventricular haemorrhage in the preterm infant. *Archives of Disease in Childhood*, **51**, 651–60.

Hasegawa, M., Houdou, S., Mito, T., Takashima, S., Asanuma, K. & Ohno, T. (1992). Development of myelination in the human fetal and infant cerebrum: a myelin basic protein immunohistochemical study. *Brain and Development*, **14**, 1–6.

Hittmair, K., Kramer, J., Rand, T., Bernert, G. & Wimberger, D. (1996). Infratentorial brain maturation: a comparison of MRI at 0.5 and 1.5T. *Neuroradiology*, **38**, 360–6.

Hughes, P., Weinberger, E. & Shaw, D. W. (1991). Linear areas of echogenicity in the thalami and basal ganglia of neonates: an expanded association. *Radiology*, **179**, 103–5.

Ishikawa, A., Murayama, T. & Sakuma, N. (1982). Computed cranial tomography in congenital rubella syndrome. *Archives of Neurology*, **39**, 420–2.

Keeney, S., Adcock, E. W. & McArdle, C. B. (1991). Prospective observations of 100 high-risk neonates by high field (1.5 Tesla) magnetic resonance imaging of the central nervous system: II, lesions associated with hypoxic–ischemic encephalopathy. *Pediatrics*, **87**, 431–8.

Kinnala, A., Suhonen Pollvi, H., Aarimaa, T. et al. (1996). Cerebral metabolic rate for glucose during the first six months of life: an FDG positron emission tomography study. *Archives of Disease in Childhood. Fetal and Neonatal Edition*, **74**, F153–7.

Kreis, R., Ernst, T. & Ross, B. D. (1993). Development of the human brain: in vivo quantification of metabolite and water content with proton magnetic resonance spectroscopy. *Magnetic Resonance Medicine*, **30**, 424–37.

Krägeloh-Mann, I., Hagberg, G., Meisner, C. et al. (1995). Bilateral spastic cerebral palsy – a collaborative study between South West Germany and Western Sweden III: Aetiology. *Developmental Medicine and Child Neurology*, **37**, 191–203.

Kuenzle, C., Baenziger, O., Martin, E. et al. (1994). Prognostic value of early MR imaging in term infants with severe perinatal asphyxia. *Neuropediatrics*, **25**, 191–200.

Levine, D., & Barnes, P. D. (1999). Cortical maturation in normal and abnormal fetuses as assessed with prenatal MR imaging. *Radiology*, **210**, 751–8.

Martin, E., Krassnitzer, S., Kaelin, P. & Boesch, C. (1991). MR imaging of the brainstem: normal postnatal development. *Neuroradiology*, **33**, 391–5.

Mathews, V. P., Kuharik, M. A., Edwards, M. K. et al. (1988). Gd-DTPA enhanced MR imaging of experimental bacterial meningitis: evaluation and comparison with CT. *American Journal of Neuroradiology*, **9**, 1045–50.

Merrill, J. D., Piecuch, R. E., Fell, S. C., Barkovich, A. J. & Goldstein, R. B. (1998). A new pattern of cerebellar haemorrhages in preterm infants. *Pediatrics*, **102**(6), p62.

Miller, E., Craddock-Watson, J. E. & Pollock, T. M. (1982). Consequences of confirmed maternal rubella at successive stages of pregnancy. *Lancet*, **ii**, 781–2.

Naidich, T. P., McLone, D. G. & Yamanouchi, Y. (1983). Periventricular white matter cysts in a murine mode of gram-negative ventriculitis. *American Journal of Neuroradiology*, **4**, 461–5.

Noorbehesht, B., Enzmann, D. R., Sullinder, W., Bradley, J. S. & Arvin, A. M. (1987). Neonatal herpes simplex encephalitis: correlation of clinical and CT findings. *Radiology*, **162**, 813–9.

Olsén, P., Vainiopää, L., Pääkkö, K., Korkman, M., Pyhtinen, J. & Järvelin, M. R. (1998). Psychological findings in preterm children related to neurologic status and magnetic resonance imaging. *Pediatrics*, **102**, 329–36.

Papile L. A., Burstein, J., Burstein, R. et al. (1978). Incidence and evolution of subependymal and intraventricular hemorrhage: a study of infants with birth weight less than 1500 gm. *Journal of Pediatrics*, **92**, 529–35.

Parisi, J. E., Collins, G. H., Kim, R. C. & Crossley, C. J. (1983). Prenatal symmetrical thalamic degeneration with flexion spasticity at birth. *Annals of Neurology*, **13**, 94–6.

Pasternak, J. F. & Gorey, M. T. (1998). The syndrome of acute near total intrauterine asphyxia in the term infant. *Pediatric Neurology*, **18**, 391–8.

Pasternak, J. F., Predley, T. A. & Mikhael, M. A. (1991). Neonatal asphyxia: vulnerability of basal ganglia, thalamus and brainstem. *Pediatric Neurology*, **7**, 147–9.

Phillips, R., Brandenberg, G., Hill, A., Roland, E. & Poskitt, K. (1993). Prevalence and prognostic value of abnormal CT findings in 100 term asphyxiated newborns. *Radiology*, **189P**, 287.

Pikus, H. J., Levy, M. L., Gans, W., Mendel, E. & McComb, J. G. (1997). Outcome, cost analysis and long-term follow-up in preterm infants with massive grade IV germinal matrix hemorrhage and progressive hydrocephalus. *Neurosurgery*, **40**, 983–9

Preblud, S. E. & Alford, C. A. (1990). In *Infectious Diseases of the Fetus and Neonate*, ed. J. S. Remington & J. O. Klein, pp. 155–64. Philadelphia: Saunders Co.

Rao, K. C. V. G., Knipp, H. C. & Wagner, E. J. (1981). The findings in cerebral sinus and venous thrombosis. *Radiology*, **140**, 391–8.

Raybaud, C., Girard, N., Svely, A. & Leboucq., N. (1996). Neuroradiologie pediatrique (1). In *Radiodiagnostic Neuroradiologie-Appariel locomoteur*, ed. C. Raybaud, N. Girard, A. Svely & N. Leboucq, p. 26. Paris: Elsevier.

Ringelberg, J. & van de Bor, M. (1993). Outcome of transient periventricular echodensities in preterm infants. *Neuropediatrics*, **24**, 269–73.

Robertson, J. S. (1962). Toxoplasmosis. *Developmental Medicine and Child Neurology*, **4**, 507–12.

Roland E. H., Hill, A., Norman, M. G., Flodmark, O. & MacNab, A. J. (1988). Selective brainstem injury in asphyxiated newborn. *Annals of Neurology*, **23**, 89–92.

Roland, E. H., Poskitt, K., Rodriguez, E., Lupton, B. A. & Hill, A. (1998). Perinatal hypoxic–ischemic thalamic injury: clinical features and neuroimaging. *Annals of Neurology*, **44**, 161–6.

Rutherford, M. A., Pennock, J. M. & Dubowitz, L. M. S. (1994). Cranial ultrasound and magnetic resonance imaging in hypoxic ischemic encephalopathy: a comparison with outcome. *Developmental Medicine and Child Neurology*, **36**, 813–25.

Schultz, P. & Leeds, N. E. (1973). Intraventricular septations complicating neonatal meningitis. *Journal of Neurosurgery*, **38**, 620–6.

Shuman, R. M. & Seludnik, L. J. (1980). Periventricular leukomalacia: a one year autopsy study. *Archives in Neurology*, **37**, 231–5.

Sie, L. T. L., van der Knaap, M. S., van Wezel-Meijler, G. & Valk, J. (1997). MRI assessment of myelination of motor and sensory pathways in the brain of preterm and term-born infants. *Neuropediatrics*, **28**, 97–105.

Siebert, J. J., Avva, R., Hronas, T. N. et al. (1998). Use of power Doppler in pediatric neurosonography: a pictorial essay. *Radiographics*, **18**, 879–90.

Siegel, M., Shackelford, G., Perlman, J. & Fulling, K. (1984). Hypoxic–ischemic encephalopathy in term infants: diagnosis and prognosis evaluated by ultrasound. *Radiology*, **152**, 395–9.

Snyder, R. D. (1992). Bacterial infections of the nervous system. In *Neurological Aspects of Pediatrics*, ed. B. O. Berg, pp. 195–226. Boston: Butterworth-Heinemann.

Spar, J. A., Lewine, J. D. & Orrison, W. W. Jr (1994). Neonatal hypoglycaemia: CT and MR findings. *Americal Journal of Neuroradiology*, **15**, 1477–8.

Stark, J. E. & Siebert, J. J. (1994). Cerebral artery Doppler ultrasonography for prediction of outcome after perinatal asphyxia. *Journal of Ultrasound in Medicine*, **13**, 595–600.

Steinlin, M., Dirr, R., Martin, E. et al. (1991). MRI following severe perinatal asphyxia: preliminary experience. *Pediatric Neurology*, **7**, 164–70.

Sudakoff, G. S., Mitchell, D. G., Stanley, C. & Graziani, L. J. (1991). Frontal periventricular cysts in the first day of life: a one year clinical follow-up and its significance. *Journal of Ultrasound in Medicine*, **10**, 25–30.

Taylor, G. A. (1995). Effect of germinal matrix hemorrhage on the terminal vein position and patency. *Pediatric Radiology*, **25**, 37–40.

Teele, R., Hernanz-Schulman, M. & Sotrel, A. (1988). Echogenic vasculature in the basal ganglia of neonates: a sonographic sign of vasculopathy. *Radiology*, **169**, 423–7.

Tokumaru, A. M., Barkovich, A. J., O'uchi, T., Matsuo, T. & Kusano, S. (1999). The evolution of cerebral blood flow in the developing brain: evaluation with Iodine-123 Iodoamphetamine SPECT and MR imaging correlation. *American Journal of Neuroradiology*, **20**, 845–52.

Van de Bor, M., Ens-Dokkum, M., Schreuder, A. M., Veen, S., Brand, R. & Verloove-Vanhorick, S. P. (1993). Outcome of periventricular–intraventricular haemorrhage at five years of age. *Developmental Medicine and Child Neurology*, **35**, 33–41.

Van der Knaap, M. S., Valk, J., de Neeling, N. & Nauta, J. J. P. (1991). Pattern recognition in MRI of white matter disorders in children and young adults. *Neuroradiology*, **33**, 478–93.

Vannucci, R. C., Nardis, E. E., Vannucci, S. J. & Campbell, P. A. (1981). Cerebral carbohydrate and energy metabolism during hypoglycemia in newborn dogs. *American Journal of Physiology*, **240**, 192–8.

Vannucci, R. C., Christensen, M. A. & Yager, J. Y. (1993). Nature, time-course, and extent of cerebral edema in perinatal hypoxic–ischemic brain damage. *Pediatric Neurology*, **9**, 29–34.

Van Wezel-Meijler, G., van der Knaap, M. S., Sie, L. T. L. et al. (1998). Magnetic resonance imaging of the brain in premature infants during the neonatal period. *Neuropediatrics*, **29**, 89–96.

Virapongse, C., Cazenave, C., Quisling, R., Sarwar, M. & Hunter, S. (1987). The empty delta sign: frequency and significance in 76 cases of dural sinus thrombosis. *Radiology*, **162**, 779–85.

Volpe, J. J. (1995a). Intracranial infections. In *Neurology of the Newborn*, 3rd edn, pp. 675–766. Philadelphia: Saunders Co.

Volpe, J. J. (1995b). Hypoxic–ishemic encephalopathy: neuropathology and pathogenesis. In *Neurology of the Newborn*, 3rd edn, pp. 279–313. Philadelphia: Saunders Co.

Volpe, J. J. (1995c). Intracranial hemorrhage: germinal matrix – intraventricular hemorrhage of the premature infant. In *Neurology of the Newborn*, 3rd edn, pp. 403–9. Philadelphia: Saunders Co.

Volpe, J. J. (1995d). Hypoglycaemia and brain injury. In *Neurology of the Newborn*, 3rd edn, pp. 467–86. Philadelphia: Saunders Co.

Volpe, J. J. (1995e). Bilirubin and brain injury. In *Neurology of the Newborn*, 3rd edn, pp. 490–514. Philadelphia: Saunders Co.

Whitley, R. J. & Hutto, C. (1985). Neonatal herpes simplex virus infections. *Pediatric Reviews*, 7, 119–26.

Wigglesworth, J. S. & Pope, K. E. (1978). An integrated model for haemorrhage and ischaemic lesions in the newborn brain. *Early Human Development*, 2, 1719–99.

Yamashita, Y., Matsuishi, T., Murakami, Y. et al. (1991). Neuroimaging findings (ultrasonography, CT, MRI) in 3 infants with congenital rubella syndrome. *Pediatric Radiology*, 21, 547–9.

Yow, M. D. (1989). Congenital cytomegalovirus disease: a now problem. *Journal of Infectious Diseases*, 159, 163–7.

15

Non-invasive techniques to investigate the newborn brain

John S. Wyatt

Department of Paediatrics, Royal Free and University College Medical School, London, UK

Introduction

Advances in technology and bioengineering have raised the prospect of being able to obtain detailed quantitative functional information from the human newborn brain without the use of ionising radiation or invasive procedures. The potential of this approach is obvious, although progress over the last decade has been frustratingly slow – technical promise has not always converted readily into practical value in clinical neonatal practice. This chapter will discuss the application of non-invasive techniques to the newborn brain, with particular attention to magnetic resonance spectroscopy and near infrared spectroscopy.

Potential of non-invasive techniques

Perinatal brain injury, frequently leading to death or permanent disability, is possibly the major unsolved problem of clinical neonatology. Non-invasive techniques have the potential to play a critical role in the introduction of novel clinical strategies to minimize the incidence and severity of this form of brain damage.

First, by obtaining measurements from the brain both before and during birth and in the critical first days of life, non-invasive techniques may allow the pathophysiological mechanisms underlying ischemic and hemorrhagic brain injury to be unravelled. If quantitative and reproducible data can be obtained from human infants, then both longitudinal and cross-sectional studies of babies at risk of injury are feasible. Secondly, these techniques offer the potential of early detection of injury, enabling those infants to be identified who may benefit from new neural rescue treatments. Thirdly, these techniques may allow continuous or intermittent surveillance of cerebral perfusion and oxidative metabolism in critically ill infants undergoing intensive care. This approach, sometimes described as 'brain-orientated intensive care', offers the theoretical potential for manipulating ventilator therapy and pharmacological interventions, in order to optimize cerebral perfusion and oxygen delivery throughout the period of intensive hospital care.

Fourthly, following intensive treatment in the neonatal period, non-invasive techniques may provide early outcome markers, so that the efficacy of different treatments may be compared at an early stage. In this chapter the main focus will be on neonatal data obtained by the two techniques of magnetic resonance spectroscopy and near infrared spectroscopy. For reasons of space, a comprehensive review of these rapidly developing techniques is not possible and only selective references can be quoted.

Magnetic resonance spectroscopy

Magnetic resonance spectroscopy (MRS) has the unique potential of allowing the oxidative metabolic processes of the living cell to be interrogated without direct interference or manipulation. The technique depends on the magnetic properties of certain nuclei (including protons (^{1}H), phosphorus (^{31}P), carbon (^{13}C), fluorine (^{19}F) and sodium (^{23}Na)). When placed within a constant magnetic field, the resonant frequencies of the nuclei depend upon their precise chemical environment. By comparing the signal intensity obtained from nuclei in different chemical compounds, the relative abundance of various biologically important compounds can be determined in vivo. In particular, ^{31}P MRS allows the detection of intracellular nucleotide triphosphate (mainly adenosine triphosphate (ATP)), phosphocreatine (PCr), inorganic phosphate (Pi), phosphodiesters and phosphomonoesters. In addition, the intracellular pH can be derived from the chemical shift of the Pi peak. ^{1}H spectroscopy enables the detection of lactate (Lac), N-acetyl aspartate (Naa), choline and creatine-containing compounds and a range of other compounds including glutamate, glutamine and other neurotransmitters.

The clinical role of MRS is limited by the complexity of the apparatus and the need for physical isolation because of intense magnetic fields. In order to study sick newborn infants in safety, it is generally necessary to employ a specialized non-ferromagnetic transport incubator equipped with facilities for maintaining intensive support and physiological monitoring. The incubator is inserted into the bore of the spectrometer, and intensive monitoring must be maintained throughout the procedure. The head rests on or within a radiofrequency coil which transmits and receives signals from the interrogated tissue.

The earliest ^{31}P MRS studies employed surface coils which received signals from a large and ill-defined area of temporoparietal cortex and subcortical white matter. Normal developmental changes have been demonstrated in phosphorus metabolite ratios (e.g. Azzopardi et al., 1989a; Boesch et al., 1989; Buchli et al., 1994) with an increase in the ratio of PCr/Pi and of the phosphodiester signal in healthy newborns with increasing gestational age. A corresponding decline in the signal from phosphomonoesters also occurs with increasing maturity. Studies using localized

^{1}H MRS, in which spectra are obtained from precisely defined anatomical volumes, provide more detailed regional information (e.g. Van der Knapp et al., 1990; Huppi et al., 1991; Penrice et al., 1996). Naa has been detected in the fetal brain at 16 weeks gestation and the Naa ratio rises with gestational age from 24 weeks to term and further during the first year of life. Naa occurs mainly in neurones (although it is also present in oligodendrocyte progenitor cells), and it seems likely that the rise in concentration largely reflects neuronal development.

Most MRS studies have employed concentration ratios but recently absolute quantification (in mmol/kg) of both phosphorus and proton metabolites has become possible. Either external reference solutions are used or brain water may be utilized as an internal concentration reference (e.g. Cady et al., 1996a,b). In a group of normal infants, the concentrations of choline, creatine and Naa were consistently higher in the thalamic region, which consisted mainly of grey matter, compared with a voxel centred on the occipito-parietal region which consisted mainly of unmyelinated white matter. Lactate concentrations were similar in the two regions, but were elevated in the preterm brain compared with term infants and older subjects (Cady et al., 1996a). These data are consistent with a range of other findings suggesting that the immature brain may depend more on glycolytic rather than oxidative ATP production (e.g. Altman et al., 1993).

MRS in perinatal asphyxia

^{31}P MRS studies of newborn infants with acute early onset encephalopathy and a clinical history suggestive of intrapartum asphyxia have shown a consistent pattern of acute derangement of oxidative metabolism (Younkin et al., 1984; Azzopardi et al., 1989b; Laptook et al., 1989). Spectra are frequently normal within the first hours following resuscitation, but after 12–24 hours a progressive decline in the PCr/Pi ratio is observed (Wyatt et al., 1989; Roth et al., 1992). In the most severely affected infants, a delayed decline in ATP signal can also be detected. The maximum energetic derangements are generally seen at 48–72 hours. This phenomenon, which has been termed 'secondary' or delayed energy failure, is observed despite the maintenance of systemic circulatory and metabolic homeostasis. Studies using ^{1}H MRS in asphyxiated infants have demonstrated an associated rise in cerebral lactate concentrations (Peden et al., 1993; Groenendaal et al., 1994; Penrice et al., 1996), and a correlation between the rise in cerebral lactate within the first 18 hours and the subsequent fall in PCr/Pi ratio has been documented (Hanrahan et al., 1996). In severely affected infants, cerebral lactate elevation persisted and became more marked after 24 hours, despite the presence of normal blood lactate concentrations, suggesting that anerobic glycolysis was occurring within the brain simultaneously with the delayed derangement in oxidative phosphorylation (Penrice et al., 1996).

In addition, lactate elevation was much more marked within the thalamic region compared with the occipito-parietal white matter (Penrice et al., 1996). It is of interest that, despite the marked elevation of cerebral lactate, intracellular pH during secondary energy failure has been found to remain within normal limits or even to show a slight alkalotic shift.

Preliminary data providing concentrations of ^{1}H and ^{31}P metabolites in severely asphyxiated infants have become available (Martin et al., 1996; Cady et al., 1996a,b). The results are broadly consistent with studies employing metabolite ratios. In one study, measurements from the thalamic region demonstrated an elevated lactate concentration of median 5.4 mmol/kg (compared with 2.8 mmol/kg in control infants), and a reduced Naa of 5.2 mmol/kg (compared with 10.3 mmol/kg). Phosphocreatine, ATP and total phosphorus concentrations in the asphyxiated infants were markedly reduced compared with control infants whereas inorganic phosphate was elevated.

In asphyxiated infants studied somewhat later (1–3 weeks) after delivery, a significant decline in Naa has been observed (Peden et al., 1993, Groenendaal et al., 1994). As Naa is thought to be present primarily within the neuronal cytoplasm, this late decline may provide a quantitative measure of permanent neuronal loss following asphyxia.

Prognosis in perinatal asphyxia

The detection of secondary energy failure has important prognostic implications. Follow-up studies of encephalopathic infants have demonstrated a close relationship between minimum PCr/Pi and adverse neurodevelopmental outcome and reduced head growth (Azzopardi et al., 1989b; Roth et al., 1992, 1997; Martin et al., 1996). Similarly elevation of lactate/creatine or lactate/Naa ratios is associated with a poor prognosis (Peden et al., 1993; Groenendaal et al., 1994; Penrice et al., 1996). These studies provide convincing evidence that the development of secondary energy failure is associated with brain cell death, leading to permanent neurological and developmental sequelae.

The complex temporal sequence of metabolic and pathophysiological changes following perinatal asphyxia has been reproduced in a neonatal piglet model which employed continuous ^{31}P and ^{1}H spectroscopy maintained over a period of more than 48 hours (Lorek et al., 1994). During transient cerebral hypoxia–ischemia, acute 'primary' depletion of cerebral PCr and ATP occurred within 60–120 minutes. Phosphorus metabolites returned rapidly to normal following reperfusion and reoxygenation of the brain. After a few hours, a progressive secondary fall in PCr/Pi and in ATP was observed. Cerebral lactate levels demonstrated a similar biphasic pattern with rapid elevation during the acute hypoxic–ischemic episode, recovery within 1–2 hours of resuscitation, followed by progressive elevation during the phase of delayed energy failure (Penrice et al., 1997). Metabolite spin–spin relaxation times (T_2 values) were markedly elevated during delayed energy failure. This may reflect neuronal swelling and increased cytoplasmic water following failure of the ATP-dependent sodium/potassium pump.

A fundamental limitation in both ^{1}H and ^{31}P MRS is low spatial resolution. It is necessary to collect signals from a substantial volume of tissue if the signal-to-noise ratio is to be acceptable. ^{1}H MRS chemical shift imaging has the potential to display spectra which have been collected simultaneously from multiple areas within the tissue of interest. If this technique can be successfully applied to the neonatal brain following perinatal asphyxia, there is likely to be a substantial improvement in the spatial localization of metabolic derangement. The technical problems are substantial and, to date, no neonatal data have been published.

Use of diffusion-weighted imaging to assess cerebral energetics

An alternative approach to provide improved spatial resolution of disturbances in cerebral energetics is to employ diffusion-weighted MRI. Several studies have documented an acute reduction in the apparent diffusion coefficient (ADC) of water, which occurs within minutes following the onset of cerebral ischemia (e.g. Busza et al., 1992). The physical mechanisms underlying this reduction in water diffusion are not fully understood, although there is evidence that it reflects, at least in part, the microscopic redistribution of tissue water from the extracellular to the intracellular compartment. A very close correlation between a fall in ADC and reductions in the ATP concentration reflecting the phosphorylation potential of the tissue has been demonstrated. As a result a two-dimensional map of ADC values may provide information about disturbances in cerebral energetics with a much higher spatial resolution (1 mm or less) than is possible with conventional localized spectroscopy.

Measurements of ADC values during the development of secondary energy failure in the piglet model have shown a progressive decrease, which mirrors the decline in ATP and PCr. Of particular interest is the observation that highly localized ADC abnormalities were observed initially in either the parasagittal cortex or the thalamic region before spreading throughout the cerebral hemispheres over the succeeding 24–48 hours (Thornton et al., 1996). These observations demonstrate the power of magnetic resonance techniques to provide novel insights into the temporal and spatial evolution of cellular injury following an acute hypoxic–ischemic insult.

MRS in other forms of brain injury

Although most studies employing MRS in the neonatal brain have been carried out in asphyxiated infants, changes indicating energy failure and tissue loss have also been observed in other pathological conditions. A progressive rise in cerebral lactate and fall in Naa has been observed in the shaken baby syndrome (Haseler et al., 1997) and a reduction in Naa has been detected in preterm infants with cystic leukomalacia (Groenendaal et al., 1997). Infants with an adverse neurodevelopmental outcome had the lowest Naa/Choline values. In another study of neonates and infants with a range of central nervous system disorders ^{1}H MRS provided valuable prediction of neurodevelopmental outcome (Holshouser et al., 1997).

In summary, localized and quantitative spectroscopy has the potential to provide detailed early assessment of the infant at risk of perinatal brain injury (Novotny et al., 1998). These methods may allow the anatomical localization and the severity of permanent cellular injury to be identified within the first few days of life. Reductions in Naa may provide a quantitative index of neuronal loss. Similarly, increases in Naa T_2 may indicate edema and impaired membrane ATPase activity in injured neurons which have not yet undergone autolysis. ^{1}H chemical shift imaging or the measurement of ADC values may provide early detailed definition of the anatomical pattern of injury. It seems likely that a combination of these measurements will lead to marked improvements in the accuracy of early predictions of long-term neurological impairments or death.

MRS in neurometabolic disorders

MRS may also have a unique role in the investigation and management of a number of congenital neurometabolic disorders. Elevated cerebral lactate has been observed in a variety of congenital mitochondrial disorders (Cross et al., 1993). ^{1}H spectra obtained from the basal ganglia of newborn patients, who were encephalopathic as a result of propionic acidemia, showed marked abnormalities, with a decrease in Naa and an elevation of glutamate/glutamine. ^{31}P MRS has demonstrated a marked reduction of high energy phosphates in a newborn infant with isovaleric acidemia, and it is particularly interesting that the cerebral energetic derangement reversed following therapeutic intervention (Lorek et al., 1996). Although limited data have as yet been published, there is little doubt that MRS has a unique role in assessing the functional impact of neurometabolic disorders and monitoring the response to therapy (Novotny et al., 1998).

Finally, MRS may play a crucial role in the investigation of moderate hypothermia as a neuroprotective intervention. Although clinical trials of brain cooling have recently commenced, a major unsolved problem is the measurement of deep brain temperature in infants undergoing different forms of intervention. ^{1}H MRS has the potential to provide valuable information in this situation as local brain temperature can be measured in anatomically defined regions, using the temperature-dependent chemical shift of water spin–spin relaxation times (Cady et al., 1995b).

Because of its complexity and expense, MRS is confined to a few research centres at present. ^{31}P MRS is likely to remain of research interest only because of the extreme technical demands. Similarly, MRS employing other nuclei like ^{13}C or ^{23}Na is unlikely to be of clinical significance in the forseeable future. On the other hand, ^{1}H MRS may be performed on commercial MR imaging systems with relatively minor software modifications, and has the potential to be more widely utilized. A major problem is the lack of standardized normal data from infants of different gestational and postnatal ages. Differences in the precise sequences and techniques employed lead to marked variations in spectral characteristics, and standardized approaches to the collection of clinical data are urgently required.

Near infrared spectroscopy

Near infrared spectroscopy (NIRS) can be regarded as a complementary technique to MRS. By supplying information on cerebral oxyhemoglobin delivery, oxygen extraction and cytochrome oxidase redox level, it has the potential to provide insights into cerebral oxidative metabolism and intracellular oxygen availability at the bedside.

Principles of NIR spectroscopy

NIRS depends on the property of light in the near infrared region (700–1000 nm) to penetrate biological tissue for distances of up to 7 or 8 cm. As the light passes through the head, it is attenuated due to a combination of absorption and scattering. The only NIR absorbers (chromophores) which are present in variable concentrations are oxy- and deoxyhemoglobin, (HbO_2 and Hb) and the oxidized form of the copper A moiety of cytochrome oxidase (Cu_A), the terminal member of the mitochondrial respiratory chain. Although other chromophores are known to be present within biological tissue (water, bilirubin, etc.), it is assumed that their concentration is constant during the period of optical transillumination.

In many respects the neonatal brain is an ideal organ for study by NIRS. This is because optical access and penetration is facilitated by the thinness of the skull and extracranial tissues and by the optical properties of the immature brain itself. During continuous transillumination of the brain, changes in optical attenuation may be converted into changes in the concentration of one or more of the chromophores using a modification of the Lambert–Beer law. As there are three variable chromophores within brain tissue (HbO_2, Hb, Cu_A), it is necessary to make measurements at a minimum of three different wavelengths.

Optical path length estimation

Quantification of NIRS measurements requires knowledge of the average path length of the photons traversing the tissue. Because of multiple scattering, this path length is considerably longer than the distance between the sites of light entry and exit. A number of optical techniques are now becoming available to allow this important variable to be measured in the newborn brain. The first technique involves the use of a pulsed laser and high-speed detector to measure the 'time of flight' of an ultrashort pulse of infrared light as it traverses the head. As the speed of light is known, it is possible to obtain the mean optical pathlength. In postmortem studies of infants, time of flight measurements have given mean values for optical path length of approximately four to five times the distance between the optical fibres (the differential path length factor) (van der Zee et al., 1991). This factor has been found to be relatively constant, provided that the distance between the transmitting and receiving fibres is greater than 2.5 cm. Because of the size and complexity of the equipment required to make time of flight measurements, this technique cannot, as yet, be employed within a neonatal intensive care unit. However, the optical pathlength can be estimated in any individual by measuring the distance between the transmitting and receiving optical fibres and multiplying this distance by a mean value for the differential path length factor.

Secondly, it is possible to use the infrared absorption of water molecules in the brain to obtain the optical path length. As the concentration of water within brain tissue is known to a reasonable degree of accuracy, it can be employed as a calibration compound and hence provide the optical path length in each baby (Cooper et al., 1996). To use this method, it is necessary to employ light at a wide range of infrared wavelengths in order to detect the water absorption peak. Preliminary data in a range of newborn infants have been obtained. This technique has the advantage that continuous path length measurements can be obtained at the cot-side.

Thirdly, if the transmitted infrared light is modulated by a very high frequency signal, the phase shift between the transmitted and received light can be measured in order to obtain both the optical path length and concentration information simultaneously (Duncan et al., 1996). Prototype instruments are now becoming available to enable these measurements to be obtained at the cot-side. Preliminary results using these new techniques suggest that there is a significant variation in optical path length between different individuals. It is therefore likely that, in the future, it will be necessary to use techniques that allow the direct determination of optical path length at the cot-side, if a high level of quantitative accuracy is required.

Several groups have reported results from studies using NIRS in newborn infants undergoing intensive care. Relative changes in $[HbO_2]$, $[Hb]$ and $[Cu_A]$ have been observed with crying, episodes of apnoea and bradycardia, and nursing procedures including endotracheal suctioning (Brazy, 1988; Livera et al., 1991; Shah et al., 1992). Spontaneous fluctuations in arterial blood pressure have been associated with changes in CBV and $[Cu_A]$ (Tsuji et al., 1998).

Quantification of hemodynamic variables

Methods have been developed for the quantification of a range of hemodynamic variables, including cerebral blood flow (CBF), cerebral blood volume (CBV) and its response to changing arterial carbon dioxide tension, mixed cerebral venous saturation and cerebral oxygen extraction.

Cerebral blood flow

Global cerebral blood flow (CBF) may be obtained by employing a version of the Fick principle which employs oxyhemoglobin as an endogenous intravascular tracer molecule (Elwell et al., 1992; Edwards et al., 1993). A rapid transient increase in the arterial saturation is induced by manipulation of the inspired oxygen concentration. Global CBF in ml $100g^{-1}$ min^{-1} is then obtained from the rise in cerebral $[HbO_2]$. Cerebral oxygen delivery (COD) can also be derived, if the small quantity of oxygen dissolved in plasma is ignored. Two studies in newborn infants undergoing intensive care have shown a good correlation between CBF measurements obtained by NIRS and by the intravenous [133]xenon technique (Skov et al., 1992; Bucher et al., 1993). An optimal computerized methodology for calculating CBF from NIRS data has been described (Wolf et al., 1996). Methodological problems have been described when this technique was compared with microspheres employed in the adult dog (Newton et al., 1997), but the relevance of this to the neonatal brain is questionable.

Measurements of CBF in very preterm infants undergoing intensive care have shown a remarkably wide range of values, from 5 to 30 ml $100g^{-1}$ min^{-1}. Although some of this variability may reflect methodological problems, a test–retest variability of 15–20% has been recorded (Wolf et al., 1996), which is similar to that of equivalent methods, and the degree of biological variability in this population is consistent with data obtained using the intravenous [133]xenon technique.

In one recent study of very preterm infants, no relationship between CBF and mean arterial blood pressure was found, suggesting that autoregulation of cerebral perfusion remained intact at mean arterial blood pressures as low as 24 mm of Hg (Tyszczuk et al., 1998). Appropriately grown very preterm infants demonstrated a consistent rise in CBF over the first 3 days of life, probably representing a normal adaptive response of the cerebral circulation to birth (Meek et al., 1998a). By contrast, there was no evidence of a similar pattern in a group of infants with objective evidence of intrauterine growth failure. Some of these growth-retarded infants had an elevated CBF on the first day of life, possibly indicating cerebral vasodilatation secondary to prolonged intrauterine hypoxia.

Although it remains likely that there is a critical lower limit of CBF required to maintain cellular integrity, in follow-up studies no clear relationship between CBF measurements and long-term neurodevelopmental outcome has, as yet, been demonstrated. In one study, however, infants who went on to develop major periventricular hemorrhage had lower CBF on the first day of life compared with controls (Meek et al., 1999a). A marked reduction in CBF and CBV in very preterm infants has been observed following administration of indomethacin for closure of a patent ductus arteriosus, whereas only minimal changes have been observed following ibuprofen. A significant reduction in CBF has also been observed following intravenous aminophylline infusion.

A major limitation of this method for CBF measurement is the need to induce a rapid change in arterial saturation. In infants with normal lungs, satisfactory measurements may be impossible. Conversely, in infants with severe lung disease or other conditions associated with right-to-left shunting of blood, arterial saturation may be fixed at a low level. As a result, satisfactory measurements may not be possible in a significant proportion of infants. In addition, changes in arterial saturation are sometimes associated with unpredictable changes in the total cerebral hemoglobin concentration leading to inaccuracy in the measurement. Finally, deficiencies in the quality of the pulse oximetry data may also lead to errors in the determination of CBF.

An alternative NIRS technique uses indocyanine green (a dye which has an intense absorption peak in the near infrared region) as an exogenous tracer. Preliminary results have been obtained in infants during cardiopulmonary bypass and in mechanically ventilated newborns undergoing intensive care (Patel et al., 1998). Blood indocyanine green concentrations were measured using a specially adapted umbilical arterial catheter. This technique might overcome many of the limitations of the oxyhemoglobin method.

Cerebral blood volume

Global cerebral blood volume (CBV) is obtained by observing the effect on cerebral $[HbO_2]$ of a small and gradual change in arterial saturation induced over several minutes by a gradual change of inspired oxygen concentration. Total cerebral hemoglobin concentration and CBV may be obtained from the change in

$[HbO_2]$, using a modification of a standard indicator dilution technique (Wyatt et al., 1990). CBV was measured in 12 term and preterm infants, who were undergoing intensive care but who were thought to have normal brains. Mean CBV was 2.2 ± 0.4 ml $100g^{-1}$, similar to values obtained previously by positron emission tomography. Further studies have suggested that CBV is relatively constant in newborn infants of varying gestational ages, but significant increases in CBV have been observed in newborn infants with acute encephalopathy following a presumed asphyxial insult. In a study investigating the relationship between early hemodynamic changes and longterm outcome in encephalopathic infants following perinatal asphyxia, elevated CBV and CBF were associated with an increased risk of adverse outcome (Meek et al., 1999b). A novel method for validation of NIRS data employing jugular venous plethysmography and simultaneous measurements from the head using NIRS and a conventional mercury strain gauge has been described (Wickramsinghe et al., 1992). A close correlation between the two methods was obtained.

CBV response to changing arterial carbon dioxide tension

The response of CBV to carbon dioxide (CBVR – measured in ml $100g^{-1}$ kPa^{-1}) may be observed if a change in arterial carbon dioxide tension is induced by a small change in ventilator rate, or, in more mature infants who are clinically stable, by adding a small amount of exogenous carbon dioxide to the inspired air. Measurements have given values ranging from 0.1 to 0.7 ml $100g^{-1}$ kPa^{-1} in term and preterm infants undergoing intensive care (Pryds et al., 1990; Wyatt et al., 1991). An attenuation of CBVR has been observed in encephalopathic infants following perinatal asphyxia (Meek et al., 1999b) indicating disruption of normal vascular control mechanisms. Some discrepancies in NIRS meaurements induced by changing arterial carbon dioxide tension in preterm infants have been reported (Brun & Greisen, 1994). The reasons are not clear, and similar studies in the newborn piglet have failed to demonstrate any systematic inaccuracy (Firbank et al., 1998). Further fundamental studies on photon migration within the neonatal brain are required to clarify this issue. Nonetheless NIRS provides a valuable tool to observe the physiological response of the neonatal cerebral circulation to changing arterial carbon dioxide tension and its alteration under pathological or pharmacological influences.

Cerebral venous oxygen saturation

An estimate of cerebral venous oxygen saturation may be obtained by investigating the effect of briefly tilting the infant head-down or by the technique of partial jugular venous occlusion. If it is assumed that the increase in cerebral blood volume is dominated by changes in the venous compartment, then the venous saturation is obtained from the ratio of the change in $[HbO_2]$ compared to $[Hb_{tot}]$ (Yoxall et al., 1995). A good correlation with invasive measurements using jugular bulb samples has been demonstrated, and this technique has been employed to estimate cross brain oxygen extraction and oxygen consumption in infants of different ages (Yoxall & Weindling, 1997).

An earlier study using the tilting technique showed that venous saturation was significantly elevated in encephalopathic term infants compared with controls. This indicated reduced cerebral oxygen extraction probably due to a combination of cerebrovascular vasodilatation and impaired cerebral oxygen consumption following hypoxic–ischemic brain injury. Similar findings have been observed in a newborn piglet model during secondary energy failure following an acute transient episode of hypoxia–ischemia.

Measurement of cerebral functional activation in response to stimulation

NIRS provides a powerful tool for investigation of the cortical vasodilatory response to functional activation. When the optical fibre bundles are positioned on the occipital scalp overlying the visual cortex, a significant rise in both $[HbO_2]$ and $[Hb]$ is observed in response to observation of a computer-generated stimulus (Meek et al., 1998b). In a study of infants in the first 3 months of life, the mean magnitude of the response represented an increase in local CBV of approximately 5%. No response was observed when the optodes were positioned over the frontal cortex. This hemodynamic response is detectable in most healthy newborn infants at term, but preliminary findings suggest that it is markedly attenuated in preterm infants and in those with underlying injury to the visual cortex and its connections. These early results demonstrate the remarkable ability of NIRS to investigate the development of cortical responses to varying forms of sensory stimulation in awake newborns. The technique is likely to play an important role in providing new insights into the ontogeny of cortical function, as well as possibly providing a sensitive means for the early detection of perinatal cortical injury.

Measurements of the redox state of cytochrome oxidase

The fact that mitochondrial cytochrome oxidase displays an absorption peak within the near infrared region was central to the initial development of NIRS. It offers the possibility that previously inaccessible information on intracellular oxygen concentration and electron flux can be obtained by a non-invasive optical method. The absorption is due to a copper-containing moeity within the cytochrome molecule termed Cu_A and changes in the redox state of this centre can thus be detected. Although several workers have published data on changes in Cu_A observed in newborn infants, the subject has been bedevilled by problems of data interpretation and questions as to whether the observed signals really arise from cytochrome oxidase or are artefacts of the mathematical algorithms used to isolate the cytochrome redox changes from the stronger hemoglobin signals (for review, see Cooper & Springett, 1997). Recent work in the neonatal piglet has clarified this issue. Using exchange transfusion with a perfluorocarbon blood substitute, the in vivo cytochrome NIR spectrum was obtained in the absence of hemoglobin. It was found to be indistinguishable from that obtained from adult animals and from in vitro analysis of the purified enzyme (Cooper et al., 1999). The response of the Cu_A signal to mitochondrial inhibition with cyanide was demonstrated in both normal and hemoglobin-free animals using multiple wavelength NIRS. These studies demonstrated that, provided appropriate NIRS techniques are employed, changes in cytochrome oxidase redox state can be determined with reasonable accuracy in the neonatal brain.

Preliminary studies have demonstrated that the Cu_A redox state does not become signifcantly reduced from baseline until the mean cerebral hemoglobin saturation falls to low levels. This supports the concept that, in the baseline normoxic state, the Cu_A centre is highly oxidized, due to a relative excess in oxygen delivery to the mitochondria compared with the metabolic demand. It is only when cerebral tissue oxygen delivery is significantly impaired that Cu_A reduction is observed, and hence observations of Cu_A in vivo may allow early detection of inadequate cerebral oxygen delivery. Observations in newborn piglets with graded hypoxia–ischemia have confirmed a close correlation between cerebral high energy phosphates measured by ^{31}P MRS and cytochrome redox state measured by NIRS (Tsuji et al., 1995). Measurements of cerebral cytochrome redox state during hypothermic cardiopulmonary bypass may also provide important information on the adequacy of cerebral oxygen delivery during different phases of the procedure (Nomura et al., 1996). It is of special interest that an increase in carbon dioxide tension has been associated with an significant oxidation in Cu_A above baseline values, but the fundamental biophysical processes underlying this observation remain unclear (Cooper et al., 1999).

Measurements from the fetal brain during labour

Using a specially designed flexible optical probe, which is inserted through the cervix and positioned on the fetal scalp, it is possible to obtain continuous NIRS measurements from the fetal brain during labour (Peebles et al., 1992; Aldrich et al., 1995). A rubber moulding ensures that the sites of light entry and exit are maintained at a constant and known separation from one another. The moulding also ensures that good apposition of the optodes to the fetal scalp is maintained throughout the monitoring process, by the continuous application of mild negative pressure, aided by pressure from the surrounding maternal tissues. Once the cervix is dilated by 2 cm, the probe is easily applied to the fetal scalp, and observations may be continued throughout labour and, where feasible, continued until the point of delivery and beyond.

Effect of uterine contractions

Large fluctuations in $[HbO_2]$ and $[Hb]$ are routinely observed during each uterine contraction due to changes in cerebral blood volume as the fetal head is mechanically compressed against the maternal perineum. When both $[HbO_2]$ and $[Hb]$ change in the same direction during a contraction, it is possible to calculate the mean cerebral oxygen saturation ($SmcO_2$) from the ratio between the changes in $[HbO_2]$ and total cerebral hemoglobin (Peebles et al., 1992).

A study of $SmcO_2$ in 33 fetuses undergoing labour gave values within a surprisingly wide range of 21–72% (Aldrich et al., 1995). A strong correlation was found between $SmcO_2$ measured within 30 minutes of delivery and measurements of umbilical artery and vein pH immediately after delivery. A further study demonstrated that fetal cerebral oxygenation during labour is influenced by the rapidity of uterine contractions with very rapid contractions leading to a progressive deoxygenation of the fetal brain. Another study investigated the effect of maternal oxygen administration during labour. A small but significant increase in fetal $SmcO_2$ was detected. Maternal posture and pushing during the second stage of labour have also been shown to influence fetal cerebral oxygenation, and an association between late fetal heart rate decelerations and a fall in fetal oxygenation after the uterine contraction has been demonstrated (for review, see Wyatt, 1997). Although studies are still at an early stage, NIRS performed during labour has obvious potential as a research tool for exploring the effects of normal and abnormal labour on fetal cerebral oxygenation, and for investigating the adaptation of the cerebral circulation to labour and delivery.

Fetal animal studies using NIRS

Studies using fibre optic probes chronically implanted on the head of fetal sheep in utero demonstrate that NIRS is a powerful tool for the investigation of fetal hemodynamic and metabolic responses to oxygen deprivation. In one study, which investigated the effects of different types of insult on the fetal brain, an episode of hypoxia of moderate severity, induced by lowering the maternal inspired oxygen concentration, caused peripheral vasoconstriction, an increase in CBF and a rise in mean arterial pressure (Bennett et al., 1998). This was coincident with a rise in CBV, reflecting cerebral vasodilatation. In contrast, a more severe insult, caused by 10 minutes of complete umbilical cord occlusion, led to a fall in both arterial blood pressure and CBF. After an initial rise, CBV, measured by NIRS, also fell or remained at baseline levels. This study suggested that it was possible, using NIRS, to discriminate between a situation where cerebral perfusion was maintained during a hypoxic challenge and one where hypoperfusion resulted. The significance of this observation lies in the fact that the severity of brain injury has been shown to correlate closely with the degree of hypoperfusion (Gunn et al., 1992).

NIRS has also been used to measure changes in the redox state of cytochrome oxidase in the ovine fetus. Occlusion of the maternal common internal iliac artery caused a fall in oxygen delivery to, and oxygen consumption by, fetal hindlimb muscle and a reduction of the Cu_A moiety of cytochrome oxidase (Newman et al., 2000). Data obtained simultaneously from the brain showed a similar fall in oxygen consumption, but an oxidation in cytochrome oxidase. The significance of these findings has not been fully clarified, but it would appear that, in the fetal brain, in contrast to hindlimb muscle, it is not oxygen deprivation at the cytochrome oxidase binding site that leads to alterations in cell metabolism, but that these may form part of a compensatory response to match oxygen supply and demand.

The ability to make continuous measurements over long periods using NIRS was exploited by Marks et al. (1996) who continued observations for 72 hours after a 1 hour bilateral carotid artery occlusion in the near term ovine fetus in utero. They reported a secondary rise in CBV starting approximately 12 hours postinsult, which mirrored changes in cortical impedance, an indirect marker of secondary energy failure. This response was attenuated by pretreatment with the nitric oxide synthase inhibitor L-NAME, resulting in a worsening of the degree of brain injury. NIRS therefore has the potential to provide non-invasive assessment of the hemodynamic consequences of perinatal hypoxia–ischemia at the bedside.

Developments in NIRS methodology

The field is changing rapidly, and a number of technical advances in NIRS will be mentioned briefly.

Wideband continuous wave spectroscopy

Although most studies with NIRS have employed spectrometers with a small number of discrete NIR wavelengths, it is possible to transilluminate the infant brain using an intense white light source and a wideband spectrometer coupled to a sensitive light detector (Cope et al., 1989). This technique has several advantages. First, because data are obtained simultaneously at a large number of wavelengths, curve-fitting techniques can be used to reduce measurement errors. This is a particular advantage in the measurement of cytochrome oxidase redox changes.

Second, the optical path length can be measured continuously using the absorption peak of water, thus allowing more accurate determination of chromophore concentration changes. Thirdly, by using curve fitting to detect the unique spectral features of the deoxyhemoglobin spectrum, it is possible to obtain continuous absolute quantification of deoxyhemoglobin concentration without the need to manipulate SaO_2 (Cooper et al., 1996). Preliminary measurements using this technique are promising and suggest that it may extend the accuracy and range of measurements which can be obtained by NIRS in the neonatal brain.

Frequency resolved spectroscopy

This employs continuous laser light, which is intensity modulated by a very high frequency sine wave. By measuring the phase shift between the incident and transmitted light, it is possible to obtain continuous optical path length information, together with measurements of light attenuation. Preliminary data using a prototype instrument have been obtained, including pilot studies in newborn infants (Duncan et al., 1996) and in the fetus during labour. In addition to providing improved accuracy of hemoglobin concentration measurements, frequency resolved spectroscopy may eventually enable direct detection of electrical activation of the cortex which is associated with small scattering changes in the activated brain region.

Spatially resolved spectroscopy

This employs multiple detectors at a fixed spacing relative to an optical transmitter, and a variety of modifications have been employed. The technique is capable of providing absolute quantification of the ratio of oxy- and deoxyhemoglobin in the brain without the need for any physiological manipulation. This offers the possibility of continuous measurement and real-time display of cerebral oxygenation in babies undergoing intensive care.

Near infrared imaging of the brain

In order to obtain two- or three-dimensional images of the brain, it is necessary to use an array of optical fibres for transmitting and detecting light coupled with complex image reconstruction computer algorithms (Hebden & Delpy, 1997). Apart from the obvious practical problems, spatial resolution is very poor with conventional image reconstruction because of the intense scattering of light within the brain. If the time of flight of light across the tissue is measured, rather than attenuation changes, better spatial resolution is attainable. Despite the considerable logistical difficulties, several groups are currently working on these devices and preliminary results have been published (Sevick et al., 1994; van Houten et al., 1996; Wells et al., 1997). Because of its size and optical properties, the neonatal brain represents an ideal target for optical transillumination and imaging. If the problems can be overcome, this approach offers information on the spatial distribution of oxy and deoxyhemoglobin and Cu_A redox level within the cranial compartment, enabling regional cerebral oxygenation to be assessed in babies undergoing intensive care (Hebden & Delpy, 1997). The adequacy of regional perfusion may be assessed by observing the inflow of an infrared absorbing dye such as indocyanine green, and alterations in the scattering properties of the brain may allow early detection and localization of cerebral injury.

Conclusion

NIRS has enormous potential for providing non-invasive information about cerebral oxygenation and hemodynamics in the newborn infant undergoing intensive care. NIR spectrometers, which are currently available can provide valuable, research information, but they have a limited role as practical clinical tools on the neonatal intensive care unit. Technical developments are now occurring at a rapid pace and, if their potential can be realized, NIRS may play an important role in future in neonatology, providing detailed quantitative and regional information about brain oxygenation and perfusion at the cotside.

SPECT imaging of the neonatal brain

Single photon emission computer tomography (SPECT) has been used to obtain unique data on regional blood flow distribution in the human preterm brain (Børch & Greisen, 1998). A technetium-labelled tracer was injected intravenously and a specialized portable detector system allowed reconstruction of an image from the entire brain at the cotside. In a group of healthy preterm infants with gestational ages between 25 and 32 weeks, the regional CBF in the subcortical white matter was found to be approximately one-fifth of that in the basal ganglia, indicating very low blood flow to white matter in the immature brain. Cortical blood flow was approximately twice that of the subcortical white matter, and the regional distribution of cerebral blood flow was found to be independent of arterial carbon dioxide tension.

Conclusion

Despite the frustratingly slow progress, non-invasive methods currently in use are able to provide novel functional information about cerebral oxidative energy metabolism and perfusion in the neonatal brain. There is little doubt that the conversion of these techniques into routine clinical tools will make a major contribution both to basic scientific understanding and to the practical intensive care of term and preterm newborn infants.

REFERENCES

Aldrich, C. A., D'Antona, D., Spencer, J. A. D. & Wyatt, J. S. (1995). Near infrared spectroscopy used in the assessment of intrapartum fetal cerebral oxygenation. *Contemporary Reviews in Obstetrics and Gynaecology*, 7, 71–6.

Altman, D. I., Perlman, J. M., Volpe, J. J. & Powers, W. J. (1993). Cerebral oxygen metabolism in newborns. *Pediatrics*, **92**, 99–104.

Azzopardi, D., Wyatt, J. S., Hamilton, P. A., Cady, E. B., Delpy, D. T. & Reynolds E. O. R. (1989a). Phosphorus metabolites and intracellular pH in the brains of normal and small-for-gestational-age infants investigated by magnetic resonance spectroscopy. *Pediatric Research*, **25**, 440–4.

Azzopardi, D., Wyatt, J. S., Cady, E. B. et al. (1989b). Prognosis of newborn infants with hypoxic–ischaemic brain injury assessed by phosphorus magnetic resonance spectroscopy. *Pediatric Research*, **25**, 445–51.

Bennett, L., Peebles, D. M., Edwards, A. D., Rios, A. & Hanson, M. A. (1998). The cerebral hemodynamic response to asphyxia and hypoxia in the near term fetal sheep as measured by near infrared spectroscopy. *Pediatric Research*, **44**, 1–7.

Boesch, C., Gruetter, R., Martin, E. et al. (1989). Variations in the in-vivo 31-phosphorus magnetic resonance spectra of the developing human brain during postnatal life. *Radiology*, **172**, 197–9.

Børch, K. & Greisen, G. (1998). Blood flow distribution in the normal human preterm brain. *Pediatric Research*, **43**, 28–33.

Brazy, J. E. (1998). Effects of crying on cerebral blood volume and cytochrome aa3. *Journal of Pediatrics*, **112**, 457–61.

Brun, N. C. & Greisen, G. (1994). Cerebrovascular responses to carbon dioxide as detected by near infrared spectrophotometry: comparison of three different measures. *Pediatric Research*, **36**, 20–4.

Bucher, H. U., Edwards, A. D., Lipp, A. E. & Duc, G. (1993). Comparison between near infrared spectroscopy and Xenon clearance for estimation of cerebral blood flow in critically ill preterm infants. *Pediatric Research*, **33**, 56–60.

Buchli, R., Martin, E., Boesiger, P. & Rumpel, H. (1994). Developmental changes of phosphorus metabolite concentrations in the human brain: a ^{31}P magnetic resonance spectroscopy study in vivo. *Pediatric Research*, **35**, 431–5.

Busza, A. L., Allen, K. L., King, M. D., van Bruggen, N., Williams, S. R. & Gaddian, G. D. (1992). Diffusion-weighted imaging studies of cerebral ischemia in gerbils: potential relevance to energy failure. *Stroke*, **23**, 1602–12.

Cady, E. B., D'Souza, P., Lorek, A. & Penrice, J. (1995). The estimation of local brain temperature by in-vivo ^{1}H magnetic resonance spectroscopy. *Magnetic Resonance in Medicine*, **33**, 862–7.

Cady, E. B., Penrice, J., Amess, P. N. et al. (1996a). Lactate, *N*-acetyl aspartate, choline and creatine concentrations, and spin–spin relaxation in thalamic and occipito-parietal regions of developing human brain. *Magnetic Resonance in Medicine*, **36**, 878–86.

Cady, E. B., Wylezinska, M., Penrice, J., Lorek, A. & Amess, P. (1996b). Quantitation of phosphorus metabolites in newborn brain using internal water as a reference standard. *Magnetic Resonance Imaging*, **14**, 293–304.

Cooper, C. E. & Springett, R. (1997). Measurement of cytochrome oxidase and mitochondrial energetics by near infrared spectroscopy. *Philosophical Transactions of Royal Society of London B*, **352**, 669–76.

Cooper, C. E., Elwell, C. E., Meek, J. H. et al. (1996). The noninvasive measurement of absolute cerebral deoxyhemoglobin concentration and mean optical pathlength in the neonatal brain by second derivative near infrared spectroscopy. *Pediatric Research*, **39**, 32–8.

Cooper, C. E., Cope, M., Springett, R. et al. (1999). Use of mitochondrial inhibitors to demonstrate that cytochrome oxidase near infrared spectroscopy can measure mitochondrial dysfunction noninvasively in the brain. *Journal of Cerebral Blood Flow and Metabolism*, **19**, 27–38.

Cope, M., Delpy, D. T., Wyatt, J. S., Wray, S. C. & Reynolds, E. O. R. (1989). A CCD spectrometer to quantitate the concentration of chromophores in living tissue utilising the absorption peak of water at 975 nm. *Advances in Experimental Medicine and Biology*, **247**, 33–41.

Cross, J. H., Gadian, D. G., Connelly, A. & Leonard, J. V. (1993). Proton magnetic resonance spectroscopy studies in lactic acidosis and mitochondrial disorders. *Journal of Inherited Metabolic Disorders*, **16**, 800–11.

Duncan, A., Meek, J. H., Clemence, M. et al. (1996). Measurement of cranial optical path length as a function of age using phase resolved near infrared spectroscopy. *Pediatric Research*, **39**, 889–94.

Edwards, A. D., Richardson C, van der Zee, P. et al. (1993). Measurement of haemoglobin flow and blood flow by near infrared spectroscopy. *Journal of Applied Physiology*, **75**, 1884–9.

Elwell, C. E., Cope, M., Edwards, A. D., Wyatt, J. S., Reynolds, E. O. R. & Delpy, D. T. (1992). Measurement of cerebral blood flow in adult humans using near infrared spectroscopy – methodology and possible errors. *Advances in Experimental Medicine and Biology*, **317**, 235–45.

Firbank, M., Elwell, C. E., Cooper, C. E. & Delpy, D. T. (1998). Experimental and theoretical comparison of NIR spectroscopy measurements of cerebral hemoglobin changes. *Journal of Applied Physiology*, **85**, 1915–21.

Groenendaal, F., Veenhoven, R. H., van der Grond, J., Jansen, G. H., Witkamp, T. D. & de Vries, L. S. (1994). Cerebral lactate and *N*-acetylaspartate/choline ratios in asphyxiated full-term neonates demonstrated in vivo using proton magnetic resonance spectroscopy. *Pediatric Research*, **35**, 148–51.

Groenendaal, F., van der Grond, J., Eken, P et al. (1997). Early cerebral proton MRS and neurodevelopmental outcome in infants with cystic leukomalacia. *Developmental Medicine and Child Neurology*, **39**, 373–9.

Gunn, A. J., Parer, J. T., Mallard, E. C., Williams, C. E. & Gluckman, P. D. (1992). Cerebral histological and electrophysiological changes after asphyxia in fetal sheep. *Pediatric Research*, **31**, 486–91.

Hanrahan, J. D., Sargentoni, J., Azzopardi, D. et al. (1996). Cerebral metabolism within 18 hours of birth asphyxia: a proton magnetic resonance spectroscopy study. *Pediatric Research*, **39**, 584–90.

Haseler, L. J., Arcinue, E., Danielsen, E. R., Bluml, S. & Ross, B. D. (1997). Evidence from proton magnetic resonance spectroscopy for a metabolic cascade of neuronal damage in shaken baby syndrome. *Pediatrics*, **99**, 4–14.

Hebden, J. C. & Delpy, D. T. (1997). Diagnostic imaging with light. *British Journal of Radiology*, **70**, S206–14.

Holshouser, B. A., Ashwal, S., Luh, G. Y. et al. (1997). Proton MR spectroscopy after acute CNS injury: outcome prediction in neonates, infants and children. *Radiology*, **202**, 487–96.

Huppi, P. S., Fusch, C., Boesch, C., Burri, R., Bossi, E. & Herschkowitz, N. (1991). Magnetic resonance in preterm and term newborns: ^{1}H-spectroscopy in developing human brain. *Pediatric Research*, **30**, 574–8.

Laptook, A. R., Corbett, R. J., Uauy, R. et al. (1989). Use of ^{31}P magnetic resonance spectroscopy to characterize evolving brain damage after perinatal asphyxia. *Neurology*, **39**, 709–12.

Livera, L. N., Spencer, S. A., Thorniley, M. S., Wickramsinghe, Y. A. B. D. & Rolfe, P. (1991). The effects of hypoxaemia and bradycardia on neonatal cerebral haemodynamics. *Archives of Diseases in Childhood*, **66**, 376–80.

Lorek, A., Takei, Y., Cady, E. B. et al. (1994). Delayed cerebral energy failure following acute hypoxia-ischaemia in the newborn piglet: continuous 48-hour studies by phosphorus magnetic resonance spectroscopy. *Pediatric Research*, **36**, 699–706.

Lorek, A. K., Penrice, J., Cady, E. B. et al. (1996). Cerebral energy metabolism in isovaleric acidaemia. *Archives of Disease in Childhood*, **74**, F211–13.

Marks, K. A., Mallard, E. C., Roberts, I. et al. (1996). Delayed vasodilation and altered oxygenation following cerebral ischaemia in fetal sheep. *Pediatric Research*, **39**, 48–54.

Martin, E., Buchli, R., Ritter, S. et al. (1996). Diagnostic and prognostic value of cerebral 31P magnetic resonance spectroscopy in neonates with perintal asphyxia. *Pediatric Research*, **40**, 749–58.

Meek, J. H., Tyszczuk, L. T., Elwell, C. E. & Wyatt, J. S. (1998a). Cerebral blood flow increases over the first three days of life in extremely preterm neonates. *Archives of Disease in Childhood*, **78**, F33–7.

Meek, J. H., Firbank, M., Elwell, C. E., Atkinson, J., Braddick, O. & Wyatt, J. S. (1998b). Regional hemodynamic responses to visual stimulation in awake infants. *Pediatric Research*, **43**, 840–3.

Meek, J. H., Tyszczuk, L. T., Elwell, C. E. & Wyatt, J. S. (1999a). Low cerebral blood flow is a risk factor for severe intraventricular haemorrhage. *Archives of Disease in Childhood*, **81**, F15–18.

Meek, J. H., Elwell, C. E., McCormick, D. C. et al. (1999b). Abnormal cerebral haemodynamics in perinatally asphyxiated neonates related to outcome. *Archives of Disease in Childhood*, **81**, F110–15.

Newman, J. P., Peebles, D. M., Harding, S., Springett, R. & Hanson, M. A. (2000). Haemodynamic and metabolic responses to moderate asphyxia in brain and skeletal muscle of the late gestation fetal sheep. *Journal of Applied Physiology*, **88**(1), 82–90.

Newton, C. R. J. C., Wilson, D. A., Gunnoe, E., Wagner, B., Cope, M. & Traystman, R. J. (1997). Measurement of cerebral blood flow in dogs with near infrared spectroscopy in the reflectance mode is invalid. *Journal of Cerebral Blood Flow and Metabolism*, **17**, 695–703.

Nomura, F., Naruse, H., duPlessis, A. et al. (1996). Cerebral oxygenation measured by near infrared spectroscopy during cardiopulmonary bypass and deep hypothermic circulatory arrest in piglets. *Pediatric Research*, **40**, 790–6.

Novotny, E., Ashwal, S. & Shevell, M. (1998). Proton magnetic resonance spectroscopy: an emerging technology in pediatric neurology research. *Pediatric Research*, **44**, 1–10.

Patel, J., Marks, K., Roberts, I., Azzopardi, D. & Edwards, A. D. (1998). Measurement of cerebral blood flow in newborn infants using near infrared spectroscopy with indocyanine green. *Pediatric Research*, **43**, 34–9.

Peden, C. J., Rutherford, M. A., Sargentoni, J., Cox, I. J., Bryant, D. J. & Dubowitz, L. M. S. (1993). Proton spectroscopy of the brain following hypoxic–ischaemic injury. *Developmental Medicine and Child Neurology*, **35**, 502–10.

Peebles, D. M., Edwards, A. D., Wyatt, J. S. et al. (1992). Changes in human fetal cerebral hemoglobin concentration and oxygenation during labor measured by near infrared spectroscopy. *American Journal of Obstetrics and Gynaecology*, **166**, 1369–73.

Penrice, J., Cady, E. B., Lorek, A. et al. (1996). Proton magnetic resonance spectroscopy of the brain in normal preterm and term infants and early changes following perinatal hypoxia–ischaemia. *Pediatric Research*, **40**, 6–14.

Penrice, J., Lorek, A., Cady, E. B. et al. (1997). Proton magnetic resonance spectroscopy of the brain during acute hypoxia–ischemia and delayed cerebral energy failure in the newborn piglet. *Pediatric Research*, **41**, 795–802.

Pryds, O., Greisen, G., Skov, L. L. & Friis-Hansen, B. (1990). Carbon dioxide related changes in cerebral blood volume and cerebral blood flow in mechanically ventilated preterm neonates. Comparison of near infrared spectrophotometry and 133 Xenon clearance. *Pediatric Research*, **27**, 445–9.

Roth, S. C., Edwards, A. D., Cady, E. B. et al. (1992). Relation between cerebral oxidative metabolism following birth asphyxia and neurodevelopmental outcome at one year. *Developmental Medicine and Child Neurology*, **34**, 285–95.

Roth, S. C., Baudin, J., Cady, E. B. et al. (1997). Relation of deranged neonatal cerebral oxidative metabolism with neurodevelopmental outcome and head circumference at 4 years. *Developmental Medicine and Child Neurology*, **39**, 718–25.

Sevick, E. M., Burch, C. L. & Chance, B. (1994). Near-infrared optical imaging of tissue phantoms with measurement in the change of optical path lengths. *Advances in Experimental Medicine and Biology*, **345**, 815–23.

Shah, A. R., Kurth, C. D. & Gwiazdowski, S. G. (1992). Fluctuations in cerebral oxygenation and blood volume during endotracheal suctioning in premature infants. *Journal of Pediatrics*, **120**, 769–74.

Skov, L., Pryds, O. & Greisen, G. (1991). Estimating cerebral blood flow in newborn infants: comparison of near infrared spectroscopy and [133]Xenon clearance. *Pediatric Research*, **30**, 570–3.

Skov L., Pryds, O., Greisen, G. & Lou, H. (1993). Estimation of cerebral venous saturation in newborn infants by near infrared spectroscopy. *Pediatric Research*, **33**, 52–5.

Tsuji, M., Naruse, H., Volpe, J. & Holtzman, D. (1995). Reduction of cytochrome aa3 measured by near-infrared spectroscopy predicts cerebral energy loss in hypoxic piglets. *Pediatric Research*, **37**, 253–9.

Tsuji, M., Du Plessis, A., Taylor, G., Crocker, R. & Volpe, J. J. (1998). Near infrared spectroscopy detects cerebral ischemia during hypotension in piglets. *Pediatric Research*, **44**, 591–5.

Tyszczuk, L. T., Meek, J. H., Elwell, C. E. & Wyatt, J. S. (1998). Cerebral blood flow is independent of mean arterial blood pressure in preterm infants undergoing intensive care. *Pediatrics*, **102**, 337–41.

Van der Knaap, M. S., Van der Grond, J., Van Rijen, P. C., Faber, J. A. J., Valk, J. & Willemse, J. (1990). Age-dependent changes in localised proton and phosphorus MR spectroscopy of the brain. *Radiology*, **176**, 509–15.

Van Houten, J. P., Benaron, D. A., Spilman, S. & Stevenson, D. K. (1996). Imaging brain injury using time-resolved near infrared light scanning. *Pediatric Research*, **39**, 470–6.

Van der Zee, P., Cope, M., Arridge, S. R. et al. (1991). Experimentally measured optical pathlengths for the adult head, calf and forearm and the head of the newborn infant as a function of inter optode spacing. *Advances in Experimental Medicine and Biology*, **316**, 143–53.

Wells, K., Hebden, J. C., Schmidt, F. E. W. & Delpy, D. T. (1997). The UCL multichannel time-resolved system for optical tomography. *Proceedings of SPIE*, **2979**, 599–607.

Wickramsinghe, Y. A. B. D., Livera, L. N., Spencer, S. A., Rolfe, P. & Thorniley, M. S. (1992). Plethysmographic validation of near infrared spectroscopic monitoring of cerebral blood volume. *Archive of Diseases in Childhood*, **67**, 407–11.

Wolf, M., Brun, N., Greisen, G., Keel, M., von Siebenthal, K. & Bucher, H. (1996). Optimising the methodology of calculating the cerebral blood flow of newborn infants from near infra-red spectrophotometry data. *Medical Biological Engineering and Computing*, **34**, 221–6.

Wyatt, J. S. (1997). Cerebral oxygenation and haemodynamics in the foetus and newborn infant. *Philosophical Transactions of the Royal Society of London, Series B* 352, 697–700.

Wyatt, J. S., Edwards, A. D., Azzopardi, D. & Reynolds, E. O. R. (1989). Magnetic resonance and near infrared spectroscopy for the investigation of perinatal hypoxic-ischaemic brain injury. *Archives of Diseases of Childhood*, **64**, 953–63.

Wyatt, J. S., Cope, M., Delpy, D. T. et al. (1990). Quantitation of cerebral blood volume in newborn human infants by near infrared spectroscopy. *Journal of Applied Physiology*, **68**, 1086–91.

Wyatt, J. S., Edwards, A. D., Cope, M. et al. (1991). Response of cerebral blood volume to changes in arterial carbon dioxide tension in preterm and term infants. *Pediatric Research*, **29**, 553–7.

Younkin, D. P., Delivoria-Papadopoulos, M., Leonard, J. C. et al. (1984). Unique aspects of human newborn cerebral metabolism evaluated with phosphorus nuclear magnetic resonance spectroscopy. *Annals of Neurology*, **16**, 581–6.

Yoxall, C. W. & Weindling, A. M. (1997). Measurement of cerebral oxygen consumption (CVO_2) in the neonate: CVO_2 increases with advancing gestational age. *Pediatric Research*, **44**, 283–90.

Yoxall, C. W., Weindling, A. M., Dawani, N. H. & Peart, I. (1995). Measurement of cerebral venous oxyhaemoglobin saturation in children by near infrared spectroscopy and partial jugular venous occlusion. *Pediatric Research*, **38**, 319–23.

16

Electroencephalography

Anne Marie D'Allest[1] and Monique André[2]

[1]Service de Pédiatrie et Réanimation Néonatales, Hôpital Antoine Béclère, Clamart, France
[2]Service de Médecine et Réanimation Néonatales – Génétique, Maternité Régionale A Pinard, Nancy, France

Introduction

Electroencephalography is a non-invasive method used for the investigation of the functional state of the brain. It complements the information provided by the clinical neurological examination of the newborn. Since 1952, Dreyfus-Brisac and Monod have solved the main technical problems involved in recording EEGs in neonates and have studied neonatal brain electrophysiology in normal as well as in pathological conditions. They have described age-specific EEG patterns and demonstrated the value of the EEG in the assessment of brain integrity. Following the first steps, many other authors have published data concerning EEG maturation, diagnostic and prognostic significance of abnormal patterns, which means that extensive information is now available for full-term and prematurely born neonates.

Neurophysiological data

The spontaneous electrical activity of the brain results from a spatio-temporal average of synchronous postsynaptic potentials arising in radially oriented pyramidal cells of cortical gyri. These synaptic potentials are the responses of the cortical cells synchronized by other cellular groups, such as the thalamus. In a normal brain, these responses are based on the equilibrium between excitatory and inhibitory processes.

EEG is recorded by electrodes placed on the surface of the scalp. The amplitude of the EEG signal depends on the generator and on the conductivity of the structures between brain and scalp.

Some characteristics of the EEG in full-term and preterm neonates are linked to immaturity. Maturation of synapses and fibres can explain the evolution from a discontinuous tracing to a continuous one. Deep neuronal structures generate electrical activity which can also be recorded on the scalp, because the short distances between subcortex and scalp, as well as a smooth brain without secondary sulci and gyri until 28 weeks GA, make the spread of electrical activity to the scalp easy.

Myelinization of the subcortical white matter allows the synchronization of the cortical potentials. The synchrony between the two hemispheres is linked to the maturity of the corpus callosum, which occurs only near the end of the gestation.

Immaturity of the excitatory–inhibitory system can enhance seizure initiation and maintenance: this could be due to a high density of excitatory receptors and synapses, paucity of inhibitory receptors, or to changing functions of neurotransmitters in an immature brain (Mizrahi & Kellaway, 1998).

Recording methods

Multichannel EEG recording is the classical method used in the newborn.

Material

The recordings are still often performed on paper with conventional machines, using bipolar, longitudinal and transverse montages. Digital systems are more and more frequently used. The miniaturization of computers has made this system easy to use with the newborn, especially in intensive care units.

Sterilized silver–silver chloride cup electrodes are either attached by rubber helmet, or secured on the scalp with conductive adhesive paste. Ultralow-profile disposable electrodes are also available. Needles are to be avoided. Because of the small circumference of the head, 8 to 11 electrodes are placed in accordance with the 10–20 international placement system. EEG is recorded with a time constant of at least 0.3 s, high pass filters >30 Hz and a gain of 10 μV per millimetre.

The recording of the electrocardiogram and of the respiratory rate is necessary to determine sleep states and to recognize artefacts.

Conditions

The EEG is recorded at the bedside, especially in neonates undergoing intensive care. The technician must be specifically trained in the techniques of neonatal EEG and in the procedures of the care unit. It is the responsibility of the technician to categorize states of sleep and wakefulness, to record behavioural disturbances of the infant and to designate artefacts.

The duration of a standard recording varies from 45 to 90 minutes, because at least one whole cycle of sleep needs to be recorded. Recognition of different states of wake–sleep cycles, including active and quiet sleep, is an important aspect of the interpretation of the neonatal tracing. During active sleep, the child has eye and limb movements, and an irregular respiratory rate. During quiet sleep, there are no eye or body movements; and respiratory and heart rates are regular. Epochs which

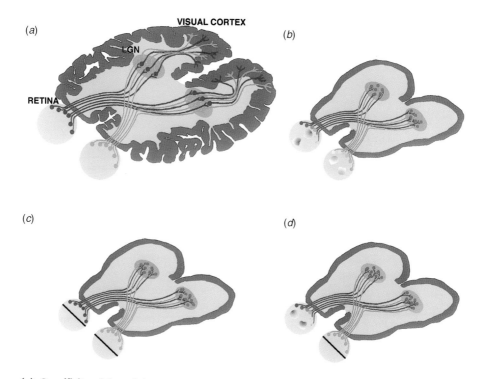

Fig. 10.1. (*a*). Specificity of the adult mammalian visual pathway. RGC axons project to the LGN topographically. The nasal axons cross over at the optic chiasm to the contralateral side of the brain, whereas the temporal axons project to the LGN on their own side of the brain. In the LGN, the RGC axons terminate in discrete eye-specific layers (only two are shown schematically here). The LGN neurons in turn project to the primary visual cortex, maintaining the retinotopic map. The LGN axons terminate in layer IV of the primary visual cortex where they are segregated into alternating eye-specific regions that form the basis of the ODC. (*b*). Developing visual pathway. During development, the projection from the retina to the LGN is not segregated into eye-specific layers. The retinal axons from the two eyes initially overlap substantially (only the binocular portion of the LGN is shown). Refinement of this projection into the precise, mature pattern of connections requires neural activity (Shatz & Stryker, 1986). During this process of segregation, waves of spontaneous, correlated activity that vary in location and direction spread through the developing retina (shown schematically in the eyes as coloured patches representing the activity of groups of RGC; the gradation in intensity from dark to light indicates the direction of propagation over time) (Feller et al., 1996). After the layers in the LGN have formed, the LGN neuron axons will segregate from an initially diffuse projection into the ODC of the visual cortex (not shown). (*c*) and (*d*). Disruption or imbalance of retinal activity blocks the development of the visual pathway. (*c*). When the RGC waves of activity are blocked during RGC axon segregation in the LGN, then the layers in the binocular region of the LGN fail to form. When the RGC activity in both eyes is blocked, segregation does not occur; both sets of axons expand the LGN territory that they fill. (*d*). When the balance of competition is disrupted by blocking the activity in only one eye, the active eye (red) gains most of the binocular territory in the LGN and many of the axons from the inactive eye (blue) are driven out (Penn et al., 1998).

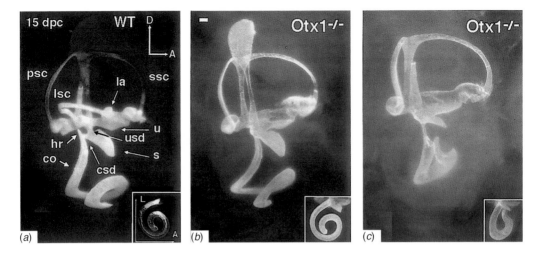

Fig. 11.7.   Lateral views of paint-filled membranous labyrinths of wild-type (*a*) and Otx1-/- mutant mice (*b*) and (*c*). The lateral canal and ampulla are missing in Otx1 mutants. In addition, an incomplete separation of the utricle and saccule, and malformations of the cochlea are often associated with these mutants. In panel (*c*), both the endolymphatic duct and sac were present but did not fill with paint. csd, cochleosaccular duct; dpc, days postcoitum; hr, hook region; la, lateral ampulla; lsc, lateral semicircular canal; psc, posterior semicircular canal; s, saccule; ssc, superior semicircular canal; u, utricle; usd, utriculosaccular duct. Orientation: (*a*), anterior; (*d*), dorsal. Scale bar, 100 μm. (Adapted with permission, Morsli et al., 1999.)

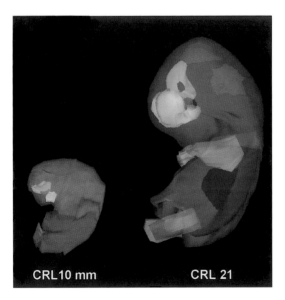

Fig. 13.7.   Three-dimensional reconstructions from ultrasound recordings made of a 7-week-2-day (CRL 10 mm) and an 8-week-6-day (CRL 21.5 mm)-old embryo. The significant changes of the form and the size of the brain cavities, which occur within a few days, can be seen. Hemispheres = yellow, diencephalon = green, mesencephalon = red, rhombencephalon = blue.

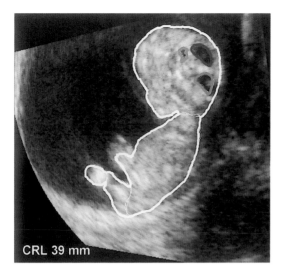

Fig. 13.8.   Sagittal section through a 10-week-5-day-old fetus, CRL 39 mm. This is a so-called 'anyplane slice' through the 3D volume. The drawing of the 'segmentation' lines in parallel tomograms through the object of interest is the first step to reconstruct a volume. Here, the third ventricle (green), the mesencephalon (red) and the fourth ventricle (blue) are outlined.

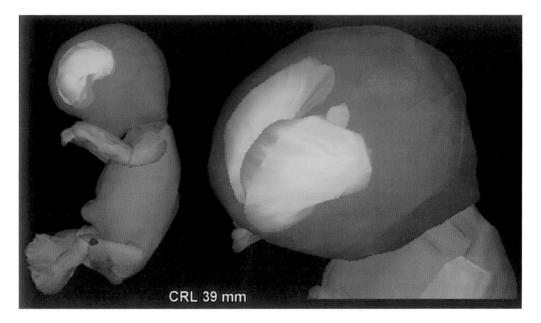

Fig. 13.9.   Three-dimensional reconstruction of the same fetus as in Fig. 13.8. The brain cavities are shown in an oblique angle. The hemispheres (lateral ventricles = yellow) conceal most of the diencephalon with its third ventricle (green). Cavity of the mesencephalon = red, cavity of the rhombencephalon = blue.

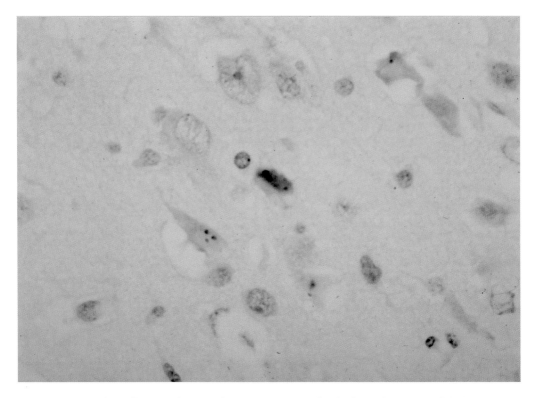

Fig. 18.2.　Histological section from the brain of an infant who died after hypoxic–ischemic encephalopathy, stained using an *in situ* technique for detecting fragmented DNA. The brown stain near the centre of the image demonstrates positive staining, showing that DNA fragments are present in the cell. The fragmented nucleus of this and another apoptotic cell nearby are clearly seen.

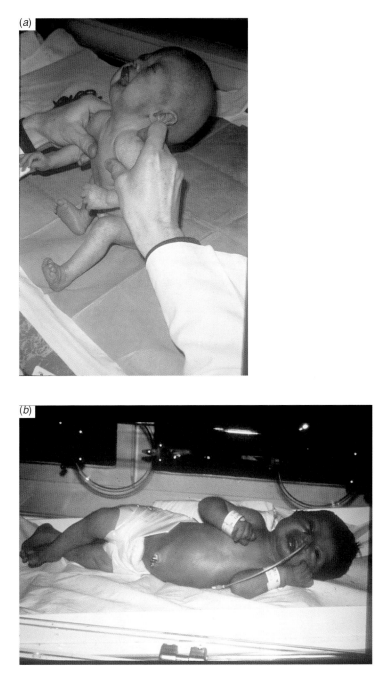

Fig. 19.2.   (a). An infant with neck extensor hypertonia. (b). An infant with moderate HIE. The legs are held extended and adducted (scissor position).
The hands are held fisted and the head is slightly extended. The eyes
are open but without fixation or following.

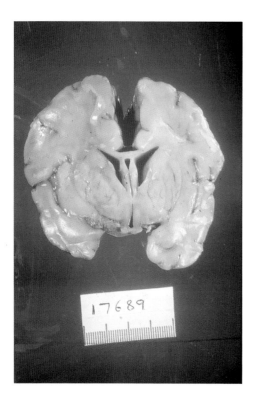

Fig. 19.8.   Postmortem brain after severe HIE. The hemispheres
are swollen, the surfaces being flattened.

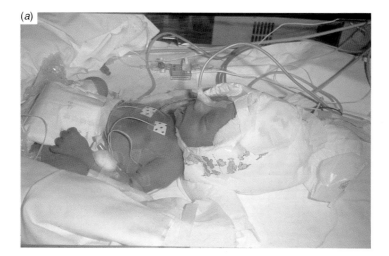

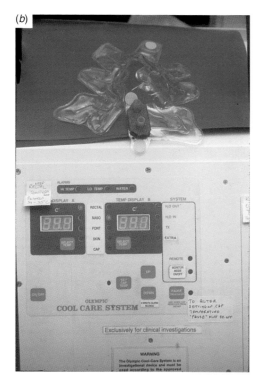

Fig. 19.9.   (*a*). An infant with moderate HIE at Southmead Hospital, Bristol, October, 1998. The head is in a cooling cap through which cold water is circulated. (*b*). An empty cooling cap on top of the control unit. The water-filled cap is still round the baby's head and the rectal temperature is registering 34.1 °C.

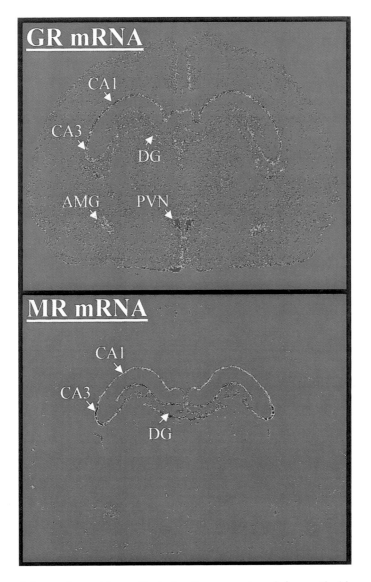

Fig. 22.3.   Colour-enhanced image illustrating the expression of glucocorticoid receptor (GR) and mineralocorticoid receptor (MR) mRNA in coronal sections of the fetal guinea-pig brain. Receptor mRNA was determined by *in situ* hybridization using ^{35}S-labelled oligonucleotide probes specific for GR and MR. GR mRNA is present at high levels in the CA1–CA4 fields of the hippocampus, the dentate gyrus (DG), paraventricular nucleus (PVN) and amygdala (AMG). Lower levels of GR mRNA are present in other brain regions. In contrast, MR mRNA is confined almost exclusively to the limbic system. Red: high expression; yellow: moderate expression; green: low expression; blue: no expression.

do not fit the criteria for active or quiet sleep are termed indeterminate. A video recording represents an important aid for the diagnosis of seizures or other abnormal movements.

The conventional EEG may be used to monitor cerebral electrical activity. With classical machines, paper speed is slowed to 5 mm/s; computer technology makes the process particularly easy. Other methods have been developed for the application of EEG monitoring to the newborn. The most widely used cerebral function monitoring (CFM) and compressed spectral array (CSA) are detailed in Chapter 17.

Normal EEG

EEG maturation and organization according to wakefulness and sleep states evolves progressively from the premature to the full-term neonate. During the first weeks of life of premature infants, sleep and EEG patterns mature practically in the same way as in utero. However, spectral EEG measures demonstrate regional differences between healthy term infants and preterm studied at term conceptional age; the preterm infants exhibit particular asymmetries (Scher et al., 1997). A new technique of analysis of self-referential neural network (Holthausen et al., 2000) establishes a brain dysmaturity index in healthy preterm neonates. This index will allow the detection of high-risk infants. The sleep–wakefulness states of the full-term newborn include wakefulness, active sleep, quiet sleep, and indeterminate or transitional sleep. The main characteristics of EEG maturation in the neonate are summarized in Table 16.1 and are illustrated in Figs. 16.1 to 16.3.

Differentiation based on EEG and rapid eye movements (REM) in active and quiet sleep states is sometimes observed as early as 27 weeks of gestational age (w GA)(Curzi-Dascalova et al., 1993), and it is consistently observable in normal neonates at 30–31 wGA. Sleep cycle organization is acquired at the same gestational age. Sleep cycle duration increases with gestational age (45 minutes at 31–34 wGA to 50–70 minutes at term) (Curzi-Dascalova & Mirmiran, 1996).

Abnormal EEG

Identification of the range of normal EEG patterns according to gestational age is essential in order to assess the significance of abnormalities. EEG disturbances should be interpreted in relation to the sleep state of the newborn: for example, some abnormalities appear only in quiet sleep. The choice of technique (continuous recording or serial EEGs) depends on several factors: maturity (preterm or full-term infants), clinical signs (seizures, coma) or whether or not a standardized intensive care neurological surveillance is being used.

Table 16.1. EEG maturational synopsis

GA (weeks)	Sleep	EEG characteristics	Reactivity
24–27	No sleep organization	Very discontinuous, but labile background activity Short bursts of diffuse, very high amplitude (> 300 μV) delta waves 0.3–1 Hz Some high voltage theta rhythms Interhemispheric synchrony	EEG reactivity not usual
28–29	Differentiation in AS and QS just outlined	Discontinuous background activity, longer bursts of activity, inactive intervals of variable duration (up to 40 s) Delta waves 0.3–1 Hz (sometimes > 300 μV): smooth or outlined delta-brushes High voltage theta rhythms in QS, isolated and diffuse; or combined with delta waves predominant on anterior and temporal areas	
30–31	AS and QS present Good concordance between EEG and sleep states	Continuous or nearly continuous tracing in AS Discontinuous tracing in QS – hypoactive periods ≦20 s Delta-brushes (0.5–1.5 Hz), 100–200 μV, posterior or temporo-occipital predominance in AS and QS Temporal theta rhythms in AS and QS	EEG reactivity outlined
32–34	W, AS and QS easily distinguished	Continuous tracing in W and AS, discontinuous tracing in QS – hypoactive periods ≦15 s at 32 w GA, ≦10 s at 34 w GA. Delta-brushes (1–2 Hz) of lower amplitude, localized on occipital channels, very numerous and characteristic Temporal theta rhythms disappear at 33–34 w GA	EEG reactivity present
35–36	AW, QW, AS and QS	*Activité moyenne* (diffuse low-voltage EEG pattern of 4–7 Hz rhythms) at 36 w GA in QW Monophasic frontal sharp transients	EEG reactivity present

GA	Stages	EEG characteristics	
		Good synchronization of occipital delta waves on both hemispheres in *AS* Discontinuous or nearly discontinuous pattern in QS Delta-brushes still observed in QS	EEG reactivity present
37–38	AS differentiated in: AS1 preceding QS AS2 following QS	*Activité moyenne* tracing in AW, QW, AS2 Higher amplitude slow activity in AS1 Synchronous and diphasic frontal transients Slow anterior dysrythmia (bilateral anterior slow waves) in AS1 Nearly continuous or continuous tracing (*tracé alternant* – see 39–41 w) in QS	
39–41	AW, QW, AS1, QS and AS2	Typical pattern of QS is *tracé alternant*: bilaterally synchronous bursts in slow waves (1–3 Hz, 50–100 μV) interrupted by an interburst activity similar to *activité moyenne*. Bursts and interbursts have an average duration of 5 to 6 s Very good synchronization of rhythms on both hemispheres	Electroclinical reactivity marked by a desynchronized pattern during 6 to 8 s

Notes:

GA: gestational age, AS: active sleep, QS: quiet sleep, AW: active wakefulness, QW: quiet wakefulness, W: wakefulness, w: weeks

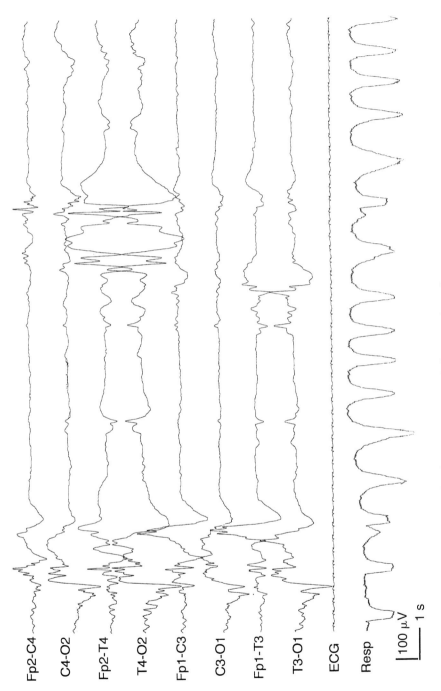

Fp2-C4

C4-O2

Fp2-T4

T4-O2

Fp1-C3

C3-O1

Fp1-T3

T3-O1

ECG

Resp

100 μV

1 s

Fig. 16.1.   Normal EEG activity of a 25 weeks and 4 days GA premature infant at 8 days of age.

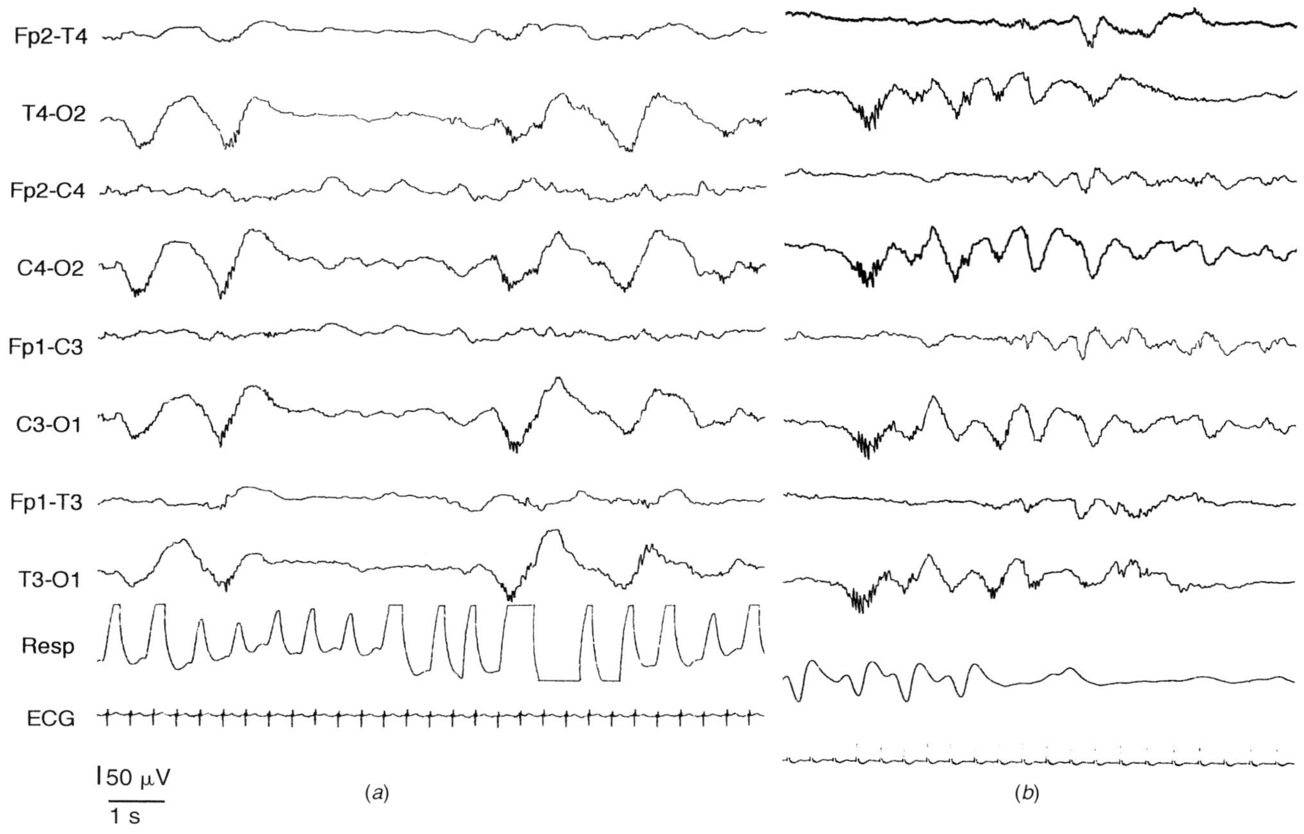

Fp2-T4

T4-O2

Fp2-C4

C4-O2

Fp1-C3

C3-O1

Fp1-T3

T3-O1

Resp

ECG

$|50\ \mu V$

1 s

(a)

(b)

Fig. 16.2.   Normal EEG activity in active sleep. (a) 31 weeks and 4 days GA premature infant at 5 days of life; (b) 34 weeks GA premature at 1 day of life.

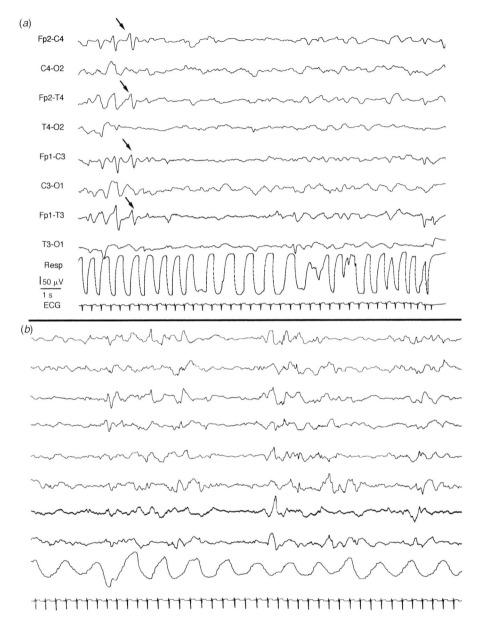

Fig. 16.3. Normal EEG in full-term newborn. (*a*) continuous tracing in active sleep (AS 1); arrows indicate frontal sharp transients; (*b*) *tracé alternant* in quiet sleep.

EEG abnormalities in premature neonates

Neurological evaluation concerning the preterm infant is difficult because of the frequent specific constraints imposed by intensive care conditions, rare or subtle clinical manifestations such as abnormal eye movements, chewing, jerking movements, autonomic manifestations, tonic posturing; clonic movements are observed in near term premature infants.

It is for this reason that EEG recorded during the first days of life and repeated during hospitalization can provide a good tool for the assessment of cerebral function. It reveals a number of different abnormal patterns.

Ictal discharges

These are rare, often brief, monorhythmic, of slow frequency (delta 1–2 Hz, Fig. 16.4) observed as early as 25 wGA (Radvanyi-Bouvet et al., 1985). After 32–33 wGA they are more polyrhythmic and comparable to those of full-term infants. They are not frequent: 3.3% in Marret's study (1997), 2.4% in D'Allest's (1992) for prematures at less than 33 wGA. In most immature babies, they appear very early in the first 2 or 3 days of life and are observed in the case of neonates with intraventricular and/or periventricular hemorrhages (IVH–PVH) (personal data). Scher et al. (1993) reported that 45% of preterm infants with seizures have IVH–PVH. Their prognosis is generally unfavourable (Marret et al., 1997).

Positive rolandic sharp waves (PRSW)

First described by Cukier et al. (1972), these are surface-positive, broad-based sharp transients with a duration of 100 to 500 ms, localized over the rolandic or central areas (C3, C4, Cz); they have since been classified as type A (Fig. 16.5), isolated and clearly differentiated from the background activity, with an amplitude between 25 and 200 μV, and type B, occurring in bundles of lower amplitude, less well differentiated, according to the Blume and Dreyfus-Brisac criteria (1982).

Initially related to intraventricular or periventricular hemorrhages (Clancy & Tharp, 1984), PRSWs have been reported to correlate better with the development of periventricular white matter lesions (Marret et al., 1989). These PRSWs appear early, during the first week of life in 78% of premature infants born before 32 weeks whose tracings include them (D'Allest et al., 1992). They always precede the ultrasonic detection of cysts (Baud et al., 1998). They can also be observed with very premature neonates (<28 wGA). Their density has also been studied: PRSWs are numerous ($\geq$ 1/min) or rare (<1/min).

PRSWs are very specific markers of periventricular leukomalacia (PVL) with a positive predictive value of 99%, but their sensitivity is GA dependent: 33% with very premature infants compared to 88% with prematures born before 33 weeks

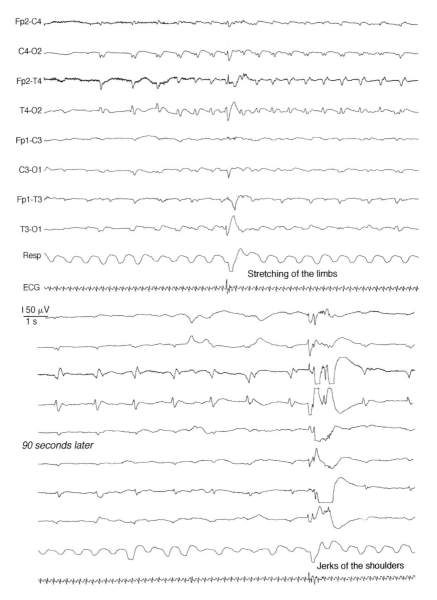

Fig. 16.4.   Abnormal EEG. Ictal discharge at day 2 in a 27 weeks and 4 days GA premature infant.

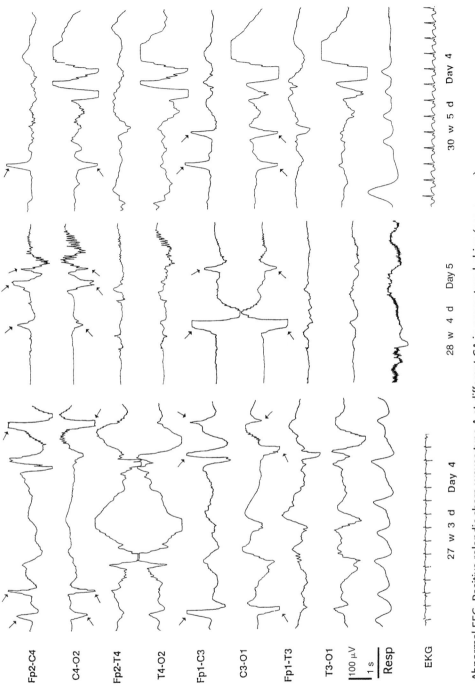

Fig. 16.5.   Abnormal EEG. Positive rolandic sharp waves type A at different GA in premature babies (see arrows).

(Baud et al., 1998). They have a strong prognostic value in indicating major neurological sequelae when they are numerous (≥ 1/min), present on both rolandic regions (C3 and C4), and/or present on two successive recordings (Marret et al., 1989; D'Allest et al., 1992).

PRSWs are recorded bilaterally on C3, C4 in most cases, but can be present only on Cz in 12% (Novotny et al., 1987) or in 13.5% of recordings (Vecchierini-Blineau et al., 1996).

In very preterm infants having initially normal EEGs and ultrasound scans, PRSWs can appear after 4 or 5 weeks of life after an infectious pathology (septicemia, enterocolitis) and correspond to late PVL or subcortical leukomalacia. This consideration justifies a prolonged EEG surveillance in very immature infants.

Background activity

This has to be in conformity with GA; the absence of typical patterns for the GA is a criterion of major cerebral injury (Dreyfus-Brisac, 1979). Excessive discontinuity for GA is difficult to appreciate, but some authors (Connell et al., 1987; Benda et al., 1989) reported that excessively discontinuous EEGs (interburst intervals > 60 seconds) were associated with poor outcomes in preterm neonates.

The presence of sleep organization in prematures at 29–30 w GA is a good criterion for favourable outcome, but it is not sufficient if PRSWs are present and numerous on the same recording, since the bad prognostic value of the latter is important. Discordance between cerebral and non-cerebral components of sleep states (dysmaturity of the EEG-sleep background) suggests a high risk of neurological sequelae (Tharp et al., 1989).

Hayakawa et al. (1997) focused on the bad prognostic value of 'disorganized EEG patterns' concerning early preterm infants after a marked EEG depression in the first 2 days of life. Recently, Biagioni et al. (2000) investigated a group of preterm infants. They find that, in the early postnatal period, background EEG 'dysmaturity' is significantly more apparent in infants with cystic periventricular leukomalacia than in control groups.

Drug effects

Antiepileptic drugs (phenobarbitone and diazepam) can increase the discontinuity of EEG background in very preterm neonates (Hellström-Westas et al., 1991). Similarly, sedatives such as short duration benzodiazepines or analgesics such as synthetic opioids (pethidine, fentanyl) can modify EEG background, increasing discontinuity (Murdoch Eaton et al., 1992) and reducing physiological fluctuations (Magny et al., 1994). Young and da Silva (2000) in a prospective study, show that morphine produces reversible alterations as prolonged periods of inactivity in neonatal EEGs at various postconceptional ages. It is thus highly important to take drugs into account when interpreting EEGs. EEG can also help to appreciate the cerebral tolerance of new treatments. Discontinuity is linked to acute cerebral blood velocity changes during and after administration of exogenous surfactants (Hascoët et al., 1995).

Abnormal EEG in full-term neonates

EEG is a sensitive indicator in real time of the functional state of the brain; it provides essential additional information to that provided by morphological imaging. The severity of EEG abnormalities is often clearly correlated with immediate and long-term outcome, especially in hypoxic–ischemic encephalopathy (HIE) secondary to perinatal asphyxia, in neonatal seizures or in abnormal states of consciousness.

Hypoxic–ischemic encephalopathy

HIE remains the most frequent cause of cerebral impairment in the newborn. This situation constitutes a kind of paradigm of neurological distress and will be discussed in detail.

Seizures are frequently observed during the first days of life. Clinical manifestations vary from typical clonic multifocal convulsions to subtle and subclinical crises. In all cases, EEG ictal patterns are characteristic (Fig. 16.6), but they may vary considerably at different times during the course of one event or from one to the next. It is very important to recognize all the seizures so that the best treatment can be prescribed; but misdiagnosis can lead to unjustified, and even noxious, drug prescription.

The most common pattern is that of a discharge of regular spikes or sharp and slow waves, repetitive with frequency varying from 1 to 10 Hz, shifting from one area of the scalp to another. This pattern is often associated with clonic multifocal seizures. The beginning and termination of the discharge are usually abrupt, but the duration and the amplitude of the waves often increase and their frequency decreases at the end of the discharge. Spike and interspike interval durations increase when the clinical status worsens.

Monorhythmic discharges consist of repetitive waves of a single frequency. They do not have a sharp appearance. Alpha-like discharges are generally of low amplitude (Engel, 1975).

A sudden and diffuse attenuation of background activity has been described as the EEG pattern accompanying some tonic seizures (Watanabe et al., 1984).

The minimum duration of ictal discharges is still the object of a certain amount of debate, but a 10-second duration was proposed by Dreyfus-Brisac et al. (1981) and is usually accepted (Lombroso & Holmes, 1993). Some discharges may be prolonged, lasting several minutes.

EEG discharges and clinical seizures are unifocal and concordant in the presence

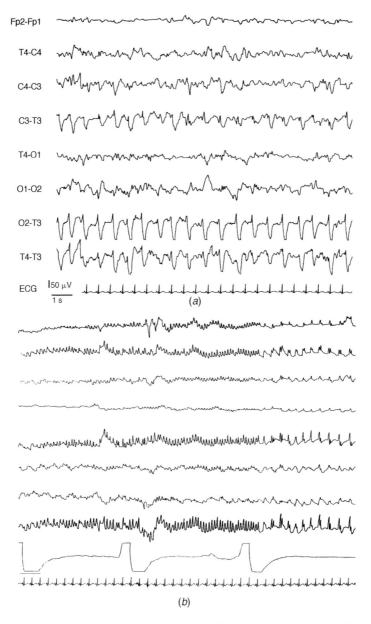

Fp2-Fp1

T4-C4

C4-C3

C3-T3

T4-O1

O1-O2

O2-T3

T4-T3

ECG $50\ \mu V$ / $1\ s$

(a)

(b)

Fig. 16.6.   Abnormal EEG. Two patterns of seizures in full-term neonates during hypoxic–ischemic encephalopathy. (a) Rhythmic sharp delta waves localized on the left temporal region (T3). (b) 'Pseudo-alpha' discharge followed by rhythmic sharp waves.

of a localized underlying cerebral lesion. Simultaneous recording of EEG and videotape allows a more accurate identification of doubtful ictal manifestations. EEG is essential to the diagnosis of subclinical or 'occult seizures', whatever the origin of the absence of symptoms may be: drugs that paralyse or sedate the infant (curare, benzodiazepines, synthetic opioids), clinical seizures already controlled by antiepileptic drugs (Scher et al., 1994), very severe brain damage which may impede the discharges from reaching the effector structures, or discharges arising from apparently 'silent' areas. Continuous EEG monitoring makes it possible to recognize all the ictal events, which are more frequent than the clinical ones (Fig. 16.7). In a study of 41 neonates, Clancy et al. (1988) demonstrated that only 21% of 393 seizures were associated with clinical activity.

Some infants with severe encephalopathy exhibit clinical symptoms such as myoclonias and tonic postures which mimic seizures in the absence of EEG ictal discharges, but with profoundly abnormal background EEG activity. This dissociation has been analysed by Mizrahi and Kellaway (1987) using EEG/video monitoring. They proposed that abnormal behaviours with no relationship to EEG ictal discharges represent 'brainstem release phenomena' resulting from functional decortication and are not convulsive. Careful clinical observation, videotaping, and EEG performed before institution of any treatment can help to distinguish ictal and non-ictal events.

EEG is also a good indicator for prognosis (André et al., 1988). The prognosis is better after infrequent seizures than after status epilepticus. The prognosis is poor when there is an electroclinical discordance: EEG discharges without clinical seizures, and appearance of clinical seizures without EEG discharges. In both situations, the encephalopathy is severe and the background EEG activity is profoundly impaired.

Background activity is permanent or interictal. Its particularities are often very helpful in predicting outcome. The background activity may be normal during the first days of life. In these cases, the long-term neurological prognosis is always favourable (Monod et al., 1972). In the neonatal period, a normal EEG predicts the absence of seizures in the subsequent 18–24 hours (Laroia et al., 1998). Some abnormal background patterns are very severe, always associated with a poor prognosis, death or sequelae. They are termed:

(a) *inactive EEG*, i.e. activity nearly isoelectric, with amplitude lower than $5\,\mu V$. Some of the general recommendations for the recording of inactive EEG are common to all neonatal EEGs: (i) check on electrodes and material; (ii) use at least eight electrodes; (iii) use long duration (>30 min); (iv) use a time constant of at least 0.3 s; (v) electrode impedance should be between 100 and 10 000 ohms. In addition the activity must be recorded with (vi) wide separation of electrodes (>10 cm); (vii) a high gain ($2\,\mu V$/mm); (viii) after intensive sensory stimulation.

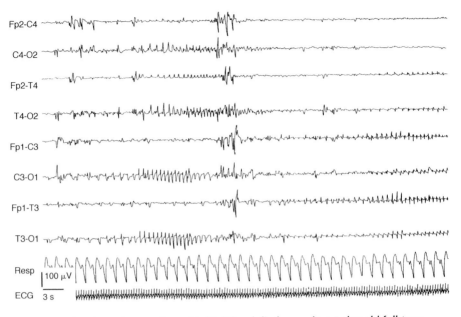

Fig. 16.7.   EEG monitoring (speed paper 5 mm/s). Multifocal discharges in a 1-day-old full-term newborn with hypoxic–ischemic encephalopathy.

(b) *Paroxysmal EEG* (Fig. 16.8)

(c) *Discontinuous EEG 'poor plus theta'.*

These three patterns are most often observed over a short period: 1 or 2 days for inactive tracings, less than a week for the two others. Scavone et al. (1985) have shown that the tracing has the most significant prognostic value when it is recorded before 2 days of postnatal life. Nevertheless, Pezzani et al. (1986) showed that an EEG which is inactive before 10 hours of life but which recovers rapidly can be followed by a favourable outcome.

To provide accurate prognosis, then, EEG needs to be monitored over the whole period between 10 and 48 hours of postnatal life since it is very important to discover or exclude the patterns discussed above.

EEGs termed 'intermediate' may be permanent or transitory discontinuous (Scavone et al., 1985; Selton & André, 1997) (Table 16.2):

(d) *Discontinuous A* (Fig. 16.8)

(e) *Discontinuous B* (Fig. 16.8)

In the same group, Pezzani et al. (1986) described continuous tracings:

(f) *Hyperactive and rapid EEGs.* The background activity is composed of normal patterns and of many spikes and waves of 4 to 8 Hz, diffuse, with high amplitude, often asynchronous.

Sometimes, these EEGs only include diffuse alpha and theta waves, with a poor

Table 16.2. Discontinuous patterns

Pattern	Circumstances	Bursts	Intervals and other characteristics
Physiological discontinuity	Normal premature infants	See Table 16.1	See Table 16.1
Paroxysmal	HIE FT	Short:1 to 10 s Morphology and amplitude variable from one burst to another, containing spikes, theta and delta waves, no normal features	Silent periods 10 to 60 s Interhemispheric asynchrony No lability, no reactivity
Discontinuous 'poor plus theta'	HIE FT	Theta rhythms Low amplitude 5 to 30 μV	No spatial organization No reactivity, no lability
Discontinuous B	HIE FT	Theta rhythms Last <10 s Amplitude 30 to 50 μV	Amplitude <15 μV
Discontinuous A	HIE FT	Near normal activity last at least 10 s	<10 s Amplitude <10 μV
Suppression-burst	EME EIEE Pyridoxine deficiency Cerebral malformations	Complex bursts: spikes, sharp waves and slow waves irregularly intermingled, synchronous or not over both hemispheres Last 1 to 5 s	Inactivity 3 to 10 s
Periodic	Amino-acidopathies Herpetic meningo-encephalitis	Repeated stereotyped complexes: slow delta waves and high theta sharp waves associated with rapid rhythms Variable amplitude	Very low activity, fixed duration

Notes:

HIE: hypoxo-ischemic encephalopathy, FT: full-term newborn, EME: early myoclonic encephalopathy, EIEE: early infantile epileptic encephalopathy.

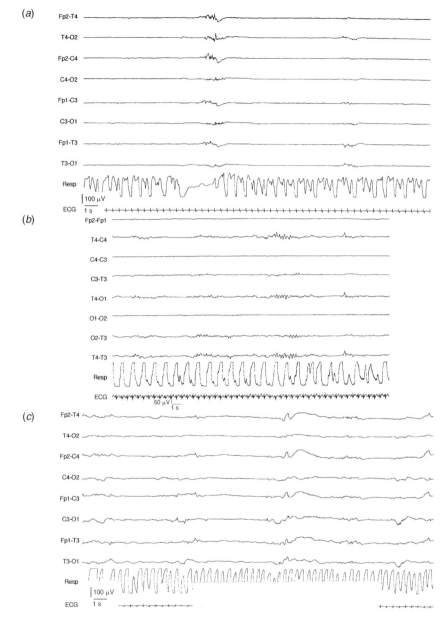

Fig. 16.8.   Background activity in full-term newborns with hypoxic–ischemic encephalopathy.
Discontinuous patterns (Table 16.2). (*a*): paroxysmal; (*b*): discontinuous (*A*); (*c*):
discontinuous (*B*).

lability. D'Allest et al. (1995) have shown that these intermediate EEGs do not allow an early prognosis before 2 days of postnatal life. With intermediate EEGs, it is necessary to record at least one more EEG between 2 and 6 days. The prognosis is good if there is an improvement. Conversely, if there is no change in EEG, or even a worsening, the prognosis is poor.

Other abnormalities of the background activity have a prognostic value only if they are observed after 1 week of life. They are slow EEG with only delta (0.5 to 1 Hz) waves, without lability or sleep organization, and low amplitude EEG, 5 to 15 µV during wakefulness and active sleep, 10 to 25 µV during quiet sleep.

Takeuchi and Watanabe (1989) described five stages of EEG depression, which corroborate the above descriptions. The prognostic significance is the same. Biagioni et al. (1998) studied constantly discontinuous tracings and showed that the maximum interburst interval duration was significantly related to neurological outcome.

Other abnormal patterns

These are superimposed over the background activity. Some non-physiological patterns have no prognostic value: slow anterior dysrhythmia, short bursts of high waves or spikes, numerous non-rolandic theta rhythms. After the first week, slow spikes during wakefulness are always very abnormal. McCutchen et al. (1985) described periodic lateralized epileptiform discharges (PLEDS). They resemble those observed in neonatal herpes encephalitis. They are very unusual in HIE, and always of poor prognosis.

Chung and Clancy (1991) found positive temporal sharp waves in neonates with cerebral lesions. Persistent focal sharp waves are usually associated with localized lesion.

However, unfavourable outcome has been observed in cases of thalamic lesions detected by ultrasound, whatever the severity of background EEG abnormality may be. But numerous and long-lasting spikes were overimposed (Lamblin et al., 1996). A study by Gire et al. (2000) emphasizes that the association of EEG tracings and MRI has a reliable prognostic value in the HIE, except in lesions of basic ganglia where MRI alone is better.

Organization and sleep states

Absence of lability, i.e. absence of modification of amplitude, morphology, or frequency of the waves during the whole recording, is in all cases a sign of severity (Monod et al., 1972). Constant asynergy or asynchrony between the two hemispheres or the anterior and posterior areas, which are frequently observed on paroxysmal EEG, are signs of unfavourable outcome during the first 2 weeks of life. The loss of sleep organization is always associated with severe neurological distress.

Influence of drugs

Classical anticonvulsant drugs, such as phenytoin or phenobarbital, only account for slight decrease of continuity. They do not modify the predictive value of the tracings. After intravenous infusion of benzodiazepines, there is a considerable, but short-lasting increase of discontinuity. High dosages of midazolam cause numerous theta rhythms to appear. Discontinuous tracings become paroxysmal after lidocaine infusion (Radvanyi-Bouvet et al., 1990). Synthetic opioids depress background activity and modify sleep. For these reasons, EEG needs to be recorded before beginning a treatment, and must be repeated over the following days.

Other conditions

Serial EEGs recorded in the case of infants with severe respiratory failure treated by venoarterial extracorporeal membrane oxygenation (ECMO) have shown an ominous predictive value of two or more recordings that disclose electrographic seizures or discontinuity (Graziani et al., 1994). These patterns occur more frequently in infants who needed cardiopulmonary resuscitation before ECMO, revealing fetal or neonatal distress responsible in large part for the neurological sequelae in ECMO survivors (Hahn et al., 1993). EEG abnormalities may be taken into account when taking the decision whether or not to initiate ECMO.

Loss of brainstem reflexes, cerebral blood flow and EEG are major criteria for diagnosis of brain death (Ashwal, 1997). As EEG is not always isoelectric, and CBF study shows no flow, the observation period can be shortened to 24 hours.

Epileptic syndromes

EEG is essential to the diagnosis of epilepsy. As in HIE, when the clinical manifestations are not sufficient, ictal EEG, associated with videotape if possible, is essential for recognizing and classifying the crises. Interictal EEG will help to identify the epileptic syndrome, in order to choose an appropriate treatment and determine a prognosis.

Benign idiopathic neonatal convulsions (BINC) were first described in 1977 as fifth day fits (Dehan et al., 1977). Multifocal seizures occur in otherwise healthy full-term neonates at 4 or 5 days, leading to a status epilepticus. After a mean duration of 20 hours, the seizures stop and the child returns progressively to a normal status. The interictal EEG often comprises a characteristic pattern, *theta pointu alternant*, which is a dominant theta activity, alternating or discontinuous, unreactive, with sharp waves and frequent interhemispheric asynergy. Nevertheless, this is not quite specific to BINC. The ictal EEG shows short discharges or rhythmic spikes or slow waves at a theta or delta frequency, lasting one or two minutes; the crises can be localized in any area, especially on the rolandic one (Navelet, 1981).

In benign familial neonatal convulsions (BFNC), seizures occur in normal neo-

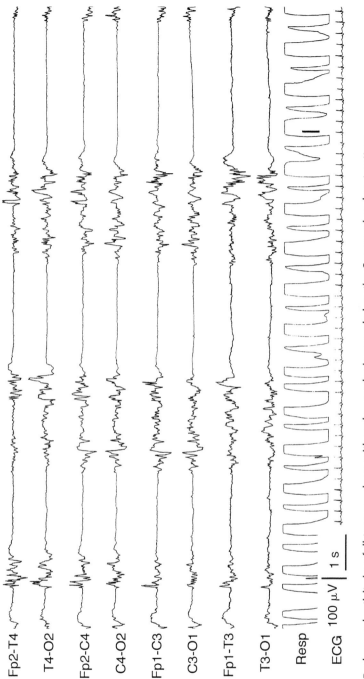

Fp2-T4

T4-O2

Fp2-C4

C4-O2

Fp1-C3

C3-O1

Fp1-T3

T3-O1

Resp

ECG 100 μV | 1 s

Fig. 16.9.   Background activity in a full-term newborn with early myoclonic encephalopathy. Suppression–burst pattern.

nates at 2 or 3 days of age. A family history of benign neonatal seizures is constant, with a dominant inheritance. One responsible gene is located on the long arm of chromosome 20. Secondary epilepsy will occur in 11 to 15% of patients. The crises are always electroclinical, of clonic type, sometimes with apnoeic spells. The ictal EEG shows a flattening of activity, followed by rhythmic slow waves lasting 1 or 2 minutes. The interictal EEG is normal.

Early myoclonic encephalopathy (EME) indicates very severe neonatal epilepsy, first described by Aicardi and Goutières (1978). It combines erratic, fragmentary myoclonus, partial motor seizures, massive myoclonia and, after the first months of life, spasms. In addition to the usual polygraphy, it is useful to record the deltoid EMG to detect massive myoclonia or spasms, and a distal EMG (fingers, face) to detect erratic myoclonus. The interictal EEG is very abnormal, showing the suppression-burst pattern (Fig. 16.9). The erratic myoclonus is not related to the bursts. Conversely, the paroxysmal bursts occur synchronously with massive myoclonus. The partial seizures have the usual features of neonatal ones, without any change of the suppression-burst pattern occurring.

Early infantile epileptic encephalopathy (EIEE), or Ohtahara syndrome (1976) begins during the first month of life and is characterized by tonic spasms, occasional unilateral partial seizures, without myoclonus. Brain malformations, often unilateral, are responsible for this syndrome in more than half of the cases. As with EME, it is useful to record electromyogram during EEG. Interictal EEG is of the suppression-burst type. Bursts are longer and intervals are shorter than in EME. Epileptic spasms are associated with a specific pattern consisting in a slow, high and diphasic wave, followed by rapid rhythms, then flattening. The suppression-burst pattern is not observed during the sequences of spasms. Ictal EEG is often asymmetrical. Partial seizures are often occipital alpha or theta discharges.

Other neonatal diseases

Here, EEG appearances are known with regard to the full-term newborn, but they have not yet been described for the premature infant.

Metabolic disturbances

Hypocalcemia occurs frequently during other causes of cerebral distress, such as HIE, which determine EEG appearance. When hypocalcemia is isolated, the EEG is normal, or contains very high spikes or sharp waves, sometimes localized. During seizures, the discharges are of very high amplitude. Reactivity is increased, flattening is longer than usual.

Pyridoxine deficiency is the cause of very early crises, sometimes in utero, which are most often myoclonia, or spasms. EEG is always severely abnormal, with a suppression-burst pattern. The bursts are very high, more than 75 μV, made up of slow waves, slow and rapid spikes, and rapid rhythms. Interburst intervals last 1 to 10 seconds. Bursts can also be made up of very high delta waves, very long periods of flattening, focal spikes, alpha sequences. Mikati et al. (1991) reported discharges, either generalized, or alternating from one hemisphere to the other.

Intravenously injected pyridoxine constitutes a diagnostic tool. Simultaneous recording of EEG is recommended. The seizures stop and the EEG improves rapidly. The procedure must be carried out with caution regarding respiration since severe depression may occur as a result of an increase in GABA.

Other inborn metabolism errors

EEGs in amino acidopathies have common characteristics. The background activity is periodic. Ictal discharges are infrequent, brief, polymorphic, of a low frequency, subclinical, or with atypical manifestations. Background activity is not influenced by the crises.

In some situations, the EEG is more specific. During non-ketotic hyperglycinemia, the periodic aspect is observed as early as the second day of life, is very characteristic and persists during the whole course of the disease. During maple syrup urine disease, at 5 to 10 days of life, there appear sharp and high fast rhythms, and spindle-like bursts of 7–13 Hz, located in rolandic areas, lasting 1 to 4 seconds. These rhythms disappear at 1 month of life (Mises et al., 1983).

Perinatal infections

During the herpetic meningo-encephalitis, seizures are partial and multifocal. The interictal EEG is characterized by stereotyped periodic complexes, separated by intervals of very low amplitude. The complexes do not vary on the same tracing. They consist of slow waves (200 or 400–500 μV in amplitude and 1.5 or 1 second duration) recurring every 2 to 3 seconds; or of sharp diphasic (negative–positive) slow waves occurring every 1.3 to 3 seconds; or of sharp slow-waves (75 to 100 μV in amplitude and 800 ms in duration), recurring every 2 to 4 seconds (Mikati et al., 1990). In the newborn, this abnormal activity is not localized on the temporal areas, but may be recorded everywhere on the hemispheres. Pettay et al. (1972) reported multifocal periodic complexes. These characteristic aspects are infrequent during the first days of the disease, but the EEG is always very abnormal. Owing to very early diagnosis and antiviral therapy, this severe disease is rarely observed. The other infections of the central nervous system are not associated with specific EEG appearances.

EEG abnormalities are linked to the extension and the intensity of the lesions (meningitis, abscesses). The abnormalities associated with abscesses due to gram negative bacteria are sometimes mild, discordant with cerebral extensive lesions. The long-term outcome is usually in agreement with the EEG characteristics.

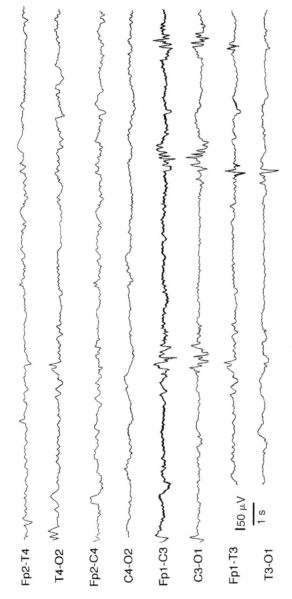

Fp2-T4

T4-O2

Fp2-C4

C4-O2

Fp1-C3

C3-O1

Fp1-T3

T3-O1

50 μV

1 s

Fig. 16.10.   Left ischemic stroke. Left rolandic and temporal interictal abnormalities.

Focal cerebral lesions

These are usually either cerebral infarction due to vascular obstruction of the middle cerebral artery or of its branches, or intracerebral hemorrhages. They can also be from abscesses, Sturge–Weber disease, or abnormalities associated with incontinentia pigmenti.

Ischemic strokes manifest themselves clinically as isolated or serial focal seizures. Ictal EEG shows focal rhythmic discharges in agreement with clinical seizures. Interictal EEG often shows sharp waves or spikes on the same area as ictal discharges (Fig. 16.10).

Intraventricular hemorrhages in the full-term newborn can be uni- or bilateral. Manifestations occur when the hemorrhage is massive and/or associated with parenchymal lesions. Interictal EEG abnormalities are positive rolandic or temporal sharp waves, or persistent rapid spikes (D'Allest et al., 1997). The long-term prognosis can be predicted from background activity.

Cerebral malformations

In migration disorders, the most severe appearances are those of Ohtahara syndrome. Other patterns are frequent, such as focal monorhythmic alpha, theta or delta sequences. These sequences are frequent on the frontal areas; they have variable amplitude and duration. They may be difficult to distinguish from ictal monorhythmic discharges. In this latter case the frequency is slower at the end of the discharge. The alpha discharges of high amplitude, which have been described in cases involving lissencephaly are not present during the neonatal period.

During Aicardi syndrome, the abnormalities vary from suppression-burst patterns to mild ones, but the independence of both hemispheres is constant. Children with hemimegalencephaly exhibit asymmetrical traces, and the abnormalities are often of the suppression-burst type, less severe on the side which seems undamaged.

Neuro-muscular diseases

The EEG may also be essential for ruling out non-cerebral causes in some neurological disturbances, such as spinal amyotrophies, congenital myopathies; in these cases, in spite of clinical difficulties, the EEG is normal.

Conclusions

EEG must be considered as a basic examination in neonates with neurological disorders, or with high risks of sequelae. It is easy to record, non-invasive and inexpensive. The conditions of recording must respect the neonatal particularities and the reading must be carried out by a skilled electroencephalographer.

These descriptions may appear too complicated but, as seen above, precise analysis of EEG – also taking into account gestational age, clinical data (seizures) postnatal age and drugs – is a dramatically efficient mean of predicting outcome in the majority of cases, and of ascertaining the etiology in some doubtful situations. For example, if all the discontinuous tracings are termed suppression-burst, etiology and prognosis are both very uncertain. The characterization of the different patterns of discontinuous activity, on the other hand, makes it possible to recognize underlying diseases accurately and precisely.

In many cases, serial recordings are necessary. The other electroencephalographic methods that can be used in the neonate, such as CFM, are complementary, making it possible to watch continuously over the child between two conventional recordings. Digital EEG offers a dual system: a continuous recording is possible, as for monitoring and, at the same time, precise data are available. New advances in software will make this increasingly simple.

REFERENCES

Aicardi, J. & Goutières, F.(1978). Encéphalopathie myoclonique néonatale. *Electro-encephalography and Clinical Neurophysiology*, **8**, 99–101.

André, M., Matisse, N., Vert, P. & Debruille, C. (1988). Neonatal seizures. Recent aspects. *Neuropediatrics*, **19**, 201–7.

Ashwal, S. (1997). Brain death in the newborn. Current perspectives. *Clinics in Perinatology*, **24**, 859–82.

Baud, O., D'Allest, A. M., Lacaze-Masmonteil, T. et al. (1998). The early diagnosis of periventricular leukomalacia in premature infants with positive rolandic sharp waves on serial electroencephalography. *Journal of Pediatrics*, **132**, 808–12.

Benda, G. I ., Engel, R. C. H. & Zhang, Y. (1989). Prolonged inactive phases during the discontinuous pattern of prematurity in the electroencephalogram of very low birth weight infants. *Electroencephalography and Clinical Neurophysiology*, **72**, 189–197.

Biagioni, E., Biver, P., Pieri, R. & Cioni, G. (1998). Prognostic value of selected EEG features in constantly discontinuous tracings of asphyxiated full-term neonates. *Brain and Development*, **20**.

Biagioni, E., Bartalena, L., Boldrini, A., Pieri, R. & Cioni, G. (2000). Electroencephalography in infants with periventricular leukomalacia: prognostic features at preterm and term age. *Journal of Child Neurology*, **15**, 1–6.

Blume, W. T. & Dreyfus-Brisac, C. (1982). Positive rolandic sharp waves in neonatal EEG. Type and significance. *Electroencephalography and Clinical Neurophysiology*, **53**, 277–82.

Chung, H. J. & Clancy, R. R. (1991). Significance of positive temporal sharp waves in the neonatal electroencephalogram. *Electroencephalography and Clinical Neurophysiology*, **79**, 256–63.

Clancy, R. & Tharp, B. R. (1984). Positive rolandic sharp waves in the electroencephalograms of premature neonates with intraventricular haemorrhage. *Electroencephalography and Clinical Neurophysiology*, 57, 395–404.

Clancy, R. R., Legido, A. & Lewis, D. (1988). Occult neonatal seizures. *Epilepsia*, 29, 256–61.

Connell, J., Oozeer, R., Regev, R. et al. (1987). Continuous four-channel EEG monitoring in the evaluation of echodense ultrasound lesions and cystic leucomalacia. *Archives of Disease in Childhood*, 62, 1019–24.

Cukier, F., André, M., Monod, N. & Dreyfus-Brisac, C. (1972). Apport de l'EEG au diagnostic des hémorragies intraventriculaires du prématuré. *Revue d'EEG et de Neurophysiologie Clinique*, 2, 318–22.

Curzi-Dascalova, L. & Mirmiran, M. (1996). *Manual of Methods for Recording and Analyzing Sleep Wakefulness States in Pre-term and Full-term Infants*, ed. INSERM, Paris, 180 pp.

Curzi-Dascalova, L., Figueroa, J. M., Eiselt, M. et al. (1993). Sleep state organization in premature infants of less than 5 weeks' gestational age. *Pediatric Research*, 34, 624–8.

D'Allest, A. M., Dworzak, P., Nedelcoux, H. et al. (1992). EEG and periventricular leukomalacia in the premature infant. *Biology of the Neonate*, 62, 301.

D'Allest, A. M., Radvanyi, M. F., André, M. et al. (1995). Prognostic value of the EEG in perinatal hypoxic–ischaemic encephalopathy of the term infant. *Developmental Medicine and Child Neurology*, 37, supp 72, 27.

D'Allest, A. M., Navelet, Y., Nedelcoux, H., Dehan, M. & Huault, G. (1997). Hémorragie intra-ventriculaire et ischémie parenchymateuse chez le nouveau-né à terme. *Neurophysiologie Clinique*, 27, 129–38.

Dehan, M., Quillerou, D., Navelet, Y. et al. (1977). Les convulsions du cinquième jour de vie: un nouveau syndrôme? *Archives Françaises de Pédiatrie*, 34, 730–42.

Dreyfus-Brisac, C. (1979). Neonatal electroencephalography. In *Reviews in Perinatal Medicine*, Vol. 3, ed. E. M. Scarpelli & E. V. Cosmi, pp. 397–471. New York: Raven Press.

Dreyfus-Brisac, C., Peschanski, N., Radvanyi, M. F., Cukier-Hemeury, F. & Monod, F. (1981). Convulsions du nouveau-né. Aspects clinique, électroencéphalographique, étiopathogénique et pronostique. *Revue d'EEG et de Neurophysiologie Clinique*, 11, 367–78.

Engel, R. C. H. (1975). *Abnormal Electroencephalograms in the Neonatal Period.* Springfield, IL: Thomas C. C.

Gire, C., Nicaise, C., Roussel, M. et al. (2000). Encéphalopathie hypoxo-ischémique du nouveau-né à terme. Apport de l'électroencéphalogramme et de l'IRM ou de la TDM à l'évaluation pronostique. A propos de 26 observations. *Neurophysiologie Clinique*, 30, 97–107.

Graziani, L. J., Streletz, L. J., Baumgart, S., Cullen, J. & McKee, L. M. (1994). Predictive value of neonatal electroencephalograms before and during extracorporeal membrane oxygenation. *Journal of Pediatrics*, 125, 969–7.

Hahn, J. S., Vaucher, Y., Bejar, R. & Coen, R. W. (1993). Electroencephalographic and neuro-imaging findings in neonates undergoing extracorporeal membrane oxygenation. *Neuropediatrics*, 24, 19–24.

Hascoët, J. M., André, M., Didier, F., Le Courtois, I., Dalati, M. & Buchweiller, M. C. (1995). Acute cerebral blood velocity and EEG changes during and after natural versus synthetic surfactant. *Pediatric Research*, 37, 211A.

Hayakawa, F., Okumura, A., Kato, T., Kuno, K. & Watanabe, K. (1997). Dysmature EEG pattern in EEG of preterm infants with cognitive impairment: maturation arrest caused by prolonged mild CNS depression. *Brain and Development*, **19**, 122–5.

Hellström-Westas, L., Rosen, I. & Svenningsen, N. W. (1991). Cerebral function monitoring during the first week of life in extremely small low birthweight (ESLBW) infants. *Neuropediatrics*, **22**, 27–32.

Holthausen, K., Breidbach, O., Scheidt, B. & Frenzel, J. (2000). Brain dysmaturity index for automatic detection of high-risk infants. *Pediatric Neurology*, **22**, 187–91.

Lamblin, M. D., Racoussot, S., Pierrat, V. et al. (1996) Encéphalopathie anoxo-ischémique du nouveau-né à terme. Apport de l'électroencéphalogramme et de l'échographie transfontanellaire à l'évaluation pronostique. A propos de 29 observations. *Neurophysiologie Clinique*, **26**, 369–78.

Laroia, N., Guillet, R., Burchfield, J. & McBride, M. C. (1998). EEG background as predictor of electrographic seizures in high-risk neonates. *Epilepsia*, **39**, 545–51.

Lombroso, C. T. & Holmes, G. L. (1993). Value of the EEG in neonatal seizures. *Journal of Epilepsy*, **6**, 39–70.

McCutchen, C. B., Coen, R. & Iragui, V. J. (1985). Periodic lateralized epileptiform discharges in asphyxiated neonates. *Electroencephalography and Clinical Neurophysiology*, **6**, 210–17.

Magny, J. F., D'Allest, A. M., Nedelcoux, H., Zupan, V. & Dehan, M. (1994). Midazolam and myoclonus in neonate. *European Journal of Pediatrics*, **153**, 389.

Marret, S., Jeannot, E., Parain, D., Samson-Dollfus, D. & Fessard, C. (1989). Pointes positives rolandiques ischémie périventriculaire et devenir neurologique. Etude prospective chez 66 prématurés. *Archives Françaises de Pédiatrie*, **46**, 249–54.

Marret, S., Parain, D., Menard, J. F., Blanc, T. et al. (1997). Prognostic value of neonatal electroencephalography in premature newborns less than 33 weeks of gestational age. *Electroencephalography and Clinical Neurophysiology*, **102**, 178–85.

Mikati, M. A., Peraru, E., Krishnamoorthy, K., Lombroso, C. T. (1990). Neonatal herpes simplex meningoencephalitis: EEG investigations and clinical correlates. *Neurology*, **40**, 1433–7.

Mikati, M. A., Trevathan, E., Krishnamoorthy, K. S. & Lombroso, C. T. (1991). Pyridoxine-dependent epilepsy: EEG investigations and long-term follow-up. *Electroencephalography and Clinical Neurophysiology*, **78**, 215–21.

Mises, J., Moussalli-Salefranque, F., Hagenmuller, M. P. & Plouin, P. (1983). Les rythmes rapides dans les maladies métaboliques chez l'enfant. *Revue d'EEG et de Neurophysiologie Clinique*, **13**, 61–7.

Mizrahi, E. M. & Kellaway, P. (1987). Characterization and classification of neonatal seizures. *Neurology*, **37**, 1837–44.

Mizrahi, E. M. & Kellaway, P. (1998). Diagnosis and management of neonatal seizures. Lippincott-Raven, Philadelphia.

Monod, N., Pajot, N. & Guidasci, S. (1972). The neonatal EEG: statistical studies and prognostic value in full-term and pre-term babies. *Electroencephalography and Clinical Neurophysiology*, **32**, 529–44.

Murdoch Eaton, D. G., Wertheim, D., Oozeer, R., Royston, P., Dubowitz, L. & Dubowitz, V. (1992). The effect of pethidine on the neonatal EEG. *Developmental Medicine and Child Neurology*, **34**, 155–63.

Navelet, Y., D'Allest, A. M., Dehan, M. & Gabilan, J. C. (1981). A propos du syndrome des convulsions néonatales du cinquième jour. *Revue d'EEG et de Neurophysiologie Clinique*, 11, 390–6.

Novotny, E. J., Tharp, B. R., Coen, R. W., Bejar, R., Enzmann, D. & Vaucher, Y. E. (1987). Positive rolandic sharp waves in the EEG of the premature infant. *Neurology*, 37, 1481–6.

Ohtahara, S., Ishida, T., Oka, E. et al. (1976). On the age-dependent epileptic syndromes: the early infantile encephalopathy with suppression-burst. *Brain and Development*, 8, 270–88.

Pettay, O., Leinikki, P., Doinner, M. & Lapinlimer, K. (1972). Herpes simplex virus infection in the newborn. *Archives of Disease in Childhood*, 47, 97–103.

Pezzani, C., Radvanyi-Bouvet, M. F., Relier, J. P. & Monod, N. (1986). Neonatal electroencephalography during the first twenty-four hours of life in full-term newborn infants. *Neuropediatrics*, 17, 11–18.

Radvanyi-Bouvet, M. F., Vallecalle, M. H., Morel-Kahn, F., Relier, J. P. & Dreyfus-Brisac, C. (1985). Seizures and electrical discharges in premature infants. *Neuropediatrics*, 16, 143–8.

Radvanyi-Bouvet, M. F., Torricelli, A., Rey, E., Bavoux, F. & Walti, H. (1990). Effects of lidocaine on seizures in the neonatal period: some electroclinical aspects. In *Neonatal Seizures*, eds. C.G. Wasterlain & P. Vert. pp 275–83. Raven, New York.

Scavone, C., Radvanyi-Bouvet, M. F., Morel-Kahn, F. & Dreyfus-Brisac, C. (1985). Coma après souffrance foetale aigüe chez le nouveau-né à terme: évolution électroclinique. *Revue d'EEG et de Neurophysiologie Clinique*, 15, 279–88.

Scher, M. S., Kosaburo, A., Beggarly, M. E., Hamid, M. Y., Steppe, D. A. & Painter, M. J. (1993). Electrographic seizures in preterm and full-term neonates: clinical correlates, associated brain lesions, and risk for neurologic sequelae. *Pediatrics*, 91, 128–34.

Scher, M. S., Alvin, J. & Gaus, L. (1994). Uncoupling of electrical and clinical expression of neonatal seizures after antiepileptic drug administration. *Pediatric Neurology*, 11, 83.

Scher, M. S., Steppe, D. A., Sclabassi, R. J. & Banks, D. L. (1997). Regional differences in spectral EEG measures between healthy term and preterm infants. *Pediatric Neurology*, 17, 218–23.

Selton, D. & André, M. (1997). Prognosis of hypoxic–ischaemic encephalopathy in full-term newborns – value of neonatal electroencephalography. *Neuropediatrics*, 28, 276–80.

Takeuchi, T. & Watanabe, K. (1989). The EEG evolution and neurological prognosis of perinatal hypoxia in neonates. *Brain and Development*, 11, 115–20.

Tharp, B. R., Scher, M. S. & Clancy, R. R. (1989). Serial EEGs in normal and abnormal infants with birth weights less than 1200 grams – a prospective study with long term follow-up. *Neuropediatrics*, 20, 64–72.

Vecchierini-Blineau, M. F., Nguyen The Tich, S., Debillon, T., Fleury, M. A. & Roze, J. C. (1996). Leucomalacies périventriculaires graves: à propos de quelques aspects électroencéphalographiques particuliers. *Neurophysiologie Clinique*, 26, 102–8.

Watanabe, K., Negoro, T., Inokuma, K. & Yamazaki, T. (1984). Subclinical delta status in the newborn – an unfavourable prognostic sign. *Revue d'EEG et de Neurophysiologie Clinique*, 15, 125–31.

Young, G. B. & Da Silva, O. P. (2000). Effects of morphine on the electroencephalograms of neonates: a prospective, observational study. *Clinical Neurophysiology*, 111, 1955–60.

17

Cerebral function monitoring

Lena Hellström-Westas

Department of Paediatrics, University Hospital, Lund, Sweden

Continuous electrophysiologic monitoring of cerebral activity is relatively new in neonatal intensive care. Since 1990, the quality of neonatal intensive care has improved. Medical care is for some infants still a matter of survival, but there is also concern for the neurological quality of life in survivors. One of the more important issues in neonatal care is to develop methods for on-line monitoring of cerebral function and early intervention in order to reduce risks for subsequent neurological handicap.

It is not possible to monitor overall brain function in a newborn infant. However, electrocortical function, as recorded with EEG, closely reflects the functional state of the brain (Ingvar et al., 1976). In newborn infants, the electrocortical background activity during the acute phase of illness has been shown to be a sensitive predictor of later neurological outcome (Holmes & Lombroso, 1990; Lombroso & Holmes, 1993; Monod et al., 1972). In both full-term and premature infants, postmortem neuropathological examinations have shown a direct relation between the number of damaged neurons and EEG background activity (Aso et al., 1989, 1993).

Continuous EEG monitoring is a development of the standard EEG. Standard EEG can be used for long-term monitoring, but for practical reasons simplification and time-compression of the EEG has to be accomplished. As a consequence, the possibility of detailed diagnosis is lost. At the same time, however, another important feature is gained – the possibility to continuously follow long-term trends and changes in cerebroelectrical activity on-line.

EEG monitoring systems

There are various types of EEG monitoring systems, the majority constructed for use after the neonatal period. Some EEG monitoring devices have been developed in combination with video techniques, which are commonly used in epilepsy investigations in older patients. Such EEG video monitoring techniques have been used in neonates and have contributed much to our knowledge of the clinical behaviour of neonatal seizures (Mizrahi & Kellaway, 1987). Other techniques have also been successfully used in newborn infants, e.g. the cerebral function monitor (CFM), the Oxford Medilog EEG (tape-recorded EEG), the Cerebro-Trac, and systems utilizing compressed spectral array (CSA) (Archbald et al., 1984; Connell et al., 1987a,b; Eyre et al., 1983; Hellström-Westas et al., 1985; Murdoch-Eaton et al., 1994a; Talwar & Torres 1988). This chapter on cerebral function monitoring will deal mainly with the amplitude-integrated EEG (aEEG) as recorded by the cerebral function monitor (CFM).

The cerebral function monitor (CFM 4640 and CFM Multitrace 2, Lectromed Devices Ltd.) records a single-channel (optional 2 channels) EEG from a pair of parietal electrodes. The EEG is first amplified and passed through an asymmetric band pass filter which strongly attenuates activity below 2 Hz and above 15 Hz in order to minimize artefacts from, e.g. sweating, ECG and electrical interference (Prior & Maynard, 1986). The EEG processing also includes semilogarithmic amplitude compression, rectifying, smoothing and time compression. The bandwidth in the output reflects variations in minimum and maximum EEG amplitude. The semilogarithmic output allows changes in background activity with very low voltage ($<5\,\mu V$) to be identifiable. The signal is written out on slow speed paper (paper speed 6 cm/h or 30 cm/h in the CFM 4640, or changeable from 1 mm/min to 100 mm/s in the CFM Multitrace 2). The electrode impedance is recorded continuously, in parallel with the EEG, in order to supervise the technical quality of the recording. Fig. 17.1 shows examples of normal CFM tracings from newborn infants of different gestational ages (Thornberg & Thiringer, 1990). The cerebral function analysing monitor (CFAM, RDM Consultants Ltd) is a development of the CFM and includes 2-channel EEG, computerized storage of the signal, frequency analysis and a possibility of performing evoked potentials (Maynard & Jenkinson, 1984). Critikon made a similar instrument without the possibility of performing evoked potentials during the 1980s.

Prior and Maynard created the cerebral function monitor (CFM) in the UK in the late 1960s. According to Prior, a clinical neurophysiologist, a brain monitoring system should have the following features: simplicity, reasonable cost, reliability, direct information about neuronal function, non-invasiveness and wide applicability, quantification and output, automatic operation, and flexibility (Prior & Maynard, 1986). The CFM was developed accordingly. The device was constructed for adult patients in intensive care, e.g. after cardiac arrest, during status epilepticus and after heart surgery (Maynard et al., 1969). The technique has been evaluated in several studies under various clinical circumstances in both children and adults (Prior & Maynard, 1986; Stidham et al., 1980; Viniker et al., 1984). The CFM has also been compared with other EEG monitoring techniques. There is a good correlation between findings in the CFM and the tape-recorded EEG; however, some very short (duration <30 s) seizures may not be detectable with the CFM (Hellström-

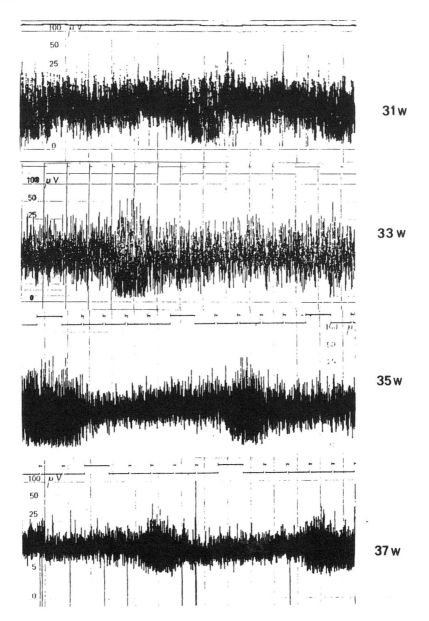

Fig. 17.1.   Normal CFM tracings from infants with gestational ages 31 to 37 weeks. The bandwidth reflects minimum and maximum voltage. As the infants mature and the EEG becomes more continuous, a rise in the level of the background activity can be seen in the CFM. Smooth cyclical changes of the bandwidth are due to sleep–wake cycling. The EEG during quiet sleep shows periods with high voltage slow activity or discontinuous acitivity (tracé alternant) which corresponds to the broad bandwidth pattern. Active sleep and awake periods, relatively narrow bandwidth, cannot be distinguished from each other in the CFM. (From Thornberg & Thiringer, 1990, with permission.)

Westas, 1992; Thiringer et al., 1986). The number of EEG channels necessary for detection of epileptiform activity was also evaluated (Hellström-Westas, 1992). When five channels of tape-recorded EEG were recorded simultaneously with the biparietal single-channel CFM, all seizures (duration > 30 s) were identifiable in the CFM tracing. However, later studies have shown that, with a reduced number of EEG channels, some seizures may be missed (Bye & Flanagan, 1995). The output from compressed spectral array (CSA) systems gives an evaluation of both EEG frequency and amplitude. Various systems for CSA are available, some have also been compared with the CFM (Aziz et al., 1986; Glaria & Murray, 1985; Grundy et al., 1981; Talwar & Torres, 1988). The CSA and CFM techniques were considered to be equal in detecting seizure activity, and changes in background activity but the CFM was considered to be somewhat easier to interpret.

Another system, the Oxford Medilog-system (Oxford 9000 system) has also been used for monitoring of newborn infants. This system, which is now replaced by a 16-channel digital storing equipment, utilizes a battery-powered EEG 4–8 channel tape-recorder for recording of raw EEG. Twenty-four hours of EEG is recorded on a 60-minute standard cassette tape and later replayed in a special monitoring unit (Connell et al., 1987a, b; Eyre et al., 1988). One or two channels can also be used for recording electrocardiography (ECG) and respiration. For research purposes, the Medilog tape-recorder has also been connected to a computer which enabled on-line monitoring of newborn infants (Wertheim et al., 1991).

Reliable interpretation of EEG monitoring recordings is dependent on adequate training in a certain technique, and that is probably the reason why different monitoring techniques may be equally efficient for detecting abnormalities. Further development of EEG monitoring systems will probably include automated computer processing and provide alarms for epileptic seizure activity or deterioration of background activity, which will result in increased accuracy in interpretation. An example of a developed computerized EEG monitoring system, based on aEEG technique, is shown in Fig. 17.2.

Indications for EEG monitoring

EEG monitoring should be viewed as part of other clinical monitoring in the neonatal intensive care unit (NICU). There are several situations when EEG monitoring will add information to the clinical evaluation of a sick newborn baby and guide medical decisions.

(i) Most newborn infants who require intensive care are at risk of developing cerebral complications (Hellström-Westas et al., 1990). Clinical neurological examinations are often of limited value under these conditions, due to, e.g. sedation for mechanical ventilation.

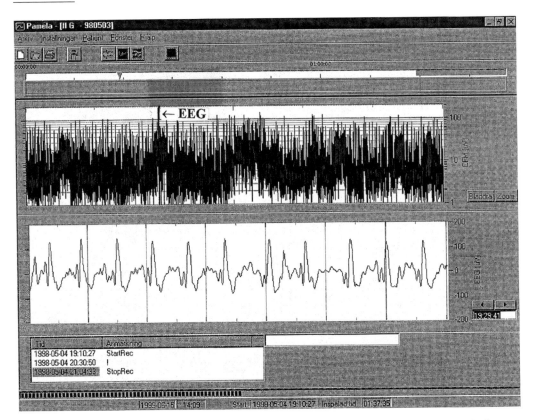

Fig. 17.2.   Computerized aEEG showing sawtooth pattern, representing recurrent seizures, in the aEEG (upper tracing) and epileptic seizure activity in the simultaneously recorded EEG (lower tracing). (Previously not published.)

(ii) **Early diagnosis of seizures.** Seizures are relatively common in distressed and sick newborn infants. The seizures are often subclinical or subtle, and therefore difficult to diagnose (Clancy et al., 1988; Hellström-Westas et al., 1985; Mizrahi & Kellaway, 1987).

(iii) **Prognosis.** Cerebroelectrical background activity in the EEG is a sensitive predictor of later neurological outcome in newborn babies, see below (Archbald et al., 1984; Eken et al., 1995; Hellström-Westas et al., 1995b; Thornberg & Ekström-Jodal 1994; Wertheim et al., 1995).

Interpretation of amplitude-integrated EEG (aEEG/CFM)

Infants with different maturity and with various medical problems are treated in NICUs. Clinical interpretation of both EEG and aEEG relies mainly on pattern recognition (Thornberg & Thiringer 1990; Verma et al., 1984). The EEG/aEEG background in newborn infants is characterized by a gradual change from discontinuous, in the very premature infant, to continuous in the more mature infant. The normal discontinuous background pattern of premature infants is called *tracé discontinu*, and includes an intermittent pattern with periods of low voltage intermixed with periods with more continuous activity of various amplitudes and frequencies. Burst suppression is a pathological discontinuous pattern including periods with electrocerebral silence (inactivity) and high voltage burst activity and can also be seen in full-term infants (Holmes & Lombroso, 1990). Since the aEEG is a development of the EEG, knowledge from standard EEG can be incorporated directly when interpreting aEEG. Quantification for comparative evaluation of time-periods or recordings can be done by, for instance, counting burst activity over a certain predefined amplitude or by measuring interburst intervals (Connell et al., 1987a,b; Thornberg & Thiringer, 1990).

Factors which may affect and depress the EEG/aEEG background include sedative and antiepileptic medications. Transient depression of shorter duration can be seen after surfactant treatment, during hypoxia, hypoglycemia and acidosis (Bell et al., 1993; Hellström-Westas et al., 1990, 1992; Murdoch-Eaton et al., 1994b). The amplitude of the background pattern may be affected by several factors, one being the distance between the recording electrodes, as the amplitude increases with the distance between the electrodes (Prior & Maynard, 1986). Specific neonatal artefacts include cephalic hematoma, which may render falsely low amplitude of the EEG/aEEG. The most important factor for the amplitude is, however, the state of the brain, e.g. a newborn infant with severe brain damage after birth asphyxia usually shows low-voltage or discontinuous background activity (Hellström-Westas et al., 1995b). In asymmetrical cerebral lesions, e.g. middle cerebral artery infarction, asymmetry of cerebroelectrical background activity is a common finding but requires recording from more than one single EEG/aEEG channel to be discovered (Mercuri et al., 1999).

Epileptic seizure activity in the aEEG is characterized by a sudden rise of the cerebroelectrical background level. Repeated seizure activity in the aEEG looks like a saw-tooth when the epileptic seizure activity is recurrently waxing and waning (see Figs. 17.3 and 17.4(*a*)). However, if an infant has continuous epileptic seizure activity, the characteristic 'saw-tooth pattern' may not be evident, since the background pattern will be continuously high voltage. In these instances, the seizure activity may easily be overlooked unless a standard EEG is recorded simultaneously.

In healthy premature infants, sleep–wake cycling can be identified in aEEG from around 30 weeks postconceptional age (Greisen et al., 1985). Also, in some very premature infants, with gestational age as low as 25–26 weeks, cyclical changes of the background activity can be seen (see Fig. 17.4(*d*)) (Hellström-Westas et al., 1991). Sick or prematurely born infants treated in NICUs may suffer from repeated

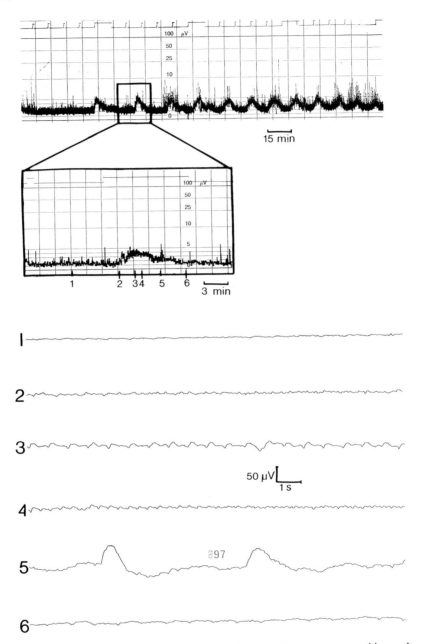

Fig. 17.3.   Continuous recording of CFM and tape recorded Medilog EEG. Repeated low voltage epileptic seizure activity (saw-tooth pattern) on an inactive background in a full-term infant who died from birth asphyxia. (Hellström-Westas, 1992, with permission.)

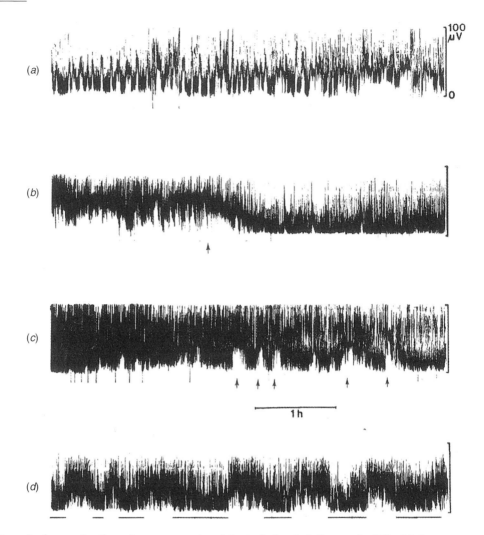

Fig. 17.4.   Background patterns in very premature infants during their first week of life. (*a*) Preterm
infant with gestational age (ga) 28 weeks, recurrent epileptic seizure activity during
development of IVH-PVH. (*b*) Preterm infant, ga 26 weeks, initially a mixture of
continuous/discontinous activity changing into a discontinuous burst–suppression pattern
after phenobarbital and intubation. (*c*) Discontinuous background pattern in a
mechanically ventilated and sedated infant, ga 30 weeks. Arrows indicate reactivity to
handling during nursing care procedures. (*d*) Cyclical changes in background activity in a
preterm infant, ga 26 weeks. Periods resembling quiet sleep periods in more mature
infants are underlined. (Hellström-Westas et al., 1991, with permission.)

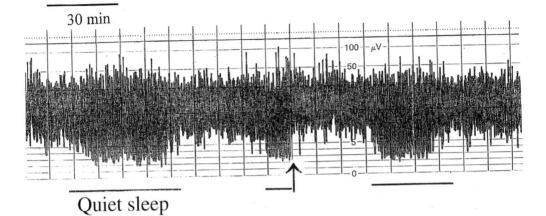

Fig. 17.5.   Interrupted quiet sleep during nursing care procedure in a premature infant with postconceptional age 32 weeks. (Previously not published.)

handling. Fig. 17.5 shows an example of interrupted quiet sleep for a routine care procedure in a premature infant.

Localization of abnormal activity, e.g. epileptic foci, sharp-wave activity or localized delta activity requires several channels of EEG to be recorded and is usually not possible with EEG monitoring systems. The aEEG output includes a weighted signal of the major EEG frequencies and additional information on EEG frequencies is only given in the computerized CFAM and the Critikon-CFM. Although EEG monitoring systems are usually constructed to reject artefacts, these may sometimes disturb the recordings. We have not been able to record reliable aEEG with the CFM in babies on high-frequency ventilation.

Diagnosing neonatal seizures

Epileptic seizures are sometimes difficult to diagnose in the neonatal period. A majority of seizures are subclinical (Clancy et al., 1988), and a majority of clinically suspected seizures do not have corresponding electrographic seizure activity (Mizrahi & Kellaway, 1987). In order to diagnose neonatal seizures correctly, a combined approach using EEG and EEG monitoring is probably optimal. The detailed information obtained by the standard EEG is essential, but still the recording is limited to a certain time period when the infant may not have any seizures.

Neonatal seizures are probably more common than previously believed, however, the exact prevalence is not known. The incidence of seizures in a NICU population is very much related to the diagnostic technique used and also varies depending on the population studied. In NICU populations the incidence of epileptic seizures may range from 2.3%, if EEG-verified clinical seizures are required for diagnosis, up to 20% in high-risk populations supervised with EEG monitoring (Connell et al., 1989; Helmers et al., 1997; Legido et al., 1991). In selected populations of high-risk infants, an even higher incidence of seizure can be found. Among premature infants, developing intraventricular–periventricular hemorrhage (IVH–PVH) epileptic seizure activity can be detected with EEG monitoring in 65–75% of infants (Greisen et al., 1987; Hellström-Westas et al., 1991). We used a combination of standard EEG and aEEG to identify infants with seizures in our NICU and obtained an incidence of 4.5% of neonatal seizures in our patient population during a 2-year period (Hellström-Westas et al., 1995a). The reason why this combined diagnostic approach did not reveal a higher incidence is that most infants with seizures have a combination of clinical and subclinical seizures and therefore will be recognized because of their clinical seizures at some time, even if the majority of seizures are subclinical.

The view that all infants with neonatal seizures need continuing long-term prophylactic antiepileptic treatment (AET) has recently been challenged. The risk for seizure recurrence is probably not as high as previously believed, but may still be rather high in some populations (Clancy & Legido, 1991). A normal EEG and a normal neurological examination have been considered to be good markers for low risk of seizure recurrence. With the guidance of aEEG, we have treated neonatal seizures for shorter time periods with very few relapses. In 36 surviving children (from a population of 58 infants with neonatal seizures), closely followed for at least 1 year, only three infants had recurrence of seizures in spite of a median antiepileptic treatment time of 4.5 days. Of these three infants, one was already on prophylactic medication, one was treated for 65 days and the third child had been treated for 6 days (Hellström-Westas et al., 1995a). A possible explanation of why so few children had recurrence of seizures is that, with aEEG monitoring, AET was more efficiently used and a majority of subclinical seizures were also treated (Hellström-Westas et al., 1988). A common finding in EEG monitoring, after a loading dose of antiepileptic medication, is that clinical seizures disappear while subclinical seizures persist (Hellström-Westas et al., 1988, 1995a; Hakeem & Wallace 1990).

Prediction of outcome

The electrocortical background activity in EEG/aEEG is a highly sensitive predictor of later neurological outcome in newborn infants if recorded early in the clinical course after, e.g. a severe hypoxic–ischemic incident (Bjerre et al., 1983). The main type of background activity is the most sensitive feature. In full-term asphyxiated infants, aEEG has been shown to give accurate prognostic information in around 90% of infants at 6 hours postnatal age (Hellström-Westas et al., 1995b;

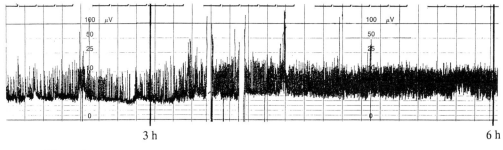

3 h   6 h

Discontinuous   Continuous

Fig. 17.6.   CFM tracing in severely asphyxiated full-term infant with good outcome. Background
activity at 3 hours postnatal age is discontinuous with burst-suppression pattern. At 6
hours the background pattern has changed into a continuous normal voltage pattern
(Previously not published.)

Eken et al., 1995). Infants with inactive or very low voltage activity tracings all had
a poor outcome (death or severe handicap), while almost all (25/26) with continuous normal voltage activity had a good outcome (healthy or minor handicap). In
infants with burst suppression background during the first 6 hours after birth
asphyxia the prognosis was more uncertain. A majority (11/14) of the infants had
a poor outcome, however, three infants actually developed well (Hellström-Westas
et al., 1995b). Recently, we have examined aEEG tracings at a postnatal age of 3
hours in full-term babies with birth asphyxia. Even at this very early postnatal age,
the outcome in over 80% of infants was correctly predicted by the background
pattern (Toet et al., 1999). Even if the early EEG is severely abnormal, the EEG background normalizes in many infants within 1–2 weeks after the asphyxic incident.
The speed with which the EEG background recovers seems to be directly related to
the severity of the asphyxtic insult, see Fig. 17.6 (Gunn et al., 1992; Hellström-
Westas et al., 1995b; Toet et al., 1999; Williams et al., 1992). In the next few years,
this information may aid medical decisions and identify high-risk infants who
might benefit from early therapeutic intervention (al Nageeb et al., 1999). The
neurophysiology behind the various background patterns in newborn infants is not
entirely known. Burst-suppression is usually a marker of severe brain damage in
full-term infants and seems to constitute a total disconnection in brain circuits
between cerebral cortex and deeper layers, e.g. thalamus (Grigg-Damberger et al.,
1989; Steriade et al., 1994). In asphyxiated fetal sheep, return of EEG with a continuous low voltage seizure pattern seems to be a marker of parasagittal injury
(Williams et al., 1992; Gunn et al., 1992). In postmortem studies of newborn
infants, Aso and colleagues found that isoelectric EEG was correlated with widespread encephalomalacia involving the cerebral cortex, corpus striatum, thalamus,

midbrain and pons (Aso et al., 1989). Burst suppression was also related to multi-focal severe brain damage but no common damaged brain structures were identified in these infants (Aso et al., 1989).

In some very premature infants, repeated EEG examinations during the neonatal period are necessary for prediction of later outcome (Tharp et al., 1989). In spite of previous findings, we found that aEEG during the first week of life in very premature infants had the same accuracy for prediction of outcome as ultrasonography for diagnosing IVH–PVH (Hellström-Westas et al., 1991). In well infants with gestational age as low as 26 weeks, the presence of a cyclical pattern in the aEEG, resembling sleep–wake cycling in more mature premature infants was predictive of good neurological outcome (see Fig. 17.4(*d*)). Preliminary studies also show that gross neurological outcome can be predicted by aEEG very early during the neonatal period in premature infants with large IVH–PVH (Hellström-Westas et al., 1998). The number of bursts per hour during the first days of life was predictive of later outcome and could distinguish infants with 'good' outcome (healthy or minor handicap) from infants with 'poor' outcome (severe cerebral palsy, multihandicap).

EEG monitoring in premature infants with IVH–PVH and PVL

In premature infants, the development of IVH–PVH and periventricular leukomalacia (PVL) is associated with depressed EEG background and presence of epileptic seizure activity. The degree of EEG background depression is related both to the size of the IVH–PVH and to the number of damaged brain structures (Aso et al., 1993; Bunt et al., 1996; Connell et al., 1987a,b, 1988; Greisen et al., 1987; Hellström-Westas et al., 1991, 1998; Watanabe et al., 1983). The EEG depression often precedes ultrasound findings (Connell et al., 1987a,b). The degree of depression of the EEG background activity is subsequently related to the degree of brain damage in premature infants and has also proved to contain early prognostic information (see above).

Epileptic seizure activity is a common finding in EEG monitoring recordings during the development of IVH–PVH and during the acute phase of PVL (Connell et al., 1987a,b, 1988; Greisen et al., 1987; Hellström-Westas et al., 1991; Watanabe et al., 1983). In around 65–75% of these infants, epileptic seizure activity, often entirely subclinical, can be identified. In a population of premature infants born before 32 weeks (mean 28 weeks) gestational age and with aEEG recorded during their first 50 hours of life, seizure activity was detected in two-thirds of infants developing IVH–PVH (Greisen et al., 1987). In a somewhat more immature population with mean gestational age 26 weeks, epileptic seizure activity, which was usually subclinical or subtle, was found in around 75% of infants developing IVH–PVH during their first week of life (Hellström-Westas et al., 1991). Presence of subclinical seizure activity during development of large IVH/PVH does not seem to be a marker of poor outcome; however, clinical convulsions seem to be predictors of poor outcome in these infants (Hellström-Westas et al., 1998).

Conclusions

The EEG monitoring systems that are commercially available today have not been developed specifically for neonatal use. However, some devices have worked very well, in this context. The available techniques for EEG monitoring need further development. Some infants may be more sensitive than others to transient hypoxia and hypoglycemia, but with the present techniques we may only detect marked abnormalities (Bunt et al., 1996; Hellström-Westas et al., 1990). It is clear that more subtle physiological changes, which might affect brain function adversely, can be detected using more sophisticated systems (Murdoch-Eaton et al., 1994a).

EEG monitoring has been applied in neonatal intensive care for at least 20 years (Bjerre et al., 1983; Eyre et al., 1983; Verma et al., 1984). The use of EEG monitoring systems for supervision of brain function in severely ill newborn infants is increasing, and in the near future will probably constitute part of standard monitoring in many neonatal units. We have used the CFM for cerebral monitoring since 1978 and presently we monitor around 15–20% of all newborn infants in our NICU for clinical reasons. The main indications for EEG monitoring are long-term supervision of the functional state of the brain in severely ill neonates, prediction of neurological outcome and seizure detection. With developed EEG monitoring systems, possibilities for automatic alarms, e.g. when background activity deteriorates or when epileptiform seizure activity appears, will further increase the clinical usefulness. EEG monitoring can never substitute for the standard EEG, but the two techniques should be used as complements to each other. In order to use EEG monitoring in a rational way, close collaboration should be established with clinical neurophysiologists.

REFERENCES

al Naqeeb, N., Edwards, A. D., Cowan, F. M. & Azzopardi, D. (1999). Assessment of neonatal encephalopathy by amplitude-integrated electroencephalography. *Pediatrics*, **103**, 1263–71.

Archbald, F., Verma, U. L., Tejani, N. A & Handwerker, S. M. (1984). Cerebral function monitor in the neonate. II. Birth asphyxia. *Developmental Medicine and Child Neurology*, **26**, 162–8.

Aso, K., Scher, M. S. & Barmada, M. A. (1989). Neonatal electroencephalography and neuropathology. *Journal of Clinical Neurophysiology*, **6**, 103–23.

Aso, K., Abdad-Barmada, M. & Scher, M. (1993). EEG and the neuropathology in premature neonates with intraventricular hemorrhage. *Journal of Clinical Neurophysiology*, **10**, 304–13.

Aziz, S., Wallace, S., Murphy, J., Sainsbury, C. & Gray, O. (1986). Cotside EEG monitoring using computerized spectral analysis. *Archives of Disease in Childhood*, **61**, 242–6.

Bell, A. H., Greisen, G. & Pryds, O. (1993). Comparison of the effects of phenobarbitone and morphine administration on EEG activity in preterm babies. *Acta Paediatrica*, **82**, 35–9.

Bjerre, I., Hellström-Westas, L., Rosén, I. & Svenningsen, N. W. (1983). Monitoring of cerebral function after severe birth asphyxia in infancy. *Archives of Disease in Childhood*, **58**, 997–1002.

Bunt, J. E., Gavilanes, A. W., Reulen, J. P., Blanco, C. E. & Vles, J. S. (1996). The influence of acute hypoxemia and hypovolemic hypotension on neuronal brain activity measured by the cerebral function monitor in new-born piglets. *Neuropediatrics*, **27**, 260–26

Bye, A. M. & Flanagan, D. (1995). Spatial and temporal characteristics of neonatal seizures. *Epilepsia*, **36**, 1009–16.

Clancy, R. R. & Legido, A. (1991). Postnatal epilepsy after EEG-confirmed neonatal seizures. *Epilepsia*, **32**, 61–76.

Clancy, R. R., Legido, A. & Lewis, D. (1988). Occult neonatal seizures. *Epilepsia*, **29**, 256–61.

Connell, J. A., Oozeer, R. & Dubowitz, V. (1987a). Continuous 4-channel EEG monitoring: a guide to interpretation, with normal values, in preterm infants. *Neuropediatrics*, **18**, 138–45.

Connell, J., Oozeer, R., Regev, R., de Vries, L.S., Dubowitz, L. M. S. & Dubowitz, V. (1987b). Continuous four-channel EEG monitoring in the evaluation of echodense ultrasound lesions and cystic leukomalacia. *Archives of Disease in Childhood*, **62**, 1019–24.

Connell, J., de Vries, L., Oozeer, R., Regev, R., Dubowitz, L. M. S. & Dubowitz, V. (1988). Predictive value of early continuous electroencephalogram monitoring in ventilated preterm infants with intraventricular hemorrhage. *Pediatrics*, **82**, 337–43.

Connell, J. A., Oozeer, R., de Vries, L., Dubowitz, L. M. S. & Dubowitz, V. (1989). Clinical and EEG response to anticonvulsants in neonatal seizures. *Archives of Disease in Childhood*, **64**, 459–64.

Eken, P., Toet, M. C., Groenendaal, F. & de Vries, L. S. (1995). Predictive value of early neuro-imaging, pulsed Doppler and neurophysiology in full term infants with hypoxic-ischaemic encephalopathy. *Archives of Disease in Childhood*, **73**, F75–F80.

Eyre, J. A., Oozeer, R. & Wilkinson A. R. (1983). Diagnosis of neonatal seizure by continuous recording and rapid analysis of the electroencephalogram. *Archives of Disease in Childhood*, **58**, 785–90.

Eyre, J. A., Nanei, S. & Wilkinson, A. R. (1988). Quantification of changes in normal neonatal EEGs with gestation from continuous five-day recordings. *Developmental Medicine and Child Neurology*, **30**, 599–607.

Glaria, A. P. & Murray, A. (1985). Comparison of EEG monitoring techniques: an evaluation during cardiac surgery. *Electroencephalography and Clinical Neurophysiology*, **61**, 323–30.

Greisen, G., Hellström-Westas, L., Lou, H., Rosén, I. & Svenningsen, N. W. (1985). Sleep-waking shifts and cerebral blood flow in stable preterm infants. *Pediatric Research*, **19**, 1156–9.

Greisen, G., Hellström-Westas, L., Lou, H., Rosén, I. & Svenningsen, N. W. (1987). EEG depression and germinal layer haemorrhage in the new-born. *Acta Paediatrica Scandinavica*, **76**, 519–25.

Grigg-Damberger, M. M., Coker, S. B., Halsey, C. L. & Anderson, C. L. (1989). Neonatal burst-suppression: its developmental significance. *Pediatric Neurology*, **5**, 84–92.

Grundy, B. L., Sanderson, A. C., Webster, M. W., Rickey, E. T., Procopio, P. & Kavanjia, P. N. (1981). Hemiparesis following carotid endarterectomy: comparison of monitoring methods. *Anesthesiology*, **55**, 462–6.

Gunn, A. J., Parer, J. T., Mallard, C. E., Williams, C. E. & Gluckman, P. D. (1992). Cerebral histologic and electrocorticographic changes after asphyxia in fetal sheep. *Pediatric Research*, **31**, 486–91.

Hakeem, V. F. & Wallace, S. J. (1990). EEG monitoring of therapy for neonatal seizures. *Developmental Medicine and Child Neurology*, **32**, 858–64.

Hellström-Westas, L. (1992). Comparison between tape-recorded and amplitude-integrated EEG monitoring in sick newborn infants. *Acta Paediatrica*, **81**, 812–19.

Hellström-Westas, L., Rosén, I. & Svenningsen, N. W. (1985). Silent seizures in sick infants in early life. *Acta Paediatrica Scandinavica*, **74**, 741–8.

Hellström-Westas, L., Westgren, U., Rosén, I. & Svenningsen, N. W. (1988). Lidocaine treatment of severe seizures in newborn infants. I. Clinical effects and cerebral electrical activity monitoring. *Acta Paediatrica Scandinavica*, **77**, 79–84.

Hellström-Westas, L., Rosén, I. & Svenningsen N. W. (1990). Cerebral complications detected by EEG-monitoring during neonatal intensive care. *Acta Paediatrica Scandinavica*, Suppl. **360**, 83–6.

Hellström-Westas, L., Rosén, I. & Svenningsen, N. W. (1991). Cerebral function monitoring in extremely small low birthweight (ESLBW) infants during the first week of life. *Neuropediatrics*, **22**, 27–32.

Hellström-Westas, L., Bell, A. H., Skov, L., Greisen, G. & Svenningsen, N. W. (1992). Cerebroelectrical depression following surfactant treatment in preterm neonates. *Pediatrics*, **89**, 643–7.

Hellström-Westas, L., Blennow, G., Lindroth, M., Rosén, I. & Svenningsen, N. W. (1995a). Low risk of seizure recurrence after early withdrawal of antiepileptic treatment in the neonatal period. *Archives of Disease in Childhood*, **72**, F97–F101.

Hellström-Westas, L., Rosén, I. & Svenningsen, N. W. (1995b). Predictive value of early continuous amplitude integrated EEG recordings on outcome after severe birth asphyxia in full term infants. *Archives of Disease in Childhood*, **72**, F34–F38.

Hellström-Westas, L., Klette, H., Thorngren-Jerneck, K., Rosén, I. & Svenningsen, N. W. (1998). Prognostication of neurological outcome during the first days of life in preterm infants with large IVH's. *Pediatric Research*, **43**, 319A.

Helmers, S. L., Constantinou, J. E., Newburger, J. W. et al. (1997). Perioperative electroencephalographic seizures in infants undergoing repair of complex congenital cardiac defects. *Electroencephalography and Clinical Neurophysiology*, **102**, 27–36.

Holmes, G. L., & Lombroso, C. T. (1990). Prognostic value of background patterns in the neonatal EEG. *Journal of Clinical Neurophysiology*, **10**, 323–52.

Ingvar, D. H., Sjölund, B. & Ardö, A. A. (1976). Correlation between dominant EEG frequency, cerebral oxygen uptake and blood flow. *Electroencephalography and Clinical Neurophysiology*, **41**, 268–276.

Legido, A., Clancy, R. R. & Berman, P. H. (1991). Neurologic outcome after electroencephalographic proven neonatal seizures. *Pediatrics*, **88**, 583–96.

Lombroso, C. T. & Holmes, G. L. (1993).Value of the EEG in neonatal seizures. *Journal of Epilepsy*, **6**, 39–70.

Maynard, D. E. & Jenkinson, J. L. (1984). The cerebral function analysing monitor. *Anaesthesia*, **39**, 678–90.

Maynard, D., Prior, P. F. & Scott, D. F. (1969). Device for continuous monitoring of cerebral activity in resuscitated patients. *British Medical Journal*, **4**, 545–6.

Mercuri, E., Rutherford, M., Cowan, F. et al. (1999). Early prognostic indicators of outcome in infants with neonatal cerebral infarction: a clinical, electroencephalogram, and magnetic resonance imaging study. *Pediatrics,* **103**, 39–46.

Mizrahi, E. M. & Kellaway, P. (1987). Characterization and classification of neonatal seizures. *Neurology*, **37**, 1837–44.

Monod, N., Pajot, N., & Guidasci, S. (1972). The neonatal EEG: Statistical studies and prognostic value in full-term and pre-term babies. *Electroencephalography and Clinical Neurophysiology*, **32**, 529–44.

Murdoch-Eaton, D., Toet, M., Livingston, J., Smith, I. & Levene, M. (1994a). Evaluation of the Cerebro Trac 2500 for monitoring of cerebral function in the neonatal intensive care. *Neuropediatrics*, **25**, 122–8.

Murdoch-Eaton, D. G., Wertheim, D., Oozeer, R., Dubowitz, L. M. S. & Dubowitz, V. (1994b). Reversible changes in cerebral activity associated with acidosis in preterm neonates. *Acta Paediatrica*, **83**, 486–92.

Prior, P. & Maynard, D. E. (1986). *Monitoring Cerebral Function. Long-term Recordings of Cerebral Electrical Activity and Evoked Potentials*, pp. 1–441. Amsterdam: Elsevier.

Steriade, M., Amzica, F. & Contreras, D. (1994). Cortical and thalamic cellular correlates of electroencephalographic burst-suppression. *Electroencephalography and Clinical Neurophysiology*, **90**, 1–16.

Stidham, G. L., Nugent, S. K. & Rogers, M. C. (1980). Monitoring cerebral electrical function in the ICU. *Critical Care Medicine*, **8**, 519–23.

Talwar, D. & Torres, F. (1988). Continuous electrophysiologic monitoring of cerebral function in the pediatric intensive care unit. *Pediatric Neurology*, **4**, 137–47.

Tharp, B. R., Scher, M. S. & Clancy, R. R. (1989). Serial EEGs in normal and abnormal infants with birthweights less than 1200 grams – a prospective study with long term follow-up. *Neuropediatrics*, **20**, 64–72.

Thiringer, K., Connell, J., Carter, E. & Levene, M. (1986). Comparison between Medilog EEG and Cerebral Function Monitor recordings on infants in neonatal intensive care. *Early Human Development*, **14**, 150 (abstract).

Thornberg, E. & Ekström-Jodal, B. (1994). Cerebral function monitoring: a method of predicting outcome in term neonates after severe perinatal asphyxia. *Acta Paediatrica*, **83**, 596–601.

Thornberg, E. & Thiringer, K. (1990). Normal patterns of cerebral function monitor traces in term and preterm neonates. *Acta Paediatrica Scandinavica*, **79**, 20–5.

Toet, M. C., Hellström-Westas, L., Groenendaal, F., Eken, P. & de Vries, L. S. (1999). Amplitude integrated EEG at 3 and 6 hours after birth in fullterm neonates with hypoxic ischaemic encephalopathy. *Archives of Disease in Childhood. Fetal Neonatal Education*, **81**, F19–23.

Verma, U. L., Archbald, F., Tejani, N. & Handwerker, S. M. (1984). Cerebral function monitor in the neonate. I. Normal patterns. *Developmental Medicine and Child Neurology*, **26**, 154–61.

Viniker, D. A., Maynard, D. E. & Scott, D. F. (1984). Cerebral function monitor studies in neonates. *Clinical Electroencephalography*, **15**, 185–92.

Watanabe, K., Hakamada, S., Kuroyanagi, M., Yamazaki, T. & Takeuchi, T. (1983). Electroencephalographical study of intraventricular hemorrhage in the preterm infant. *Neuropediatrics*, **14**, 225–30.

Wertheim, D. F. P., Murdoch Eaton, D. G., Oozeer, R. C. et al. (1991). New system for cotside display and analysis of the preterm neonatal electroencephalogram. *Developmental Medicine and Child Neurology*, **33**, 1080–6.

Wertheim, D., Mercuri, E., Faundez, J. C., Rutherford, M., Acolet, D. & Dubowitz, L. (1995). Prognostic value of continuous electroencephalographic recording in full term infants with hypoxic ischaemic encephalopathy. *Archives of Disease in Childhood*, **71**, F97–F102.

Williams, C. E., Gunn, A. J., Mallard, C. & Gluckman, P. D. (1992). Outcome after ischemia in the developing brain: an electroencephalographic and histological study. *Annals of Neurology*, **31**, 14–21.

18

Hypoxic–ischemic encephalopathy

A. David Edwards[1], Huseyin Mehmet[1] and Henrik Hagberg[2]

[1]Weston Laboratory, Imperial College School of Medicine, Hammersmith Hospital, London, UK
[2]Perinatal Center, Sahlgrenska University Hospital, Östra, Göteborg, Sweden

The role of hypoxia–ischemia in perinatal brain injury

Injury to the brain depends not only on the type and severity of insult, but also on the maturity of the tissue. Hypoxic–ischemic encephalopathy is generally considered to be characteristic of the term infant who has suffered a severe perinatal deficit in cerebral oxygen delivery leading to disruption of cerebral energy metabolism (Volpe, 1994). This is frequently followed by a global hypoxic–ischemic injury, with a widespread, although not uniform, distribution of apoptotic and necrotic cell death. Nevertheless, focal cerebral infarction is also seen in term infants, and may be underdiagnosed unless sophisticated techniques such as diffusion-weighed magnetic resonance imaging (MRI) are employed (Cowan et al., 1994). Hypoxic–ischemic changes are also seen in many stillbirths, although in these infants apoptotic death may be particularly prominent (Edwards et al., 1997).

Recently doubt has been cast on the primary or unique etiological role of hypoxia–ischemia in neonatal encephalopathy, and other causes, such as intrauterine or neonatal inflammation have been emphasized. For example, cerebral palsy is associated with maternal fever even when there is little clinical evidence of impaired intrauterine gas exchange (Grether & Nelson, 1997), and meningitis caused by group B streptococci can lead to both necrosis and apoptosis in brain cells (Leib et al., 1996). Cerebral palsy is also associated with maternal thyroid disease (Badawi et al., 1998) and possibly with abnormalities of the clotting cascade and immune systems (Nelson et al., 1998).

Uncertainty about the role of intrauterine hypoxemia or cerebral ischemia is exacerbated by the imprecise measures of fetal oxygenation or cerebral blood flow available to clinicians. Observations of clinical variables such as cardiotocography or meconium staining of the liquor may mislead if interpreted as precise measures of fetal cerebral hypoxia and ischemia (Nelson et al., 1996). However, more accurate techniques such as magnetic resonance spectroscopy (MRS) have defined at least a subgroup of infants with characteristic hypoxic–ischemic injury, and it is clear that cerebral hypoxia and/or ischemia is involved in a significant proportion of neonatal encephalopathy (Azzopoardi et al., 1989).

Basic research into the mechanisms of cerebral injury is beginning to suggest that the apparent distinction between hypoxic–ischemic and other forms of cerebral damage may be less clear that has previously been thought. It is now apparent that not only does infection and sepsis often cause cerebral hypoxia, but hypoxia–ischemia triggers inflammatory cascades within the brain. Different pathologies can activate common cell death pathways. This chapter will focus upon these processes in the developing brain, examining first the pathophysiology of brain damage, then discussing the mode of death and mechanisms of cell injury.

The pathophysiology of hypoxic–ischemic cerebral injury

Initial and delayed injury after perinatal hypoxia–ischemia

MRS has permitted non-invasive observation of intracellular pH (pHi), and the cerebral concentrations of adenosine triphosphate (ATP), phosphocreatine (PCr), inorganic phosphate (Pi) and lactate in association with cerebral hypoxia–ischemia. When ATP generation is impaired, energy flux is maintained by the breakdown of PCr while Pi increases, so that a decline in the ratio [PCr]/[Pi] is a valuable indicator of impaired energy metabolism, even in the presence of normal or near normal concentrations of ATP. Impaired oxidative phosphorylation is also associated with increased intracerebral lactate (Cady, 1990).

Infants with hypoxic–ischemic encephalopathy show characteristic abnormalities. Cerebral energy metabolism is frequently normal soon after birth, but shows a progressive decline in [PCr]/[Pi] and increase in lactate some hours later. Infants displaying this phenomenon develop severe neurodevelopmental impairment or die and there is a close relationship between the magnitude of the late decline in [PCr]/[Pi], reduced brain growth and the severity of neurodevelopmental impairment 1 and 4 years later (Roth et al., 1992, 1997; Hanrahan et al., 1999).

These findings suggested the concept of 'secondary energy failure', which has been developed and extended by several groups (Hope et al., 1984; Martin et al., 1996; Hanrahan et al., 1996). Delayed declines in [PCr]/[Pi] beginning some 8–12 hours after birth asphyxia have been confirmed and quantitated in a number of studies. It was found that delayed disruption of cerebral energy metabolism is associated with a normal or increased pHi, in clear contrast to acute hypoxia–ischemia when pHi characteristically falls.

These data led to the hypothesis that hypoxic–ischemic injury occurred in at least two main phases, with a primary defect in cerebral energy production during hypoxia-ischemia precipitating the later events. This has been supported by studies of global hypoxia–ischemia in the newborn piglet (Lorek et al., 1994), and in focal

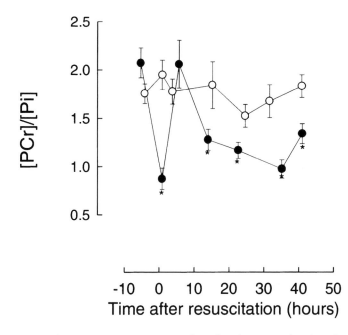

Fig. 18.1.   Magnetic resonance spectroscopy data showing secondary impairment of energy metabolism following unilateral carotid artery occlusion and reduced inspired oxygen concentration for 90 minutes in 14-day-old rat pups (closed circles), compared to sham operated controls (open circles). The cerebral concentration ratio of phosphocreatine to inorganic phosphate ([PCr]/[Pi]) is observed as a measure of cerebral energy metabolism. The effect of hypoxia–ischemia is seen, with a reduction in [PCr]/[Pi] that recovers after resuscitation, but then declines again after 10 hours. (Reproduced from Blumberg et al., 1996.)

stroke in rat pups (Blumberg et al., 1996, Palmer et al., 1990a,b). During hypoxia–ischemia intracerebral [PCr]/[Pi] and pHi fall, and lactate increases. Eventually [ATP] declines, but even if this transiently falls to undetectable levels, the reprovision of substrate usually causes the metabolites to return to normal values within an hour or two. Some hours later, [PCr]/[Pi] again declines (Fig. 18.1), lactate increases and pHi becomes alkaline. There is a dose–response relationship between the severity of the hypoxic–ischemic insult and the magnitude of the secondary changes in cerebral energy metabolism (Lorek et al., 1994). Equally, the more severe the cerebral metabolic impairment, the more extensive the histological injury (Blumberg et al., 1996). Electrophysiological studies of fetal sheep have provided further evidence for a biphasic model of cerebral injury (Williams et al., 1992).

It is unlikely that delayed hypoperfusion explains the fall in high energy phosphates during secondary energy failure. Simultaneous measurements of cerebral energy metabolism and blood flow have not been made in infants following peri-natal hypoxia–ischemia, but the delayed changes in metabolism occur at a time when cerebral blood flow and volume are increased (Wyatt et al., 1990; Pryds et al., 1990). Nevertheless, cerebral perfusion is not completely normal during secondary energy failure, as loss of both the normal response to changes in arterial carbon dioxide tension, and blood pressure autoregulation have been reported (Pryds et al., 1990; Wyatt et al., 1991).

However, although it has been useful, the concept of biphasic cerebral damage is an oversimplification. Diffusion-weighted MRI studies in piglets have shown that, although changes in the apparent diffusion coefficient of brain (an index of the restriction of movement of water, and thus of cell membrane integrity) closely par-allel changes in [PCr]/[Pi] during secondary energy failure, the changes are not uniform throughout the brain. Rather, abnormal diffusion frequently begins later-ally and then progresses towards the parasagittal and central regions (Thornton et al., 1998). A change in global [PCr]/[Pi] obscures considerable complexity of regional response.

MRI of infants with hypoxic–ischemic encephalopathy confirms that damage is distributed heterogenously throughout the brain, although injury to the basal ganglia and deep structures of the brain seems to predict adverse neurological outcome most accurately (Rutherford et al., 1998). Localized MRS measurements also show that metabolite concentration abnormalities differ in different regions of the brain; for example, lactate seems to be higher in the thalamus than the occipi-tal region (Penrice et al., 1996).

Abnormal cerebral energy metabolism also continues for much longer than was previously thought. In children who are neurologically normal 1 year following birth asphyxia, cerebral lactate concentrations rapidly fall. However, in those who develop neurodevelopmental impairment by lactate, an increased pHi can be detected in the brain for many months (Hanrahan et al., 1998; Robertson et al., 1999). The mechanism is unknown, but in adult rats moderate hypoxia–ischemia is followed by a very prolonged period of increased apoptotic death in affected areas (Du et al., 1996).

The mode of cell death in hypoxic–ischemic injury: apoptosis and necrosis

Cell death is conventionally classified as apoptotic or necrotic. In necrosis, death is triggered by an overwhelming insult resulting in the catastrophic loss of membrane integrity and leaking of cytoplasmic contents into the extracellular matrix. In con-trast, cells dying by apoptosis carry out a highly conserved and regulated genetic pro-gramme. They do not lose membrane integrity until very late on, and the organelles remain largely intact until the final stages when cell fragments are 'shrink-wrapped' in the contracting plasma membrane and bud off as apoptotic bodies which are subsequently phagocytozed by healthy neighbouring cells. Apoptosis requires time, energy and, in some cases, gene transcription and translation (Wyllie & Duvall, 1992).

Apoptosis involves a recently described class of enzymes, the caspases, which are cysteine proteases requiring a specific aspartate residue at the cleavage site. They form a highly regulated amplification and effector system central to cellular execution. Caspases can be activated by a wide variety of internal and external factors including: specific receptor-mediated stimuli such as the binding of Fas-ligand or pro-apoptotic cytokines; by non-specific insults like hypoxia, particularly those affecting mitochondrial function; or by a variety of genetic triggers (Thornberry & Lazebnik, 1998).

The observation of delayed injury after hypoxia–ischemia prompted the search for apoptosis in damaged tissue. Apoptotic cells have now been reported following hypoxic–ischemic injury in both the immature (Mehmet et al., 1994; Beilhartz et al., 1995) and adult animal brain (Linnik et al., 1993), and in the brains of infants who die after intrauterine injury (see Fig. 18.2 in colour plate section), either with or without evidence of hypoxia–ischemia (Edwards et al., 1997; Scott & Hegyi, 1997).

Although apoptosis and necrosis are often considered distinct, they are perhaps better seen as available routes to extinction for damaged or unwanted cells, and the cellular choice will depend on a variety of internal and external influences. Both apoptotic and necrotic cells are found after hypoxia–ischemia in direct proportion to the severity of the disruption to cerebral energy metabolism (Yue et al., 1997). Many necrotic cells are probably already triggered to apoptosis, but run out of energy and necrose before the programme is complete.

The close relation between apoptotic and necrotic death is demonstrated by the involvement of the nuclear repair enzyme, poly (ADP ribose) polymerase (PARP) in hypoxic–ischemic damage. Damage to DNA activates PARP, which utilizes NAD^+. ATP is consumed in NAD regeneration, and consequent energy depletion may induce necrosis (Bolanas et al., 1997). PARP is induced by hypoxia–ischemia, and genetic disruption of PARP provides profound protection against cell death in vitro and in vivo (Eliasson et al., 1997b). As the susceptibility of primary neurons towards apoptosis is unaffected in PARP−/− mice, PARP activation is not necessary for apoptosis (Leist et al., 1997). Thus in cerebral ischemia PARP activation probably leads to cell death without involvement of apoptotic pathways (Endres et al., 1997).

However, both caspase activity and PARP cleavage increase immediately following ischemic injury in vivo (Namura et al., 1998; Joashi et al., 1999), and inhibition of caspase activity reduces cell death and PARP cleavage in the 7-day-old rat (Cheng et al., 1998). PARP does have a role in apoptosis: specific proteolytic cleavage of PARP by caspase 3 is an important event in at least one pathway to apoptosis

(Lazebnik et al., 1994), probably as a mechanism to maintain the ATP needed for successful completion of the apoptotic programme.

A number of different factors influence whether a cell will undergo apoptosis or necrosis. Apoptosis seems to be prominent during development. Following excitotoxic injury to the newborn rat striatum, neuronal death occurs by apoptosis, while in the adult the same insult produces necrosis (Portera-Cailliau et al., 1997b). Similarly, cerebellar Purkinje cells differentiate early in brain morphogenesis and in the piglet are induced to undergo necrosis but not apoptosis by hypoxia–ischemia, while in contrast, cerebellar granule cells (which continue to divide after birth) undergo apoptosis (Yue et al., 1997). The degree of cell differentiation can also affect the response to injury: dividing progenitor cells are particularly sensitive to apoptotic stimuli since the cell cycle machinery is intimately linked to the mechanisms of apoptosis (Ross, 1996). Apoptosis may thus be a particularly important factor in perinatal cerebral injury, and the impressive degree of protection seen with many antiapoptotic trophic factors in immature animal models of injury (see below) supports this idea. The severity of hypoxia–ischemia is also important: the same cell type can be triggered to undergo apoptosis following mild injury but necrosis if the damage is severe (Ankarcrona et al., 1995). This may reflect injury to organelles, but the availability of ATP directly affects cellular fate.

Mitochondrial function and cell death

Mitochondria play a central role in cell death, and the severity of mitochondrial damage may be the most important deciding factor between apoptosis and necrosis (Kroemer et al., 1998). It is suggested that a small increase in mitochondrial membrane permeability can result in the controlled release of apoptogenic factors, while severe mitochondrial damage releases a flood of calcium and oxygen free radicals (OFR) into the cytosol, leading to the disruption of plasma membrane integrity and cell necrosis (Fig. 18.3).

The basis for this current hypothesis lies in the suggestion that the mitochondrial megachannel or permeability transition (PT) pore is involved in preventing OFR accumulation (Skulachev, 1996, 1998). In the normal homeostatic situation, increased concentrations of OFRs in the mitochondria would trigger opening of the pore, allowing release of these species into the cytosol, thus decreasing mitochondrial OFR concentrations to a safe level and allowing pore closure. Persistent free radical accumulation (such as might occur in hypoxia–ischemia – see below) would prevent pore closure with disruption of membrane potential and energy production, and might lead to the release of the apoptosis-inducing proteins. More severe damage by whatever means would drastically disrupt energy metabolism and may lead to necrosis due to acute energy depletion.

There is evidence to support this theory. PT is indeed activated by OFRs (Chernyak, 1997) and by other potentially damaging events (Kroemer et al., 1997).

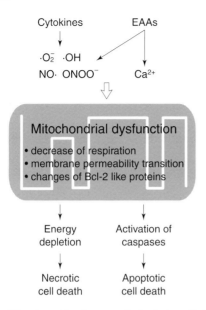

Fig. 18.3.   Mitochondria play a central role in cell death. Multiple stimuli such as free radicals,
excitatory amino acids or ATP depletion lead to mitochondrial dysfunction. Severe
disruption leads to failure of ATP generation and if this cannot be compensated from
other sources such as PCr it will lead to rapid necrosis. Less severe damage may induce
the secretion of proapoptotic factors into the cytosol, activation of caspases and apoptotic
execution. (For abbreviations see main text.)

Transient opening of the PT pore increases the permeability of the inner mitochondrial membrane to small molecules, but sustained PT causes uncoupling of the respiratory chain enzymes, failure of ATP generation and the release of specific
apoptosis-initiating proteins such as cytochrome-c, dATP and APAF-1(Liu et al.,
1996; Zou, Henzel Liu et al., 1997) into the cytosol. Mitochondrial changes precede
the activation of cytosolic enzymes involved in apoptotic execution, and inhibitors
of the permeability transition pore can prevent apoptosis (Hirsh et al., 1998).

Much of the information regarding the identity of mitochondrial factors
involved in apoptosis has been obtained from cell-free systems established to reproduce the apoptotic programme in vitro (Ellerby et al., 1997). In one such model,
apoptosis could be initiated by addition of dATP but also required cytochrome-c.
Intact cells undergoing apoptosis showed a translocation of cytochrome-c (which
normally functions as an electron carrier in the respiratory chain) from mitochondria to the cytosol (Liu et al., 1996) which, in turn, results in the activation of specific caspases (Bossy-Wetzel et al., 1998), particularly caspase-3 which is pivotal in
apoptotic execution (Li et al., 1997).

Cytochrome-c release is an important link between mitochondria and apoptosis in at least some neural systems. However, it is not universally required (Chauhan

et al., 1997): apoptosis induced by branched chain amino acids or their metabolites is preceded by a fall in oxygen consumption without cytochrome-c release, and in this situation apoptosis proceeds in the absence of cytosolic translocation of cyto-chrome-c (Jouvet et al., 1998).

The integration of mitochondrial control of apoptosis into overall cellular function is imperfectly understood, but involves members of the Bcl-2 family of proteins. Bcl-2 is a mitochondrial membrane protein that blocks the apoptotic death of many cell types (Hockenbery et al., 1990) and has been shown to protect neurons from death if overexpressed following cerebral ischemia (Martinou et al., 1994). Other Bcl-2 family members have a variety of anti-or proapoptotic actions.

The precise mechanism of Bcl-2 protection is unclear but members of the Bcl-2 family form part of the PT pore (Kroemer et al., 1998). Bcl-2 regulates an antioxidant pathway at sites of free radical generation (Hockenbery et al., 1993), and Bcl-2 family members can prevent the mitochondrial PT (Van der Heiden et al., 1997). In some cell types, Bcl-2 cannot prevent or delay the decrease of the cellular ATP level subsequent to metabolic inhibition, so it seems to block apoptosis at a point downstream of the collapse of cellular energy homeostasis (Marton et al., 1997).

Cellular and molecular mechanisms of hypoxic–ischemic brain injury

The deficit in ATP induced by hypoxia–ischemia leads to a failure to maintain transmembrane ionic gradients, release of neuroactive compounds into the extra-cellular compartments and the activation of a series of mechanisms that, if sustained, will lead to immediate cell necrosis. If the individual is resuscitated, these acute alterations are completely or partly reversed, but the complex process has been started in which multiple interrelated factors may produce secondary brain injury with necrotic and apoptotic cell death.

The precise mechanisms of damage are incompletely understood but some components of the process have been elucidated. Excitatory amino acids (EAA), intra-cellular calcium regulation, OFR generation, nitric oxide (NO), specific gene activation, changes in the availability of trophic factors and the immuno-inflammatory system are all implicated in the process, as are other factors. The entire process is extremely temperature dependent, and a reduction in brain temperature of only 3–4 °C either during or after hypoxia–ischemia dramatically reduces the amount of cell death, offering a potentially important method of neuroprotective therapy (Edwards et al., 1998).

Excitatory amino acids

Glutamate and aspartate are the main excitatory transmitters in the brain, but they have been known for a long time to exert toxic effects (excitotoxicity) if applied in

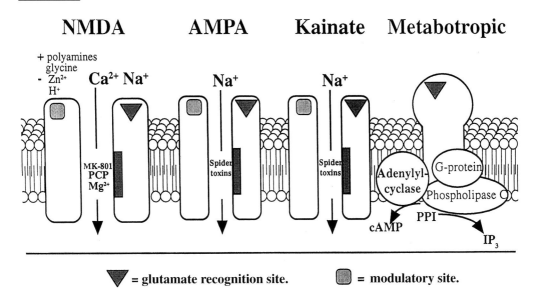

Fig. 18.4.   Glutamate receptor subtypes. NMDA, AMPA and kainate receptors are ion channels, and the metabotropic receptor activates second messengers in the inosine triphosphate (IP_3) and cyclic AMP (cAMP) pathways. The ion channels have glutamate recognition sites and modulatory sites. The NMDA receptor is activated by unbinding of magnesium (Mg^{2+}) which blocks the ion channel, and can be blocked by binding of drugs such as MK-801 and PCP. NMDA activity is modulated by multiple factors such as zinc ions (Zn^{2+}), hydrogen ions (H^+), polyamines, glycine and membrane potential. AMPA and Kainate receptors can be antagonized by specific toxins.

excess to the nervous system (Lucas & Newhouse 1957; Olney & Ho, 1970). EAA receptors are present on virtually all neurons (Lodge & Collinridge, 1991; Wong & Kemp, 1991). There are three ionotropic EAA receptor subclasses: the N-methyl-D-aspartate (NMDA), the α-amino-3-hydroxy-5-methyl-4-isoxazole-propionic acid (AMPA) and the kainate receptors that are named after their respective most selective receptor agonist. A fourth subclass of metabotropic receptors are coupled to G proteins and stimulate phosphoinositide hydrolysis or decrease cAMP formation (Michaelis,1998) (Fig. 18.4).

The expression of EAA receptors is upregulated in the immature human brain, which reflects the critical role of these receptors for neuronal development (McDonald & Johnston, 1990). Hence, the immature brain is also more vulnerable to excitotoxicity (especially NMDA) than the adult (McDonald et al., 1988). Glutamate is the main excitotoxin in vivo, although microglia may produce a compound with NMDA receptor agonistic properties (Giulian and Vaca, 1993), and quinolinic acid (Heyes et al., 1997; Sinz et al., 1998) which may have significant excitotoxic actions.

There is considerable evidence for a role of EAAs in the process leading to hypoxic–ischemic brain injury. There is a high density of NMDA and other EAA receptors in regions vulnerable to hypoxia–ischemia (Silverstein et al., 1987). Extracellular concentrations of EAAs and glycine increase during neonatal hypoxia–ischemia (Hagberg et al., 1987; Andiné et al., 1991) followed by a secondary increase during reperfusion (Tan et al., 1996; Thoresen et al., 1997). Blocking NMDA receptors before or after hypoxia–ischemia reduces subsequent brain damage in most animal models (McDonald et al., 1987; Andiné,et al., 1988; Hattori et al., 1989; Tan et al., 1992, Hagberg et al., 1994). The results with AMPA blockade have been more equivocal: in immature rats, the AMPA receptor antagonist NBQX reduced brain damage moderately when given after hypoxia–ischemia (Hagberg et al., 1994) but another AMPA receptor antagonist (LY293558) did not provide neuroprotection in the newborn pigs (Le Blanc et al., 1995).

The mechanism of excitotoxicity in response to hypoxia–ischemia is unclear. Previously, accumulation of EAAs during hypoxia–ischemia was thought to lead to overactivation of EAA receptors leading to postsynaptic overload of calcium and neuronal death (Fig. 18.5). However, EAA concentrations are not as high extracellularly after hypoxia–ischemia in the immature brain (Hagberg et al., 1987; Cherici et al., 1991) as in the adult brain (Hagberg et al., 1985). NMDA receptor antagonists reduce cell death even if administered an hour after hypoxia–ischemia when extracellular EAA levels are not particularly raised (Hattori et al., 1989), suggesting that other mechanisms are at play. Glutamate appears to induce both apoptosis and necrosis in the immature brain (Portera-Cailliau et al., 1997a; Martin et al., 1998), which can be blocked by NMDA receptor antagonists. However these antagonists can also induce apoptosis in the immature brain (Ikonomidou et al., 1999), which would complicate the use of such drugs for cerebroprotection.

Calcium homeostasis

Calcium (Ca^{2+}) ions are ubiquitous intracellular second messengers, acting as key regulators of numerous cellular functions (Miller, 1987). In order to allow efficient Ca^{2+}-dependent signalling, the intracellular Ca^{2+} concentration ($Ca^{2+}ic$) is strictly regulated at a low level of 100 nM, i.e. 10 000 times lower than the extracellular concentration (Miller, 1991), and the large electrochemical gradient created imposes an obligatory requirement for ATP upon the cell (Miller, 1991). In the adult brain, even a few minutes of complete anoxia or ischemia causes a rise in $Ca^{2+}ic$ (Silver & Erecinska,1990; Siesjö, 1986), which may trigger a number of toxic processes such as activation of calpains, OFR, apoptosis, phospholipases, endonucleases and NO production (Fig. 18.5).

Intracellular calcium regulation may thus play an important role in the cellular response to injury (Choi, 1995). However, its significance in immature brain injury

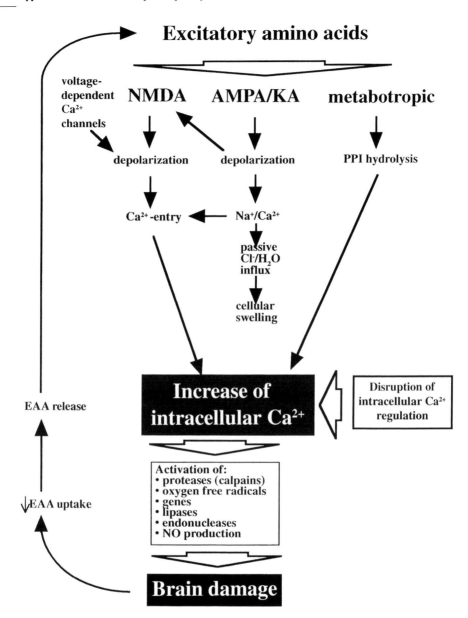

Fig. 18.5.   Possible mechanism for the pathological effects of excitatory amino acids on neural cells. Excess excitatory amino acid (EAA) secretion stimulates glutamate receptors allowing ion transport and depolarization, and activation of second messenger systems which increase intracellular calcium concentrations. Cellular mechanisms are activated and EAA uptake hindered, producing a cycle of cell damage.

is less clear. In studies in vitro, the rise of $Ca^{2+}ic$ tends to be slower and less pronounced in immature neurons (Bickler et al., 1993; Bickler and Hansen, 1998). However, Ca^{2+} accumulates to some extent in the brain tissue during hypoxia–ischemia (Stein and Vannucci, 1988), and calcium-dependent enzymes like calpains and phospholipase C are activated (Blomgren et al., 1995a,b; Chen et al., 1988) which offers some indirect information in support of an increase of $Ca^{2+}ic$ in the immature brain during hypoxia–ischemia.

It is also unclear exactly what happens to $Ca^{2+}ic$ during delayed injury, when there is an accumulation of calcium in regions with brain injury (Stein & Vannucci, 1988), but it is not known whether this accumulation is cause or consequence of brain injury. The calcium entry blocker flunarizine administered prior to (but not after) hypoxia–ischemia attenuated brain injury in 7-day-old rats (Silverstein et al., 1986; Chumas et al., 1993), but high doses were administered and non-selective effects of the drug make the interpretation difficult.

Oxygen free radicals

OFRs are atoms or molecules that contain one or more unpaired electrons, which makes the free radicals highly reactive and able to disrupt the molecular structure of lipids and proteins with devastating consequences for cellular function (Halliwell, 1992). OFRs can induce necrosis directly, but may also cause apoptosis by mechanisms such as the effects on mitochondrial PT.

There are several pathways whereby OFRs are produced in the brain (Fig. 18.6) (Halliwell, 1992). The superoxide radical ($\cdot O_2^-$) is produced by: (i) electron leakage from the electron transport chain in mitochondria; (ii) oxidation of hypoxanthine to xanthine and urate by xanthine oxidase (mainly in endothelial cells); (iii) degradation of free fatty acids by phospholipase A_2 into arachidonic acid and subsequent oxidation of arachidonic acid by cyclo-oxygenase and lipo-oxygenase; and (iv) NADPH oxidase activity in macrophages, neutrophils and microglia (Fig. 18.6).

The $\cdot O_2^-$ radical has a relatively low reactivity and does not easily cross cell membranes. However $\cdot O_2^-$ can react with Fe^{2+} ions and form hydroxyl radicals ($\cdot OH$) (Fig. 18.6), which react with almost every molecule at diffusion limited speed in the presence of transition metals such as Fe^{2+} ions and exert toxic effects on DNA, activating PARP and depleting cellular NAD^+ and ATP. The $\cdot OH$ radical initiates lipid peroxidation in a self-perpetuating reaction, which disrupts membrane function. Thiol groups on enzymes and structural proteins are oxidized with loss of enzyme function and cytoskeletal disruption (Halliwell 1992; Palmer, 1995).

There are several defence systems in the brain to reduce the formation of OFRs and several pathways for their inactivation. The $\cdot O_2^-$ adduct is dismutated by superoxide dismutase (SOD) into hydrogen peroxide (H_2O_2), which is converted to water and oxygen by either of the two enzymes, catalase or glutathione peroxidase.

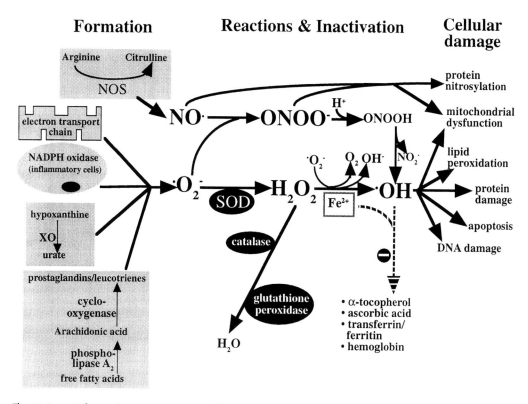

Fig. 18.6.   Schematic representation of the role of free radicals in neural cell damage. Superoxide
($\cdot O_2^-$) is generated by several reactions, and nitric oxide (NO·) by conversion of arginine
to citrulline. Complex interactions generate hydrogen peroxide (H_2O_2), peroxynitrite
(ONOO⁻) and the highly reactive hydroxyl radical (·OH) which affect a variety of cellular
functions. The cell has a series of antioxidant defences including superoxide dismutase
(SOD), ascorbic acid and iron chelators.

Compounds such as ascorbic acid and α-tocopherol act as scavengers which inhibit
lipid peroxidation. Chelation of transition metals such as iron by ferritin or trans-
ferrin is another endogenous protective mechanism against excessive formation of
OFRs (Palmer, 1995). Intracellular concentrations of glutathione may be particularly important, and immature oligodendrocytes are especially prone to OFR-
induced death because of limited glutathione stores (Back et al., 1998).

Immature brain probably has major differences in the handling of free radicals
from adults. Scavenging systems may be less developed (Saugstad, 1996) and therapeutic free radical scavengers may sometimes exacerbate brain injury, perhaps by
upsetting the balance of a complex but underdeveloped endogenous system
(Ditelberg et al., 1996).

There is evidence for increased hypoxanthine levels, free radical formation and lipid peroxidation during reperfusion after hypoxia–ischemia in neonatal mice, newborn piglets, immature rats and fetal sheep (Kjellmer et al., 1989; Hasegawa et al., 1991, 1993; Armstead et al., 1988; Bågenholm et al., 1996, 1998). Treatment with the 21-aminosteroid tirilazad mesylate, a lipid peroxidation inhibitor, after hypoxia–ischemia in 7-day-old rats reduces brain damage (Bågenholm et al., 1996). Allopurinol and oxypurinol, being inhibitors of xanthine oxidase and OFR scavengers in high concentrations, reduce brain damage when administered before or after hypoxia–ischemia (Palmer et al., 1993). Furthermore, the iron chelator deferoxamine attenuates hypoxic–ischemic brain damage (Palmer et al., 1994).

All these pharmacologic agents penetrate poorly across the blood–brain barrier and it has been suggested that OFR production is initiated in endothelial and immuno-inflammatory cells from within the vascular compartment (Palmer et al., 1994; Rosenberg et al., 1989; Armstead et al., 1992; Matsumiya et al., 1991). In adult ischemia neutrophils are a major source of free radical production following hypoxia–ischemia and the major site of action for some neuroprotective free radical scavengers appears to be at the blood–brain barrier (Hall, 1995).

Nitric oxide

The hypothesis that NO, a free radical, is involved in brain injury was supported by the demonstration that inhibition of NO synthesis attenuated NMDA neurotoxicity (Dawson et al., 1993). Production of NO occurs through conversion of arginine to citrulline by three different nitric oxide synthases (NOS): neuronal NOS (nNOS), endothelial NOS (eNOS) and macrophage or inducible NOS (iNOS) (Jaffrey and Snyder, 1995). Both eNOS and nNOS are expressed constitutively, but all types of NOS can be induced in response to a variety of stimuli. eNOS and nNOS are dependent upon Ca^{2+} binding for activation and nNOS is activated by NMDA receptor stimulation (Eliasson et al., 1997). The activity of iNOS is mainly expressed in inflammatory cells and produces large amounts of NO and its activity is Ca^{2+} independent (Iadecola & Ross, 1997). NO binds to iron and thiol groups including metabolic enzymes and can induce apoptotic and necrotic cell death, with different redox states of NO (NO^+, $NO\cdot$ and NO^-) having different effects; NO^+ and $NO\cdot$ probably inducing predominantly apoptotic death, while NO^- precipitates necrosis (Khan et al., 1997). $NO\cdot$ and $\cdot O_2^-$ react very quickly to form peroxynitrite ($ONOO^-$) which is freely diffusible and oxidizes thiol groups, induces protein nitrosylation and mitochondrial impairment (Crow & Beckman 1995) (Fig. 18.6).

Investigations on the role of NO in hypoxic–ischemic brain injury have yielded conflicting results, and the effects of different subtypes of NOS have to be considered separately (Huang, et al., 1994; Iadecola & Ross, 1997). In many studies, eNOS confers protection through a beneficial vasodilator effect improving perfusion, while nNOS and iNOS enhances injury in response to focal ischemia.

Recent data also suggest that immature brain behaves differently from adult tissue. As in the adult, NO is produced in increasing amount during reperfusion (Tan et al., 1996; Thoresen et al., 1997), and some data support a role for NO and NOS in hypoxic–ischemic injury to the developing brain. Selective lesioning of cells with NOS activity prior to an hypoxic–ischemic insult decreased brain injury (Ferriero et al., 1995); neonatal mice lacking the gene for nNOS develops smaller brain injury than wild-type mice following hypoxia–ischemia (Ferriero et al., 1996); and non-specific NOS inhibitors provide neuroprotection if administered before the insult (Trifiletti, 1992; Hamada et al., 1994; Ashwal et al., 1995). However, tissue concentrations of iNOS are very low in immature rat brain and do not appear to be induced within 36 hours of hypoxia–ischemia (Blumberg et al., 1996), and both broad spectrum and specific NOS inhibition after hypoxia–ischemia is less effective at reducing injury in immature sheep, rats and mice than in most studies of adult brain (Marks et al., 1999; Blumberg et al., 1996, Ferriero et al., 1995). NOS inhibition was unable to prevent the secondary energy failure developing after hypoxia–ischemia in immature rats (Blumberg et al., 1996). Equally, intracerebral injection of the NO donor nitroprusside at doses which inflict damage in the adult brain is not toxic to the neonatal brain (Maragos & Silverstein 1994) suggesting that the immature brain may be more resistant to NO toxicity. Further work is needed to understand the role of NO in hypoxic–ischemic encephalopathy.

Specific gene activation

In spite of a general reduction of gene transcription after ischemia, more than 80 different mRNAs are induced by an ischemic insult (Koistinaho and Hökfelt, 1997). Some of these are induced to promote survival or repair, other gene products are involved in the apoptotic process, whereas some may never result in bioactive proteins due to inhibition of protein translation after hypoxia–ischemia (Dwyer et al., 1987).

Immediate early genes (IEGs) constitute some of the earliest transcriptional responses to a wide variety of stimuli including hypoxia–ischemia. The products are themselves transcription factors which act as nuclear messengers that couple extracellular stimuli to the regulation of target genes (Hughes & Dragunow, 1995). Many studies indicate that IEG expression is triggered by events associated with cell death in the neonatal brain (Smeyne et al., 1993). A large number of IEGs, e.g. *c-fos, fos-B, c-jun, jun-B, jun-D, NGFI-A, TIS-1, TIS 11* and *TIS 21* (Gunn et al., 1990; Gubits et al., 1993; Ådén et al., 1994) are activated in response to neonatal hypoxia–ischemia. Many form active heterodimers, so the situation is complex and the role of most of these genes in neural cell death is unknown.

Other potentially important genes are expressed and lead to protein synthesis.

The β amyloid precursor protein is expressed in both human infant and rodent brain after hypoxia–ischemia (Baden Amissah et al., 1998). This has also been seen after head injury in adults, and although its function is unclear it may predispose to long-term cerebral dysfunction in susceptible individuals.

Calpains

Calpains are cysteine proteases involved in signal transduction cascades which differ from caspases as their proteolytic activity is calcium dependent and their substrate specificity does not require an aspartic acid residue (Croall & DeMartino, 1991). Calpains have been implicated in apoptosis and necrosis (Nath et al., 1996), axonal degeneration and cytoskeletal disruption (Nath et al., 1996; Leist & Nicotera, 1998). Calpain inhibitors reduce brain injury in adult models of ischemia.

Calpain activity is high in the developing brain, especially in the white matter (Croall & DeMartino, 1991). In immature rats, hypoxia–ischemia activates and relocates calpain activity to the membrane (Ostwald et al., 1993) and inactivates the endogenous calpain inhibitor calpastatin in vulnerable brain regions (Blomgren et al., 1997). Calpain cleavage products accumulate during delayed cerebral injury, especially in white matter (Blomgren et al., 1995a).

Growth factors

Growth or survival factors are constitutively required by all cells, which undergo apoptosis by default if appropriate factors are withdrawn. Growth factors are often upregulated during development (Lindsay, 1994), and selective availability of growth factors in part controls the pattern of brain morphogenesis. Growth factor expression both modulates and is modulated by brain injury.

mRNA or protein of transforming growth factor-b1 (TGF-b1), calcitonin-gene-related peptide (CGRP), basic fibroblast growth factor (bFGF), insulin-like growth factor-1 (IGF-1) and insulin-like growth factor-2 (IGF-2) are all upregulated after an hypoxic–ischemic insult, although the neurotrophins brain-derived neurotrophic factor (BDNF) and nerve growth factor (NGF) are less affected (Klempt et al., 1992; Lee et al., 1996; Gluckman et al., 1998). However, the process is complex, as has been demonstrated in studies of the IGF system, which includes two active proteins (IGF-1 and IGF-2), two receptors (type I and type II) and six binding proteins (IGFBP1–6). In 21-day-old rats, hypoxia–ischemia upregulates IGF-1 (mRNA and protein), IGFBP2 mRNA and IGFBP3 mRNA 3 days and IGF-2 mRNA from 7 days after the insult (for review, see Gluckman et al., 1998). In 7-day-old rats the pattern was somewhat different with a general suppression of all IGF system components (mRNA of IGF-1, IGF-1 receptor, IGFBP-2 and IGFBP5) (Lee et al., 1996) followed by an upregulation of IGF-1 mRNA and IGFBP5 mRNA in astrocytes after 3–5 days of recovery.

Nevertheless, administration of trophic factors may be particularly effective in reducing damage in the immature brain. Intracerebroventricular administration of IGF-1 after hypoxia–ischemia reduces brain injury more significantly in fetal lambs than in adult rodents (Guan et al., 1993; Johnston et al., 1996). BDNF also provided a considerable degree of neuroprotection in the 7-day-old rat, whereas the effect was less marked in the 21-day-old rat (Cheng et al., 1997). Neonatal brain injury is also attenuated by other trophic factors like NGF (Holtzman et al., 1996) and bFGF (Nozaki et al., 1993). These results have led to the suggestion that expression of growth factors following hypoxia–ischemia is part of an endogenous brain rescue response to injury, which may be more effective in immature brain.

Vascular and immunoinflammatory mechanisms in cerebral damage

Pathological processes in the brain often involve the endothelium and its interactions with circulating blood elements. Neutrophils, monocytes and platelets are activated by the endothelium, and immunoinflammatory cells activate the endothelium to produce humoral factors and to express adhesion molecules (Akopov et al., 1996). These processes have been implicated in adult neurological diseases (Kochanek & Hallenbeck, 1992) and are likely to play a role in the pathogenesis of injury in the immature brain (Palmer, 1995).

Immunoinflammatory cells

The immune response of the adult brain to an inflammatory stimulus is characterized by a minimal infiltration of polymorphonuclear leukocytes and a delay before monocytic cells are activated (Lawson and Perry, 1995; Andersson et al., 1991). Major insults with vast destruction of tissue components are needed to elicit an acute inflammatory reaction such as occurs in other tissues.

The immature brain, however, is different. Injection of endotoxin into the 7-day-old mouse brain induces a considerable recruitment of polymorphs and a rapid mononuclear response (Lawson & Perry, 1995; Perry et al., 1995). Microglial activation occurs early following hypoxia–ischemia or excitotoxicity in the immature rat CNS, and is more rapid in white than in grey matter (McRae et al., 1995). Polymorphonuclear cells accumulate in capillaries and postcapillary venules (Hudome et al., 1997) and a limited recruitment of lymphocytes (CD4+ and CD8+) occurs (Bona et al., 1999). The mechanisms whereby these cells are activated is not known, but cytokines and chemokines are believed to be involved.

Cytokines and chemokines

Cytokines constitute a large and heterogeneous group of proteins with multiple actions within the nervous and the immune systems. Among the activities of different cytokines relevant to neurological injury are pro- and anti-inflammatory actions, activation of microglia and macrophages, triggering of apoptosis through cell surface receptors, stimulating production of adhesion molecules on endothelium and neutrophil surface and direct neuroprotective effects (Thomson, 1998; Akopov, 1996).

Chemokines are a subgroup of cytokines with chemotactic activity for specific types of leukocytes. The α-chemokines mainly attract polymorpholeukocytes whereas β-chemokines attract and activate macrophages, microglia and other immune cells. IL-8, MIP-2 and GRO are examples of α-chemokines and MCP-1, RANTES, MIP-1α/β are β-chemokines.

The effects of chemokines and cytokines are interrelated and, in some cases, very different in immature and adult brain. For example, a 500 times higher dose of IL-1β is required to elicit an inflammatory response in adult rat brain as compared to juvenile or neonatal rats, whereas the response to TNF-α is not as dependent on stage of postnatal development (Anthony et al., 1997). This maturational effect is mediated by CXC chemokines (Anthony et al., 1998).

Cytokines and chemokines are expressed in the immature brain in response to a variety of insults. IL-1β and MCP-1 are expressed after intracerebral injection of NMDA (Hagan et al., 1996; Szaflarski et al., 1998), and IL-1α, IL-1β, TNF-α, IL-6, MIP-1α, MIP-1β, MIP-2, RANTES, GRO and MCP-1 are all induced after hypoxia–ischemia in 7-day-old rats (Szaflarski et al., 1995; Hagberg et al., 1996; Szaflarski et al., 1998; Bona et al., 1999), although expression for TNF-α and MIP-2 in the white matter may be slower and less pronounced after hypoxia–ischemia than endotoxin (H. Hagberg et al., unpublished data).

IL-6, IL-8 and, in some infants, IL-1β immunoreactive proteins were increased in the CSF during hypoxic–ischemic encephalopathy, and the levels correlated to the degree of newborn encephalopathy (Sävman et al., 1998), whereas TNF-α, IL-10 and GM-CSF were unaffected.

The role of cytokines and chemokines in perinatal brain injury is highly complex, as the example of TNF-α demonstrates. TNF-α has two receptors (p55 and p75), and can be toxic to neurons (Gelbard et al., 1993) and oligodendroglia (Selmaj & Raine, 1988), inducing apoptosis in oligodendroglia (Leist & Nicotera, 1998) by receptor-mediated activation of caspase-8 (Cohen, 1997), probably mediated by the p75 receptor (Bruce et al., 1996). However, in different conditions TNF-α can protect against cell death, probably through the p55 receptor (Liu et al., 1998).

Other cytokines are less well studied, but IL-1β (combined with interferon-γ) induces apoptosis in fetal neurons incubated in vitro (Hu et al., 1997). Administration of the endogenous IL-1 receptor antagonist (IL-1 ra) systemically

(Martin et al., 1994) intracerebrally (Hagberg et al., 1996) or by adenovirus-mediated overexpression (Hagan et al., 1996) reduces brain injury in immature rats.

Conclusion

The mechanisms of cerebral injury in hypoxic–ischemic encephalopathy are multiple and complex, and the infant brain is different from the adult in many ways. The realization that brain injury develops over a considerable period of time and that active cell processes such as apoptosis are important has led to important advances, not least the belief that treatment of hypoxia–ischemia might be successfully initiated after resuscitation from the insult. Clinical trials of neural rescue therapies are beginning, and although potential treatments have yet to prove themselves, further advances in basic understanding of the mechanisms, such as inflammatory responses, may significantly improve our chances of developing successful treatments for hypoxic–ischemic encephalopathy.

REFERENCES

Aden, U., Bona, E., Hagberg, H. & Fredholm, B. B. (1994). Changes in c-fos mRNA in the neonatal rat brain following hypoxic ischemia. *Neuroscience Letters*, **180**(2) 91–5.

Akopov, S., Sercombe, R. & Seylaz, J. (1996). Cerebrovascular reactivity: role of endothelium/platelet/leucocyte interactions. *Cerebrovascular and Brain Metabolism Reviews*, **8**, 11–94.

Andersson, P. B., Perry, V. H. & Gordon, S. (1991). The CNS acute inflammatory response to excitotoxic neuronal cell death. *Immunology Letters*, **30**, 177–81.

Andine, P., Lehmann, A., Ellren, K. et al. (1988). The excitatory amino acid antagonist kynurenic acid administered after hypoxic–ischemia in neonatal rats offers neuroprotection. *Neuroscience Letters*, **90**, 208–12.

Andine, P., Sandberg, M., Bagenholm, R., Lehmann, A. & Hagberg, H. (1991). Intra- and extracellular changes of amino acids in the cerebral cortex of the neonatal rat during hypoxic-ischemia. *Brain Research and Developmental Brain Research*, **64**, 115–20.

Ankarcrona, M., Dypbukt, J. M., Bonfoco, E. et al. (1995). Glutamate-induced neuronal death: a succession of necrosis or apoptosis depending on mitochondrial function. *Neuron*, **15**(4), 961–73.

Anthony, D. C., Bolton, S. J., Fearn, S. & Perry, V. H. (1997). Age-related effects of interleukin-1 beta on polymorphonuclear neutrophil-dependent increases in blood–brain barrier permeability in rats. *Brain*, **120**, 435–44.

Anthony, D., Dempster, R., Fearn, S. et al. (1998). CXC cytokines generate age-related increases in neutrophil-mediated brain inflammation and blood–brain barrier breakdown. *Current Biology*, **8**, 923–6.

Armstead, W. M., Mirro, R., Busija, D. W. & Leffler, C. W. (1988). Postischemic generation of superoxide anion by newborn pig brain. *American Journal of Physiology*, **255**, H401–3.

Armstead, W. M., Mirro, R., Thelin, O. P. et al. (1992). Polyethylene glycol superoxide dismutase and catalase attenuate increased blood–brain barrier permeability after ischemia in piglets. *Stroke*, **23**(5), 755–62.

Ashwal, S., Cole, D. J., Osborne, S., Osborne, T. N. & Pearce, W. J. (1995). L-NAME reduces infarct volume in a filament model of transient middle cerebral artery occlusion in the rat pup. *Pediatric Research*, **38**, 652–6.

Azzopardi, D., Wyatt, J. S., Cady, E. B. et al. (1989). Prognosis of newborn infants with hypoxic–ischemic brain injury assessed by phosphorus magnetic resonance spectroscopy. *Pediatric Research*, **25**, 445–51.

Back, S. A., Gan, X., Li, Y., Rosenberg, P. A. & Volpe, J. J. (1998). Maturation-dependent vulnerability of oligodendrocytes to oxidative stress-induced death caused by glutathione depletion. *Journal of Neuroscience*, **18**(16), 6241–53.

Badawi, N., Kurinczuk, J. J., Keogh, J. M. et al. (1998). Intrapartum risk-factors for newborn encephalopathy: the Western Australia case-control study. *British Medical Journal*, **317**, 1554–8.

Bågenholm, R., Andine, P. & Hagberg, H. (1996). Effects of the 21-amino steroid tirilazad mesylate (U-74006F) on brain damage and edema after perinatal hypoxia–ischemia in the rat. *Pediatric Research*, **40**(3), 399–403.

Bågenholm, R., Nilsson, U. A., Götberg, C. W. & Kjellmer, I. (1998). Free radicals are formed in the brain of fetal sheep during reperfusion after cerebral ischemia. *Pediatric Research*, **43**, 271–5.

Beilharz, E. J., Bassett, N. S., Sirimanne, E. S., Williams, C. E. & Gluckman, P. D. (1995). Insulin-like growth factor II is induced during wound repair following hypoxic–ischemic injury in the developing rat brain. *Brain Research Molecular Brain Research*, **29**(1), 81–91.

Bickler, P. E. & Hansen, B. M. (1998). Hypoxia-tolerant neonatal CA1 neurons: relationship of survival to evoked glutamate release and glutamate receptor-mediated calcium changes in hippocampal slices. *Brain Research Developmental Brain Research*, **106**(1–2), 57–69.

Bickler, P., Gallego, S. & Hansen, B. (1993). Developmental changes in intracellular calcium regulation in rat cerebral cortex during hypoxia. *Journal of Cerebral Blood Flow and Metabolism*, **13**, 811–19.

Blomgren, K., Kawashima, S., Saido, T. C., Karlsson, J. O., Elmered, A. & Hagberg. H. (1995a). Fodrin degradation and subcellular distribution of calpains after neonatal rat cerebral hypoxic–ischemia. *Brain Research*, **684**(2), 143–9.

Blomgren, K., McRae, A., Bona, E., Saido, T. C., Karlsson, J. O. & Hagberg, H. (1995b). Degradation of fodrin and MAP 2 after neonatal cerebral hypoxic-ischemia. *Brain Research*, **684**(2), 136–42.

Blomgren, K., McRae, A., Elmered, A., Bona, E., Kawashima, S., Saido, T. C., Ono, T. & Hagberg, H. (1997). The calpain proteolytic system in neonatal hypoxic–ischemia. *Annals of the New York Academy of Science*, **825**, 104–19.

Blumberg, R. M., Cady, E. B., Wigglesworth, J. S., McKenzie, J. E. & Edwards, A. D. (1996). Relation between delayed impairment of cerebral energy metabolism and infarction following transient focal hypoxia–ischemia in the developing brain. *Experimental Brain Research*, **113**, 130–7.

Bolanas, J. P., Almeida, A., Stewart, V., Peuchen, S. L., Clark, J. B. & Heales, S. J. R. (1997). Nitric oxide-mediated mitochondrial damage in the brain: mechanisms and implication for neurodegenerative diseases. *Journal of Neurochemistry*, **68**, 2227–40.

Bona, E., Andersson, A. L., Blomgren, K. et al. (1999). Chemokine and inflammatory cell response to hypoxia–ischemia in immature rats. *Pediatric Research* **45**, 500–9.

Bossy-Wetzel, E., Newmeyer, D. D. & Green, D. R. (1998). Mitochondrial cytochrome c release in apoptosis occurs upstream of DEVD-specific caspase activation and independently of mitochondrial transmembrane depolarization. *EMBO Journal*, **17**(1), 37–49.

Bruce, A. J., Boling, W., Kindy, M. S. et al. (1996). Altered neuronal and microglial responses to excitotoxic and ischemic brain injury in mice lacking TNF receptors. *Nature Medicine*, **2**(7), 788–94.

Cady, E. B. (1990). *Clinical Magnetic Resonance Spectroscopy*. New York: Plenum.

Chauhan, D., Pandey, P., Ogata, A. et al. (1997). Cytochrome c-dependent and independent induction of apoptosis in multiple myeloma cells. *Journal of Biological Chemistry*, **272**(48), 29995–7.

Chen, C-K., Silverstein, F. S., Statman, D. & Johnston, M. V. (1988). Perinatal hypoxic–ischemic brain injury enhances quisqualic acid-stimulated phosphoinositide turnover. *Journal of Neurochemistry*, **51**, 353–9.

Cheng, Y., Gidday, J. M., Yan, Q., Shah, A. R. & Holtzman, D. M. (1997). Marked age-dependent neuroprotection by brain-derived neurotrophic factor against neonatal hypoxic–ischemic brain injury. *Annals of Neurology*, **41**, 521–9.

Cheng, Y., Deshmukh, M., D'Costa, A. et al. (1998). Caspase inhibitor affords neuroprotection with delayed administration in a rat model of neonatal hypoxic–ischemic brain injury. *Journal of Clinical Investigation*, **101**, 1992–9.

Cherici, G., Alesiani, M., Pellegrini-Giampietro, D. E. & Moroni, F. (1991). Ischemia does not induce the release of excitotoxic amino acids from the hippocampus of newborn rats. *Pediatric Research*, **60**, 235–40.

Chernyak, B. V. (1997). Redox regulation of the mitochondrial permeability transition pore. *Bioscience Reports*, **17**(3), 293–302.

Choi, D. W. (1995). Calcium: still center-stage in hypoxic–ischemic neuronal death. Trends. *Neuroscience*, **18**, 58–60.

Chumas, P. D., Del Bigio, M. R., Drake, J. M. & Tuor, U. I. (1993). A comparison of the protective effect of dexamethasone to other potential prophylactic agents in a neonatal rat model of cerebral hypoxia–ischemia. *Journal of Neurosurgery*, **79**, 414–20.

Cohen, G. M. (1997). Caspases: the executioners of apoptosis. *Biochemical Journal*, **326**(1), 1–16.

Cowan, F., Pennock, J. M., Hanrahan, D., Manji, K. & Edwards, A. D. (1994). Early detection of infarction and hypoxic–ischaemic encephalopathy in neonates using diffusion weighted magnetic resonance imaging. *Neuropediatrics* **25**, 172–5.

Croall, D. E. & DeMartino, G. N. (1991). Calcium-activated neutral protease (calpain) system: structure, function, and regulation. *Physiological Reviews*, **71**(3), 813–47.

Crow, J. P. & Beckman, J. S. (1995). The role of peroxynitrite in nitric oxide-mediated toxicity. *Current Topics in Microbiology and Immunology*, **196**(57), 57–73.

Dawson, V. L., Dawson, T. M., Bartley, D. A., Uhl, G. R. & Snyder, S. H. (1993). Mechanisms of nitric oxide-mediated neurotoxocity in primary brain cultures. *Journal of Neuroscience*, **13**(6), 2651–61.

Ditelberg, J. S., Sheldon, R. A., Epstein, C. J. & Ferriero, D. M. (1996). Brain injury after perinatal hypoxia-ischemia is exacerbated in copper/zinc superoxide dismutase transgenic mice. *Pediatric Research*, **39**(2), 204–8.

Du, C., Hu, R., Csernansky, C. A., Hsu, C. Y. & Choi, D. W. (1996). Very delayed infarction after mild focal cerebral ischemia: a role for apoptosis? *Journal of Cerebral Blood Flow and Metabolism*, **16**, 195–201.

Dwyer, B. E., Nishimura, R. N., Powell, C. L. & Mailheau, S. L. (1987). Focal protein synthesis inhibition in a model of neonatal hypoxic-ischaemic brain injury. *Experimental Neurology*, **95**, 277–89.

Edwards, A. D., Yue, X., Cox, P. et al. (1997). Apoptosis in the brains of infants suffering intrauterine cerebral injury. *Pediatric Research*, **42**, 684–9.

Edwards, A. D., Wyatt, J. S. & Thoresen, M. (1998). Treatment of hypoxic–ischaemic brain damage by moderate hypothermia. *Archives of Disease in Childhood*, **78**, F85–8.

Eliasson, M. J. L., Blackshaw, S., Schell, M. J. & Snyder, S. H. (1997a). Neuronal nitric oxide synthase alternatively spliced forms: prominent functional localizations in the brain. *Proceedings of the National Academy of Sciences, USA*, **94**, 3396–401.

Eliasson, M. J., Sampei, K., Mandir, A. S. et al. (1997b). Poly(ADP-ribose) polymerase gene disruption renders mice resistant to cerebral ischemia. *Nature Medicine*, **3**(10), 1089–95.

Ellerby, H. M., Martin, S. J., Ellerby, L. M. et al. (1997). Establishment of a cell-free system of neuronal apoptosis: comparison of premitochondrial, mitochondrial, and postmitochondrial phases. *Journal of Neuroscience*, **17**(16), 6165–78.

Endres, M., Wang, Z. Q., Namura, S., Waeber, C. & Moskowitz, M. A. (1997) Ischemic brain injury is mediated by the activation of poly(ADP-ribose)polymerase. *Journal of Cerebral Blood Flow & Metabolism*, **17**(11), 1143–51.

Ferriero, D. M., Sheldon, R. A., Black, S. M. & Chuai, J. (1995). Selective destruction of nitric oxide synthase neurons with quisqualate reduces damage after hypoxia-ischemia in the neonatal rat. *Pediatric Research*, **38**, 912–918.

Ferriero, D. M., Holtzman, D. M., Black, S. M. & Sheldon, R. A. (1996). Neonatal mice lacking neuronal nitric oxide synthase are less vulnerable to hypoxic–ischemic injury. *Neurobiology of Disease*, **3**, 64–71.

Gelbard, H. A., Dzenko, K. A., DiLoeto, D., del Cerro, C., del Cerro, M. & Epstein, L. G. (1993). Neurotoxic effects of tumor necrosis factor alpha in primary human neuronal cultures are mediated by activation of the glutamate AMPA receptor subtype: implications for AIDS neuropathogenesis. *Developmental Neuroscience*, **15**, 417–422.

Giulian, D. & Vaca, K. (1993). Inflammatory glia mediate delayed neuronal damage after ischemia in the central nervous system. *Stroke*, **24**(Suppl. 1), 184–90.

Gluckman, P. D., Guan, J., Williams, C. et al. (1998). Asphyxial brain injury – the role of the IGF system. *Molecular and Cellular Endocrinology*, **40**(1–2), 95–9.

Grether, J. K. & Nelson, K. B. (1997). Maternal infection and cerebral palsy in infants of normal birth weight. *Journal of the American Medical Association*, **278**, 207–11.

Guan, J., Williams, C., Gunning, M., Mallard, C. & Gluckman, P. (1993). The effect of IGF-1 treatment after hypoxic–ischemic brain injury in adult rats. *Journal of Cerebral Blood Flow and Metabolism*, **13**(4), 609–16.

Gubits, R., Burke, R., Casey-McIntosh, G., Bandele, A. & Munell, F. (1993). Immediate early gene induction after neonatal hypoxia–ischemia. *Molecular Brain Research*, **18**, 228–238.

Gunn, A. J., Dragunow, M., Faull, R. L. M. & Gluckman, P. D. (1990). Effects of hypoxia-ischemia and seizures on neuronal and glial-like c-*fos* protein levels in the infant rat. *Brain Research*, **531**, 105–16.

Hagan, P., Poole, S., Bristow, A. F., Tilders, F. & Silverstein, F. S. (1996). Intracerebral NMDA injection stimulates production of interleukin-1 beta in perinatal rat brain. *Journal of Neurochemistry*, **67**(5), 2215–18.

Hagberg, H., Lehmann, A., Sandberg, M., Nyström, B., Jacobson, I. & Hamberger, A. (1985). Ischemia-induced shift of inhibitory and excitatory amino acids from intra- to extracellular compartments. *Journal of Cerebral Blood Flow and Metabolism*, **5**, 413–19.

Hagberg, H. Andersson, P., Kjellmer, I., Thiringer, K. & Thordstein, M. (1987). Extracellular overflow of glutamate, aspartate, GABA and taurine in the cortex and basal ganglia of fetal lambs during hypoxia–ischemia. *Neuroscience Letters*, **78**, 311–17.

Hagberg, H., Gilland, E., Diemer, N. H. & Andiné, P. (1994). Hypoxia-ischemia in the neonatal rat brain: histopathology after post-treatment with NMDA and non-NMDA receptor antagonists. *Biology of the Neonate*, **66**, 206–213.

Hagberg, H., Gilland, E., Bona, E. et al. (1996). Enhanced expression of interleukin (IL)-1 and IL-6 messenger RNA and bioactive protein after hypoxia–ischemia in neonatal rats. *Pediatric Research*, **40**(4), 603–9.

Hall, E. D. (1995). Inhibition of lipid peroxidation in central nervous system trauma and ischemia. *Journal of the Neurological Sciences*, **134**, 79–83.

Halliwell, B. (1992). Reactive oxygen species and central nervous system. *Journal of Neurochemistry*, **59**, 1609–23.

Hamada, Y., Hayakawa, T., Hattori, H. & Mikawa, H. (1994). Inhibitor of nitric oxide synthesis reduces hypoxic–ischemic brain damage in the neonatal rat. *Pediatric Research*, **35**(1), 10–14.

Hanrahan, D., Sargentoni, J., Azzopardi, D. et al. (1996). Cerebral metabolism within 18 hours of birth asphyxia: a proton magnetic resonance spectroscopy study. *Pediatric Research* **39**(4), 584–90.

Hanrahan, D., Cox, I. J., Edwards, A. D. et al. (1998). Persistent increases in cerebral lactate concentration after birth asphyxia. *Pediatric Research*, **44**, 304–11.

Hanrahan, D., Cox, I. J., Azzopardi, D. et al. (1999). Relation between proton magnetic resonance spectroscopy within 18 hours of birth asphyxia and neurodevelopment at one year of age. *Developmental Medicine and Child Neurology*, **41**, 76–82.

Hasegawa, K., Yoshioka, H., Sawada, T. & Nishikawa, H. (1991). Lipid peroxidation in neonatal mouse brain subjected to two different types of hypoxia. *Brain Development*, **13**(2), 101–3.

Hasegawa, K., Yoshioka, H., Sawada, T. & Nishikawa, H. (1993). Direct measurement of free radicals in the neonatal mouse brain subjected to hypoxia: an electron spin resonance spectroscopic study. *Brain Research*, **607**(1–2), 161–6.

Hattori, H., Morin, A. M., Schwartz, P. H., Fujikawa, D. G. & Wasterlain, C. G. (1989). Posthypoxic treatment with MK-801 reduces hypoxic–ischemic damage in the neonatal rat. *Neurology*, **39**, 713–18.

Heyes, M. P., Saito, K., Chen, C. Y. et al. (1997). Species heterogeneity between gerbils and rats: quinolinate production by microglia and astrocytes and accumulations in response to ischemic brain injury and systemic immune activation. *Journal of Neurochemistry*, **69**, 1519–29.

Hirsch, T., Susin, S. A., Marzo, I., Marchetti, P., Zamzami, N. & Kroemer, G. (1998). Mitochondrial permeability transition in apoptosis and necrosis. *Cell Biology and Toxicology*, **14**(2), 141–5.

Hockenbery, D. M., Nunez, G., Milliman, C., Schreiber, R. D. & Korsmeyer, S. J. (1990). Bcl-2 is an inner mitochondrial membrane protein that blocks programmed cell death. *Nature*, **348**(6299), 334–6.

Hockenbery, D. M., Oltvai, Z. N., Yin , X. M., Milliman, C. L. & Korsmeyer, S. J. (1993). Bcl-2 functions in an antioxidant pathway to prevent apoptosis. *Cell*, **75**, 241–51.

Holtzman, D. M., Sheldon, R. A., Jaffe, W., Cheng, Y., Ferriero, D. (1996). Nerve growth factor protects the neonatal brain against hypoxic–ischemic injury. *Annals of Neurology*, **39**, 114–122.

Hope, P. L., Costello, A. M., Cady, E. B. et al. (1984). Cerebral energy metabolism studied with phosphorus NMR spectroscopy in normal and birth-asphyxiated infants. *Lancet*, **2**, 66–370.

Hu, S., Peterson, P. K. & Chao, C. C. (1997). Cytokine-mediated neuronal apoptosis. *Neurochemistry International*, **30**(4–5), 427–31.

Huang, Z., Huang, P. L., Panahian, N., Dalkara, T., Fishman, M. C. & Moskowitz, M. A. (1994). Effects of cerebral ischemia in mice deficient in neuronal nitric oxide synthase. *Science*, **265**, 1883–5.

Hudome, S., Palmer, C., Roberts, R. L., Mauger, D., Housman, C. & Towfighi, J. (1997). The role of neutrophils in the production of hypoxic–ischemic brain injury in the neonatal rat. *Pediatric Research*, **41**, 607–16.

Hughes, P. & Dragunow, M. (1995). Induction of immediate-early genes and the control of neurotransmitter- regulated gene expression within the nervous system. *Pharmacological Reviews*, **47**(1), 133–78.

Iadecola, C. & Ross, M. E. (1997). Molecular pathology of cerebral ischemia: delayed gene expression and strategies for neuroprotection. *Annals of the New York Academy of Sciences*, **835**, 203–17.

Ikonomidou, C., Bosch, F., Bittigau, P., Miksa, M., Turski, L. & Olney, J. W. (1999). NMDA antagonists induce massive apoptotic neurodegeneration in the developing rat CNS. *Society of Neurosciences*, **24**, 274.

Jaffrey, S. R. & Snyder, S. H. (1995). Nitric oxide: A neural messenger. *Annual Review of Cell and Developmental Biology*, **11**, 417–40.

Joashi, U., Greenwood, K., Taylor, D. L. et al. (1999). Poly(ADP ribose) polymerase cleavage precedes neuronal death in the hippocampus and cerebellum following injury to the developing rat forebrain. *European Journal of Neuroscience*, **11**, 91–100

Johnston, B. M., Mallard, E. C., Williams, C. E. & Gluckman, P. D. (1996). Insulin-like growth factor-1 is a potent neuronal rescue agent after hypoxic–ischemic injury in fetal lambs. *Journal of Clinical Investigation*, **97**, 300–8.

Jouvet, P., Rustin, P., Felderhoff, U. et al. (1998). Maple syrup urine disease metabolites induce apoptosis in neural cells without cytochrome c release or changes in mitochondrial membrane potential. *Biochemical Society Transactions*, **26**, S341.

Khan, S., Kayahara, M., Joashi, U. et al. (1997). Differential induction of apoptosis in Swiss 3T3 cells by nitric oxide and the nitrosonium cation. *Journal of Cell Science*, **110**(18), 2315–22.

Kjellmer, I., Andiné, P., Hagberg, H. & Thiringer, K. (1989). Extracellular increase of hypoxanthine and xanthine in the cortex and basal ganglia of fetal lambs during hypoxia–ischemia. *Brain Research*, **478**, 241–7.

Klempt, N., Sirimanne, E., Gunn, A. J. et al. (1992). Hypoxia–ischemia induces transforming growth factor β_1 mRNA in the infant rat brain. *Molecular Brain Research*, **13**, 93–101.

Kochanek, P. M. & Hallenbeck, J. M. (1992). Polymorphonuclear leukocytes and monocytes/macrophages in the pathogenesis of cerebral ischemia and stroke. *Stroke*, **23**, 1367–79.

Koistinaho, J. & Hökfelt, T. (1997). Altered gene expression in brain ischemia. *Neuroreport*, **8**, I–VIII.

Kroemer, G., Zamzami, N. & Susin, S. A. (1997). Mitochondrial control of apoptosis. *Immunology Today*, **18**(1), 44–51.

Kroemer, G., Dallaporta, B. & Resche-Rigon, M. (1998). The mitochondrial death/life regulator in apoptosis and necrosis. *Annual Review of Physiology*, **60**, 619–42.

Lawson, L. J. & Perry, V. H. (1995). The unique characteristics of inflammatory responses in mouse brain are acquired during postnatal development. *European Journal of Neurosciemce*, **7**, 1584–95.

Lazebnik, Y. A., Kaufmann, S. H., Desnoyers, S., Poirier, G. G. & Earnshaw, W. C.(1994). Cleavage of poly(ADP-ribose) polymerase by a proteinase with properties like ICE. *Nature*, **371**, 346–7.

LeBlanc, M. H., Li, X. Q., Huang, M., Patel, D. M. & Smith, E. E. (1995). AMPA antagonist LY293558 does not affect the severity of hypoxic–ischemic injury in newborn pigs. *Stroke*, **26**(10), 1908–14.

Lee, W.-H., Wang, G-M., Seaman, L. B., & Vannucci. S. J. (1996). Coordinate IGF-I and IGFBP5 gene expression in perinatal rat brain after hypoxia–ischemia. *Journal of Cerebral Blood Flow and Metabolism*, **16**, 227–36.

Leib, S. L., Kim, Y. S., Chow, L. L., Sheldon, R. A. & Tauber, M. G. (1996). Reactive oxygen intermediates contribute to necrotic and apoptotic neuronal injury in an infant rat model of bacterial meningitis due to group B streptococci. *Journal of Clinical Investigation*, **98**(11), 2632–9.

Leist, M. & Nicotera, P. (1998). Apoptosis, excitotoxicity, and neuropathology. *Experimental Cell Research*, **239**, 83–201.

Leist, M., Single, B., Kunstle, G., Volbracht, C., Hentze, H. & Nicotera, P. (1997). Apoptosis in the absence of poly-(ADP-ribose) polymerase. *Biochemical Biophysical and Research Communication*, **233**(2), 518–22.

Li, F., Srinivasan, A., Wang, Y., Armstrong, R. C., Tomaselli, K. J. & Fritz, L. C. (1997). Cellspecific induction of apoptosis by microinjection of cytochrome c. Bcl-xL has activity independent of cytochrome c release. *Journal of Biology and Chemistry*, **272**(48), 30299–305.

Lindsay, R. M. (1994). Neurothrophic growth factors and neurodegenerative diseases: therapeutic potential of the neurotrophins and ciliary neurotrophic factor. *Neurobiology of Aging*, 4(15), 249–51.

Linnik, M. D., Zorbrist, R. H. & Hatfield, M. D. (1993) Evidence supporting a role for programmed cell death in focal cerebral ischemia in rats. *Stroke*, **24**, 2002–8.

Liu, J., Marino, M. W., Wong, G. et al. (1998). TNF is a potent anti-inflammatory cytokine in autoimmune-mediated demyelination. *Nature Medicine*, **4**(1), 78–83.

Liu, X., Kim, C. N., Yang, J., Jemmerson, R. & Wang, X. (1996). Induction of apoptotic program in cell-free extracts: requirement for dATP and cytochrome c. *Cell*, **86**(1), 147–57

Lodge, D. & Collinridge, G. L. (1991). The pharmacology of excitatory amino acids. *Trends in Pharmacological Science,* **Special Report**, 1–89.

Lorek, A., Takei, Y., Cady, E. B. et al. (1994). Delayed ('secondary') cerebral energy failure following acute hypoxia–ischaemia in the newborn piglet: continuous 48-hour studies by 31P magnetic resonance spectroscopy. *Pediatric Research*, **36**, 699–706.

Lucas, D. R. & Newhouse, J. P. (1957). The toxic effect of sodium-L-glutamate on the inner layers of retina. *Annals of American Ophthalmology*, **58**, 193.

McDonald, J. W. & Johnston, M. W. (1990). Physiological and pathophysiological roles of excitatory amino acids during central nervous system development. *Brain Research Reviews*, **15**, 41–70.

McDonald, J. W., Silverstein, F. S. & Johnston, M. V. (1987). MK-801 protects the neonatal brain from hypoxic–ischemic damage. *European Journal of Pharmacology*, **140**, 359–61.

McDonald, J. W., Silverstein, F. S. & Johnston, M. V. (1988). Neurotoxicity of *N*-methyl-D-aspartate is markedly enhanced in developing rat central nervous system. *Brain Research*, **459**, 200–3.

McRae, A., Gilland, E., Bona, E. & Hagberg, H. (1995). Microglia activation after neonatal hypoxic–ischemia. *Developmental Brain Research*, **84**, 245–52.

Maragos, W. F. & Silverstein, F. S. (1994). Resistance to nitroprusside neurotoxicity in perinatal rat brain. *Neuroscience Letters*, **172**, 80–4.

Marks, K.A., Mallard, C., Roberts, I., Williams, C. E., Gluckman, P. D. & Edwards, A. D. (1999). Nitric oxide synthase inhibition and delayed cerebral injury following severe cerebral ischemia in sheep. *Pediatric Research*, **46**, 8–13.

Martin, D., Chinookoswong, N. & Miller, G. (1994). The interleukin-1 receptor antagonist (rhIL-1ra) protects against cerebral infarction in a rat model of hypoxia–ischemia. *Experimental Neurology*, **130**, 362–7.

Martin, E., Buchli, R., Ritter, S. et al. (1996). Diagnostic and prognostic value of cerebral 31P magnetic resonance spectroscopy in neonates with perinatal asphyxia. *Pediatric Research*, **40**, 749–58.

Martin, L. J., Al-Abdulla, N. A., Brambrink, A. M., Kirsch, J. R., Sieber, F. E. & Portera-Cailliau, C. (1998). Neurodegeneration in excitotoxicity, global cerebral ischemia, and target deprivation: a perspective on the contributions of apoptosis and necrosis. *Brain Research Bulletin*, **46**(4), 81–309.

Martinou, J. C., Dubois-Dauphin, M., Staple, J. K. et al. (1994). Overexpression of BCL-2 in

transgenic mice protects neurons from naturally occurring cell death and experimental ischemia. *Neuron* **13**(4), 1017–30.

Marton, A., Mihalik, R., Bratincsak, A. et al. (1997). Apoptotic cell death induced by inhibitors
of energy conservation–Bcl-2 inhibits apoptosis downstream of a fall of ATP level. *European
Journal of Biochem*istry, **250**(2), 467–75.

Matsumiya, N., Koehler, R. C., Kirsch, J. R & Traytsman, R. J. (1991). Conjugated superoxide dismutase reduces extent of caudate injury after transient focal ischemia in cats. *Stroke*, **22**,
11983–2000.

Mehmet, H., Yue, X., Squier, M. V et al. (1994). Increased apoptosis in the cingulate sulcus of
newborn piglets following transient hypoxia–ischaemia is related to the degree of high energy
phosphate depletion during the insult. *Neuroscience Letters*, **181**, 121–5.

Michaelis, E. K. (1998). Molecular biology of glutamate receptors in the central nervous system
and their role in excitotoxicity, oxidative stress and aging. *Progress in Neurobiology*, **54**(4),
369–415.

Miller, R. J. (1987). Multiple calcium channels and neuronal function. *Science*, **235**(4784), 46–52.

Miller, R. J. (1991). The control of neuronal Ca^{2+} homeostasis. *Progress in Neurobiology*, **37**(3),
255–85.

Namura, S., Zhu, J., Fink, K. et al. (1998). Activation and cleavage of caspase-3 in apoptosis
induced by experimental cerebral ischemia. *Journal of Neuroscience*, **18**(10), 3659–68.

Nath, R., Raser, K. J., Stafford, D. et al. (1996). Non-erythroid a-spectrin breakdown by calpain
and interleukin-1b-converting-enzyme-like protease(s) in apoptotic cells: contributory roles
of both protease families in neuronal apoptosis. *Biochemical Journal*, **319**, 683–90.

Nelson, K. B., Dambrosia, J. M., Ting, T. Y. & Grether, J. K. (1996). Uncertain value of electronic
fetal monitoring in predicting cerebral palsy [see comments]. *New England Journal of
Medicine*, **334**(10), 613–18.

Nelson, K. B., Dambrosia, J. M., Grether, J. K. & Phillips, T. M. (1998). Neonatal cytokines and
coagulation factors in children with cerebral palsy. *Annals of Neurology*, **44**(4), 665–75.

Nozaki, K., Finklestein, S. P. & Beal, M. F. (1993). Basic fibroblast growth factor protects against
hypoxia–ischemia and NMDA neurotoxicity in neonatal rats. *Journal of Cerebral Blood Flow
and Metabolism*, **13**, 221–8.

Olney, J. W. & Ho, O. L. (1970). Brain damage in infant mice following oral intake of glutamate,
aspartate and cysteine. *Nature*, **227**, 609–11.

Ostwald, K., Hagberg, H., Andiné, P. & Karlsson, J-O. (1993). Upregulation of calpain activity in
neonatal rat brain after hypoxic–ischemia. *Brain Research*, **630**, 289–94.

Palmer, C. (1995). Hypoxic–ischemic encephalopathy. Therapeutic approaches against microvascular injury, and role of neutrophils, PAF, and free radicals. *Clinical Perinatology*, **22**,
481–517.

Palmer, C., Brucklacher, R. M., Christensen, M. A. & Vannucci, R. C. (1990a). Carbohydrate and
energy metabolism during the evolution of hypoxic–ischemic brain damage in the immature
rat. *Journal of Cerebral Blood Flow and Metabolism*, **10**, 227–35.

Palmer, C., Vannucci, R. C. & Towfighi, J. (1990b). Reduction of perinatal hypoxic–ischemic
brain damage with allopurinol. *Pediatric Research*, **27**, 332–6.

Palmer, C., Towfighi, J., Roberts, R. & Heitjan, D. F. (1993). Allopurinol administered after inducing hypoxic–ischemia reduces brain injury in 7-day-old rats. *Pediatric Research*, **33**(4), 405–11.

Palmer, C., Roberts, R. L. & Bero, C. (1994). Deferoxamine posttreatment reduces ischemic brain injury in neonatal rats. *Stroke*, **25**, 1039–45.

Penrice, J., Cady, E., Lorek, A. et al. (1996). Proton magnetic resonance spectroscopy of the brain in normal preterm and term infants, and early changes after perinatal hypoxia–ischaemia. *Pediatrics Research*, **40**, 6–14.

Perry, V. H., Bell, M. D., Brown, H. C. & Matyszak, M. K. (1995). Inflammation in the nervous system. *Current Opinion in Neurobiology*, **5**(5), 636–41.

Portera-Cailliau, C., Price, D. L. & Martin, L. J. (1997a). Excitotoxic neuronal death in the immature brain is an apoptosis–necrosis morphological continuum. *Journal Comparative Neurology*, **378**, 70–87.

Portera-Cailliau, C., Price, D. L. & Martin, L. J. (1997b). Non-NMDA and NMDA receptor-mediated excitotoxic neuronal deaths in adult brain are morphologically distinct: further evidence for an apoptosis–necrosis continuum. *Journal of Comparative Neurology*, **378**(1), 88–104.

Pryds, O., Greisen, G., Lou, H. & Friis Hansen, B. (1990). Vasoparalysis associated with brain damage in asphyxiated term infants. *Journal of Pediatrics*, **117**, 119–25.

Robertson, N.J., Cox, I.J., Cowan, F.M., Counsell, S., Azzopardi, D. & Edwards, A.D. (1999). Cerebral intracellular lactic alkalosis persisting months after neonatal encepalopathy measured by magnetic resonance spectroscopy. *Pediatric Research*, **46**, 287–97.

Rosenberg , A. A., Murdaugh, E. & White, C. W., (1989). The role of oxygen free radicals in post-asphyxia cerebral hypoperfusion in newborn lambs. *Pediatric Research*, **26**, 215–19.

Ross, M. E. (1996). Cell division and the nervous system: regulating the cycle from neural differentiation to death. *Trends in Neurosci*ence, **19**(2), 62–8.

Roth, S. C., Edwards, A. D., Cady, E. B. et al. (1992). Relation between cerebral oxidative metabolism following birth asphyxia and neurodevelopmental outcome and brain growth at one year. *Developmental Medicine and Child Neurology*, **34**, 285–95.

Roth, S. C., Baudin, J., Cady, E. et al. (1997). Relation of deranged neonatal cerebral oxidative metabolism with neurodevelopmental outcome and head circumference at 4 years. *Developmental Medicine and Child Neurology*, **39**, 718–25.

Rutherford, M. A., Pennock, J., Counsell, S. et al. (1998). Abnormal magnetic resonance signal in the internal capsule predicts poor outcome in infants with hypoxic–ischaemic encephalopathy. *Pediatrics*, **102**, 323–8.

Saugstad, O. D. (1996). Mechanisms of tissue injury by oxygen radicals: implications for neonatal disease. *Acta Pediatrica*, **85**, 1–4.

Sävman, K., Blennow, M., Gustafson, K., Tarkowski, E. & Hagberg, H. (1998). Cytokine response in cerebrospinal fluid after birth asphyxia. *Pediatric Research*, **43**(6), 746–51.

Scott, R. J. & Hegyi, L. (1997). Cell death in perinatal hypoxic–ischaemic brain injury. *Neuropathology and Applied Neurobiology*, **23**(4), 307–14.

Selmaj, K. & Raine, C. S. (1988). Tumor necrosis factor mediates myelin and oligodendrocyte damage in vitro. *Annals of Neurology*, **23**, 339–46.

Siesjö, B. K. (1986). Calcium and ischemic brain damage. *European Neurology*, **25**, 45–56.

Silver, I. A. & Erecinska, M. (1990). Intracellular and extracellular changes of [Ca^{2+}] in hypoxia and ischemia in rat brain in vivo. *Journal of General Physiology*, **95**(5), 837–66.

Silverstein, F. S., Buchanan, K., Hudson, C. & Johnston, M. V. (1986). Flunarizine limits hypoxia–ischemia induced morphologic injury in immature rat brain. *Stroke*, **17**, 477–82.

Silverstein, F., Torke, L., Barks, J. & Johnston, M. V. (1987). Hypoxia–ischemia produces focal disruption of glutamate receptors in developing brain. *Developmental Brain Research*, **34**, 33–9.

Sinz, E. H., Kochanek, P. M., Heyes, M. P et al. (1998). Quinolinic acid is increased in CSF and associated with mortality after traumatic brain injury in humans. *Journal of Cerebral Blood Flow amd Metabolism*, **18**, 610–15.

Skulachev, V. P. (1996). Why are mitochondria involved in apoptosis? Permeability transition pores and apoptosis as selective mechanisms to eliminate superoxide-producing mitochondria and cell. *FEBS Letters*, **397**(1), 7–10.

Skulachev, V. P. (1998). Cytochrome c in the apoptotic and antioxidant cascades. *FEBS Letters* **423**(3), 275–80.

Smeyne, R. J., Vendrell, M., Hayward, M. et al. (1993). Continuous c-*fos* expression precedes programmed cell death *in vivo*. *Nature*, **363**, 166–9.

Stein, D. T. & Vannucci, R. C. (1988). Calcium accumulation during the evolution of hypoxic–ischemic brain damage in the immature rat. *Journal of Cerebral Blood Flow and Metabolism*, **8**, 834–42.

Szaflarski, J. Burtrum, D. & Silverstein, F. S. (1995). Cerebral hypoxia-ischemia stimulates cytokine gene expression in perinatal rats. *Stroke*, **26**, 1093–100.

Szaflarski, J., Ivacko, J., Liu, X. H., Warren, J. S. & Silverstein, F. S. (1998). Excitotoxic injury induces monocyte chemoattractant protein-1 expression in neonatal rat brain. *Molecular Brain Research*, **55**, 306–14.

Tan, W. K. M., Williams, C. E., Gunn, A. J., Mallard, C. E. & Gluckman, P. D. (1992). Suppression of postischemic epileptiform activity with MK-801 improves neural outcome in fetal sheep. *Annals of Neurology*, **32**, 677–82.

Tan, W. K. M., Williams, C. E., During, M. J. et al. (1996). Accumulation of cytotoxins during the development of seizures and edema after hypoxic–ischemic injury in late gestation fetal sheep. *Pediatric Research*, **39**(5), 791–7.

Thomson, A. W. (1998). *The Cytokine Handbook*. San Diego: Academic Press.

Thoresen, M., Satas, S., Puka-Sundvall, M. et al. (1997). Post-hypoxic hypothermia reduces cerebrocortical release of NO and excitotoxins. *Neuroreport*, **8**(15), 3359–62.

Thornberry, N. A. & Lazebnik, Y. (1998). Caspases: enemies within. *Science*, **281**, 1312–16.

Thornton, J. S., Ordidge, R. J., Penrice, J. et al. (1998). Temporal and anatomical variations of brain water apparent diffusion coefficient in perinatal cerebral hypoxic–ischemic injury: relationships to cerebral energy metabolism. *Magnetic Resonance in Medicine*, **39**, 920–7.

Trifiletti, R. (1992). Neuroprotective effects of N^{G}-nitro-L-arginine in focal stroke in the 7-day old rat. *European Journal of Pharmacology*, **218**, 197–8.

Van der Heiden, M. G., Chandel, N. S., Williamson, E. K., Schumacker, P. T. & Thompson, C. B.

(1997). Bcl-xL regulates the membrane potential and volume homeostasis of mitochondria. *Cell*, **91**(5), 627–37.

Volpe, J. J. (ed.) (1994). Hypoxic–ischemic encephalopathy: neuropathology and pathogenesis. In *Neurology of the Newborn*, ed. J. J. Volpe, pp. 279–314. Philadelphia: W. B. Saunders Co.

Williams, C., Gunn, A., Mallard, C. & Gluckman, P. (1992). Outcome after ischemia in developing sheep brain: an electroencephalographic and histological study. *Annals of Neurology*, **31**, 14–21.

Wong, E. H. F. & Kemp, J. A. (1991). Sites for antagonism on the N-methyl-D-aspartate receptor channel complex. *Annual Review of Pharmacology and Toxicology*, **31**, 401–25.

Wyatt, J. S., Cope, M., Delpy, D. T. et al. (1990). Quantitation of cerebral blood volume in newborn infants by near infrared spectroscopy. *Journal of Applied Physiology*, **68**, 1086–91.

Wyatt, J. S., Edwards, A. D., Cope, M. et al. (1991). Response of cerebral blood volume to changes in arterial carbon dioxide tension in preterm and term infants. *Pediatric Research*, **29**, 553–7.

Wyllie, A. H. & Duvall, E. (1992) Cell injury and death. *Oxford Textbook of Pathology*, ed. J. McGee, P. G. Isacsson & N. A. Wright, pp. 141–93. Oxford: Oxford University Press.

Yue, X., Mehmet, H., Penrice, J. et al. (1997). Apoptosis and necrosis in the newborn piglet brain following transient cerebral hypoxia–ischaemia. *Neuropathology and Applied Neurobiology*, **23**(1), 16–25.

Zou, H., Henzel, W. J., Liu, X., Lutschg, A. & Wang, X. (1997). Apaf-1, a human protein homologous to *C. elegans* CED-4, participates in cytochrome c-dependent activation of caspase-3. *Cell*, **90**(3), 405–13.

19

Clinical assessment and therapeutic interventions for hypoxic–ischemic encephalopathy in the full-term infant

Andrew Whitelaw and Marianne Thoresen

Division of Child Health, University of Bristol Medical School, Southmead Hospital, Bristol, UK

Definition and diagnostic criteria

The term hypoxic–ischemic encephalopathy (HIE) implies a clinically apparent acute disturbance in brain function resulting from a period of critical deprivation of cerebral oxygen delivery and/or blood supply. For the diagnosis of HIE following intrapartum asphyxia to be upheld, there needs to have been obstetric evidence of risk of hypoxia/ischemia to the fetus (e.g. prolapse of the umbilical cord, late decelerations of the fetal heart, fresh meconium, placental abruption, etc.) after which the infant is born in poor condition, is resuscitated and is then observed to have cerebral dysfunction (e.g. hypotonia, inability to suck, abnormal posture, clonic movements). The finding of metabolic acidosis or raised lactate levels in cord blood or blood taken within 30 minutes of birth provides important supporting evidence that there has been acute hypoxia–ischemia at or shortly before delivery. Further support for a global hypoxic–ischemic episode is provided by deranged liver function (raised transaminases or ammonia), a period of renal impairment with oliguria (and raised serum creatinine), cardiac dysfunction and changes of disseminated intravascular coagulation. The diagnosis of HIE also requires that steps have been taken to rule out other causes of cerebral dysfunction such as infection, preexisting anatomical abnormalities of the brain or an inherited metabolic disease.

Clinical assessment of HIE

Clinical features

During resuscitation after acute asphyxia, the infant is typically hypotonic, apnoeic and unresponsive. The initial response is in the heart rate and blood pressure followed by improvement in skin colour. Following resuscitation there may be a period of mild to moderate neurological signs but severe neurological dysfunction may also be apparent from the start. There is usually a sequence of clinical features, and it is possible to grade the severity over a period of 48 hours. Clinical assessment of the neurological status of sick newborn infants is based on the following.

 (i) Observation of spontaneous movements.

Respiration, regular/ irregular/apnoea.

Eyes open/closed, eye movements.

Posture. Is the neck held in extension? Are the legs flexed or straight?

The character and quality of limb movements, tremors? Clonic movements?

Facial expression, spontaneous crying? Does the baby seem irritable?

 (ii) Response to light and sound.

(iii) Sucking and swallowing.

(iv) Passive tone in the limbs and trunk.

 (v) Active tone in the limbs and trunk including Moro reflex, grasp and deep tendon reflexes at the knee and ankle.

One physical sign which is often observed in moderate HIE is neck extensor hypertonia (Amiel-Tison, 1995). The examiner holds the infant's shoulders and pulls the infant from the lying to the sitting position, noting the position of the head in relation to the trunk. Normally this elicits active contraction of the neck flexors with the head flexed forward onto the chest (Fig. 19.1(a)). The examiner then moves the trunk gently backwards. Normally there is contraction of the neck extensors tending to lift the head before the trunk gets to the vertical position. In the normal term infant, flexion of the neck is equally strong as extension. Fig. 19.1(b) shows the effect of global hypotonia or weakness. There is no active contraction of the neck muscles either way. In Fig. 19.1(c) the head is held extended even when the trunk is flexed forward and the chin is poking out. This is illustrated in Fig. 19.2(a) (see colour plate section). Neck extensor hypertonia can also be observed, to some extent, when one holds the infant in ventral suspension. Besides being common in moderate HIE, this finding is also frequent in full-term infants with subarachnoid hemorrhage. Figure 19.2(b) (see colour plate section) shows an infant with more signs of moderate HIE. The legs are extended and adducted (scissor position). The hands are held fisted with the thumbs adducted. The head is held slightly extended. The eyes are open, but there is no fixation or following.

It is very important to listen to the nurse's description and impression of the baby's alertness, irritability/consolability, tone and movement quality.

It is usually possible by a combination of observation and examination to see a pattern which enables one to classify the affected baby as mildly, moderately or severely encephalopathic.

Sarnat and Sarnat (1976) first classified postasphyxial encephalopathy into three grades (Table 19.1). This approach has been used with minor modifications by others such as Amiel-Tison & Ellison (1986), Finer et al. (1983), Fenichel (1983)

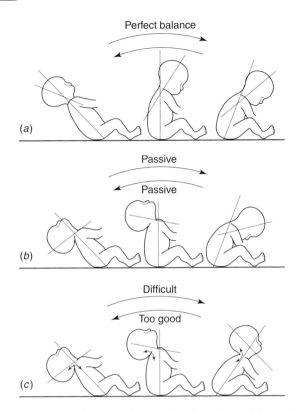

Fig. 19.1.   (*a*). Holding the shoulders and moving the trunk forwards and then backwards. Normally flexion of the neck is equally strong as is extention of the neck. (*b*). If there is global weakness or hypotonia, the head hangs back when the trunk is held back and the head hangs forward when the trunk is held forward. (*c*). When there is neck extensor hypertonia, the head is still held back even when the trunk is held forward. (From Amiel-Tison, 1995, with permission.)

and Levene et al. (1986). The clinical picture may be dominated by tachypnoea at this stage and this may be sufficient to cause hypocapnia. This may be combined with period breathing and apnoea. From the clinician's point of view, it is important to determine whether the infant is deteriorating from moderate encephalopathy to severe encephalopathy. Loss of reflex activity including respiratory failure, pooling of saliva and the loss of the doll's eye movements are important signs of severe encephalopathy.

Clinical examination and prognosis

The largest study examining the grade of HIE and neurological follow-up is by Robertson and Finer (1985). They examined survivors at 3.5 years and documented

Table 19.1. A clinical grading system for post-asphyxial encephalopathy

	Mild	Moderate	Severe
Level of consciousness	Hyperalert	Lethargic	Stuporous
Tone	Normal	Mild hypotonia	Flaccid
Posture	Mild distal flexion	Strong distal flexion	Intermittent decerebration
Stretch reflexes	Overactive	Overactive	Decreased or absent
Segmental myoclonus	Present	Present	Absent
Complex reflexes			
Suck	Weak	Weak or absent	Absent
Moro	Strong: low threshold	Weak: incomplete; high threshold	Absent
Oculovestibular	Normal	Overactive	Weak or absent
Tonic neck	Slight	Strong	Absent
Autonomic function	Generalized sympathetic	Generalized parasympathetic	Both systems depressed
Pupils	Mydriasis	Miosis	Variable; often unequal; often poor light reflex
Heart rate	Tachycardia	Bradycardia	Variable
Salivary secretions	Sparse	Profuse	Variable
Gastrointestinal motility	Normal or decreased	Increased; diarrhoea	Variable
Seizures	None	Common; focal or multifocal	Uncommon (excluding decerebration)
EEG	Normal	Early: low voltage continuous Spike and wave	Burst suppression or iso-potential

Source: From Sarnat and Sarnat (1976).

deaths among 226 infants with HIE. Of 79 infants with mild HIE, no child died or survived with disability. Of 119 with moderate HIE, 5% died and 21% of survivors were disabled. Of 28 with severe HIE, 75% died and 100% of the survivors were disabled, mostly with spastic cerebral palsy and cognitive disturbances.

The duration of encephalopathy also helps with prognosis. In Sarnat and Sarnat's 1976 study, infants who did not enter stage 3 and had signs of stage 2 for less than 5 days were normal at follow-up, but persistence of stage 2 for more than

7 days was associated with neurologic sequelae or death. Other studies have found that infants with a normal neurological examination by about 1 week were grossly normal at follow-up (Robertson & Finer, 1985; Scott, 1976).

Clinical seizures

Clinical seizures occur during the period 6–12 hours in over half of the infants who will eventually convulse (Volpe, 1995). Recognition of seizure activity in newborns can be difficult, but focal or multifocal clonic movements which are sustained and rhythmic, not stopped by restraint, have a fast component and a slow component and are accompanied by deviation of the eyes and disturbance of breathing are very likely to correlate with electrical seizure activity. It has become apparent that many episodes of seizure activity on EEG are not accompanied by clinical seizure activity (Eyre et al., 1983). Episodes of bilateral extensor tonus look very dramatic and are certainly an abnormal neurological sign, but they correlate only rarely with EEG epileptic activity (Volpe, 1995).

EEG and prognosis

Continuous 2 channel EEG recording with the Oxford Medilog system attached to a personal computer showing real time EEG on the screen is, in our experience, the best way of detecting epileptic activity in the NICU. Figure 19.3(a) shows one channel from an Oxford Medilog recording from an infant with moderate HIE. The top tracing shows normal speed EEG 30 mm/s with typical spike/wave epileptic activity. The lower trace shows the later interictal EEG printed more slowly and demonstrating good continuous activity. Fig. 19.3(b) shows one channel of EEG from an infant with severe HIE. The top trace shows typical epileptic activity, while the interictal EEG printed slowly shows virtually no activity at all. Easier and cheaper is the cerebral function monitor (CFM), which prints out at slow speed an amplitude integrated single channel EEG. The amplitude signal gives very useful information in real time on the severity of brain dysfunction and the prognosis, but it can sometimes be difficult to be certain about epileptic activity on the CFM. Nevertheless, the ease of application, relatively small size and robustness of the CFM make it acceptable to junior medical and nursing staff. The finding of continuously low amplitude EEG or burst suppression is of great importance prognostically and had a positive predictive value of 84.2% and a negative predictive value of 91.7% at 6 hours (Eken et al., 1995). A very low amplitude or isoelectric recording preceded death or disability in all cases. Figure 19.4 shows a CFM recording from an infant with severe HIE at about 6 hours. The lower margin of the trace is very low, about 1 microvolt and the activity is very intermittent. This child went on to develop severe motor problems. Burst suppression may, in a few cases, revert to continuous activity over 24 hours with the possibility of normal outcome (Hellstrom-Westas et al.,

(a)

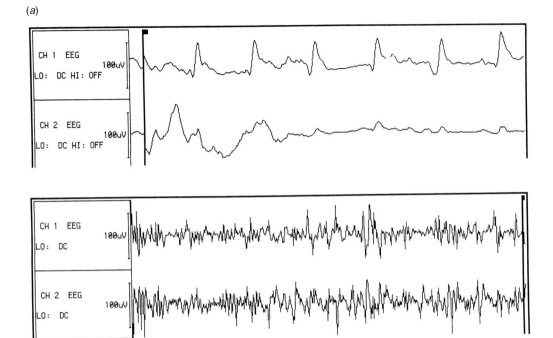

Fig. 19.3.   (a). Moderate HIE. The top panel shows two channel EEG from an Oxford Medilog recording at normal EEG speed, showing spike/wave epileptic activity. The bottom panel shows interictal EEG at four times normal speed demonstrating continuous activity.

1995). In the piglet model of global hypoxia, the severity of the hypoxic insult and the ultimate brain injury correlated with the time before spontaneous respiration and the return of EEG activity (Thoresen et al., 1996). For more details, see the chapters on electrophysiology.

Biochemical markers

Severe hypoxia produces characteristic metabolic derangements, which help in the clinical assessment if the analyses can be carried out rapidly. The magnitude of the metabolic acidosis in cord blood or in the first hour or two is confirmation of an acute intrapartum hypoxic insult. Marked neurological abnormality with normal acid–base status in cord blood is good evidence that the insult was probably a considerable time before delivery. There is an association between umbilical artery acidosis (< 7.0) and HIE (Goodwin et al., 1992) and neurological deficit at 1 year (Low et al., 1988), although it is important to point out that the majority of fetuses with umbilical artery pH < 7.0 were normal later. A number of metabolites, brain proteins and enzymes, which can be measured in blood, urine or cerebrospinal fluid, have been shown to correlate with HIE and neurological deficit but, as they

(b)

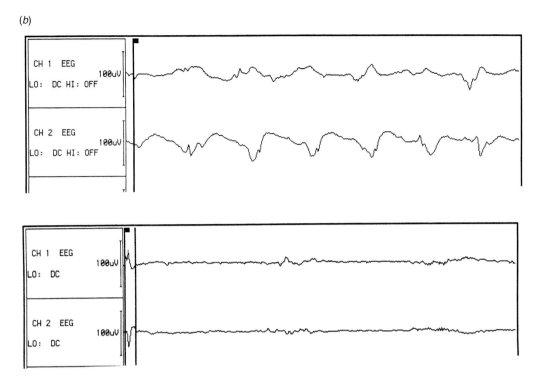

Fig. 19.3.   (b). Severe HIE. The top panel shows two channel EEG from an Oxford Medilog recording with spike/wave epileptic activity. The bottom panel shows interictal EEG at four times normal speed showing virtually no activity.

are not routinely available in clinical laboratories, they will not be considered further.

Ultrasound and prognosis

Cranial ultrasound is helpful in the assessment of hypoxic–ischemic encephalopathy as it can be carried out at the cot side with no disturbance and no ionizing radiation to the infant. Ultrasound may show increased echogenicity in the basal ganglia and thalamus as seen in Fig. 19.5 but is usually normal in the first 6 hours. If there is severe cerebral oedema, a generalized echogenicity with loss of details of the cerebral structures (bright brain) may be seen as in Fig. 19.6. This is also associated with compression of the cerebral ventricles. Another important function of an early ultrasound examination is the ruling out of gross congenital abnormalities such as holoprosencephaly or agenesis of the corpus callosum and antenatal abnormalities such as ventricular dilatation. Ultrasound is still a somewhat operator-dependent examination and, in our experience, is less helpful than clinical examination and EEG in assessing the severity and prognosis of HIE.

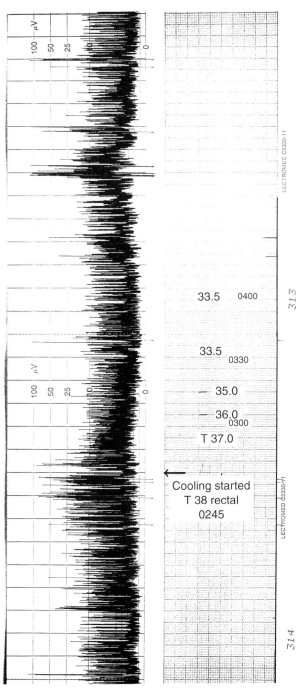

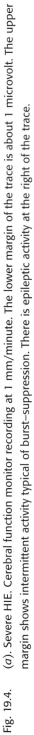

Fig. 19.4. (*a*). Severe HIE. Cerebral function monitor recording at 1 mm/minute. The upper margin of the trace is about 1 microvolt. The lower margin shows intermittent activity typical of burst–suppression. There is epileptic activity at the right of the trace.

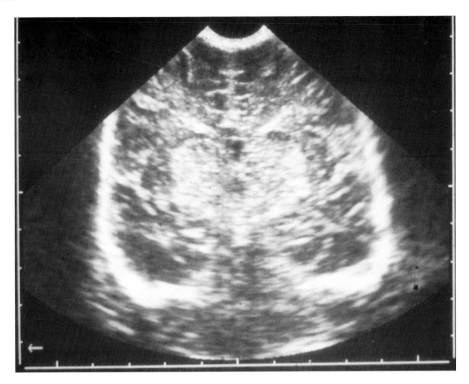

Fig. 19.5.   Severe HIE (same baby as in Fig. 19.7). Cerebral ultrasound (coronal view) showing increased echogenicity in the basal ganglia and thalamus.

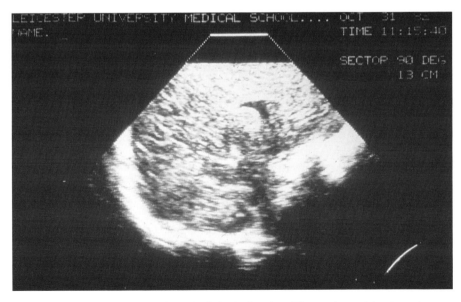

Fig. 19.6.   Severe HIE. Cerebral ultrasound (sagittal view) showing diffuse echogenicity throughout the brain substance.

Subcortical lesions can be demonstrated early in HIE but a 10 MHz transducer is required.

Cerebral Doppler and prognosis

Cerebral blood flow velocity studies of the middle cerebral artery have shown that a low resistance index (systolic velocity – diastolic velocity/systolic velocity), which is below 0.55 after 24 hours is highly predictive of poor neurological outcome (Archer et al., 1986). Rather than demonstrating a late no-reflow phenomenon, infants with severe HIE tend to show increased blood flow (luxury perfusion). Thus a low resistance index after 24 hours is a feature of cerebral vasodilatation with uncoupling of cerebral blood flow to metabolism.

Cranial CT and prognosis

CT findings in HIE are discussed in the chapter on imaging but CT, in our experience, is not helpful in assessing prognosis early.

Magnetic resonance imaging and prognosis

Magnetic resonance imaging is a challenging examination in a critically ill infant but is becoming increasingly valuable and abnormal signal density in the posterior limb of the internal capsule at about 4–17 days of age in infants with HIE was shown to be 100% predictive of neurological abnormality at 1 year of age. Negative predictive value was 0.87%. Sensitivity was 0.9 and specificity was 1.0 (Rutherford et al., 1998). This is still rather late if prognostic information is to be used for withdrawal of life support but preliminary results with diffusion-weighted imaging suggest that lesions may be shown earlier (Mary Rutherford, personal communication, 1998). An abnormal signal in the basal ganglia, thalamus and brainstem on MRI is also associated with a bad prognosis (Fig. 19.7). MRI is the best method of revealing or excluding prenatal or congenital abnormalities of the brain including migration disorders. This is extensively described in Chapter 14 on imaging.

Interventions

Mannitol

Cerebral edema often follows severe cerebral hypoxia–ischemia in adults and is common in severe HIE in infants (see Fig. 19.8 in colour plate section). Mannitol acts as an osmotic agent drawing water out of the brain and thus reducing edema. This effect has often been used in adult neurosurgical practice to reduce raised intracranial pressure. Marchal (1974) reported an uncontrolled study of 225 asphyxiated full-term infants. The infants qualified for the study if they had an Apgar score of 7 or less at 5 minutes. Others had neurological findings and many

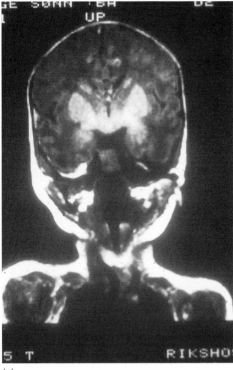

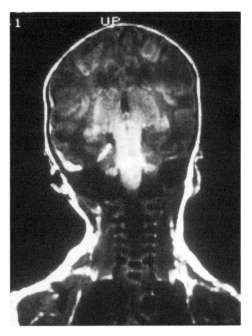

(b)

(a)

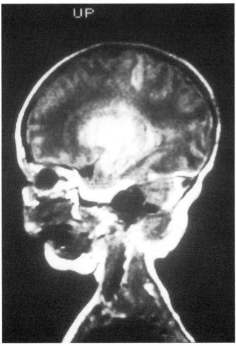

Fig. 19.7.   Severe HIE (same baby as in Fig. 19.5). Cerebral magnetic resonance image. T_1-weighted image. (a) Coronal view: abnormal bright signal in the basal ganglia and thalami. (b) Coronal view: abnormal bright signal in the brainstem and basal ganglia. (c) Sagittal view: abnormal bright signal in basal ganglia and thalamus.

(c)

of the infants had both. One hundred and thirty of the infants received 1g/kg i.v. mannitol before 2 hours and 95 received mannitol after 2 hours. There was a lower proportion of deaths and of disabled infants at 1 year in the group who received mannitol before 2 hours but, as the groups were not randomized, no conclusion about the efficacy of early mannitol is justified.

Levene and Evans (1985) studied the effect of mannitol in asphyxiated infants who developed HIE and had raised intracranial pressure (> 10 mm Hg measured by subarachnoid catheter), which had not resolved despite dexamethazone. Mannitol infusion 1g/kg i.v. produced a fall in intracranial pressure in four infants and an improvement in cerebral perfusion pressure within 60 minutes but in a larger series, all nine infants with sustained ICP > 15 mm Hg died or survived with disability in spite of mannitol. There is no randomized trial of mannitol in neonatal HIE, but the observations that some infants develop severe HIE without marked rises in ICP and the finding that raised ICP tends to occur after many hours of encephalopathy suggest that raised ICP from cerebral edema is probably a marker that severe brain damage has occurred rather than a mechanism by which damage is caused.

Mujsce et al. (1990) studied the efficacy of mannitol on 7-day-old rats subjected to unilateral carotid artery occlusion and 8% oxygen for 3 hours. 27 rats were given mannitol subcutaneously immediately after the cerebral hypoxia–ischemia and mannitol was repeated every 12 hours for a total of 4 doses. Control animals received either nothing or normal saline. Mannitol without hypoxia produced no deaths but increased serum osmolality from 287 to 361 mosm/l. The brains were examined at 48 hours. Mannitol significantly reduced brain water content but did not reduce the incidence, distribution or severity of tissue injury in the cortex, subcortical white matter, hippocampus or thalamus. Thus, the routine use of mannitol is not justified in neonatal HIE. There may be a number of infants with HIE who develop raised intracranial pressure which is reversible with mannitol therapy. At the moment, there is no objective evidence that such therapy improves long-term outcome.

Glucocorticoids

Glucocorticoids have been used to reduce edema surrounding brain tumours. Because of this, glucocorticoids, particularly dexamethazone began to be used in the management of HIE, in order to prevent or reduce cerebral oedema. No randomized trials have evaluated the effect of dexamethazone on neonatal HIE but Svenningsen et al. (1982) included 2 mg 6 hourly of dexamethazone in 'brain-oriented intensive care treatment in severe perinatal asphyxia'. Because the study used historical controls, and several interventions were introduced together, it is impossible to conclude that dexamethazone had a positive effect on outcome.

Levene and Evans (1985) measured intracranial and arterial pressure invasively in infants with HIE and gave dexamethazone 4 mg if ICP rose above 10 mm Hg. There was a fall in ICP within 1 hour, but this was accompanied by a fall in arterial pressure so that cerebral perfusion pressure was not improved.

The 7-day-old rat cerebral hypoxia–ischemia model with unilateral carotid ligation and several hours of hypoxia has been used to evaluate dexamethazone. Barks et al. (1991) found that dexamethazone given 24 hours before the insult was protective but treatment after the insult was not protective. Altman et al. (1984) showed, in the same model, that dexamethazone given immediately before the hypoxic insult did not alter the pattern of neuropathological damage or reduce the fall in high-energy phosphates. Furthermore, high dose dexamethazone (40 mg/kg) was associated with an increase in mortality when compared to low dose (4 mg/kg) or no dose dexamethazone. There is also considerable evidence that corticosteroid administration in early life restricts brain growth and development (Howard, 1968). When all the above evidence is combined with the lack of evidence that glucocorticoids improve outcome in adult patients with hypoxic–ischemic injury or head trauma (Dearden et al., 1986; Fishman, 1982), glucocorticoids cannot be recommended as therapy for neonatal HIE.

Barbiturates

Seizures are frequently present in moderate and severe HIE. Some clinical seizures cause disturbances in respiration and blood pressure, which may worsen the cerebral injury. In addition, there is evidence that prolonged seizure activity may produce cerebral injury in its own right, although the evidence for this in the newborn brain is inconsistent (Soderfeldt et al., 1990). Seizures experimentally induced in normal brain by chemicals increase cerebral lactate concentrations greatly, but posthypoxic seizures in the neonatal piglet are not accompanied by a further increase in cerebral lactate (Thoresen et al., 1998). This may be because lactate is itself used as a fuel by the neonatal brain.

In addition to anticonvulsant activity, barbiturates decrease cerebral metabolic rate and scavenge free radicals. Barbiturates have been proposed as agents which might reduce brain injury in neonatal HIE if given prophylactically without waiting for clinical seizure activity. Three randomized trials have compared prophylactic barbiturate therapy with no routine anticonvulsant therapy in full-term neonates with severe asphyxia. Goldberg et al. (1986) gave thiopentone 25 mg/kg over 20 hours as the initial intervention to infants with poor Apgar scores and early signs of HIE. Ruth et al. (1991) gave 30 mg/kg phenobarbitone i.v. then 15 mg/kg 4 hours later to infants with Apgar score <4 at 5 minutes or ventilator dependent for more than 30 minutes. Hall et al. (1998) gave 40 mg/kg i.v. on the basis of Apgar score at 10 minutes of age. The results of the three trials are shown in Table 19.2.

Table 19.2. Barbiturate vs. control after severe perinatal asphyxia

Study	Barbiturate	Control	Relative risk (95% CI)
Outcome: severe neurodevelopmental disability in survivors examined/total			
Goldberg (1986)	5/11	6/11	0.83 (0.36–1.94)
Ruth (1991)	3/16	2/14	1.31 (0.25–6.76)
Hall (1998)	1/13	6/12	0.15 (0.02–1.1)
Outcome: death or severe neurodevelopmental disability/total			
Goldberg (1986)	10/17	9/15	0.98 (0.55–1.74)
Ruth (1991)	8/21	5/17	1.3 (0.52–3.24)
Hall (1998)	3/20	10/20	0.3 (0.1–0.93)

Source: Modified from Evans & Levene (1998).

Carrying out such trials is more difficult than most clinical trials and the three studies above represent considerable achievements. Birth asphyxia is often unexpected and informed consent from a recently delivered mother when any intervention must be started as soon as possible poses great demands on the investigator and the infant's parents. Moderate to severe HIE is, itself, uncommon being approximately 1–2 per thousand live births. This means that accumulating over 20 cases takes considerable time, even in the largest obstetric service.

Close examination of the three trials does show potential sources of bias. It is important to conceal treatment allocation until the infant is irrevocably entered into the trial. This was done in Hall's trial but the method of allocation concealment is not clear in the studies by Ruth and Goldberg. None of the trials used a placebo and thus all the clinical staff knew which infants received the barbiturate, raising the possibility that infants who had received the active therapy might have been treated differently (consciously or unconsciously) in other ways, e.g. more (or less) careful attention to oxygenation, blood pressure, blood glucose sterile technique or temperature. Many infants in the control group developed clinical seizures and were then treated with anticonvulsant therapy, usually phenobarbitone initially. Thus in Hall's trial the control group received a mean of 27 mg/kg of phenobarbitone, although this was started much later than the larger dose of phenobarbitone given to the active treatment group. There was significant loss during follow-up, 3% in Goldberg's trial and 23% in Hall's trial, but Ruth did not state the number lost to follow-up. Appropriate standardized neurodevelopmental tests were used in all three studies (e.g. Bayley, Stanford-Binet, WISC), although it was not stated how blinding of outcome assessment was achieved in the studies by Hall and Ruth. Only one study (Hall et al., 1998) showed a reduction in relative risk of severe developmental disability or death in the barbiturate-treated group. The loss to follow-up detracts somewhat from the strength of the conclusion. The meta-analysis of all three trials involves only 110 infants and shows no significant effect on death or severe neurodevelopmental disability. High dose barbiturate therapy can also produce significant reductions in blood pressure in asphyxiated infants (Goldberg et al., 1986; Eyre & Wilkinson, 1986).

Thus prophylactic therapy with barbiturates cannot be recommended for infants with severe birth asphyxia or early HIE on present evidence.

Calcium channel blockers

Following hypoxia, reoxygenation is followed by a cascade of cellular reactions which may lead to death of neurones and oligodendroglial cells. These events include (i) release of oxygen free radicals, (ii) influx of calcium which activates phospholipase and causes membrane destruction, and (iii) high extracellular concentrations of excitotoxic amino acids with overstimulation of NMDA and other glutamate receptors. These processes are fully described in the chapter by Hagberg and Edwards. Calcium channel blocking agents have been used clinically as vasodilators and might be therapeutic following severe hypoxia–ischemia, by reducing calcium influx, dilating cerebral vessels and possibly by reducing platelet aggregation and improving cardiac function. Steen et al. (1983) demonstrated that the calcium channel blocker, nimodipine, given immediately after temporary aortic occlusion, improved neurologic recovery and cerebral blood flow in dogs. Vaagenes et al. (1984) showed, in a controlled trial, that the calcium channel blocker, lidoflazine, given after 10 minutes of cardiac arrest in dogs produced significantly better neurological recovery, although histopathological scoring was not significantly different. Allen et al. (1983) showed that the calcium channel blocker, nimodipine, given to adult human patients with subarachnoid hemorrhage, significantly reduced secondary cerebral vasospasm. A placebo-controlled, double-blind, randomized trial in 155 patients resuscitated after out-of-hospital ventricular fibrillation tested the effect of lidoflazine injected immediately after restoration of spontaneous circulation (Roine et al., 1990). Overall, there was no difference in survival at one year (40% with lidoflazine vs. 36% in the control group) but, in a posthoc analysis of patients with more than 10 minutes delay before advanced life support, there was a higher rate of survival in the lidoflazine group (47% vs. 8%). There was no statistically significant difference between the two treatment groups in neurological outcome.

Levene et al. (1990) reported on the use of the calcium channel blocker, nicardipine, by continuous intravenous infusion in four severely asphyxiated human neonates. The mean arterial pressure fell in three out of four cases and there was a marked drop in arterial pressure with an associated fall in cerebral blood flow velocity in two infants. We have observed a similar fall in arterial pressure and cerebral blood flow velocity when nimodipine was given to an infant with HIE. Avoidance of hypotension is one of the few principles of treatment of HIE that everyone agrees on, and calcium channel blockers have never been assessed in a large randomized trial in human newborns with asphyxia or HIE. Despite the positive results from animal models, there is doubt as to whether calcium channel blockers are safe or effective in protecting the brain after hypoxia. The time scale of calcium influx may be such that very early administration of a calcium channel blocker is necessary to have any therapeutic effect. In practice, very early administration within a few minutes is usually not possible in perinatal asphyxia.

Magnesium sulfate

Posthypoxic neuronal damage is partly caused by raised extracellular concentrations of the excitotoxic amino acids, glutamate and aspartate and the N-methyl-D-aspartate (NMDA) receptor is thought to be important in the pathogenesis of posthypoxic damage in the perinatal period. Increasing the extracellular concentration of magnesium can block the NMDA receptor by hyperpolarization. McDonald et al. (1990) were able to produce cerebral injury in a neonatal rat model by direct injection of NMDA. The extent of the cerebral damage was reduced by magnesium administration. Thordstein et al. (1993) treated 7-day-old rats with magnesium sulphate, mannitol and L-methionine after unilateral carotid ligation and 2 hours of hypoxia and demonstrated a significant reduction in cerebral damage. There is, however, no neonatal model of cerebral hypoxia–ischemia where magnesium alone has reduced the extent of brain damage. Magnesium sulfate had been widely used in obstetric practice for both pre-eclampsia and as tocolysis in preterm labour. Observational studies have reported an association between maternal magnesium sulfate treatment and a reduction in the rate of cerebral palsy in infants born prematurely (Hirtz & Nelson, 1998). This observation cannot be explained by an excess of deaths among vulnerable infants in the magnesium-treated group.

In 1993 it was suggested that clinical studies of magnesium sulfate as cerebral protection after severe birth asphyxia should begin in Europe. It had been well known for many years that high concentrations of magnesium could produce hypotonia, vasodilatation and muscle paralysis. The phase 1 study was to investigate the pharmacokinetics of magnesium and to examine the effects of two different doses of magnesium on blood pressure, heart rate, respiration and neurological function (Levene et al., 1995). Infants were eligible if (i) there was evidence of fetal distress (ii) the gestational age was 35 weeks or more (iii) Apgar score was less than 6 at 10 minutes (iv) postnatal age was less than 12 hours. Seven infants received

400 mg/kg of MgSO$_4$.7H$_2$O. (Magnesium sulfate is normally in the heptahydrate form). Eight infants received 250 mg/kg of MgSO$_4$.7H$_2$O. The serum Mg^{2+} rose from 0.79 mmol/l to 3.6 mmol/l at one hour and was still elevated at 24 hours. Mean arterial pressure fell in the first hour by an average of 6 mm Hg and, in the most seriously ill infant, already requiring an infusion of dopamine at 12 μg/kg/min, the mean arterial pressure fell from 40 to 25 mm Hg 5 minutes after the magnesium sulfate infusion was completed. After increasing the dopamine infusion to 20 μg/kg/min, the mean arterial pressure rose to 43 mm Hg by 60 minutes. Mean heart rate fell by 10 beats/min but this did not reach statistical significance. All the infants receiving 400 mg/kg were already intubated and ventilated and ceased to breathe spontaneously for 3–6 hours after the magnesium infusion. Muscle activity and tone diminished but EEG did not change.

The infants who received 250 mg/kg of MgSO$_4$.7H$_2$O showed a rise in serum concentration from 0.71 mmol/l to 2.42 mmol/l. There was no significant change in heart rate, blood pressure, muscle tone or EEG but one infant who was not initially intubated, became apnoeic and required ventilation by face mask for 5 minutes. In two infants, cerebrospinal fluid concentrations of Mg^{2+} were measured and found to be lower than the corresponding serum level (1.43 vs. 2.15 mmol/l and 1.71 vs. 1.91 mmol/l).

The experience from the phase 1 study and other anecdotal communications indicate that high doses of magnesium sulfate can produce potentially dangerous hypotension in asphyxiated infants. It is likely that the most severely asphyxiated infants, with hypoxic damage to the myocardium and endothelium are the ones that are most vulnerable to cardiovascular collapse if a large dose of magnesium is administered. There is also some doubt as to how quickly high concentrations of magnesium are achieved in the brain. Magnesium sulfate has now been tested in the newborn piglet using bilateral transient carotid occlusion and hypoxemia (Penrice et al., 1997). This study was randomized, placebo controlled and blinded. This hypoxic–ischemic insult is previously documented to give secondary energy failure in the brain with depletion of nucleotide triphosphates on magnetic resonance spectroscopy (MRS) and subsequent neuropathological changes. The maturity of the newborn piglet is roughly equivalent to a human infant of 36–40 weeks. 400 mg/kg of MgSO$_4$ intravenously had no effect on cerebral secondary energy failure or lactate/creatine or N-acetylaspartate/creatine ratios. Subsequent neuropathological examination also failed to show any effect from the magnesium sulfate (Wyatt J. personal communication, 1998). Thus on the available evidence, magnesium sulfate does not look promising as a treatment for HIE in the full-term infant. This does not mean that pathologically low levels of serum magnesium should not be corrected. Nor does it rule out the possibility that magnesium sulfate administration to women before preterm delivery may have a beneficial effect on the infant.

It is even possible that NMDA receptor-mediated damage to white matter differs substantially between the preterm infant and the full-term infant and that the consequent benefit from magnesium might only be apparent in preterm infants.

Allopurinol

Reoxygenation after hypoxia–ischemia gives rise to free radical-induced injury. Xanthine oxidase contributes to this by synthesising hypoxanthine. Palmer et al. (1990) investigated the effect of allopurinol, a xanthine oxidase inhibitor, in the 7-day-old rat unilateral carotid ligation and hypoxia model. Allopurinol treated rats had significantly less water in the ligated hemisphere at 42 hours and less severe neuropathological changes at 30 days. Van Bel et al. (1998) have studied the effect of high dose allopurinol, an inhibitor of xanthine oxidase and a free radical scavenger, on severely asphyxiated newborn infants. The study was not a randomized trial, but there was a control group. There were only 22 infants altogether. No toxic effects from allopurinol were observed. Non-protein-bound iron (a source of free radicals) rose in the control group but dropped to zero in the allopurinol treated group. Malondialdehyde (an indicator of lipid peroxidation) increased in the control group but remained stable in the allopurinol group. Electrocortical brain activity (recorded by the cerebral function monitor) decreased in the control group but remained stable in the allopurinol group during the first 8 hours. Six control and two allopurinol-treated infants died after neurological deterioration. Saugstad (1996) has pointed out that high activities of xanthine oxidase are restricted to a few organs (especially the liver) in humans. As positive effects from xanthine oxidase blockade with allopurinol have been reported even in organs containing relatively low concentrations of xanthine oxidase, allopurinol may exert its effect by (i) scavenging oxygen free radicals directly or (ii) augmenting adenine nucleotides. Another possibility considered was that hypoxic damage to the liver released large amounts of xanthine oxidase into the blood from where it could reach the brain. However, Rootwelt et al. (1995) showed that only low levels of xanthine oxidase were released into the blood after severe hypoxemia in newborn pigs. In the light of all the promising preliminary findings, there is considerable interest in a large randomized trial of allopurinol in infants with severe asphyxia or early HIE.

Hypothermia

Hypothermia at the time of hypoxia–ischemia has been well known for many years to protect the brain. This has enabled open heart surgery to be carried out and there have been numerous reports of near drownings in cold water where individuals have been submerged for up to 40 minutes in cold water with complete recovery. Cooling was first reported as treatment for birth asphyxia by the Swedish obstetrician, Bjorn

Westin (1959). He reported six neonates who failed to respond to other forms of resuscitation and were placed in a bath of cold water so that colonic temperature fell to between 23 and 30°C. The cooling began between 4 and 15 minutes after birth and was continued for up to 39 minutes. Only one of the six infants died. Similar reports have been made by Miller et al. (1964) and Cordey et al. (1973). It is important to point out that rapid cooling as a means of resuscitation of the newborn preceded the introduction of endotracheal intubation and ventilation. When effective oxygenation could rapidly be achieved by intubation, and doctors were trained to intubate in Western countries, interest in cooling evaporated after Silverman et al. (1958) reported that a cooler thermal environment for a number of days increased mortality in very low birthweight infants. Only in the Soviet Union was rapid cooling used in the resuscitation of asphyxiated neonates during the 1970s and 1980s. During this period, one of the cardinal principles of neonatal intensive care was the maintenance of normothermia throughout illness and procedures.

In 1989 Busto et al. reported that mild cooling after cerebral ischemia reduced the extent of brain damage in the CA1 region of the adult rat hippocampus. In 1992 Carroll and Beck confirmed this finding and showed a dose–response effect. The earlier the cooling started and the longer the duration of cooling, the better the cerebral protection. Two other studies in adult rats failed to confirm cerebral protection from postischemic hypothermia (Welsh & Harris, 1991; Dietrich et al., 1993). Yager et al. (1993) found no cerebral protection from postischemic hypothermia in the unilateral carotid ligation and hypoxia 7-day-old rat model. The first report showing cerebral protection in a neonatal animal model with posthypoxic hypothermia was by Thoresen et al. (1995). Twelve hours of mild hypothermia (4 degrees reduction) prevented secondary energy failure in the newborn piglet, as determined by MRS. In 1996 Thoresen showed that 3 hours of posthypoxic hypothermia (6 degrees reduction) was protective in the 7-day-old rat unilateral carotid ligation and hypoxia model as demonstrated by quantitative neuropathology at 7 days. This therapeutic effect has later been shown to persist for 6 weeks (Bona et al., 1998). Sirimanne et al. (1996) have shown that only 2 degrees of hypothermia lasting 72 hours reduced the extent of cerebral damage in the 21-day-old rat using unilateral carotid ligation and 15 minutes of 8% oxygen. Gunn et al. (1997) have developed selective head cooling in the fetal lamb. Thirty minutes of carotid occlusion was followed, 90 minutes later, by cooling via a coil around the head for 72 hours. In a randomized study, 72 hours of cooling produced a large reduction in infarction and neuronal loss. A delay in starting cooling to 5.5 hours still gave protection (Gunn et al., 1998).

Not only is there now considerable evidence that posthypoxic cooling is protective, but mild cooling by 2 to 6 degrees appears also to be safe. None of the groups working with hypothermia in neonatal animal models have documented any adverse effects. Phase 1 clinical studies have now begun with both whole body cooling and selective head cooling. Gunn et al. (1998) pioneered head cooling via a coil of tubing wrapped around the head. Cold water is pumped through the tubing, the water temperature being adjusted to keep the rectal temperature at 36.3 or 35.7 °C. A head cooling cap system made by Olympic Medical of Seattle is currently being evaluated in a pilot study in Auckland, London and Bristol. Although described as 'selective head cooling' it is in fact cooling via the head to achieve systemic cooling to a rectal temperature of 34–35 °C. This treatment system has been used for 72 hours in infants who have clinical evidence of perinatal asphyxia and show abnormal electrocortical activity (by cerebral function monitor) within the first six hours. Figure 19.9 in colour plate section shows an infant with HIE being treated with the Olympic cooling cap system at Southmead Hospital, Bristol. So far this treatment approach appears to be safe and a large multicentre trial is currently being planned to see if 72 hours of mild hypothermia can reduce death or disability at 18 months of age in the above group of infants. Whole body cooling using surface cooling with a mattress is also being evaluated in pilot studies by D. Azzopardi et al. at the Hammersmith Hospital, London (personal communication). We and others have previously carried out pilot studies of whole body cooling using rubber gloves filled with cold water placed around the infant's body. Rectal temperature was maintained at 33–34 °C for 24–72 hours without apparent adverse effects. Fig. 19.10 shows data from one asphyxiated baby, cooled systemically, in whom rectal temperature was maintained at about 34 °C for 72 hours. The heart rate fell to around 80/minute but mean arterial pressure was well maintained. One of the practical issues still unresolved is the need for sedation or analgesia, while hypothermia is used.

Current recommendations for clinical management of neonatal HIE

Maintenance of adequate ventilation and oxygenation after birth

In the current state of knowledge, this means achieving an arterial pO_2 of 8–12 kPa (60–90 mm Hg) with Hb saturation 93% or more. There is no evidence that hyperoxia is beneficial and, in theory, it might be toxic. Saugstad (1998) has presented evidence that air is as effective as 100% oxygen in the resuscitation of asphyxiated newborns and may have advantages. If mechanical ventilation is necessary, it is important to avoid hypocapnia. Hypocapnia reduces cerebral blood flow as well as altering oxygen delivery and possibly affecting a number of important pH dependent enzymes. We are willing to permit mild hypercapnia during mechanical ventilation with $paCO_2$ up to 7.0 kPa (53 mm Hg) as long as arterial pH is above 7.2. In addition to the considerable evidence linking hypocapnia with cerebral injury in preterm infants, there is an association between duration of hyperventilation and worse neurological outcome in full-term infants (Bifano & Pfannenstiel, 1988).

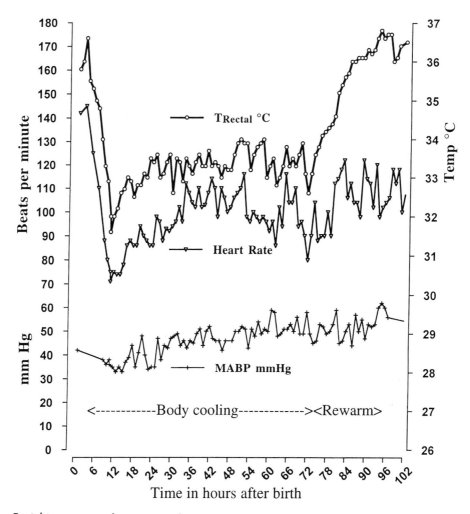

Fig. 19.10.   Rectal temperature, heart rate and mean arterial blood pressure from an asphyxiated infant during 72 hours of mild systemic hypothermia.

Maintenance of adequate cerebral perfusion

The lower limits of the accepted range for mean arterial pressure in the full-term infant is about 40 mm Hg (Versmold et al., 1981) and this figure is widely used as an indication for intervention. In many cases, the clinician will not be able to exclude hypovolemia and a rapid infusion of 10–15 ml/kg of 0.9% sodium chloride is indicated. Echocardiography is increasingly used by neonatologists to assess filling of the heart and myocardial contractility. If there is strong suspicion of blood loss or anemia, whole blood or red cells would be preferable. Despite being traditional as volume replacement for many years in neonatal medicine, albumin is not indicated and may increase the chances of fluid retention (So et al., 1997). If volume replacement does not achieve adequate blood pressure, dopamine by continuous infusion is used as the first inotropic agent. If this proves inadequate, dobutamine may be added for more inotropic effect or noradrenaline for more peripheral vaso-constriction. Avoiding hypoxaemia and circulatory impairment also involves avoiding unnecessary manipulations particularly of the airway, head or neck and also minimizing pain and compression.

Maintenance of adequate blood glucose levels

After a severe hypoxic–ischemic insult, mitochondrial function may be disturbed for many hours despite reoxygenation, and cells may be dependent on cytosolic gly-colysis for production of energy in the form of ATP. Glycolysis produces fewer molecules of ATP from one molecule of glucose than does oxidative phosphoryla-tion in the mitochondria. Thus glucose stores may easily become depleted. Hattori and Wasterlain (1990) showed that cerebral hypoxia–ischemia in the 7-day-old rat reduced brain glucose to 0.3 mmol/l. In a controlled study, these investigators showed that administration of glucose after hypoxia reduced the severity of neuro-pathological injury. In order to achieve a brain glucose of 3–5 mmol/l, we now rec-ommend maintaining blood glucose between 4 and 6 mmol/l (75–100 mg/dl) in infants developing HIE.

Avoidance of hyperviscosity

Polycythemia and hyperviscosity are not uncommon in fetuses with intrauterine growth retardation who are at increased risk of intrapartum asphyxia. Polycythemia is associated with lower IQ scores at school (Delaney-Black et al., 1989). It is still not clear how much difference dilutional exchange transfusion makes to outcome in newborn infants but the general recommendation that a venous hematocrit of 70% should be reduced even in the absence of symptoms should probably apply to an infant symptomatic with early HIE. It is relevant here to mention that hemodilution was introduced into acute stroke therapy in adults on the basis of animal modelling. Lee et al. (1994) showed in dogs with left middle cerebral artery occlusion that a 30% hematocrit gave a smaller infarct size than did hematocrit values of 40%, 35% or 25%.

Control of clinical seizures

As mentioned in the section on barbiturate therapy, it is unclear as to whether sub-clinical electrical seizures in the newborn are damaging, but there is agreement that repeated clinical seizures are likely, on balance, to be harmful. Clearly, seizures which impair respiration or circulation are potentially harmful. When seizure activity is not interfering with vital functions, it seems sensible that anticonvulsant therapy be started if a clinical seizure lasts 3 minutes or 3 briefer seizures occur within one hour (Levene, 1993).

Fluid restriction

Fluid volume is often restricted for infants with severe asphyxia but this is only really relevant (i) if the infant develops renal failure where a regime of replacing urine output + insensible loss would be indicated or (ii) where there is evidence of inappropriate antidiuretic hormone. Fluid restriction has no role in prevention of brain injury, and maintenance of perfusion and blood glucose may necessitate short periods of increased fluid administration.

Criteria for withdrawal of life support

An important part of the assessment and treatment of infants with severe HIE is the question of when withdrawal of life support is the best option. If the infant is in stage III (severe HIE) for 72 hours, and the clinical picture is supported by an EEG showing a low amplitude or burst suppression pattern and low resistance index on cerebral Doppler, the follow-up experience suggests that the chances of surviving to achieve independent existence with education, mobility and employment are vanishingly low. In our view, withdrawal of life support should be discussed between the clinical medical and nursing staff responsible for the infant after 72 hours of severe HIE. If no reversible factors emerge and no improvement has occurred by this time, we have recommended to the infant's parents that life support should be withdrawn. In our practice, it is not necessary for the infant to be clinically brain dead to make this recommendation, nor is it necessary to demonstrate total absence of cerebral blood flow or isoelectric (isopotential) EEG. The recommendation is based on the very poor quality of life if survival occurs. To withdraw life support is such a serious decision that it is essential that all the clinical team and the parents agree before support is actually withdrawn (Whitelaw, 1986). The discussions and the agreement should be noted in writing. Because the infant has been in a critical condition from early on, it will have been necessary for the neonatologist to have talked with one or both parents repeatedly during the first 3 days informing them of the evidence for brain injury, the treatment being given and the methods used to assess the infant's response. Thus the discussion on withdrawal of treatment is a natural consequence from what has been talked about before. Leaving the decision to withdraw for longer than 72 hours may, in our view, be counterproductive. Thus we would not delay the decision while waiting for an MRI examination to be arranged (after a holiday weekend, for example). Even severely damaged infants will usually eventually breathe spontaneously, and the longer one postpones extubation of an infant with HIE, the more likely it becomes that the baby will breathe or gasp spontaneously and survive. This is likely to be stressful if the baby is conscious at all and is very distressing for the parents and staff who have reluctantly come round to the view that the most humane thing is for the baby to die quickly and peacefully. In some cases, an unresponsive baby and very low amplitude EEG will prompt discussion of withdrawal of treatment by 24 hours. In such cases, it is essential that all relevant diagnostic measures have been taken (to rule out other diagnoses especially treatable conditions) and there has been enough time to see if there is a response to treatment.

REFERENCES

Allen, G. S., Ahn, H. S., Preziosi, T. J., Battye, R., Boone, S. C. & Chou, S. N. (1983). Cerebral arterial spasm – a controlled trial of nimodipine in patients with subarachnoid hemorrhage. *New England Journal of Medicine,* **17**, 619–24.

Altman, D. I., Young, R. S. & Yagel, S. K. (1984). Effects of dexamethazone in hypoxic–ischemic brain injury in the neonatal rat. *Biology of the Neonate,* **46**, 149–56.

Amiel-Tison, C. (1995). Clinical assessment of the infant nervous system. In *Fetal and Neonatal Neurology and Neurosurgery,* ed. M. I. Levene & R. J. Lilford, pp. 83–104. Edinburgh: Churchill Livingstone.

Amiel-Tison, C. & Ellison, P. (1986). Birth asphyxia in the fullterm newborn: early assessment and outcome. *Developmental Medicine and Child Neurology,* **28**, 671–82.

Archer, L. N. J., Levene, M. I. & Evans, D. H. (1986). Cerebral artery Doppler ultrasonography for prediction of outcome after perinatal asphyxia. *Lancet,* **ii**, 1116–18.

Barks, J. D., Post, M. & Tuor, U. I. (1991). Dexamethazone prevents hypoxic–ischemic brain damage in the neonatal rat. *Pediatric Research,* **29**, 558–63.

Bifano, E. M. & Pfannenstiel, A. (1988). Duration of hyperventilation and outcome in infants with persistent pulmonary hypertension. *Pediatrics,* **81**, 657–61.

Bona, E., Hagberg, H., Loberg E. M., Bagenholm, R. & Thoresen M. (1998). Protective effects of moderate hypothermia after neonatal hypoxia–ischemia: short and long-term outcome. *Pediatric Research,* **43**, 738–45.

Busto, R., Dietrich, W. D., Globus, M. Y. T. & Ginsberg, M. D. (1989). Postischemic moderate hypothermia inhibits CA1 hippocampal ischemic neuronal injury. *Neuroscience Letters,* **101**, 299–304.

Carroll, M. & Beck, O. (1992). Protection against hippocampal CA1 cell loss by post–ischemic hypothermia is dependent on delay of initiation and duration. *Metabolism and Brain Disease,* **7**, 45–50.

Cordey, R., Chiolero, R. & Miller, J. (1973). Resuscitation of neonates by hypothermia: report on 20 cases with acid-base determination on 10 cases and the long-term development of 33 cases. *Resuscitation,* **2**, 169–81.

Dearden, N. M., Gibson, J. S., McDowall, D. G., Gibson, R. M. & Cameron, M. M. (1986). Effect of high dose dexamethazone on outcome from severe head injury. *Journal of Neurosurgery*, **64**, 81–8.

Delaney-Black, V., Camp, B. W., Lubchenko, L. O. et al. (1989). Neonatal hyperviscosity association with lower achievement and IQ scores at school age. *Pediatrics*, **83**, 662–7.

Dietrich, W. D., Busto, R., Alonso, O., Globus, M. Y. T. & Ginsberg, M. D. (1993) Intraischemic but not postischemic brain hypothermia protects chronically following global forebrain ischemia in rats. *Journals of Cerebral Blood Flow and Metabolism*, **13**, 541–9.

Eken, P., Toet, M. C., Groenendal, F. & de Vries L. S. (1995). Predictive value of early neuroimaging, pulsed Doppler and neurophysiology in full term infants with hypoxic–ischemic encephalopathy. *Archives of Disease in Childhood*, **73**, F75–80.

Evans, D. J. & Levene (1998). Prophylactic neonatal anticonvulsant therapy following perinatal asphyxia in full-term new borns (Cochrane Review). In *The Cochrane Library*, Issue 4. Oxford: Update Software.

Eyre, J. A. & Wilkinson, A. R. (1986). Thiopentone induced coma after severe birth asphyxia. *Archives of Disease in Childhood*, **61**, 1084–9.

Eyre, J. A., Oozeer, R. C. & Wilkinson, A. R. (1983). Diagnosis of neonatal seizure by continuous recording and rapid analysis of the electroencephalogram. *Archives of Disease in Childhood*, **58**, 785–90.

Fenichel, G. M. (1983). Hypoxic–ischemic encephalopathy in the newborn. *Archives of Neurology*, **40**, 261–6.

Finer, N. N., Robertson, C. M., Peters, K. L. & Coward J. H. (1983) Factors affecting outcome in hypoxic–ischemic encephalopathy in term infants. *American Journal of Diseases of Children*, **137**, 21–5.

Fishman, R. A. (1982). Steroids in the treatment of brain oedema. *New England Journal of Medicine*, **306**, 359–60.

Goldberg, R. N., Moscoso, P., Bauer, C. R. et al. (1986). Use of barbiturate therapy in severe perinatal asphyxia: a randomised controlled trial. *Journal of Pediatrics*, **109**, 851–6.

Goodwin, T. M., Belai, I., Hernandez, P. et al. (1992). Asphyxial complications in the term newborn with severe umbilical acidemia. *American Journal of Obstetrics and Gynecology*, **167**, 1506–12.

Gunn, A. J., Gunn, T. R., de Haan, H. H. et al. (1997). Dramatic neuronal rescue with prolonged selective head cooling after ischemia in fetal lambs. *Journal of Clinical Investigation*, **15**, 248–56.

Gunn, A. J., Gluckman, P. G. & Gunn, T. R. (1998). Selective head cooling in newborn infants after perinatal asphyxia: a safety study. *Pediatric Research*, **41**, 803–8.

Hall, R. T., Hall, F. K. & Daily, D. K. (1998). High dose phenobarbital therapy in term newborn infants with severe perinatal asphyxia. A randomized prospective study with three year follow-up. *Journal of Pediatrics*, **132**, 345–8.

Hattori, H. & Wasterlain, C. G. (1990). Posthypoxic glucose supplement reduces hypoxic–ischemic brain damage in the neonatal rat. *Annals of Neurology*, **28**, 1228.

Hellstrom-Westas, L., Rosen, I. & Svenningsen N. W. (1995). Predictive value of early continuous amplitide integrated EEG recordings on outcome after severe birth asphyxia in full term infants. *Archives of Disease of Childhood*, **72**, F34–8.

Hirtz, D. G. & Nelson, K. (1998). Magnesium sulphate and cerebral palsy in premature infants. *Current Opinion in Pediatrics,* **10**, 131–7.

Howard, E. (1968). Reductions in size and total DNA of cerebrum and cerebellum in adult mice after corticosterone treatment in infancy. *Experimental Neurology,* **22**, 661–73.

Lee, S. H., Heroes, R. C., Mullan, J. C. & Korosue, K. (1994). Optimum degree of hemodilution for brain protection in a canine model of focal cerebral ischemia. *Journal of Neurosurgery,* **80**, 469–75.

Levene, M. I. (1993). Management of the asphyxiated full term infant. *Archives of Disease in Childhood,* **68**, 612–6.

Levene, M. I. & Evans, D. (1985). Medical management of raised intracranial pressure after severe birth asphyxia. *Archives of Disease in Childhood,* **60**, 12–6.

Levene, M. I., Sands, C., Grindulis, H. & Moore, J. R. (1986). Comparison of two methods of predicting outcome in perinatal asphyxia. *Lancet,* **i**, 67–9.

Levene, M. I., Gibson, N. A., Fenton, A. C., Papathoma, E. & Barnett, D. (1990). The use of a calcium channel blocker, nicardipine, for severely asphyxiated newborn infants. *Developmental Medicine and Child Neurology,* **32**, 567–74.

Levene, M. I., Blennow, M., Whitelaw, A., Hankø, E., Fellman, V. & Hartley, R. (1995). Acute effects of two different doses of magnesium sulphate in infants with birth asphyxia. *Archives of Disease in Childhood,* **73**, F174–7.

Low, J. A., Galbraith, R. S., Muir, D. W. et al. (1988). Motor and cognitive deficiency after intrapartum in the mature fetus. *American Journal of Obstetrics and Gynecology,* **162**, 802–6.

McDonald, J. W., Silverstein, F. S. & Johnston, M. V. (1990). Magnesium reduces N-methyl-D-aspartate (NMDA)-mediated brain injury in perinatal rats. *Neuroscience Letters,* **109**, 234–8.

Marchal, C., Costagliola, P., Leveau, P., Dulucq, P., Steckler, R. & Rouqier, F. (1974). Traitement de la souffrance cerebrale neonatale d'origine anoxique par le mannitol. *Revue de Pediatrie,* **9**, 581–9.

Miller, J., Miller, F. & Westin, B. (1964). Hypothermia in the treatment of asphyxia neonatorum. *Biology of the Neonate,* **6**, 148–63.

Mujsce, D. J., Towfighi, J., Stern, D. & Vannuci, R. C. (1990). Mannitol therapy in perinatal hypoxic–ischemic brain damage in rats. *Stroke,* **21**, 1210–14.

Palmer, C., Vannuci, R. C. & Towfighi, J. (1990) Reduction of perinatal hypoxic–ischemic brain damage with allopurinol. *Pediatric Research,* **27**, 332–6.

Penrice, J., Amess, P. N., Punwani, S. et al. (1997). Magnesium sulfate after transient hypoxia–ischemia fails to prevent delayed cerebral energy failure in the newborn piglet. *Pediatric Research,* **41**, 443–7.

Robertson, C. & Finer, N. (1985). Term infants with hypoxic-iscchaemic encephalopathy: outcome at 3.5 years. *Developmental Medicine and Child Neurology,* **27**, 473–84.

Roine, R. O., Kaste, M., Kinnunen, A., Nikki, P., Sarna, S. & Kajaste, S. (1990). Nimodipine after resuscitation from out-of-hospital ventricular fibrillation. *Journal of the American Medical Association,* **264**, 3171–7.

Rootwelt, T., Almaas, R., Oyasaeter, S., Moen, A.x & Saugstad, O. D. (1995). Release of xanthine oxidase to the systemic circulation during resuscitation from severe hypoxemia in newborn pigs, *Acta Paediatrica,* **84**, 507–11.

Ruth, V., Korkman, M., Liikanen, A. & Paetau, R. (1991). High-dose phenobarbitol treatment to prevent postasphyxial brain damage: a 6 year follow-up. *Pediatric Research*, **30**, 638 (abstract).

Rutherford, M. A., Pennock, J. M., Counsell, S. J. et al. (1998). Abnormal magnetic resonance signal in the internal capsule predicts poor neurodevelopmental outcome in infants with hypoxic–ischemic encephalopathy. *Archives of Disease in Childhood*, **102**, 323–8.

Sarnat, H. S. & Sarnat, M. S. (1976). Neonatal encephalopathy following fetal distress. *Archives of Neurology*, **33**, 696–706.

Saugstad, O. D. (1996). Role of xanthine oxidase and its inhibitor in hypoxia: reoxygenation injury. *Pediatrics*, **98**, 103–7.

Scott, H. (1976). Outcome of very severe birth asphyxia. *Archives of Disease in Childhood*. **51**, 712–16.

Silverman, W. A., Fertig, J. W. & Berger, A. P. (1958). The influence of the thermal environment upon the survival of newly born premature infants. *Pediatrics*, **22**, 876–86.

Sirimanne, E. S., Blumberg, R. M., Bossano, D. et al. (1996). The effect of prolonged modification of cerebral temperature on outcome after hypoxic–ischemic brain injury in the infant rat. *Pediatric Research*, **39**, 591–7.

So, K. W., Fok, T. F., Ng, P. C., Wong, W. W. & Cheung, K. L. (1997). Randomised controlled trial of colloid or crystalloid in hypotensive preterm infants. *Archives of Disease in Childhood*, **F76**(1), F43–6 .

Soderfeldt, B., Fujikawa, D. G. & Wasterlain, C. G. (1990). Neuropathology of status epilepticus in the neonatal marmoset monkey. In *Neonatal Seizures*, ed. C. G. Wasterlain & P. Vert, pp. 91–112. New York: Raven Press.

Steen, P. A., Newberg, L. A., Milde, J. H. et al. (1983). Nimodipine improves cerebral blood flow and neurologic recovery after complete cerebral ischemia in the dog. *Journal of Cerebral Blood Flow and Metabolism*, **3**, 38–43

Svenningsen, N. W., Blennow, G., Lindroth, M., Gaddlin, P. O. & Ahlstrom, H. (1982). Brain-oriented intensive care treatment in severe perinatal asphyxia. *Archives of Disease in Childhood*, **57**, 176–83.

Thordstein, M., Bågenholm, R., Thiringer, K. & Kjellmer, I. (1993). Scavengers of free oxygen radicals in combination with magnesium ameliorate perinatal hypoxic–ischemic brain damage in the rat. *Pediatric Research*, **34**, 23–6.

Thoresen, M., Penrice, J., Isrek, A. et al. (1995). Mild hypothermia following severe transient hypoxia–ischemia ameliorates delayed (secondary) cerebral energy failure in the newborn piglet. *Pediatric Research*, **37**, 667–70.

Thoresen, M., Haaland, K., Loberg, E. M., Whitelaw, A., Apricena, F., Hanko, E. & Steen, P.A. (1996). A piglet survival model of posthypoxic encephalopathy. *Pediatric Research*, **40**, 738–48.

Thoresen, M., Hallstrom, A., Whitelaw, A. et al. (1998). Lactate and pyruvate changes in the cerebral gray and white matter during posthypoxic seizures in newborn pigs. *Pediatric Research*, **44**, 746–54.

Vaagenes, P., Cantadore, R., Safar, P. et al. (1984). Amelioration of brain damage by lidoflazine after prolonged ventricular fibrillation in cardiac arrest in dogs. *Critical Care Medicine*, **12**, 846–55.

Van Bel, F., Shadid, M., Moison, R. M. et al. (1998). Effect of allopurinol on postasphyxial free radical formation, cerebral hemodynamics and electrical brain activity. *Pediatrics,* **101**, 185–93.

Versmold, H. T., Kitterman, J. A., Phibbs, R. H., Gregory, G. A. & Tooley, W. H. (1981). Aortic blood pressure during the first 12 hours of life in infants with birthweight 610 to 4220 grams. *Pediatrics,* **67**, 607–13.

Volpe J. J. (1995). *Neurology of the Newborn.* Philadelphia: Saunders.

Welsh, F. A. & Harris, V. A. (1991). Postischemic hypothermia fails to reduce ischemic injury in gerbil hippocampus. *Journal of Cerebral Blood Flow and Metabolism,* **11**, 617–20.

Westin, B., Miller, J., Nyberg, R. & Wedenberg, E. (1959). Neonatal asphyxia pallida treated with hypothermia alone or with hypothermia and transfusion of oxygenated blood. *Surgery,* **45**, 868–79.

Whitelaw, A. (1986). Death as an option in neonatal intensive care. *Lancet,* **ii**, 328–31.

Yager, J., Towfighi, J. & Vannucci, R. C. (1993). Influence of mild hypothermia on hypoxic–ischemic brain damage in the immature rat. *Pediatric Research,* **34**, 525–9.

20

Clinical aspects of brain injury in the preterm infant

Michael Weindling

Neonatal Unit, Liverpool Women's Hospital, UK

Introduction

Brain damage in the preterm infant born before 32 weeks' gestation mainly causes motor disability. Depending on the extent of the injury, there may also be associated cognitive loss. The motor disability is usually manifest as spasticity (stiffness) affecting the legs more than the arms. This condition is known as spastic diplegia. Sigmund Freud appropriately called it 'spasticity of prematurity'. Its neuropathological correlate is periventricular leukomalacia (PVL). Because PVL affects the periventricular white matter, usually bilaterally although not necessarily evenly, it is likely that it is caused by a generalized brain injury.

The other pathological entity, which causes brain damage in preterm infants and which attracted the early attention of pathologists and ultrasonographers because of its dramatic appearance, is periventricular hemorrhage (PVH). This condition arises in the germinal matrix and, in its minor and commoner forms when it affects only the germinal matrix or the cerebral ventricles, it has such little clinical effect that it is considered to be benign. It is only when the bleeding involves the adjacent brain parenchyma that there may be clinical effects. Because the condition is often unilateral, the clinical presentation usually takes the form of a hemiplegia – spasticity affecting one side of the body more than the other, and usually the arm more than the leg (Fig. 20.1).

Although PVH and PVL affect the same group of infants, namely those born 2 or more months prematurely, the conditions should be considered as being separate. Their etiologies and their clinical effects are different. However, both conditions affect the brain during its early development, and both are probably due in part to disturbances of the cerebral circulation. An awareness of the relevant development, anatomy and physiology of the cerebrovasculature is therefore central to an understanding of PVH and PVL, and this chapter considers these aspects first. Then PVH and PVL are considered separately and in more detail. Finally, the chapter looks at procedures that are currently used to prevent PVH and PVL, strategies that have been investigated to diminish the effects of these brain-damaging

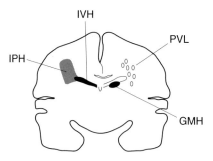

Fig. 20.1.   Diagram of a coronal section of the immature brain showing the sites of germinal matrix (GMH), intraventricular (IVH) and intraparenchymal (IPH) hemorrhages and periventricular leukomalacia (PVL).

conditions and their implications for the concept of neuronal plasticity, and finally some approaches that may have a place in the future.

The cerebral circulation – anatomy and physiology

Anatomy

The embryology of the developing brain has been considered in detail by Pape and Wigglesworth (1979), who have also reviewed the work of others. Some features are particularly relevant to the present discussion.

The basic pattern of the external cerebral vessels (the internal carotid artery and branches of the anterior, middle and posterior cerebral arteries) is established by 7 weeks' postconceptional age, and the postembryonic period is characterized by the growth and development of the cerebral hemispheres. This is reflected by the pattern of development of the internal cerebral vessels. Between about 24 and 32 weeks there is a watershed area between centrifugal and centripetal vessels (Fig. 20.2). This is relevant to the development of PVL, which is characterized by ischemic lesions. By contrast, PVH is due to bleeding in the germinal matrix and then into the lateral cerebral ventricles with blood tracking into the subarachnoid space (Fig. 20.3). PVH is a disorder that uniquely affects the brain during its early development.

An understanding of the way in which the brain develops during postembryonic life is helpful to an appreciation of the etiologies of PVH and PVL. The wall of the earliest cerebral hemisphere consists of a pseudostratified epithelium. First, neuronal percursors proliferate and migrate radially towards the pial surface. The peripheral migration of these neurons is guided by glial cell processes that stretch radially across the full thickness of the wall of the telencephalon and provide contact guide paths; these glial cells are characterized by the presence of glial fibrillary acidic protein (Collins, 1995). Then, deep progenitor cells migrate to the superficial layers

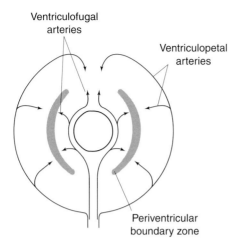

Fig. 20.2.   Diagram of the arterial pattern of the brain. (Redrawn from Pape & Wigglesworth, 1979.)

with the oldest cells taking up the deepest positions and being bypassed, or 'leap-frogged', by younger cells, the youngest making up the neocortex after the neuro-blasts have passed through the older layers. The proceses of proliferation, neurogenesis and gliogenesis are not necessarily sequential, but the effect is that astrocytes and oligodendrocytes have taken up their final positions by about 28 weeks post conception (Dobbing & Sands, 1970). An important consequence of this process that is very relevant to the development of GMH–IVH (germinal matrix hemorrhage–intraventricular hemorrhage) is the relative, but temporary, prominence of the subependymal germinal matrix between the postembryonic period and about 30 weeks post conception. ('Germinal matrix' is a term favoured by clinicians, although the Boulder Committee, 1970, preferred to call the region the 'ventricular zone' (Collins, 1995).)

The germinal matrix is situated in the floor of the lateral cerebral ventricles over the head and body of the caudate nucleus and in the notch between this nucleus and the thalamus; it is 'densely packed' with glioblasts, which take part in the migratory process (Pape & Wigglesworth, 1979). After about 30 weeks, the germi-nal matrix becomes progressively thinner. This metabolically active area is supplied by the recurrent artery of Heubner, a branch of the anterior cerebral artery that is relatively insignificant in the adult but prominent during this period of fetal life. The germinal matrix comprises an extensive capillary bed and is reckoned to be the source of about 80% of subependymal and intraventricular hemorrhages (Pape & Wigglesworth, 1979). After 30 weeks PVH becomes increasingly less likely because of regression of this area.

An appreciation of the formation of the blood supply to the cortex and subcor-tical white matter is also important for an understanding of the distribution of the

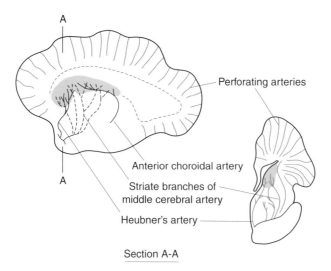

Section A-A

Fig. 20.3.   Arterial supply to the basal ganglia at 29 weeks' gestation. (From Hambleton & Wigglesworth, 1976.)

lesions of PVL. The subject has been reviewed by Collins (1995) and by Pape and Wigglesworth (1979), amongst others. Blood vessels first form because of sprouting of vessels in the pial plexus around the neural tube (Collins, 1995). These sprouts then extend between the ventricular and marginal zones. Meningeal perforating branches pass into the brain parenchyma as cortical, medullary and striate branches. The short cortical branches supply a peripheral part of the cerebrum and are termed 'ventriculopetal'; medullary branches supply the white matter. The more central part of the cerebrum is supplied by the longer striate branches that arborize near the ventricles and then send branches back out towards the cortex, the 'ventriculofugal' arteries (Fig. 20.2). The inner centrifugal and outer centripetal vessels run towards each other, but there are no connections. The boundary region between these two arterial systems is therefore particularly vulnerable to ischemia, and this is where the lesions of PVL are located.

Between 32 and 34 weeks' gestation there is involution of the germinal matrix and Heubner's artery eventually supplies just a small area at the head of the caudate nucleus (Collins, 1995). As the cortex becomes more complex and its gyral pattern becomes more pronounced, the balance of the blood supply moves away from the germinal matrix to the cortex. By the end of the third trimester the blood supply has shifted from a circulation that is mainly central to one where most of the supply is to the cortex and subcortical white matter, a similar situation to that of the adult. The change in the position of the boundary or watershed areas explains the different distributions of ischemic brain lesions in babies. In the premature brain (i.e. before about 34 weeks' postconception) the periventricular white matter in the watershed between the centripetal and centrifugal arteries is particularly vulnerable. In the infant at or near to term the area of vulnerability has changed to the cortical and subcortical region.

As development advances, there are also changes in the morphology of blood vessels. Before about 30 weeks, vessels in the germinal matrix are immature: there is no complex basal lamina or glial sheet, the endothelium is thinner than in cortical vessels and there is no smooth muscle, collagen or elastic fibres, with relatively little reticulin (Collins, 1995). The lack of smooth muscle is likely to interfere with the ability of these vessels to change diameter and take part in autoregulation, and the lack of other components may make them particularly vulnerable to changes in intraluminal pressure.

Mechanisms of cortical development will be considered later in the section on 'neuronal plasticity'.

Physiology

Three features are relevant here. The relative resistance of the preterm brain to hypoxia, the ability to divert blood to essential organs (the diving reflex), and the concept of autoregulation.

First, resistance to hypoxia. The fetus is hypoxemic compared to the baby after birth, the PaO_2 being about 20 to 25 mm Hg (Teitel, 1998), but not hypoxic. The pH of fetal blood is between 0.1 and 0.15 units below the pH of maternal blood in late gestation, and the fetus is about 0.5 °C warmer than the mother is. These factors have the effect of shifting the oxygen dissociation curve to the right, facilitating the release of oxygen from the hemoglobin molecule to the fetal tissues. However, the high proportion of HbF, particularly at earlier gestations, ensures that fetal red cell oxygen affinity is greater than that of the maternal blood. A hematocrit that is significantly higher in the fetus than after birth also has an effect in preserving oxygen delivery to fetal tissues. The net effect of these factors is that fetal arterial blood oxygen content and oxygen saturation are similar to those of the human adult (Delivoria-Papadopoulos & McGowan, 1998).

Second, the diving reflex. This is well established in the term infant, although the degree to which it operates in the extremely preterm infant remains uncertain, as is the degree to which it is altered by intrauterine growth restriction.

Third, autoregulation. Cerebral blood flow (CBF) is maintained provided blood pressure remains within normal limits. These have not, however, been clearly defined in the preterm infant, and are likely to vary with other factors such as the availability of metabolic substrates, e.g. glucose (Pryds, 1994) and acidemia. CBF in the preterm infant seems to be particularly susceptible to hypocarbia, which would be expected to cause cerebral vasoconstriction, and the condition is associated with the development of PVL (see below).

Periventricular hemorrhage (PVH)

In this chapter the term PVH is used to describe the conditions germinal matrix hemorrhage (GMH) or subependymal hemorrhage (SEH), intraventricular hemorrhage (IVH) and intraparenchymal hemorrhage (IPH) (Fig. 20.1). It is a disease of prematurity. PVH occurs in about 40% of infants below 35 weeks or 1500 g and in only very few babies above 37 weeks. The etiology of subependymal and intraventricular hemorrhages is rather different to that of intraparenchymal hemorrhages (see below). Infants who have had subependymal and/or intraventricular hemorrhages also have a much better neurodevelopmental outcome than those damaged by an intraparenchymal hemorrhage.

It is useful to set aside any confusion about nomenclature. The terms germinal matrix hemorrhage, subependymal hemorrhage and grade 1 periventricular hemorrhage (PVH) are interchangeable. The terms grade 2 or grade 3 describe hemorrhage into the cerebral ventricles. In the original widely used classification proposed by Papile (1978), a grade 2 hemorrhage meant that blood was confined to the lateral cerebral ventricle, while a grade 3 hemorrhage was defined as one where the ventricle had become distended. When the bleeding has caused disruption of the brain parenchyma, i.e. true brain damage, the condition is known as intraparenchymal hemorrhage or grade 4 by the Papile classification. A useful term now used for this most serious form of PVH is periventricular hemorrhagic infarction (e.g. Volpe, 1998).

Germinal matrix bleeding usually arises over the caudate nucleus. In the more immature infants the hemorrhage is over its body, but, as gestation increases, bleeding becomes more likely to occur over the head of the caudate nucleus (Leech & Kohnen, 1974; Pape & Wigglesworth, 1979). A great deal about the timing and clinical associations of PVH has been learnt from cranial ultrasound scanning, the most appropriate imaging modality. Germinal matrix and intraventricular hemorrhages become more common with increasing immaturity, and have been associated with respiratory distress and its complications (particularly pneumothorax) and asphyxia (Weindling et al., 1985a). These findings, as well as the observation that such bleeding tends to be seen within 48 hours after birth (between 40% and 50% occur within the first 8 postnatal hours (e.g. Ment et al., 1995)), suggest that maturity of the vascular bed in the germinal matrix may be important in determining whether bleeding occurs. The perception that bleeding is more likely to occur into an immature vascular bed has implications for understanding the mechanism of action of some of the successful preventative strategies that have been used.

Choroid plexus bleeding was found in 25% of autopsied neonates by Larroche (Banker & Larroche, 1977), but usually in addition to subependymal hemorrhage and only to a small extent. In general, germinal matrix and intraventricular hemorrhages are much more common that intraparenchymal hemorrhage.

In parenchymal PVH there is hemorrhagic necrosis in the periventricular white matter, usually just dorsal and lateral to the external angle of the cerebral lateral ventricles (Fig. 20.1) and usually asymmetrically (Volpe, 1998). The pathogenesis of intraparenchymal hemorrhage is rather different to that of minor germinal matrix and intraventricular hemorrhages. Here, two mechanisms may occur, probably separately, although they could coexist. Pape and Wigglesworth (1979) observed that massive germinal matrix hemorrhage was associated with congestion of the branches of the terminal vein which drains the area, and that the related white matter may also become infarcted. Thus, venous infarction will occur after the drainage of deep veins has been obstructed, perhaps as a consequence of dilatation of the lateral cerebral ventricles or because of obstruction of the terminal vein in the subependyma (Pape & Wigglesworth, 1979; Volpe, 1998). Another explanation is that bleeding may occur into parenchyma that has been injured by ischemia, i.e. when the baby has been subjected to hypoxia–ischemia around the time of birth (Weindling et al., 1985a; Volpe, 1998).

The clinical associations between prematurity, respiratory distress syndrome (hyaline membrane disease) and PVH have been known for a long time, although prematurity was not separated from low birthweight in the earlier pathology literature (for review, see Pape & Wigglesworth, 1979). The link with respiratory distress syndrome and its complications, e.g. pneumothorax, metabolic acidosis and hypercarbia, has also been seen by paediatricians and radiologists using cranial ultrasound (for review, see Levene & de Vries 1995), and Weindling et al. (1985b) also found an association with birth asphyxia. PVH usually occurs after birth, although it has been noticed in up to 6% of stillbirths (Harcke et al., 1972; Leech & Kohnen, 1974; Pape & Wigglesworth, 1979). The timing of bleeding is generally within 48 hours, although Tsiantos et al. (1974) observed that some infants develop the hemorrhage later during the first or second week after birth. Abnormalities of coagulation are not usually associated with PVH.

There is some debate about the extent to which antenatal and postnatal conditions cause severe PVH and PVL (e.g. Weindling et al., 1985a,b; Sinha et al., 1985). There is, however, no doubt that the conditions are complications of prematurity, and therefore likely to be related to the process that caused the infant to be delivered prematurely. The interactions of these various factors are summarized in Fig. 20.4.

Clinical features

Although a wide range of clinical presentations has been associated with PVH, Papile et al. (1978), using computerized tomography, found that the condition was

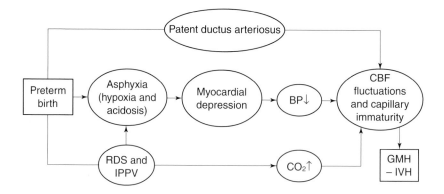

Fig. 20.4.   Diagram of the pathways relating preterm birth to GMH–IVH.

undetected by the attending clinicians about half the time. In practice, a fall in hematocrit should lead to the suspicion that there may have been an intracranial disaster, but the diagnosis is readily made at the cotside using cranial ultrasound.

The complications of PVH largely depend on the size of the hemorrhage, and whether there is associated white matter injury. At the time of a large bleed, the infant may collapse, either because of a sudden rise in intracranial hemorrhage or because of a fall in blood pressure. But, since most PVHs are small and confined to the germinal matrix or within the cerebral ventricle, such a picture is unusual. When there is hemorrhagic infarction, an affected infant may be comatose, suffer from seizures (notoriously difficult to detect and varied in manifestation in the premature neonate), or the bleeding may be entirely unnoticed by even the most vigilant and experienced clinical staff. Mostly infants are asymptomatic.

In the medium term, the main complication of PVH is posthemorrhagic hydrocephaly, particularly when there is hemorrhagic infarction of the brain parenchyma. The treatment of this has been the subject of a randomized trial that looked at the effectiveness of ventricular taps compared with the use of diuretic therapy. The outcome was that there was no clear advantage to ventricular tapping (Ventriculomegaly trial, 1990; for review, see Whitelaw et al., 1996). More recently, there has been interest in fibrinolytic therapy (for review, see Whitelaw et al., 1996). This approach is based on the hypothesis that multiple blood clots in the CSF are the initial cause of posthemorrhagic ventricular dilatation and lysis of clots might be expected to reopen the pathways of circulation and reabsorption of CSF. But when the clot-busting drug, streptokinase, was introduced into the ventricular system, and the effects were compared with conservative management of posthemorrhagic ventricular dilatation, the numbers of deaths and babies with shunt dependence were identical in both groups (Whitelaw et al., 1992; Hudgins, 1994; Whitelaw et al., 1996).

The incidence of posthemorrhagic hydrocephaly has, however, declined markedly over the last five years or so, probably because of the increased use of antenatal steroids (see below).

The long-term complications of PVH mainly affect those infants where there has been white matter destruction, i.e. those with periventricular hemorrhagic infarction, and the pattern of neurodisability is associated with the degree of white matter damage. Even when there is posthemorrhagic hydrocephaly, two separate studies 10 years apart have shown that the pattern of disability was related to the associated brain damage, rather than to the process that had led to hydrocephaly (Cooke, 1987; Fletcher et al., 1997). Since such bleeds are more usually unilateral, or at least asymmetrical, the degree of disability is generally less than that associated with periventricular leukomalacia (PVL) (see below). But children with subependymal and mild intraventricular hemorrhages have also been found to perform less well on cognitive tests than gestation-matched controls without mild PVH or term infants. Using Bayley scales, the mean $\pm$ SD Mental Development Index was 102 ± 16 for premature infants with minor PVH, 105 ± 19 for premature infants without PVH, and 109 ± 20 for term controls. The respective Psychomotor Development Indices were 98 ± 19 (preterm with minor PVH), 97 ± 16 (preterm without PVH), and 106 ± 16 (term controls) (Ross et al., 1996). About 5% of infants with isolated IVH later develop CP (Levene & de Vries, 1995), disability occurring when there is associated damage to the periventricular white matter.

In conclusion, PVH is a condition that affects premature infants, and its incidence increases with increasing prematurity. Minor degrees of PVH are relatively common, but are not associated with major neurodevelopmental disability. Severe PVH causes white matter destruction and consequent disability, and may lead to posthemorrhagic hydrocephaly. Fortunately, the incidences of intraparenchymal hemorrhage and posthemorrhagic hydrocephaly have declined over the last seven years or so. The decline occurred at about the same time – between 1990 and 1993 – as antenatal steroids and postnatal surfactant entered general clinical use in the UK, suggesting that these interventions may have had an effect.

Periventricular leukomalacia

This condition typically affects infants before 34 weeks' gestation. Although it may affect a baby at term, this is unusual, and the peak timing of this condition means that it occurs at a time of white matter development before active myelination – microscopic myelin does not occur until after the first postnatal month, and myelin tubes only appear at between 11 and 13 months post-conception (Back & Volpe, 1997). Estimates of the prevalence of PVL vary. A general figure (the median of 13 studies between 1983 and 1992, for review, see De Vries & Levene, 1995) is that it affects approximately 8% of infants below 32 weeks' gestation, and such infants comprise about 0.7% of all babies born. Ringelberg and van de Bor (1993) recorded an incidence of 5.4% in a hospital-based study in the Netherlands, but an extraordinary geographically based study in northern Finland using magnetic resonance imaging study found PVL in 32% of premature infants, and not at all in a control group of children born at term (Olsén et al., 1997).

PVL was first fully described by Banker and Larroche (1962), although Virchow described a similar condition in 1867. The basic gross appearance on sectioning the affected brain is of small white spots around the lateral cerebral ventricles, and this explains the condition's name (Gr. $\lambda\epsilon\upsilon\kappa\acute{o}s$ = white, $\mu\alpha\lambda\alpha\chi\iota\alpha$ = softness). The following description of histopathological changes is based on Kinney and Back (1998) and Back et al. (1998). Between 3 and 8 hours after injury starts, there is coagulation necrosis of all cells. Within 12 hours, astrocytes start to proliferate at the edge of the lesion and there is capillary hyperplasia. Between the next 3 and 10 days, microglia start to infiltrate the damaged area, followed by reactive hypertrophic astrocytes and there is accumulation of lipid-laden cells. As the damaged area becomes organized, reactive gliosis occurs. Then, over the next few weeks, there is cavitation and/or gliosis.

Our understanding of PVL has advanced considerably with the development of cranial ultrasound scanning using a high resolution 7.5 MHz scanhead. This is the best of the imaging modalities during the weeks after birth. Ultrasound scans have shown how the condition evolves after the causative injury. First, echodense areas appear around the ventricles. Then, between 2 and 4 weeks later, cavities, known as cysts, appear: the average time before cysts or cavities appear on ultrasound is three weeks (e.g. Weindling et al., 1985a; Trounce et al., 1986; Pierrat et al., 2001). Because the condition invariably represents white matter damage, it is much more serious than PVH. Even extensive periventricular leukomalacia is compatible with survival, and, typically, signs of spasticity affecting the legs more than the arms are not manifest until the baby is 6 or 8 months old.

The pathogenesis of the condition is interesting. Pape and Wigglesworth (1979) described PVL as the most common ischemic lesion of the preterm brain, although the etiology is now thought to be more complicated than just ischemia, and the lesion may affect some infants around term and even adults (e.g. Ginsberg et al., 1976). Nevertheless, the distribution of the lesions, which are mainly in the periventricular watershed area, strongly suggests that hypoxia and ischemia are important but the story has become more complicated. Three factors have emerged. The first relates to hemodynamics and the striking observation that the lesions of PVL are in an area of the developing brain that is particularly vulnerable to ischemia. There is an association with hypocapnia (e.g. Calvert et al., 1986; Greisen et al., 1987). Since a low carbon dioxide tension has a powerful cerebral vasoconstrictor effect, the link is plausible and ties in with the watershed distribution of PVL. Hypocarbia leads to cerebral vasoconstriction (and possible loss of the ability to autoregulate) and hence to hypoperfusion of the vulnerable periventricular region. A direct link with hypotension is less clear, although there is an association (summarized by Rennie, 1997). Using near infrared spectroscopy, cerebral blood flow in low birthweight infants as low as 4.9 ml per 100 g per min may occur without apparent cerebral infarction (Tyszczuk et al., 1998), compared with about 60 ml per 100 g per min in adults. The authors of that paper observed that their study did not support the assumption that a low mean arterial blood pressure (between 24 and 30 mm Hg) was necessarily associated with reduced cerebral perfusion. They make the point that:

Although there is evidence of a statistical association between low [mean arterial blood pressure] and adverse outcome, there may not be a causal link. The statistical association may simply reflect the fact that the sickest infants tend to have the lowest blood pressures. (Tyszczuk et al., 1998).

Another observation, linked to this first one, is that an increased risk of cerebral palsy (probably due to PVL) has been noted in monochorionic twins. The likely cause is altered intrauterine hemodynamics. The evidence has been discussed by Williams et al. (1996), and summarized by Pharoah and Cooke (1997) and Landy and Keith (1998). The argument runs like this. The crude rate of cerebral palsy per 1000 survivors at 1 year rises with increasing plurality. It is 1 or 2 in singletons, between 6.7 and 12.6 in twins and between 28 and 44.8 in triplets (Grether et al., 1993; Petterson et al., 1993; Williams et al., 1996; Pharoah & Cooke, 1996). The relative risk in normal birthweight twins is 4.5 and this is not explained by their increased risk of prematurity and low birthweight (Williams et al., 1996). It is argued that, in a significant proportion of singletons, spastic cerebral palsy may be due to the death of a monochorionic cotwin (Pharoah & Cooke, 1997). The mechanism is probably through the disruption of the supply of blood and oxygen to the surviving fetus, causing damage to vulnerable areas of the brain, for example, in the watershed areas. Support for this notion comes from the observation that cerebral palsy is more likely to affect a surviving twin if the cotwin died during the third trimester: Yoshida and Matayoshi (1990) observed that, when a monozygotic twin died early in pregnancy, the survivor survived without cerebral palsy. What probably happens is that there is blood loss from the survivor through artery-to-artery or vein-to-vein anastomoses into the lower resistance circulation of the dead monochorionic twin (Benirschke, 1993; Grafe, 1993). In a series of 39 children with cerebral palsy resulting from 30 twin births, PVL was observed in 19 (79%) of the 24 babies who were born prematurely (Shimogaki et al., 1998). A similar mechanism may cause cortical blindness (Good et al., 1996). An observation by

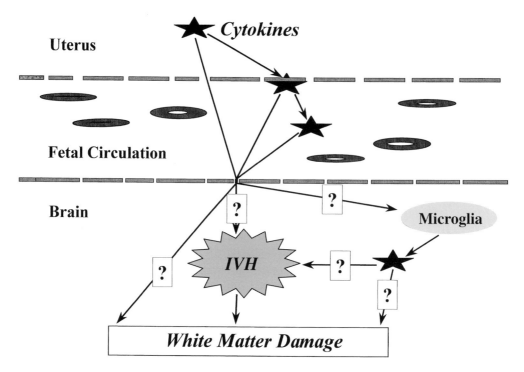

Fig. 20.5.   The proposed site of action of cytokines in the pathogenesis of PVL. (From Damann &
Leviton, 1997, with permission.)

Geva et al. (1998) is also connected with this concept: more children developed
PVL amongst infants who had been exposed to multifetal pregnancy reduction
than singletons (4/14, 29%) compared with 1.9% (OR 21, 95% CIs 6–79). The
same group also noted a significant excess of IVF (in vitro fertilization) and twinning amongst the infants who developed PVL.

Secondly, an association with chorioamnionitis, observed by Spinillo et al.
(1995) amongst others, has become established, although a single causative organism has not been identified (Romero et al., 1991). There is a persuasive argument
(summarized by Dammann & Leviton, 1997) that the action of inflammation-
related cytokines link chorioamnionitis with PVL (Fig. 20.5). The mechanism
might be through neuropeptides and neuronal gene expression, which is also influenced by glucocorticoids (see below) (Patterson & Nawa, 1993). A rabbit model
demonstrated that intrauterine infection can cause fetal brain white matter lesions
(Yoon et al., 1997), and the same group found raised interleukin-6 (IL-6) concentrations in umbilical cord plasma in infants who had PVL-associated lesions on
early cranial ultrasound scan (Yoon et al., 1996). In that latter study, however, a
cord plasma IL-6 concentration of ≤400 pg/l had only a positive predictive value
of 14% for identifying neonates with cystic PVL. In a mouse model, IL-1β, IL-6,
IL-9 or TNF-α (but not IL-4) induced white matter lesions when injected with ibot-

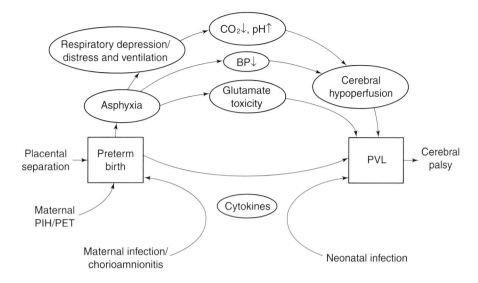

Fig. 20.6.   Diagram of the pathways relating preterm birth with PVL and cerebral palsy.

enate, a glutamatergic agonist acting on NMDA receptors (*N*-methyl-D-aspartate) receptors (Dommergues et al., 2000).

Verma et al. (1997) recorded that clinical chorioamnionitis doubled the chance of an abnormal cranial ultrasound scan during the neonatal period (odds ratio (OR) 2.03, 95% confidence interval (CI) 1.24–3.30). A recent meta-analysis found that clinical chorioamnionitis and preterm delivery was significantly associated with both cerebral palsy (relative risk (RR) 1.9%, 95% CI 1.4–2.5) and cystic PVL (RR 3.0, 95% CI 2.2–4.0) (Wu & Colford, 2000). In full-term infants, there was also a positive association between clinical chorioamnionitis and cerebral palsy (RR 2.1, 95% CI 1.5–2.9) (Wu & Colford, 2000). Since intrauterine infection causes premature labour (Goldenberg et al., 2000), it is possible that the brain damage is a consequence of the infection, and that the time of birth (prematurity) affects the pattern of injury, rather than being its cause. There is also a suggestion that delivery by caesarean section might be helpful: Baud et al. (1998) reported that, in 99 infants, 16 of whom developed cystic PVL, the risk of developing PVL was reduced significantly in those delivered by caesarean section (OR 0.15, 95% CI 0.04–0.57).

A third point is that neonatal cerebral white matter is particularly vulnerable to injury before about 34 weeks gestation. Cell culture has shown that the early differentiating oligodendrocyte is more susceptible to injury by oxygen-derived free radicals than the mature cell, possibly because of poorly developed antioxidant systems at this stage of development (Volpe, 1998; Kinney & Back, 1998). The observation that there is coagulation necrosis suggests that glutamate toxicity may play a part in perinatal white matter injury, and the evidence has been summarized by Kinney and Back (1998). The various causative factors are summarized in Fig. 20.6.

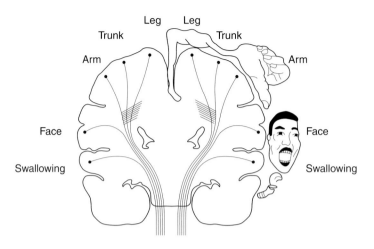

Fig. 20.7.   Figure showing the (usually) symmetrical distribution of the lesions in PVL (hatched) affecting the lower, rather than the upper, limbs or face.

There are no clinical manifestations associated with PVL during the immediate neonatal period (e.g. Amiel-Tison, 1973; Pape & Wigglesworth, 1979). Abnormal neurological features occur after several months and vary according to the regions of the brain that have been damaged. Because the sites of periventricular infarction lie in the path of the motor tracts (Fig. 20.7), PVL causes motor disability, which takes the form of spasticity. This is usually described as a diplegia (when the legs are affected more severely than the arms), but when the lesions are widespread all limbs may be affected (spastic quadriplegia). The more of the brain that is affected by the lesions of PVL, the more severe will be the ensuing disability. Very extensive damage causes severe cognitive impairment, as well as motor disability. When the lesions are posterior, the optic radiation may be affected, resulting in cortical visual impairment, sometimes with delayed visual maturation (e.g. Van den Hout et al., 1998). Even when the ultrasound appearances have not progressed beyond the appearance of transient echodensities without cavitation, there is an increased incidence of minor motor disabilities (Ringelberg & van de Bor, 1993). In their study in northern Finland, Olsén et al. (1997), studying a group of 8-year-old children who had been born prematurely, found evidence on magnetic resonance imaging of PVL in all children with cerebral palsy. There was also evidence of PVL in 25% of children with minor neurological dysfunction and in 25% of children who were clinically healthy, but in none of those who had been born at term.

In summary, PVL is the result of injury to the white matter around the lateral cerebral ventricles. Chorioamnionitis, hypocapnia and hypoperfusion seem to be implicated in its etiology. There is debate about whether the condition originates before or after birth; it is likely that the disease represents the consequence of a process, which often begins before birth but which is manifest afterwards. Infection after birth may also have an etiological role. Even though cavities in the brain parenchyma ('cystic lesions') are clearly seen on ultrasound scans during the days and weeks just after birth, it is surprisingly difficult to make reliable predictions about outcome. In one intervention study where entry depended on the presence of signs of serious brain damage on an ultrasound brain scan, cerebral palsy was only accurately predicted in 54% infants (Weindling et al., 1996). There are two possible reasons for this. One is that it is difficult to identify the precise anatomical location of the lesions. The other is that the damaging process occurs relatively early in the brain's development, and neuronal plasticity may compensate. Although it might have been hoped that a decrease in the incidence of this condition would be seen with the widespread use of antenatal steroids, this has not yet been demonstrated to be the case.

Neuronal plasticity and the effects of programmes of early interventions

The damaging processes described in the previous sections of this chapter have an effect on human brain development relatively early. Almost all of the estimated one hundred billion neurons present in the mature brain are generated during prenatal life, i.e. an average of 200 000 neurons per minute (Kandel, 2000). During the most rapid phase of synaptogenesis, 40 000 new synapses are formed every second in the striate cortex of the macaque monkey; in this animal this phase occurs around birth, which is 165 days after conception. In the macaque, during the plateau phase of synaptogenesis there are between 600 and 900 million synapses mm^{-3} of neuropil throughout infancy and adolescence (Bourgeois, this volume). The general picture of cortical development is one where input is important in securing the final hard wiring (e.g. for review see Penn & Shatz, this volume). If this is the case, the possibility arises that a child's development might be positively affected by altering inputs early during postnatal life. This next section will consider the evidence that such interventions are able to affect cognitive and motor development.

The effect of interventions on cognitive function

A newborn baby's physical environment seems to have an effect. In Nottingham, UK, Mann et al. (1986) studied the effect of alternating night and day on sleep, feeding, and weight gain by a randomized controlled trial. Babies from a nursery, where the intensity of light and noise was reduced for 12 hours at night spent longer sleeping and less time feeding and gained more weight, than those from a control nursery where the intensity of light and noise was not reduced. Differences became apparent only after discharge home and were still detectable three months after the expected date of delivery, when infants from the night and day nursery were an average of 0.5 kg heavier ($P < 0.02$). These findings suggested that physical environment has an effect (either direct or indirect) on the subsequent behaviour of preterm infants and that there is benefit from creating a separate night and day environment (Mann et al., 1986).

The environment was also studied by the newborn individualized developmental care and assessment programme (NIDCAP), a philosophy of neonatal nursing care for neonates. It involves promoting infant development and parenting and making the neonatal intensive care unit's environment less stressful to babies by reducing the levels of light and noise (Als et al., 1994). The NIDCAP approach was subjected to a small randomized controlled trial in Boston, Mass. Forty-three infants who weighed less than 1250 g at birth were entered over a 21-month period between 1984 and 1986. The infants were randomized after birth. They were either nursed by a team of specially trained nurses, or given routine care. The outcome was analysed for 18 babies in the control group and 20 in the experimental (NIDCAP) group. The results were striking. Six (33%) of the control group developed chronic lung disease, compared with none in the experimental group. Four (22%) control infants developed PVH with parenchymal involvement, compared with none in the experimental group. Babies, who received what has come to be known as individualized nursing, seemed to do much better than controls. On average, they fed by bottle sooner than controls (104 days vs. 59 days), spent less time in hospital (151 days vs. 87 days), were in oxygen for a shorter period (139 days vs. 57 days), and their hospital stay was cheaper ($189 000 vs. $98 000). At 42 weeks postconceptional age, the NIDCAP babies generally did better according to an assessment scheme (Assessment of Preterm Infants' Behaviour, APIB) in terms of their posture, tone, and movement. Significant differences in the EEGs and visual-evoked responses were also reported. At 9 months postconception, 16 babies in the control group and all 20 who had been in the experimental group were assessed using the Bayley Scales of Infant Development. The experimental group had a significantly higher mean Mental Development Index than controls (118 vs. 94, $P \leq 0.001$) and Psychomotor Developmental Index (101 vs. 84, $P \leq 0.01$). In addition, when 20 variables were measured in the 6-minute Kangaroo Box paradigm Play Episode, 17 were reported to show differences in favour of the experimental group. The paper was accompanied by a rapturous editorial (Merenstein, 1994), and followed by serious criticism in the correspondence columns of JAMA (Garland, 1995; Ohlsson, 1995; Lacy, 1995; Saigal & Streiner, 1995; Sepkowitz, 1995). The correspondents made a number of points. They pointed out that the study was carried out before artificial surfactant became available, and that the rate of severe PVH in the control group was very high. The study was also criticized on the basis that the staff would have been aware which group the infants were in, the relatively small sample size, and the wide variability of some of the results (for example, the mean

±SD number of days in oxygen was 139 ± 166). There was also a relatively long interval between finishing the study and its publication (8 years), and Saigal and Streiner (1995) described the results of this study as 'almost too good to be true'. In a robust reply the authors of the original paper commented that the last observation might be a consequence of the very rapid development of the preterm infant's brain at the time of the intervention. They called for a larger randomized controlled trial (Als et al., 1995), but this has still not been done, and, since many of the concepts advanced by Als and her colleagues have been accepted into neonatal nursing practice, are now unlikely to be tested in this way. A smaller Swedish trial showed some advantages (Westrup et al., 2000).

Psychologists describe children being 'doubly vulnerable' through both biological and environmental disadvantage (e.g. Guralnick, 1998). Separation of these two issues is sometimes difficult when assessing the effects of intervention programmes. For example, the Infant Health and Development Program was a US national collaborative study aimed at examining the efficacy of combining early child development and family support services with pediatric follow-up to reduce the incidence of health and developmental problems among low birthweight, preterm infants (Ramey et al., 1992). The outcome was affected by whether a child's mother had been to college. Only children whose mothers had a high school education or less showed significant enhancement in IQ scores at 3 years. But birthweight had an effect too: the lighter (< 2000 g) low birthweight preterm children of white mothers with some college education were less influenced by the intervention than the corresponding heavier children (Brooks-Gunn et al., 1992), suggesting that the intrauterine environment also had some effect.

The effectiveness of early intervention programmes to improve cognitive functioning has been recently reviewed by Guralnick (1998). He pointed out that children who are vulnerable through disadvantage and those who already have disabilities are likely to suffer from an increasing gap between their level of cognition and those of healthy controls during the first 5 years. This means that, if there is no intervention, children who are considered vulnerable because of their social circumstances end up with an apparent IQ between 0.5 and 1.5 standard deviations (SDs) lower at 5 years compared with earlier assessment. Children with established disabilities start at a lower level and their IQ at 5 years is approximately between 0.5 and 0.75 SDs lower, i.e. between 8 and 12 IQ points. Guralnick (1998) concludes that there is now 'unequivocal evidence' that early intervention can reduce this apparent decline.

In 1987, Shonkoff and Hauser-Cram published a meta-analysis of 31 early intervention programmes for children up to 3 years old with disability due to an acquired impairment. This showed that participation was associated with an average gain of 0.62 SD for measurements of cognitive development, and that the most effective programmes targeted both parents and children.

There is also evidence of benefit due to early intervention for infants with Down's syndrome. Guralnick (1998) reported an effect of between 0.5 and 0.75 SDs for four such intervention programmes. Gibson and Harris (1988) pooled findings from 21 early intervention studies for Down's syndrome infants and children. They found a consistency of short-term benefits in the growth of finer motor skills, simple social repertoire and DQ/IQ scores, but there was conflicting evidence about benefits in the gross motor, linguistic and intellectual fields. They were disappointed to record that there was no support for the gains remaining at follow-up to the early years of primary schooling. Neser et al. (1989) found that preschool children with Down's syndrome showed improved developmental functioning with the additional stimulation of a playgroup or preschool centre when compared to children cared for at home during the day.

There are three other randomized studies that are worth considering in some detail: the Abecedarian Project (Ramey & Campbell, 1984), the Vermont study (Rauh et al., 1988), and the Infant Health and Development Program (McCormick et al., 1991; McCarton et al., 1997). The type and frequency of intervention and the socioeconomic status of the families were rather different in each.

The Abecedarian Project (Ramey & Campbell, 1984) examined the effect of early educational intervention for children of poor families. Subjects were randomly assigned to one of four interventions: educational treatment from infancy until the age of 8 in public school; preschool treatment only (from infancy until 5 years old); primary school treatment only (age 5 to 8 years); and an untreated control group. At 4 years of age, only 3% of the group who received an intervention had an IQ below 70 compared with 18% of controls, and their IQ was on average 0.82 SD higher. The advantage was most marked amongst children whose mother's IQ was below 70 (Martin et al., 1990). The preschool intervention appeared to have a continuing positive effect on intellectual development and academic achievement, with a detectable effect at 12 years. The intervention that was undertaken only when children were at school was less effective than the preschool intervention. The authors concluded that the results generally supported the hypothesis that the duration of an intervention had an effect: cognitive and academic achievement seemed to increase with longer treatment (Campbell & Ramey, 1994). Another interpretation is that interventions applied early, when the developing brain has greatest plasticity, are more likely to have an effect than those applied when the child is older.

The Vermont study was a low intensity intervention, aimed at preterm infants of birthweight below 2200 g (Rauh et al., 1988). The programme was aimed mainly at improving maternal adjustment to caring for her low birthweight baby, but the child's development was also assessed. There were only 11 sessions, which started during the final week of hospitalization and continued for 3 months at home. Low birthweight babies were randomly assigned to experimental ($n=25$) or control conditions ($n=29$), and the results were compared with the outcome for 28 full-term, normal birthweight infants. After 6 months, the experimental group mothers reported significantly greater self-confidence and satisfaction with mothering, as well as a more favourable perception of their infant's temperament than the low birthweight control group mothers. By 36 and 48 months there were significant group differences on the McCarthy GCI: the low birthweight controls were the most disadvantaged, but the low birthweight experimental group had caught up with the normal birthweight group.

The third North American study was the Infant Health and Development Program, a remarkable randomized, controlled, multicentre trial, where the intervention was applied from birth to 3 years. There was stratification of low birthweight premature infants to below and above 2001 g (Ramey et al., 1992). The intervention group received home visits from the time of discharge from the maternity unit until they were 3 years old, as well as special schooling and parent group meetings between 1 and 3 years of age. Three hundred and seventy-seven infants were assigned to the intervention group and there were 608 controls. Cognitive development, behavioural problems, and health status were measured.

There was no difference at 12 months of age, but the cognitive and behaviour problem scores were significantly better for the intervention group at 24 and 36 months (Brooks-Gunn et al., 1993). The gains were most pronounced for receptive language and visual–motor and spatial skills (Brooks-Gunn et al, 1992). By the time the children were 5 years old, the differences were less clear. The intervention group considered as a whole had full-scale IQ scores similar to those of children in the control group, but the heavier low birthweight children who had received the intervention had average full-scale IQ scores which were 3.7 points higher ($P=0.03$) and mean verbal IQ scores which were 4.2 points higher ($P=0.02$) than those who had been lighter babies (Brooks-Gunn et al., 1994). Both groups of low birthweight infants showed no significant differences in cognitive measures at 5 years. The intervention and follow-up groups were similar in behaviour and health measures regardless of low birthweight stratum.

At 8 years, the children in the lighter low birthweight cohort were still similar to controls, and those in the heavier low birthweight group still showed advantages. The children who had been larger babies had a full scale IQ that was 4.4 points higher ($P=0.007$), a better verbal IQ score (4.2 points higher, $P=0.01$), a higher performance IQ score (3.9 points higher, $P=0.02$), and better mathematics (4.8 points higher, $P=0.04$) and receptive vocabulary scores (6.7 points higher, $P=0.001$) (McCarton et al., 1997). The general observation was that lower birthweight children do less well and this has also been found in other studies (e.g. McCormick et al., 1996). There was another interesting finding, which related to the effect of environmental stimulation: children whose mothers had attended college did not exhibit significant enhancement, but those whose mothers had had a high school education or less, benefited from the intervention (Brooks-Gunn et al., 1992).

Another study in Avon, England, also showed a small advantage for a structured developmental programme over social support, particularly for the smallest infants (birthweights <1250 g) and those with brain injuries (Anonymous, 1998). Here, a randomized controlled trial compared Portage, a home developmental education programme, with non-directional counselling by parent advisers. Social variables confounded the results, but, when linear regression analysis was applied, there was a positive effect due to Portage (+4.3 general quotient points, 95% CI 1.6–7.0) and the parent adviser group (+3.4 general quotient points, 95% CI 1.4–6.1.)

In conclusion, it seems that early interventions may result in improved cognition, but there is a powerful environmental effect. It is not easy to characterize the most effective type of intervention or the frequency at which it should be applied. Infants whose growth was restricted in utero seemed to do worst (Zeskind & Ramey, 1978, 1981).

The effect of early interventions on children with cerebral palsy

There have been a number of papers on physical therapy for children with cerebral palsy, but few randomized controlled trials. Trials carried out between 1966 and 1994 were reviewed by Hur (1995), and Turnbull (1993) also carried out a review using quantitative and qualitative analyses. There have been three trials where randomization was blind, and only one in which the control group received no intervention at all (Goodman et al., 1985; Piper et al., 1986; Weindling et al., 1996).

In 1981, Goodman et al. (1985) used a neurodevelopmental assessment at 3 months to identify babies who were considered to be likely to benefit from neurodevelopmental therapy. Infants below 34 weeks' gestation and 1700 g were eligible for the study. Forty infants were considered to be at risk of developing disabilities and 40 were considered to be normal. Children in both groups were randomly assigned to a hospital-based programme with additional home exercises. Although at-risk infants had lower developmental quotients at 1 year than normals (suggesting that the neurodevelopmental assessment scale was valid), intervention did not alter outcome. When these children were about 6 years old, 49 of the original 80 infants were reassessed. At-risk and normal children had similar mean developmental quotients, but the locomotor score of the at-risk children was significantly below that of normal children, and 6/24 of the at-risk children had cerebral palsy, compared with 0/25 of those who had been considered normal at three months. The authors concluded that early intervention had had no demonstrable benefit in this case (Rothberg et al., 1991).

In Montreal, Piper et al. (1986) also carried out a prospective, randomized, controlled trial. They also decided to study an 'at-risk' population, defined as infants with a birthweight below 1500 g and any infant, regardless of birthweight, who had been asphyxiated at birth, had had convulsions or 'CNS dysfunction' with an abnormal EEG during the neonatal period. One hundred and thirty-four infants were randomized either to neurodevelopmental therapy aimed at optimizing position and movements or to normal care. The result was that the experimental and control groups were similar at 12 months, although infants weighing below 750 g at birth, regardless of group assignment, showed poorer growth and development than their heavier peers.

Palmer et al. (1988) studied slightly older children, who were between 12 and 19 months old and who had spastic diplegia. Forty-eight infants received either 12 months of physical therapy (Group A) or 6 months of infant stimulation followed by 6 months of physical therapy (Group B). The stimulation comprised motor, sensory, language, and cognitive activities. After six months, the physical therapy infants (Group A) had a lower mean motor quotient than the infant stimulation infants in Group B (49 vs. 58, $P=0.02$) and were less likely to walk (12% vs. 35%, $P=0.07$). These differences persisted after 12 months of therapy (mean motor quotient 48 vs. 63, $P<0.01$; likelihood to walk 36% vs. 73%, $P=0.01$). There were no significant differences between the groups in the incidence of contractures or the need for orthopedic interventions. Group A also had a lower mean mental quotient than Group B after 6 months of therapy (66 vs. 76, $P=0.05$). Although those infants who had been given stimulation did rather better than those who had had physical therapy, the usefulness of the study was diminished by the absence of a no-intervention control group.

The final study to comment on was done in Liverpool. Here, we also examined the hypothesis that infants at high risk of cerebral palsy could benefit from early neurodevelopmental therapy. One hundred and five infants with abnormal cranial ultrasound scans were randomized at around term to early neurodevelopmental therapy or standard treatment (delaying physiotherapy until abnormal physical signs became apparent). There was no difference in outcome at 12 and 30 months (Weindling et al., 1996).

It is worth drawing attention to two studies, which examined the intensity of intervention. Mayo (1991) randomized 29 infants who were less than 18 months old and who mostly had cerebral palsy. Bower et al. (1996) investigated the effect of increased frequency of physiotherapy on 44 children with quadriplegic cerebral palsy aged between 3 and 11 years. Both studies found short-term benefit from more intensive therapy, although in the Bower study this was also associated with setting specific goals.

The preceding studies described in this section illustrate some of the difficulties in devising and assessing therapy programmes aimed at improving motor function. The patterns of disability of the children studied are usually heterogeneous.

The nature of the intervention varies and there is no clear guidance from the scientific literature as to which intervention is most likely to be effective. There is difficulty in defining a robust criterion-referenced outcome measure. Ideally account should be taken of confounding factors, such as social and family circumstances, although this should not matter if the intervention is randomized and controlled. The family may seek out other interventions without the knowledge of the investigator, although this effect should balance out in a randomized controlled trial. Of the above studies, only the Liverpool and the Montreal studies were randomized and compared an intervention with no intervention, although some of the control Canadian babies received some therapy. Both studies found no difference in effect.

Pharmacological interventions

There have been several pharmacological interventions particularly intended to reduce the incidence of PVH. Of these, corticosteroids given to the mother antenatally for its effect on the fetus, and indomethacin given to the neonate after birth, have an effect (Crowley et al., 1990; Crowley, 1998; Fowlie, 1996, 1997), and have found their way into routine clinical practice. Two other drugs, vitamin E and ethamsylate, have been shown by randomized trial to have some effect in reducing PVH (especially severe grades in the case of vitamin E), but have not entered general clinical practice. Vitamin E is an antioxidant (Sinha et al., 1985), and Chiswick et al. (1983) suggested that it protects endothelial cell membranes from oxidative damage and disruption, and so limits the magnitude of hemorrhage and its spread from the subependyma into the ventricles. Ethamsylate also stabilizes capillary membranes and inhibits prostaglandin synthesis (Morgan et al., 1981; Benson et al., 1986). Phenobarbitone either before or after birth (e.g. Shankaran et al., 1997) has not been found to be effective.

The most outstanding success story has been the increasingly widespread use of antenatal steroids. The drug was first used to reduce the incidence of respiratory distress in preterm infants (see overviews by Crowley et al., 1990; Crowley, 1998). This effect is certainly achieved (OR 0.53, 95% CI 0.44–0.63). The risk of dying is reduced by 40% (OR 0.60, 95% CI 0.48–0.75). It is particularly relevant to note that PVH is also significantly reduced in infants who have been exposed to steroid before delivery: there is a significant reduction in PVH at autopsy (OR 0.29, 95% CI 0.14–0.61) and on cranial ultrasound examination (OR 0.48, 95% CI 0.32–0.72). Even in premature infants treated with surfactant, antenatal exposure to dexamethasone resulted in a decrease in serious grades of PVH (Silver et al., 1996). The effect on long-term neurological abnormality just fails to reach significance (OR 0.62, 95% CI 0.36–1.08) (Crowley, 1998).

There is also convincing evidence from a rat model that corticosteroids have a remarkable brain-protective effect against hypoxia–ischemia (Barks et al., 1991). The effect of neonatal corticosteroid administration on brain damage caused by cerebral hypoxia was investigated by the administration of the various doses of dexamethasone to 7-day-old rats. These animals were subjected to a unilateral cerebral hypoxic–ischemic insult, causing a large unilateral cerebral infarct in 79% of controls, whereas all those which had been given dexamethasone for 3 days before the hypoxic–ischemic insults had no infarction. The neuroprotective effect of dexamethasone pretreatment was dose and time dependent. Treatment with dexamethasone after hypoxia or with lower doses before the insult did not prevent infarction. The neuroprotective effect was only seen when the dexamethasone was given 24 hours before hypoxia–ischemia, and not when it was given immediately before hypoxia–ischemia. The authors concluded that glucocorticoid administration in the neonatal period, even in low doses, protected the brain during subsequent periods of hypoxia–ischemia. The relevance of these observations to the human condition is that these rat experiments would seem to confirm that fetal exposure to corticosteroids has a brain-protective effect when there is subsequent (or perhaps on-going) hypoxia–ischemia.

These observations confirmed earlier work that had also demonstrated a protective effect (Pappius & Wolfe, 1983). Using a 3-day-old rat model, both dexamethasone and indomethacin had similarly sized protective effects. The experiment was designed to investigate whether the effects of dexamethasone were mediated by an inhibition of arachidonic acid in cerebral tissues or through the actions of oxygen-derived free radical. Neither seemed to be the case. Neither drug affected the thiobarbituric acid reaction as a measure of free radical formation. Nor, it seems, do prostaglandins play a part. There was a rise in $PGF_{2\alpha}$, PGE2 and PGD2 in the lesion area of untreated animals. Although indomethacin blocked this rise and dexamethasone had no effect, the protective effect of both drugs was almost equivalent. The authors speculated that the drugs might have their effects through a neurotransmitter system, such as the serotonergic system.

In spite of the evidence that antenatal steroids have a beneficial effect in protecting the brain against damage due to hypoxia and ischemia, concerns about the effect of the powerful steroids on brain growth and development are starting to emerge. These are considered fully in Chapter 22.

During hypoxia–ischemia adenosine is utilized and there is accumulation of purine metabolites. When reperfusion occurs, oxygen is again available and superoxide free radicals are produced during the oxidation of hypoxanthine by xanthine oxidase. Allopurinol inhibits xanthine oxidase. One study where allopurinol was given to preterm babies after birth did not reduce the incidence of PVL, but gave a useful insight into a causative mechanism of a number of neonatal diseases (Russell & Cooke, 1995). It has relevance to the general discussions in this chapter, and provides support to a view that hypoxia–ischemia and reperfusion are important causes of cerebral lesions during the perinatal period. In Liverpool, 400 infants between 24 and 32 weeks' gestation were randomly assigned to receive enteral allopurinol or a placebo daily for 7 days after birth. There was no difference in the primary end points of the study, the development of PVL (4.4% in the allopurinol group and 2.6% in the controls) or PVH with brain parenchymal involvement (6.8% in the allopurinol group and 5.1% in the controls). The most interesting finding was, however, that just after birth there were significantly higher plasma hypoxanthine concentrations in infants who subsequently developed PVL, chronic lung disease and retinopathy of prematurity. This lends weight to the notion that hypoxia–ischemia and the generation of oxygen-derived free radicals play a part in the etiology of PVL. It also supports a view that the etiologies of PVL and porencephaly due to parenchymal involvement by PVH might both be due in part to ischemia–reperfusion injury. The hypoxanthine concentrations (medians and interquartile ranges) for PVL and porencephaly were 13.75 (6.2–56.5) μmol/l and 12.7 (6.5–17.5) μmol/l, respectively, compared with around 7.0 μmol/l in healthy controls.

Although the precise mode of action of steroids remains uncertain, it is likely that they also affect the production of oxygen-derived free radicals. Studies of neurological trauma have also shown a protective effect by corticosteroids. Hydrocortisone seems to be relatively ineffective compared to prednisolone and methyl prednisolone (Hall, 1992). The effect seems to be due to the presence of a 1,2 double bond found in methyl prednisolone and prednisolone, but not in hydrocortisone. The efficacy of prednisolone and methyl prednisolone – and, presumably, betamethasone, which is administered to women at risk of delivering prematurely – is not related to their anti-inflammatory effect (Hall, 1992), but to the ability of the steroid to inhibit CNS membrane lipid peroxidation (Braughler, 1985). Methyl prednisolone is three times as effective as prednisolone (Hall, 1992).

Several authors have reported a reduction in the incidence of PVH in preterm infants exposed to antenatal steroids and also delivered by caesarean section, supporting a view that hypoxia–ischemia during the immediate prenatal and intrapartum period is likely to be damaging (e.g. Ment et al., 1995). One possible mechanism is that corticosteroids exercise their effect through maturation of the germinal matrix microvasculature in the preterm infant, since indomethacin has been shown to induce basement membrane production in the germinal matrix microvasculature of the newborn beagle pup and it too has a protective effect on PVH (Ment et al., 1992, 1994a,b).

The prostaglandin synthetase inhibitor, a non-steroidal anti-inflammatory drug, reduces PVH and Fowlie (1997) has reviewed its effect on infants weighing below 1750 g at birth. The clinical reason for giving indomethacin was to reduce the incidence of symptomatic patent ductus arteriosus. This was achieved in treated infants (pooled relative risk (RR) 0.35 (95% CI 0.26–0.47)). There was a trend towards reduced neonatal mortality in infants receiving prophylactic indomethacin (pooled RR 0.85 (95% CI 0.66–1.09)). Most relevant to this present discussion was the observation that prophylactic indomethacin also significantly reduced the incidence of Grade 3 and 4 intraventricular hemorrhage in treated infants (pooled RR 0.60, 95% CI 0.43–0.83). There was no evidence that prophylactic indomethacin prevented the progression of Grade 1 IVH if it was present before starting the drug.

There are fewer data about the effects of indomethacin on long-term development. Bandstra et al. (1988) found no evidence of a significant difference between the treatment and placebo groups when assessed using the Bayley Mental and Physical Developmental Index (MDI) at between 12 and 24 months. Fourteen out of sixty-four (22%) indomethacin-treated infants had an abnormal outcome compared with 15/59 (25%) control infants. There was, however, a trend toward a lower incidence of abnormal physical scores in the indomethacin group (8/64 (13%)) compared with 14/59 (24%) in the control group ($P < 0.1$). In a study by Ment (1994b) there was no difference at 36 months of age corrected for gestation between indomethacin and placebo groups in terms of blindness, deafness, general development or the incidence of cerebral palsy.

Indomethacin reduces blood flow to organs, particularly the brain (Edwards, 1990), kidneys (Cifuentes, 1979) and gut (Coombs, 1990), and it may interfere with platelet aggregation and impair hemostasis (Friedman, 1978). There is no evidence to suggest that prophylactic indomethacin is associated with any long-term adverse effects, although there was a trend in treated infants towards an increased incidence of necrotizing enterocolitis, and some evidence that treatment may transiently impair renal function (Fowlie, 1997). There was no evidence that hemostasis was disturbed (Fowlie, 1997). Fowlie (1997) calculated that 19 babies would need to be treated prophylactically with indomethacin to prevent one severe PVH, and only five infants would need treatment to prevent a symptomatic patent ductus developing. Administration of indomethacin does not, however, seem to affect the incidence of periventricular leukomalacia.

Finally, a brief mention of the nutritional role during the perinatal period of omega-3 (*n*-3) and omega-6 (*n*-6) essential fatty acids (for review, see Uauy-Dagach & Mena, 1995; Simmer, 1998). Omega-3 refers to a double bond in position three of the carbon chain, counting from the omega end of the molecule. The main omega-3 polyunsaturated fatty acids are alpha-linolenic acid, eicosapentanoic acid and docosahexanoic acid (DHA). The importance of these acids is that human tissue is unable to introduce a double bond before carbon 9. The clinical effects of omega-3 essential fatty acid deficiency are abnormal visual function and a peripheral neuropathy. There are particularly high concentrations of DHA in the cerebral cortex and retina, where DHA makes up about 50% of fatty acids in the phospholipids. Arachidonic acid is formed from the omega-6 fatty acid, linoleic acid.

Infants born significantly prematurely are particularly vulnerable to deficiencies of long chain polyunsaturated fatty acids because the placenta selectively transports arachidonic acid and DHA only during the third trimester. The assessment of vision has been considered a particularly sensitive indicator of the effects of omega-3 fatty acids, and infants fed on diets rich in DHA have been shown to have better visual acuity than those fed on infant formulae without DHA supplementation (Uauy-Dagach & Mena, 1995). Farquharson et al. (1995) studied the fatty acid composition of brain cortex phospholipids of infants dying before they were 6 months old because of sudden infant death syndrome. They found that the cerebral cortex of infants who had been breast-fed contained a higher DHA content than that of infants who had been fed on a cows' milk-based formula. This can be linked to the observation that breast-fed infants (with higher plasma and red blood cell DHA concentrations throughout the first year of life) had higher stereo acuity at 3 years (Birch et al., 1993). Add to this the observation that when low birthweight preterm infants fed human milk by gastric tube were compared with those fed milk formula by the same route, there was a mean 8.3 IQ advantage when they were 8 years old (Lucas et al., 1992), and the advantage conferred by omega-3 fatty acids seems clear. But when six randomized studies of supplementation by polyunsaturated fatty acids for term infants were critically reviewed by Simmer (1998), she was unable to show an advantage in terms of visual function, development and growth of term infants. There is, however, another down side. Lipid membranes are damaged by oxygen-derived free radicals because they are broken at the double bonds in the carbon chains of the fatty acids (Uauy-Dagach & Mena, 1995). Thus, membranes, which are rich in arachidonic acid, eicosapentanoic acid and DHA, are particularly susceptible to oxidative damage. This may be another reason for the vulnerability of the cerebral cortex and subcortical layer in term infants.

Conclusions

This chapter has reviewed the two common brain-damaging conditions that affect preterm infants, PVH and PVL. The point has been made that, although the same population of infants are vulnerable to both conditions, PVH and PVL should be viewed as separate in their etiologies. In part, the vulnerability of the premature infant to PVH and PVL is due to the characteristics of the cerebral circulation at this time, but the causes, particularly of PVL, are now understood to be complex.

The most striking benefit in reducing brain damage in premature infants has been through the use of corticosteroids administered antenatally to the mother.

The general impression is that programmes intended to improve cognitive function have been rather more effective than those aimed at motor function, and that more intensive regimes have been more effective in the short term than those where the intervention has been less frequent. There are, however, considerable methodological difficulties in assessing such programmes; these are related to the heterogeneity of the populations studied and the relatively poor discriminatory power of the tests used.

REFERENCES

Agostini, C., Trojan, S., Bellu, R., Riva E. & Giovannini, M. (1995). Neurodevelopmental quotient of healthy term infants at 4 months and feeding practice: the role of long-chain polyunsaturated fatty acids. *Pediatric Research*, **38**, 262–6.

Agostini, C., Trojan, S., Bellu, R., Riva, E., Bruzzese, M. G. & Giovannini, M. (1997). Developmental quotient at 24 months and fatty acid composition of diet in early infancy: a follow up study. *Archives of Disease in Childhood*, **76**, 421–4.

Als, H. & Gibes, R. (1986). *Newborn Individualized Developmental Care and Assessment Program (NIDCAP): Training Guide*. Boston, MA: Children's Hospital.

Als, H., Lawhon, G., Duffy, F. H., McNulty, G. B., Gibes-Grossman, R. & Blickman, J. G. (1994). Individualized developmental care for the very low-birth-weight preterm infant. *Journal of the American Medical Association*, **272**, 853–8.

Als, H., Duffy, F. H., McNulty, G. B., Gibes-Grossman, R. & Blickman, J. G. (1995). Developmental care for the very low-birth-weight preterm infant. *Journal of the American Medical Association*, **273**, 1577–8.

Amiel-Tison, C. (1973). Neurologic disorders in neonates associated with abnormalities of pregnancy and birth. *Current Problems in Pediatrics*, **3**, 3–37.

Anonymous (1998). Randomised trial of parental support for families with very preterm children. Avon Premature Infant Project. *Archives of Disease in Childhood, Fetal and Neonatal Edition*, **79**, F4–11.

Auested, N., Montalto, M. B., Hall, R. T. et al. (1997). Visual acuity, erythrocyte fatty acid composition, and growth in term infants fed formulas with long-chain polyunsaturated fatty acids for one year. *Pediatric Research*, **41**, 1–10.

Back, S. A., Gan, X., Li, Y., Rosenberg, P. A. & Volpe, J. J. (1998). Maturation-dependent vulnerability of oligodendrocytes to oxidative stress-induced death caused by glutathione depletion. *Journal of Neuroscience*, **18**, 6241–53.

Bada, H. S., Green, R. S., Pourcyrous, M. et al. (1989). Indomethacin reduces the risks of severe intraventricular hemorrhage. *Journal of Pediatrics*, **115**, 631–7.

Bandstra, E. S., Montalvo, B. M., Goldberg, R. N. et al. (1988). Prophylactic indomethacin for prevention of intraventricular hemorrhage in premature infants. *Pediatrics*, **82**, 533–42.

Banker, B. & Larroche, J. (1962). Periventricular leukomalacia of infancy: a form of neonatal anoxic encephalopathy. *Archives of Neurology*, **7**, 386–410.

Barks, J. D., Post, M. & Tuor, U. I. (1991). Dexamethasone prevents hypoxic–ischaemic brain damage in the neonatal rat. *Pediatric Research*, **29**, 558–63.

Baud, O., Ville, Y., Zupan, V. et al. (1998). Are neonatal brain lesions due to intrauterine infection related to mode of delivery? *British Journal of Obstetrics and Gynaecology*, **105**, 121–4.

Benirschke, K. (1993). Intrauterine death of a twin: mechanisms, implications for surviving twin, and placental pathology. *Seminars in Diagnostic Pathology*, **10**, 222–31.

Benson, J. W. T., Drayton, M. R., Hayward, C. et al. (1986). Multicentre trial of ethamsylate for prevention of periventricular haemorrhage in very low birth weight infants. *Lancet*, **ii**, 1297–300.

Birch, E. E., Birch, D. G., Hoffman, D. et al. (1993). Breast feeding and optimal visual development. *Journal of Pediatric Ophthalmology and Strabismus*, **30**, 33–8.

Bower, E., McLellan, D. L., Arney, A. & Campbell, M. J. (1996). A randomised controlled trial of different intensities of physiotherapy in different goal-setting procedures in 44 children with cerebral palsy. *Developmental Medicine and Child Neurology*, **38**, 226–37.

Bourgeois, J. P. (1997). Synaptogenesis, heterochrony and epigenesis in the mammalian neocortex. *Acta Paediatrica Supplement*, **422**, 27–33.

Braughler, J. M. (1985). Lipid peroxidation-induced inhibition of gamma aminobutyric acid uptake in rat brain synaptosomes: protection by glucocorticoids. *Journal of Neurochemistry*, **44**, 1282–8.

Brooks-Gunn, J., Gross, R. T., Kraemer, H. C., Spiker D. & Shapiro, S. (1992). Enhancing the cognitive outcomes of low birth weight, premature infants: for whom is the intervention most effective? *Pediatrics*, **89**, 1209–15.

Brooks-Gunn, J., Klebanov, P. K., Liaw, F. & Spiker, D. (1993). Enhancing the development of low-birthweight, premature infants: changes in cognition and behavior over the first three years. *Child Development*, **64**(3), 736–53.

Brooks-Gunn, J., McCarton, C. M., Casey, P. H. et al. (1994). Early intervention in low-birth-weight premature infants. Results through age 5 years from the Infant Health and Development Program. *Journal of the American Medical Association*, **272**(16), 1257–62.

Calvert, S. A., Hoskins, E. M., Fong, F. W. & Forsyth, S. C. (1986). Periventricular leukomalacia: ultrasonic diagnosis and neurological outcome. *Acta Paediatrica Scandinavica*, **75**, 489–96.

Calvert, S. A., Hoskins, E. M. & Fong, F. W. (1987). Etiological factors associated with the development of periventricular leukomalacia. *Acta Paediatrica Scandinavica*, **76**, 254–9.

Campbell, F. A. & Ramey, C. T. (1994). Effects of early intervention on intellectual and academic achievement: a follow-up study of children from low-income families. *Child Development*, **65**, 684–98.

Carlson, S. E., Ford, A. J., Werkman, S. H., Peeples, J. M. & Koo, W. W. K. (1996). Visual acuity and fatty acid status of term infants fed human milk and formulas with and without decosahexaenoate and arachidonate from egg yolk lecithin. *Pediatric Research*, **39**, 882–8.

Chiswick, M. L., Johnson, M., Woodhall, C. et al. (1983). Protective effect of vitamin E (DL-alpha-tocopherol) against intraventricular haemorrhage in premature babies. *British Medical Journal*, **287**, 81–4.

Cifuentes, R. F., Olley, P. M., Balfe, J. W. et al. (1979). Indomethacin and renal function in premature infants with persistent patent ductus arteriosus. *Journal of Pediatrics*, 95, 583–7.

Collins, P. (1995). Embryology and development. In *Gray's Anatomy*, 38th edn, pp. 252, 315, 316. Edinburgh: Churchill Livingstone.

Cooke, R. W. I. (1987). Determinants of major handicap in post-haemorrhagic hydrocephalus. *Archives of Disease in Childhood*, 62, 504–6.

Coombs, R. C., Morgan, M. E. I., Durbin, G. M. et al. (1990). Gut blood flow velocities in the newborn: effects of patent ductus arteriosus and parenteral indomethacin. *Archives of Disease in Childhood*, 65, 1067–71.

Couser, R. J., Ferrara, T. B., Wright, G. B. et al. (1996). Prophylactic indomethacin therapy in the first 24 hours of life for the prevention of patent ductus arteriosus in preterm infants treated prophylactically with surfactant in the delivery room. *Journal of Pediatrics*, 28, 631–7.

Crowley, P. (1998). Corticosteroids prior to preterm delivery (Cochrane Review). In *The Cochrane Library*, Issue 4, Update Software, Oxford.

Crowley, P., Chalmers, I., Keirse, M. J. N. C. (1990). The effects of corticosteroid administration before preterm delivery: an overview of the evidence from controlled trials. *British Journal of Obstetrics and Gynaecology*, 97, 11–25.

Dammann, O. & Leviton, A. (1997). Maternal intrauterine infection, cytokines, and brain damage in the preterm newborn. *Pediatric Research*, 42, 1–8.

Delivoria-Papadopoulos, M. & McGowan, J. E. (1998). Oxygen transport and delivery. In *Fetal and Neonatal Physiology*, ed. R. A. Polin and W. W. Fox. W. B. Saunders Co.

De Vries, L. & Levene, M. I. (1995). Cerebral ischaemic lesions. In *Fetal and Neonatal Neurology and Neurosurgery*, ed. M. I. Levene, R. J. Lilford, M. J. Bennet & J. Punt. Edinburgh: Churchill Livingstone.

Dobbing, J. & Sands, J. (1970). Timing of neuroblast multiplication in developing human brain. *Nature*, 226, 639–40.

Dommergues, M-A., Parkai, J., Renauld, J-C., Evrard, P. & Gressens, P. (2000). Proinflammatory cytokines and interleukin-9 exacerbate excitoxic lesions of the newborn murine neopallium. *Annals of Neurology*, 47, 54–63.

Edwards, A. D., Wyatt, J. S., Richardson, C. et al. (1990). Effects of indomethacin on cerebral haemodynamics in very preterm infants. *Lancet*, 335, 1491–5.

Encyclopaedia Britannica CD99, 1998.

Farquharson, J., Cockburn, F., Ainslie, P. W. et al. (1992). Infant cerebral cortex phospholipid fatty acid composition and diet. *Lancet*, 340, 810–13.

Farquharson, J., Jamieson, E. C., Abbasi, K. A., Patrick, W. J., Logan, R. W. & Cockburn, F. (1995). Effect of diet on the fatty acid composition of the major phospholipids of infant cerebral cortex. *Archives of Disease in Childhood*, 72, 198–203.

Fletcher, J. M., Landry, S. H., Bohan, T. O. et al. (1997). Effects of intraventricular hemorrhage and hydrocephalus on the long-term neurobehavioural development of very-low-birthweight infants. *Developmental Medicine and Child Neurology*, 39, 596–606.

Fowlie, P. W. (1996). Prophylactic indomethacin: systematic review and meta-analysis. *Archives of Disease in Childhood*, 74, F81–7.

Fowlie, P. W. (1997). Prophylactic intravenous indomethacin in very low birth weight infants. *Cochrane Review 1997.*

Friedman, Z., Whitman, V., Maisels, M. J. et al. (1978). Indomethacin disposition and indomethacin-induced platelet dysfunction in premature infants. *Journal of Clinical Pharmacology,* **18,** 272–9.

Garland, J. S. (1995). Developmental care for very-low-birth-weight preterm infants. *Journal of the American Medical Association,* **273,** 1575.

Geva, E., Lerner-Geva, L., Stavorovsky, Z. et al. (1998). Multifetal pregnancy reduction a possible risk factor for periventricular leukomalacia in premature newborns. *Fertility and Sterility,* **69,** 845–50.

Gibson, D. & Harris, A. (1988). Aggregated early intervention effects for Down's syndrome persons: patterning and longevity of benefits. *Journal of Mental Deficiency Research,* **32,** 1–17.

Ginsberg, M. D., Hedley-Whyte, E. T. & Richardson, E. P. (1976). Hypoxic–ischemic leukoencephalopathy in man. *Archives of Neurology,* **33,** 5–14.

Goldenberg, R. L., Hauth, J. C. & Andrews, W. W. (2000). Intrauterine infection and preterm delivery. *New England Journal of Medicine,* **342,** 1500–7.

Good, W. V., Brodsky, M. C., Angtuaco, T. L., Ferriero, D. M., Stephens, D. C. 3rd & Khakoo, Y. (1996). Cortical visual impairment caused by twin pregnancy. *American Journal of Ophthalmology,* **122,** 709–16.

Goodman, M., Rothberg, A. D., Houston-McMillan, J. E., Cooper, P. A., Cartwright, J. D. & van der Velde, M. A. (1985). Effect of early neurodevelopmental therapy in normal and at-risk survivors of neonatal intensive care. *Lancet,* **ii**(8468), 1327–30.

Grafe, M. R. (1993). Antenatal cerebral necrosis in monochorionic twins. *Pediatric Pathology,* **13,** 15–19.

Greisen, G., Munck, H. & Lou, H. (1987). Severe hypocarbia in preterm infants and neurodevelopmental deficit. *Acta Paediatrica Scandinavica,* **76,** 401–4.

Grether, J. K., Nelson, K. B. & Cummins, S. K. (1993). Twinning and cerebral palsy: experience in four northern California counties, births 1983 through 1985. *Pediatrics,* **92,** 854–8.

Guralnick, M. J. (1998). Effectiveness of early intervention for vulnerable children: a developmental perspective. *American Journal of Mental Retardation,* **102,** 319–45.

Hall, E. D. (1992). The Neuroprotective pharmacology of methylprednisolone. *Journal of Neurosurgery,* **76,** 13–22.

Hall, E. D. & Braughler, J. M. (1981). Acute effects of intravenous glucocorticoid pretreatment on the in vitro peroxidation of cat spinal cord tissue. *Experimental Neurology,* **73,** 321–4.

Hambleton, G. & Wigglesworth, J. S. (1976). Origin of intraventricular haemorrhage in the preterm infant. *Archives of Disease in Childhood,* **51,** 651–9.

Hanigan, W. C., Kennedy, G., Roemisch, F. et al. (1988). Administration of indomethacin for the prevention of periventricular hemorrhage in high-risk neonates. *Journal of Pediatrics,* **112,** 941–7.

Harcke, H. T., Naeye, R. L., Sturch, A. et al. (1972). Perinatal cerebral intraventricular hemorrhage. *Journal of Pediatrics,* **80,** 37–42.

Hill, A., Shackleford, G. D. & Volpe, J. J. (1984). A potential mechanism of pathogenesis for early posthemorrhagic hydrocephalus in the premature newborn. *Pediatrics,* **73,** 19–21.

Hudgins, R. J., Boydston, W. R., Hudgins, P. A. & Adler, S. R. (1994). Treatment of intraventricular hemorrhage in the premature infant with urokinase. A preliminary study. *Pediatric Neurosurgery*, **20**, 190–7.

Hur, J. J. (1995). Review of research on therapeutic interventions for children with cerebral palsy. *Acta Neurologica Scandinavica*, **91**, 423–32.

Jackson, J. & Benirschke, K. (1989). The recognition and significance of the vanishing twin. *Journal of the American Board of Family Practice*, **2**, 58–63.

Janowsky, J. S., Scott, D. T., Wheeler, R. E. & Auestad, N. (1995). Fatty acids affect early language development. *Pediatric Research*, **41**, 310A.

Kandel, E. R. (2000). *The Principles of Neural Science*. 4th edn. New York: McGraw-Hill.

Katz, H. C. & Shatz, C. (1996). Synaptic activity and the construction of cortical circuits. *Science*, **274**, 1133–8.

Kinney, H. C. & Back, S. A. (1998). Human oligodendroglial development: relationship to periventricular leukomalacia. *Seminars in Pediatric Neurology*, **5**, 180–9.

Krueger, E., Mellander, M., Bratton, D. & Cotton, R. (1987). Prevention of symptomatic patent ductus arteriosus with a single dose of indomethacin. *Journal of Pediatrics*, **111**, 749–54.

Lacy, J. B. (1995). Developmental care for very low-birth-weight preterm infants. *Journal of the American Medical Association*, **273**, 1576.

Landy, H. J. & Keith, L. G. (1998). The vanishing twin: a review. *Human Reproduction Update*, **4**, 177–83.

Leech, R. W. & Kohnen, P. (1974). Subependymal and intraventricular hemorrhage in the newborn. *Annals of Pathology*, **77**, 465–75.

Leikin, E., Verma, U., Klein, S. & Tejani, N. (1996). Relationship between neonatal nucleated red blood cell counts and hypoxic–ischemic injury. *Obstetrics and Gynecology*, **87**, 439–43.

Levene, M. I. (1981). Measurement of the growth of the lateral ventricle in preterm infants with real time ultrasound. *Archives of Disease in Childhood*, **56**, 900–4.

Levene, M. I. & de Vries, L. (1995). Neonatal intracranial haemorrhage. In *Fetal and Neonatal Neurology and Neurosurgery*, ed. M. I. Levene, R. J. Lilford, M. J. Bennet & J. Punt. Edinburgh: Churchill Livingstone.

Liggins, G. C. & Howie, R. N. (1972). A controlled trial of antepartum glucocorticoid treatment for prevention of the respiratory distress syndrome in premature infants. *Pediatrics*, **50**, 515–25.

Lipman, B., Server, G. A. & Brazy, J. E. (1982). Abnormal cerebral haemodynamics in preterm infants with patent ductus arteriosus. *Pediatrics*, **69**, 778–81.

Lucas, A., Morley, R. & Cole, T. J. (1992). Breast milk and subsequent intelligence quotient in children born preterm. *Lancet*, **339**, 261–4.

Luciano, R., Velardi, F., Romagnoli, C., Papacci, P., De Stefano, V. & Tortorolo, G. (1997). Failure of fibrinolytic endoventricular treatment to prevent neonatal post-haemorrhagic hydrocephalus. *Child's Nervous System*, **13**, 73–6.

McCarton, C. M., Brooks-Gunn, J., Wallace, I. F. et al. (1997). Results at age 8 years of early intervention for low-birth-weight premature infants. The Infant Health and Development Program. *Journal of the American Medical Association*, **277**, 126–32.

McCormick, M. C., Brooks-Gunn, J., Shapiro, S., Benasich, A. A., Black, G. & Gross, R.T. (1991).

Health care use among young children in day care. Results in a randomized trial of early intervention. *Journal of the American Medical Association*, **265**, 2212–17.

McCormick, M. C., Workman-Daniels, K. & Brooks-Gunn, J. (1996). The behavioral and emotional well-being of school-age children with different birth weights. *Pediatrics*, **97**, 18–25.

Mahony, L., Caldwell, R. L., Girod, D. A. et al. (1985). Indomethacin therapy on the first day of life in infants with very low birth weight. *Journal of Pediatrics*, **106**, 801–5.

Makrides, M., Neumann, M., Simmer, K., Pater, J. & Gibson, R. (1995). Are long-chain polyunsaturated fatty acids essential nutrients in infancy? *Lancet*, **345**, 1463–8.

Mann, N. P., Haddow, R., Stokes, L., Goodley, S. & Rutter, N. (1986). Effect of night and day on preterm infants in a newborn nursery: randomised trial. *British Medical Journal*, **293**, 1265–7.

Martin, S. L., Ramey, C. T. & Ramey, S. (1990). The prevention of intellectual impairment in children of impoverished families: findings of a randomized trial of educational day care. *American Journal of Public Health*, **80**, 844–7.

Mayo, N. E. (1991). The effect of physical therapy for children with motor delay and cerebral palsy. A randomized clinical trial. *American Journal of Physical and Medical Rehabilitation*, **70**, 258–67.

Ment, L. A., Stewart, W. B., Duncan, C. C. et al. (1983). Beagle puppy model of intraventricular haemorrhage: effect of indomethacin on cerebral blood flow. *Journal of Neurosurgery*, **58**, 857.

Ment, L. R., Duncan, C. C., Ehrenkranz, R. A. et al. (1985). Randomized indomethacin trial for prevention of intraventricular hemorrhage in very low birth weight infants. *Journal of Pediatrics*, **107**, 937–43.

Ment, L. R., Duncan, C. C., Ehrenkranz, R. A. et al. (1988). Randomized low-dose indomethacin trial for prevention of intraventricular hemorrhage in very low birth weight neonates. *Journal of Pediatrics*, **112**, 948–55.

Ment, L. R., Stewart, W. B., Ardito, T. A., Huang, E. & Madri, J. A. (1992). Indomethacin promotes germinal matrix microvessel maturation in the newborn beagle pup. *Stroke*, **23**, 1132–7.

Ment, L. R., Oh, W., Ehrenkranz, R. A., Philip, A. G. S. et al. (1994b). Low-dose indomethacin therapy and extension of intraventricular hemorrhage: a multicenter randomized trial. *Journal of Pediatrics*, **124**, 951–5.

Ment, L. R., Oh, W., Ehrenkranz, R. A., Philip, A. G. S. et al. (1994c). Low-dose indomethacin and prevention of intraventricular hemorrhage: a multicenter randomized trial. *Pediatrics*, **93**, 543–50.

Ment, L. R., Oh, W., Ehrenkranz, R. A., Philip, A. G. S., Duncan, C. S. & Makuch, R. W. (1995). Antenatal steroids, delivery mode, and intraventricular hemorrhage in preterm infants. *American Journal of Obstetrics and Gynecology*, **172**, 795–800.

Ment, L. R., Vohr, B., Oh, W. et al. (1996). Neurodevelopmental outcome at 36 months corrected age of preterm infants in the multicenter indomethacin intraventricular hemorrhage prevention trial. *Pediatrics*, **98**, 714–18.

Ment, L. R., Oh, W., Philip, A. G. S. et al. (1999). Risk factors for early intraventricular hemorrhage in low birth weight infants. *Journal of Pediatrics*, **121**, 776–83.

Merenstein, G. B. (1994). Individualized developmental care. An emerging new standard for neonatal intensive care units? *Journal of the American Medical Association*, **272**, 890–1.

Morgan, M. E. I., Benson, J. W. T. & Cooke, R. W. I. (1981). Ethamsylate reduces the incidence of periventricular haemorrhage in very low birthweight babies. *Lancet*, **ii**, 830–1.

Neser, P. S., Molteno, C. D. & Knight, G. J. (1989). Evaluation of preschool children with Down's syndrome in Cape Town using the Griffiths Scale of Mental Development. *Child: Care, Health and Development*, **15**, 217–25.

Ohlsson, A. (1995). Developmental care for very low-birth-weight preterm infants. *Journal of the American Medical Association*, **273**, 1575.

Olsén, P., Pääkkö, E., Vainionpää, L., Pyhtinen, J. & Järvelin, M-R. (1997). Magnetic resonance imaging of periventricular leukomalacia and its clinical correlation in children. *Annals of Neurology*, **41**, 754–61.

Palmer, F. B., Shapiro, B. K., Wachtel, R. C. et al. (1988). The effects of physical therapy on cerebral palsy. A controlled trial in infants with spastic diplegia. *New England Journal of Medicine*, **318**(13), 803–8.

Pape, K. & Wigglesworth, J. S. (1979). Haemorrhage, ischaemia and the perinatal brain. *Clinics in Developmental Medicine*, 69/70. Spastics International Medical Publications. London, William Heinemann Medical Books. Philadelphia: J. B. Lippincott Co.

Papile, L. A., Burstein, J., Burstein, R. & Koffler, H. (1978). Incidence and evolution of subependymal and intraventricular haemorrhage: a study of infants with birth weights less than 1500 gm. *Journal of Pediatrics*, **92**, 529–34.

Pappius, H.M. & Wolfe, L.S. (1983). Functional disturbances in brain following injury: search for underlying mechanisms. *Neurochemical Research*, **8**, 63–72.

Patterson, P. H. & Nawa, H. (1993). Neuronal differentiation factors/cytokines and synaptic plasticity. *Cell (Neuron)*, **71**(10 Suppl.), 123–37.

Petterson, B., Nelson, K. B., Watson, L. & Stanley, F. (1993). Twins, triplets, and cerebral palsy in births in Western Australia in the 1980s. *British Medical Journal*, **307**, 1239–43.

Pharoah, P. O. & Cooke, T. (1996). Cerebral palsy and multiple births. *Archives of Disease in Childhood: Fetal and Neonatal Edition*, **75**, F174–7.

Pharoah, P. O. & Cooke, R. W. (1997). A hypothesis for the aetiology of spastic cerebral palsy – the vanishing twin. *Developmental Medicine and Child Neurology*, **39**, 292–6.

Pierrat, V., Duquennoy, C., van Haastert, I. C., Ernst, M., Guilley, N. & de Vries, L. S. (2001). Ultrasound diagnosis and neurodevelopmental outcome of localised and extensive cystic periventricular leukomalacia. *Archives of Disease in Childhood*, **84**, F151–6.

Piper, M. C., Kunos, V. I., Willis, D. M., Mazer, B. L., Ramsay, M. & Silver, K. M. (1986). Early physical therapy effects on the high-risk infant: a randomized controlled trial. *Pediatrics*, **78**, 216–24.

Pryds, O. (1994). Low neonatal cerebral oxygen delivery is associated with brain injury in preterm infants. *Acta Paediatrica*, **83**, 1233–6.

Punt, J. (1995). Neurosurgical management of hydrocephalus. In *Fetal and Neonatal Neurology and Neurosurgery*, ed. M. I. Levene & R. J. Lilford, pp. 661–6. Edinburgh: Churchill Livingstone.

Ramey, C. T. & Campbell, F. A. (1984). Preventive education for high-risk children: cognitive consequences of the Carolina Abecedarian Project. *American Journal of Mental Deficiency*, **88**, 515–23.

Ramey, C. T., Bryant, D. M., Wasik, B. H., Sparling, J. J., Fendt, K. H. & LaVange, L. M. (1992). Infant health and development program for low birth weight, premature infants: program elements, family participation, and child intelligence. *Pediatrics*, **89**, 454–65.

Rauh, V. A., Achenbach, T. M., Nurcombe, B., Howell, C. T. & Teti, D. M. (1988). Minimizing adverse effects of low birthweight: four-year results of an early intervention program. *Child Development*, **59**, 544–53.

Rennie, J. M. (1997). Neonatal cerebral ultrasound. Cambridge University Press.

Rennie, J. M., Doyle, J. & Cooke, R. W. I. (1986). Early administration of indomethacin to preterm infants. *Archives of Disease in Childhood*, **61**, 233-8.

Ringelberg, J. & van de Bor, M. (1993). Outcome of transient periventricular echodensities in preterm infants. *Neuropediatrics*, **24**, 269–73.

Romero, R., Ghidini, A., Mazor, M. & Behnke, E. (1991). Microbial invasion of the amniotic cavity in premature rupture of membranes. *Clinical Obstetrics and Gynecology*, **34**, 769–78.

Ross, G., Boatright, S., Auld, P. A. M. & Nass, R. (1996). Specific cognitive abilities in 2-year-old children with subependymal and mild intraventricular haemorrhage. *Brain and Cognition*, **32**, 1–13.

Rothberg, A. D., Goodman, M., Jacklin, L. A. & Cooper, P. A. (1991). Six-year follow-up of early physiotherapy intervention in very low birthweight infants. *Pediatrics*, **88**, 547–52.

Russell, G. A. B. & Cooke, R. W. I. (1995). Randomised controlled trial of allopurinol prophylaxis in very preterm infants. *Archives of Diseases in Childhood*, **73**, F27–31.

Saigal, S. & Streiner, D. (1995). Developmental care for very low-birth-weight preterm infants. *Journal of the American Medical Association*, **273**, 157–67.

Scott, D. T., Janowsky, J. S., Hall, R. T. et al. (1997). Cognitive and language assessment of 3.25 year old children fed formulas with or without longchain polyunsaturated fatty acids in the first year. *Pediatric Research*, **41**, 240A.

Seligman, M. L., Mitamura, J., Shera, N. et al. (1979). Corticosteroid (methylprednisolone) modulation of photoperoxidation by ultraviolet light in liposomes. *Photochemistry and Photobiology*, **29**, 549–58.

Sepkowitz, S. (1995). Developmental care for very low-birthweight preterm infants. *Journal of the American Medical Association*, **273**, 1577.

Shankararn, S., Papile, L. A., Wright, L. L. et al. (1997). The effect of antenatal phenobarbital therapy on neonatal intracranial hemorrhage in preterm infants. *The New England Journal of Medicine*, **337**, 466–71.

Shimogaki, K., Koterazawa, K., Nabetani, M., Miyata, H., Kodama, S. & Nakamura, H. (1998). A study on the clinical features of cerebral palsy in twins. *No To Hattatsu*, **30**, 24–8.

Shonkoff, J. P. & Hauser-Cram, P. (1987). Early intervention for disabled infants and their families: a quantitative analysis. *Pediatrics*, **80**, 650–8.

Shinnar, S., Gammon, K., Bergman, E. W., Epstein, M. & Freedom, J. M. (1985). Management of hydrocephalus in infancy: use of acetazolamide and furosemide to avoid cerebrospinal fluid shunts. *Journal of Pediatrics*, **107**, 31–6.

Silver, R. K., Vyskocil, C., Solomon, S. L., Ragin, A., Neerhof, M. G. & Farrell, E. E. (1996). Randomized trial of antenatal dexamethasone in surfactant-treated infants delivered before 30 weeks' gestation. *Obstetrics and Gynecology*, **87** (5 Pt 1), 683–91.

Simmer, K. (1998). Longchain polyunsaturated fatty acid supplementation of term infants. *Cochrane Review 1998*.

Sinclair, J. C. & Bracken, M. B. (eds.) (1992). *Effective Care of the Newborn Infant*, pp. 285–9, 403–5, 568–71, 606–7, 624–5. New York: Oxford University Press.

Sinha, S. K., Davies, J. M., Sims, D. G. & Chiswick, M. L. (1985). Relation between periventricular haemorrhage and ischaemic brain lesions diagnosed by ultrasound in very preterm infants. *Lancet*, **ii**, 1154–5.

Spinillo, A., Capuzzo, E., Stronati, M., Ometto, A., Orcesi, S. & Fazzi, E. (1995). Effect of preterm premature rupture of membranes on neurodevelopmental outcome: follow up at two years of age. *British Journal of Obstetrics and Gynaecology*, **102**, 882–7.

Teitel, D. F. (1998). Physiologic development of the cardiovascular system in the fetus. In *Fetal and Neonatal Physiology*, ed. R. A. Polin & W. W. Fox. Philadelphia: W. B. Saunders Co.

Trounce, J. Q., Rutter, N. & Levene, M. I. (1986). Periventricular leukomalacia and intraventricular haemorrhage in the preterm neonate. *Archives of Diseases in Childhood*, **61**, 1196–202.

Tsiantos, A., Victorin, L., Relier, J. P. et al. (1974). Intracranial hemorrhage in the prematurely born infant. Timing of clots and evaluation of clinical signs and symptoms. *Journal of Pediatrics*, **85**, 854–9.

Turnbull, J. D. (1993). Early intervention for children with or at risk of cerebral palsy. *American Journal of Diseases in Children*, **147**, 54–9.

Tyszczuk, L., Meek, J., Elwell, C. & Wyatt, J. S. (1998). Cerebral blood flow is independent of mean arterial blood pressure in preterm infants undergoing intensive care. *Pediatrics*, **102**, 337–41.

Uauy-Dagach, R. & Mena, P. (1995). The nutritional role of omega-3 fatty acids during the perinatal period. *Clinics in Perinatology*, **22**, 157–75.

Van den Hout, B. M., Eken, P., Van der Linden, D. et al. (1998). Visual, cognitive, and developmental outcome at 5½ years in children with perinatal haemorrhagic–ischaemic brain lesions. *Developmental Medicine and Child Neurology*, **40**, 820–8.

Ventriculomegaly Trial Group. (1990). Randomised trial of early tapping in neonatal posthaemorrhagic ventricular dilatation. *Archives of Disease in Childhood*, **65**, 1–10,

Verma, U., Tejani, N., Klein, S. et al. (1997). Obstetric antecedents of intraventricular hemorrhage and periventricular leukomalacia in the low-birth-weight neonate. *American Journal of Obstetrics and Gynecology*, **176**, 275–81.

Vincer, V., Allen, A., Evans, J. et al. (1985). Early intravenous indomethacin prolongs respiratory support in very low birth weight infants. *Acta Paediatrica Scandinavica*, **76**, 894–7.

Volpe, J. J. (1998). Neurologic outcome of prematurity. *Archives of Neurology*, **55**, 297–300.

Weindling, A. M., Fok, T-F., Calvert, S., Rochefort, M. J. & Wilkinson, A. (1985a). Newborn babies with periventricular cysts detected ultrasonographically are likely to develop cerebral palsy. *Developmental Medicine and Child Neurology*, **27**, 806.

Weindling, A. M., Wilkinson, A. R., Cook, J., Calvert, S. A., Fok, T-F. & Rochefort, M. J. (1985b). Perinatal events which precede periventricular haemorrhage and leukomalacia in the newborn. *British Journal of Obstetrics and Gynaecology*, **92**, 1218–223.

Weindling, A. M., Hallam, P., Gregg, J., Klenka, H., Rosenbloom, L. & Hutton, J. L. (1996). A randomized controlled trial of early physiotherapy for high-risk infants. *Acta Paediatrica*, **85**, 1107–11.

Westrup, B., Kleberg, A., von Eichwald, K., Stjernqvist, K. & Lagercrantz, H. (2000). A random-ized, controlled trial to evaluate the effects of the newborn individualized developmental care and assessment program in a Swedish setting. *Pediatrics*, **105**, 66–72.

Whitelaw, A. (1997a). Intraventricular streptokinase after intraventricular hemorrhage in new-borns. *Cochrane Review 1997*.

Whitelaw, A. (1997b). Repeated lumbar or ventricular punctures in newborns with intraventric-ular hemorrhage. *Cochrane Review 1997*.

Whitelaw, A., Rivers, R., Creighton, L. & Gaffney, P. (1992). Low dose intraventricular fibrino-lytic therapy to prevent posthaemorrhagic hydrocephalus. *Archives of Disease in Childhood*, **67**, F12–4.

Whitelaw, A., Mowinckel, M-C. & Abildgaard, U. (1995). Low levels of plasminogen in cerebro-spinal fluid after intraventricular haemorrhage: a limiting factor for clot lysis? *Acta Paediatrica*, **84**, 933–6.

Whitelaw, A., Saliba, E., Fellman, V., Mowinckel, M-C., Acolet, D. & Marlow, N. (1996). Phase 1 study of intraventricular recombinant tissue plasminogen activator for treatment of post-haemorrhagic hydrocephalus. *Archives of Disease in Childhood*, **74**, F20–6.

Williams, K., Hennessy, E. & Alberman, E. (1996). Cerebral palsy: effects of twinning, birth-weight, and gestational age. *Archives of Disease in Childhood: Fetal and Neonatal Edition*, **75**, F178–82.

Wu, Y. W. & Colford, J. M. (2000). Chorioamnionitis as a risk factor for cerebral palsy. A meta-analysis. *Journal of the American Medical Association*, **284**, 1417–24.

Yoon, B. H., Romero, R., Yang, S. H. et al. (1996). Interleukin-6 concentrations in umbilical cord plasma are elevated in neonates with white matter lesions associated with periventricular leu-komalacia. *American Journal of Obstetrics and Gynecology*, **174**, 1433–40.

Yoon, B. H., Chong, C. J., Romero, R. et al. (1997). Experimentally induced intrauterine infec-tion causes fetal brain white matter lesions in rabbits. *American Journal of Obstetrics and Gynecology*, **177**, 797–802.

Yoshida, K. & Matayoshi, K. (1990). A study on prognosis of surviving cotwin. *Acta Geneticae Medicae et Gemellologiae (Roma)*, **39**, 383–8.

Yoshida, K. & Soma, H. (1986). Outcome of the surviving cotwin of a fetus papyraceus or of a dead fetus. *Acta Geneticae Medicae et Gemellologiae (Roma)*, **35**, 91–8.

Zeskind, P. S. & Ramey, C. T. (1978). Fetal malnutrition: an experimental study of its conse-quences on infant development in two caregiving environments. *Child Development*, **49**, 1155–62.

Zeskind, P. S. & Ramey, C. T. (1981). Preventing intellectual and interactional sequelae of fetal malnutrition: a longitudinal, transactional, and synergistic approach to development. *Child Development*, **52**, 213–18.

21

Development of motor functions in health and disease

Mijna Hadders-Algra[1] and Hans Forssberg[2]

[1]Department of Medical Physiology, University Hospital Groningen, The Netherlands
[2]Department of Women and Child Health, Karolinska Institute, Astrid Lindgren Children's Hospital, Stockholm, Sweden

Theories on motor development

Neural-Maturationist Theories

In the middle of the twentieth century, motor development was generally regarded as a process based on a gradual unfolding of predetermined patterns in the central nervous system. Arnold Gesell and Catherine Amatruda, for instance, claimed that 'maturation is the net sum of the gene effects operating in a self-limited time cycle', a concept which left virtually no place for interaction with the environment. The idea that behavioural patterns emerge in an orderly genetic sequence resulted in the formation of general developmental rules, such as the cephalo-caudal and central-to-distal sequences of development. These notions paved the way for the pioneering work 'Developmental Diagnosis', consisting of a neat series of tests for the assessment of developmental milestones (Gesell & Amatruda, 1947). Motor development was considered to be the result of an increasing cortical control over lower reflexes:

At birth the various brain portions do not function equally well; rather, their function starts from the midbrain and continues to the cerebral hemispheres, which at birth are still neurologically inactive. Therefore, they have no inhibitory influence on the deeper cerebral portion and as a consequence the reflexes of the midbrain are not suppressed and become manifest (Peiper, 1963, p. 149).

Another pioneering developmentalist deserving attention is Myrtle McGraw. In part, McGraw's work was inspired by the neuroembryologist Coghill, who studied the relationships between neuroanatomical and behavioural development in the salamander *Amblystomum* (Coghill, 1929). Coghill claimed, in contrast to contemporary beliefs, that the development of complex behaviour did not arise from a blend of simple reflexes, but that motor behaviour from the very onset was complex and integrated (Coghill, 1929). McGraw supplied us with a careful description of infant motor development (McGraw, 1943), and a fascinating account of the striking developmental differences between Johnny, whose motor development was stimulated excessively, and Jimmy, his 'non-trained' twin brother (McGraw, 1939). She concluded that 'a certain amount of neural maturation must take place before any function can be modified by specific stimulation', thus leaving place for environmental stimulation and experience (McGraw, 1943). This implies that McGraw is not purely a neural maturationalist.

Dynamic systems theory

Esther Thelen and coworkers were not satisfied with the neural–maturationist theories, querying 'How can the timetable of motor solutions be encoded in the brain or in the genes?' (Thelen, 1995). Instead, they embraced the ideas of Kugler and coworkers (Kugler & Turvey, 1987). The latter, who followed the lines of thought of Bernstein (1935), tried to understand how the nervous system solves the problem of motor coordination in a system with a redundancy of degrees of freedom created by the movement characteristics of hundreds of muscles and joints. The ideas of the Kugler group, at present known as the dynamic systems theory, are based on the principles of non-equilibrium thermodynamics, i.e. non-equilibrium dissipative structures. Nature is full of such complex dissipative structures, which are systems which themselves maintain energy by way of exchange with the environment and which give rise to the self-organization of globally stable structures over extended periods of time. Thelen and coworkers argue that development can be regarded as a dissipative structure, i.e. as a dynamic system, because patterns of behaviour act as collectives ('attractor states') of the component parts, such as muscle strength, body weight, postural support, the infant's mood, and brain development, within particular environmental and task contexts. The patterns arise through self-organization (Thelen, 1985; Ulrich, 1997). According to Thelen (1995, p.84):

Developmental change can be seen as a series of states of stability, instability, and phase shifts in the attractor landscape, reflecting the probability that a pattern will emerge under particular constraints.

Thus, the difference between the neural–maturationist and the dynamic systems theories, is that the former considers the maturational state of the nervous system as the main constraint for developmental progress, whereas in the latter the neural substrate plays only a subordinate role. Or, as Thelen (1995, p.86) formulates it:

The Dynamic Systems view differs sharply from the traditional maturational accounts by proposing that even the so-called 'phylogenetic' skills – the universal milestones such as crawling, reaching, and walking – are learned through a process of modulating current dynamics to fit a new task through exploration and selection of a wider space of possible configurations.

Neuronal group selection theory

One of the principal properties of normal development is variation (Touwen, 1978, 1993). The variation is present in practically all developmental parameters, such as motor performance, developmental sequence, or the duration of developmental stages. But the variation is not always equally abundant. Gerald M. Edelman forwarded an explanation for such variations in development (Edelman, 1989; Sporns & Edelman, 1993). According to his neuronal group selection theory, development starts with primary neuronal repertoires. The cells and the gross connectivity of these primary repertoires are determined by evolution. The repertoires show variation through the dynamic epigenetic regulation of cell division, adhesion, migration, death and neurite extension and retraction (Changeux & Danchin, 1976). Next, development proceeds with selection on the basis of afferent information produced by behaviour and experience. This experiential selection results in secondary, more adapted repertoires of neuronal groups. The selection process is thought to be mediated by changes in synaptic strength of intra- and intergroup connections, in which the topology of the cells (Nelson et al., 1993) and the presence or absence of coincident electrical activity in pre- and postsynaptic neurons play a role (Hebb, 1949; Changeux & Danchin, 1976). When the selection has just been accomplished, behavioural variation is slightly reduced. Soon, however, abundant variation returns, because the organism and its populations of neurons is constantly exposed to a multitude of experiences. As a result, the neural structures of the secondary repertoires are globally mapped with large collections of parallel channels. The coordination between the various maps and channels is effected by a higher-order selection process called re-entry signalling (Edelman, 1989). The presence of the global mapping in the secondary repertoires is the basis of variable behaviour which can be adapted to environmental constraints.

The neuronal group selection theory could end the continuing 'nature–nurture' debate between the neural–maturationists and the dynamic systems theoreticians. According to the neuronal group selection theory, development is not governed by either a genetically dictated neural substrate or environmental conditions. On the contrary, development is the result of a complex intertwining of information from genes and environment. Similar ideas – albeit without the concept of variation and selection – were already forwarded by Waddington (1962), who portrayed development as an 'epigenetic landscape' in which developmental processes were canalized into specific process chains ('chreods'). Waddington's concept of experiential canalization was elaborated by Gottlieb (1991). Gottlieb stressed two points. In the first place, he underlined the idea that the various organizational levels, such as genes, cells, organ systems, organisms and the interactions between organisms, can mutually influence each other. Secondly, he drew attention to the role of species- and age-specific behaviour, which could play a canalizing role by exposing the individual to specific experiences. The presence of such age-dependent canalizing behaviour was already noted by McGraw (1943), when she reported that children exhibit an indomitable urge to exercise a function as soon as it emerges. The drive to exercise a newly developing function underscores the importance of self-produced activity for the creation of optimal neuronal circuitries (cf. Hadders-Algra et al., 1996b).

Normal motor development

Non-goal directed motor behaviour

Prenatal motor behaviour

Ultrasound studies of the human fetus in utero have demonstrated that the first movements emerge at 6–7 weeks postmenstrual age (PMA). They have been called 'smooth vermicular movements' (Ianniruberto & Tajani, 1981) or 'just discernible movements' (De Vries et al., 1982). Soon thereafter, at 8–9 weeks PMA, movements involving all parts of the body appear (Ianniruberto & Tajani, 1981; De Vries et al., 1982). Two major forms of such movements can be distinguished, the startle and the general movement. The startle is a quick and phasic generalized movement during which the muscles of the body and extremities are activated in synchrony (Hadders-Algra et al., 1993). General movements (GMs) consist of series of gross movements of variable speed and amplitude, which involve all parts of the body but lack a distinctive sequencing of the participating body parts (Prechtl & Nolte, 1984). It is interesting to note that the first movements exist prior to the completion of the spinal reflex arc, which is accomplished at 8 weeks PMA (Okado & Kojima, 1984). This means that the first human movements, just like those of the chick embryo (Hamburger et al., 1966), are generated in the absence of afferent information. This underscores the spontaneous or autogenic nature of the first movements (Hall & Oppenheim, 1987) and refutes the long-held belief that all movements of the fetus and newborn are reflex in character (Humphrey, 1969).

During the following weeks, new movements are added to the fetal repertoire, such as isolated arm and leg movements, various movements of the head (rotations, ante- and retroflexion), stretches, periodic breathing movements, and sucking and swallowing movements (Fig. 21.1; De Vries et al., 1982). Arm and leg movements, just like the palmar and plantar grasp reflex (Humphrey, 1969), develop concurrently at 9–12 weeks, suggesting that fetal motility develops without a clear cranio-caudal sequence. The age at which the various movements develop shows considerable interindividual variation, but at about 16 weeks PMA all fetuses exhibit the entire fetal repertoire. The repertoire continues to be present throughout gestation.

General Movements
Startle
Hiccup
Isolated arm movements
Isolated leg movements
Head retroflexion
Head rotation
Breathing movements
Hand-face contact
Jaw opening
Head anteflexion
Stretch
Yawn
Sucking + swallowing

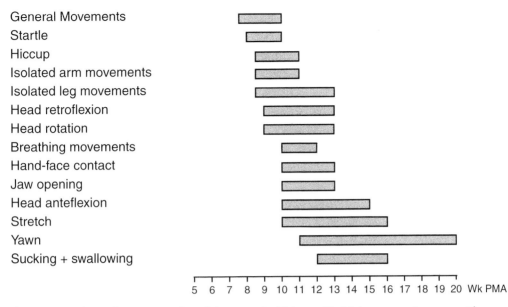

5 6 7 8 9 10 11 12 13 14 15 16 17 18 19 20 Wk PMA

Fig. 21.1.   Schematic representation of the ages at which specific fetal movements emerge. The length of the bars reflects the inter-individual variation. PMA = postmenstrual age. (Adapted from De Vries et al., 1982.)

The amount of fetal motility varies enormously, both intra- and inter-individually (De Vries et al., 1984). Still, some general characteristics can be distinguished. In the first place, GMs are the most frequently occurring movements (Roodenburg et al., 1991). Secondly, fetal motility shows during the second half of gestation a diurnal variation, with the lowest activity occurring in the morning and the highest in the evening (De Vries et al., 1987). Thirdly, the amount of motility decreases between 20 and 32 weeks PMA. This reduction is due to a gradual decrease in the number of startles and stretches, and a sudden drop in the number of GMs between 28 and 32 weeks (Roodenburg et al., 1991). According to Ten Hof & Nijhuis (1998), fetal motility continues to decrease slowly until term, a decrease which cannot be attributed to developmental changes in fetal behavioural state. The reduction in fetal motility appears to be less in female than in male fetuses (Ten Hof & Nijhuis, 1998). At present, it is not clear whether the reduction in fetal motility can be explained by the increasing spatial limitation of the growing fetus in utero, or by intrinsic neurodevelopmental processes. The demonstration of a similar reduction in motility in low-risk preterm infants would be an argument in favour of the latter explanation, but at present only conflicting evidence is available (Prechtl et al., 1979; Cioni & Prechtl, 1990).

The early presence of the fetal movement repertoire is intriguing. The movements reflect the basic characteristic of neural tissue to generate spontaneous, patterned activity (Droge et al., 1986). In addition, fetal motility can be considered as an ontogenetic adaptation as it promotes further development of various organ systems, such as the nervous and musculo-skeletal system (Oppenheim, 1984; Prechtl, 1984). For instance, it has been demonstrated that prevention of embryonic motility in the chick by blocking the neuromuscular junction results in a reduction of the normally occurring neuronal death (Okada et al., 1989) and in a malformation of the joints (Oppenheim et al., 1978; cf. arthrogryposis multiplex congenita in human infants with impaired fetal motility). Analogously, fetal breathing movements are a prerequisite for proper lung development (Prechtl, 1981). Fetal motility can also be regarded as a preparation for postnatal life, the breathing movements forming a vital case in point (Hall & Oppenheim, 1987). It means that the newborn infant immediately at birth has a repertoire of motor behaviour that is necessary for survival. To this category of so-called 'innate behaviours' belong feeding (i.e. rooting, sucking, mastication, swallowing), respiration as well as various protective reactions, such as blinking and coughing. There are also transient movement patterns, such as infant stepping and the Moro reaction, which are present for a time after birth without any obvious meaning for the individual infant. Most of these behaviours have already emerged during the fetal period. From neurobiological research in other species, it is known that central pattern generators (CPGs) underlie the generation of this type of movement (e.g. Grillner et al., 1995 (locomotion); Selverston & Moulin, 1987 (feeding); Fung & Feldman, 1995 (respiration)). The CPG neurones are coupled in networks which can generate complex basic activation patterns of the muscles without any sensory signals. Yet, sensory information about the movement is important in adapting the movement to the environment. The networks, usually located in the spinal cord or brainstem, are then controlled from cortical and subcortical centres via descending motor pathways.

Postnatal motor behaviour

At birth, be it term or preterm, minor changes in the motor repertoire occur. Breathing movements become continuous instead of periodic, the Moro-reaction can be elicited for the first time, and the infant, who is now hampered by the forces of gravity, is no longer able to anteflex the head in supine position (Prechtl, 1984). In preterm infants the extra-uterine environment also induces a change in the posture of the limbs: the flexed posture preferred in utero (Ververs et al., 1998) changes into extension (Saint-Anne Dargassies, 1974). In preterm infants younger than 32 weeks, the preferred extension posture is present in both arms and legs. From 32 weeks onwards, the extension changes into a preference for flexion, at first in the legs and from about 36 weeks onwards also in the arms (Saint-Anne

Dargassies, 1974). It should be realized, however, that the age-dependent preference postures can only be observed during the relatively short periods of active wakefulness and not during sleep (Prechtl et al., 1979; Vles et al., 1989; Cioni & Prechtl, 1990; Hadders-Algra et al., 1998a). With respect to the posture of neck and trunk, it has been reported that before 32 weeks (alternatively 2nd, after PMA) PMA antigravity postural control of the neck and trunk is entirely lacking (Saint-Anne Dargassies, 1974). During the following weeks some head control develops, so that, at term, low risk preterm infants, like full-term infants, can keep the head upright for a few seconds while in a sitting position (Prechtl, 1977).

Around 36–38 weeks PMA a transition in motor behaviour can be observed. The quality of the GMs changes from the extremely variable 'preterm' form into the more slow and forceful 'writhing' movements (Hadders-Algra et al., 1997), the fetus develops a head preference for the right side (Ververs et al., 1994), and in the arms and legs a strong flexed posture becomes dominant (Saint-Anne Dargassies, 1974). This transition in motor behaviour coincides with the emergence of clearly defined behavioural states (Nijhuis et al., 1982), suggesting that the behavioural transformation is due to changes in the neural substrate. EMG recordings of spontaneous motor behaviour (Hadders-Algra et al., 1992; 1997) and H-reflex studies (Hakamada et al., 1988) indicated that the periterm period, i.e. the period from 36–38 weeks until 6–8 weeks post-term, during which the 'writhing' GMs are present, is characterized by a temporary increased excitability of the motoneurones. This might explain why previously the motor behaviour around term was described as the phase of 'physiological hypertonia' (Peiper, 1963; Saint-Anne Dargassies, 1974). What could be the significance of this transient phase of increased motoneuronal excitability? It is conceivable that the high excitability of the motoneurones serves the sustainment of breathing movements, thereby assisting the transition from prenatal to postnatal life. This hypothesis is supported by the finding that problems in the continuation of respiration are especially encountered prior to 36 weeks (in the form of apnoeas; Prechtl et al., 1979) and around 3 months post-term (in the form of the sudden infant death syndrome; Wennergren et al., 1987).

At the end of the temporary 'writhing' phase another transformation in behaviour takes place. The infant is significantly more awake than during earlier ages (Wolff, 1984), and is able to use smiles and pleasure vocalizations in social interaction (Van Wulfften Palthe & Hopkins, 1984). Motor behaviour also shows substantial changes. The GMs lose their 'writhing' character and change into 'fidgety' GMs, which consist of a continuous stream of tiny, elegant movements occurring irregularly all over the body (Hadders-Algra & Prechtl, 1992). The predominant flexor posture of arms and legs disappears, with the flexion decreasing somewhat earlier in the arms than in the legs (McGraw, 1943; Touwen, 1976). At 2–3 months post-term, the head can be stabilized on the trunk (Touwen, 1976), vestibular responsiveness has improved (Eviatar et al., 1974), and a steady visual fixation and brisk visual orienting reactions have been developed (Atkinson & Braddick, 1989). Functional neuroimaging studies suggest that an increasing activity in the basal ganglia, the cerebellum and the parietal, temporal and occipital cortices could play a role in the transition at 2–3 months (Rubinstein et al., 1989). Hadders-Algra and Prechtl (1992) demonstrated that the transformation of 'writhing' GMs into 'fidgety' GMs was more closely related to postmenstrual than to postnatal age. This suggests that endogenous maturational processes play a major, but not exclusive, role in this transition. The minor effect of experience on the transition was indicated by Cioni and Prechtl (1990), who reported that low-risk preterms develop 'fidgety' GMs about 1 week earlier than full-term infants.

The fact that the infant first becomes a socially attractive partner at the age of 2–3 months post-term has induced speculations on the grounds for the typical term timing of human birth. Prechtl (1984) hypothesized that the 'physiological preterm birth' of the human infant could be explained by the relative large brain- and head size of the infant. A prolongation of gestation beyond term age would result in a further increase of brain- and head size, thereby creating immense energetic and mechanical problems for the mother. Nature apparently preferred the term birth solution with its transient phase of increased motoneuronal excitability.

Goal-directed motor behaviour

Motor development during infancy

Goal-directed motor behaviour develops during the final phase of general movement activity, i.e. during the phase of 'fidgety' GMs. The emergence of voluntary motor behaviour is announced by the ability of the infant to stop GM activity when it sees or hears something interesting. Next, goal-directed motility, such as mutual manipulation of the hands, and general movement activity are displayed in an alternating fashion. With increasing age, general movement activity is gradually replaced by goal-directed behaviour. In terms of neural networks this could mean that the generalized networks controlling GM activity are flexibly rearranged into multiple smaller networks, dedicated to the control of specific motor behaviour, such as goal-directed motility of the arms and the legs and postural control (cf. Simmers et al., 1995).

Infant motor development is characterized by intra- and interindividual variation (Touwen, 1976, 1978). The variation occurs, for instance, as variation in the emergence of a function, variation in the performance of a function, variation in the duration of specific developmental phases, and variation in the disappearance of infantile reactions, such as the Moro-reaction. Infancy is the period during which the fetally conceived primary neural repertoires are elaborated further. It is the phase of primary variability (Touwen, 1993; Hadders-Algra et al., 1998b) with

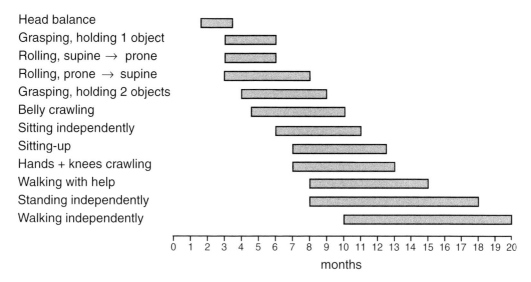

Fig. 21.2.   Schematic representation of the ages at which some motor skills emerge during infancy. The length of the bars reflect the interindividual variation. (Adapted from Touwen, 1976.)

an abundant (cortical) synaptogenesis (Huttenlocher et al., 1982). The multifarious primary networks pave the way for the selection of the most appropriate circuitries, a process which occurs especially during the second half of infancy (Hadders-Algra et al., 1996a). The variation in development includes the co-occurrence of different developmental phases. For instance, infants of a certain age can alternate belly crawling with crawling on hands and knees (McGraw, 1943; Touwen, 1976). Healthy infants can also exhibit a temporary regression, an 'inconsistency', in the development of a specific function (Touwen, 1976). As long as the regression is restricted to a single function, it can be regarded as another expression of developmental variation. The large variation in the attainment of milestones (Fig. 21.2) implies that their assessment has limited value. A slow development of a single function usually has no clinical significance but the finding of a general delay is clinically relevant. For the assessment of motor milestones in preterm infants, the age of the infant should be corrected for prematurity, i.e. functional age should be calculated from term age onwards (Touwen, 1981). This rule is especially useful during the first half year post-term, when the variation in the emergence of motor skills lies in the order of about 3 months, which is equivalent to the degree of prematurity. At later ages, the variation in motor skill attainment exceeds the degree of prematurity, thereby reducing the significance of age correction in older preterm infants.

A major accomplishment during infancy is the development of postural control, resulting in the ability to stand and walk without support. Postural control is primarily aiming at the maintenance of a vertical posture of head and trunk against the forces of gravity, because a vertical orientation of the proximal parts of the body provides an optimal condition for vision and goal-directed motility (Massion, 1998). At the age of 3 months, when the infant is able to stabilize the head in space, reaching movements emerge (Touwen, 1976). The first reaching movements are accompanied by a relatively unorganized simultaneous activation of the neck and trunk muscles. But at 4–5 months, when the reaching movements result in actual grasping, the variable neck and trunk muscle activity shows distinct organization: the postural activity is direction specific, i.e. the forward sway of the body induced by the reaching movement elicits a primary activation of the dorsal postural muscles, and it shows a top-down recruitment, meaning that the neck muscles are activated prior to the trunk muscles (Van der Fits et al., 1999b). With increasing age, the postural muscles are less often activated, so that at 5–6 months the combination in which the muscles are activated is very variable. This temporary phase of little postural activity probably serves as a transition phase, as after the transition the process of selection starts – heralding the development of adaptive postural strategies (Hadders-Algra et al., 1996a; Van der Fits et al., 1999c). The selection, which is experience dependent and which takes place during the phase that infants learn to sit independently, favours the pattern in which all direction-specific muscles are activated ('complete pattern', Hadders-Algra et al., 1996b). After the selection of the complete pattern, i.e. from 8–9 months onwards, infants obtain the ability to modulate the quantity of the postural muscle activity with respect to specific conditions, such as the pelvis position during sitting. Also this ability, the capacity to adapt postural muscle activity to environmental conditions, can be facilitated by training (Hadders-Algra et al., 1996b). From about 15 months of age, feedforward motor control processes become increasingly important. This is reflected by the development of postural muscle activity preceding muscle activity in the reaching arm. The development of this type of anticipatory postural control is related to the development of independent walking (Van der Fits et al., 1999c).

Successful reaching is preceded by various forms of pre-reaching activity. For instance, Von Hofsten (1982) demonstrated that newborn infants move their hands closer to a nearby object when they visually fixate it, than when they do not pay visual attention to the object. Reaching results in actual grasping of an object from 4 months onwards (Touwen, 1976). At this age, reaching movements have an irregular and fragmented trajectory consisting of multiple movement units, which underlines the heavy reliance of the first reaching movements on feedback control mechanisms (Von Hofsten, 1979). During the following months, the reaching movement becomes increasingly fluent and straight, and the orientation of the hand gets increasingly adapted to the object (Von Hofsten & Fazal-Zandy, 1984; Konczak et al., 1995). Infants start to grasp with the palmar grasp, in which they use the whole palmar surface of the hand and fingers. With increasing age, the prehensile activities move to the radial part of the hand: the palmar grasp is succeeded by the radial palmar grasp, the scissor grasp (grasping with extended index finger and thumb), the inferior pincer grasp (flexed index finger and extended thumb), and finally by the pincer grasp, in which the object is held between the tips of the flexed index finger and the flexed thumb (Touwen, 1976). Thus, gradually the ability to use independent finger movements develops. From monkey studies it is known that the ability to produce discrete finger movements requires the function of the motor cortex and the corticospinal pathways (Lawrence & Hopkins, 1976). Concurrent with the development of a more accurate grasping technique, the grasping reaction – one of the infantile reactions, which in the past were inadequately labelled as 'primitive reflexes' (Touwen, 1984) – disappears. Interestingly, the two processes, the development of the precision grip and the disappearance of the palmar grasp reaction, are not related (Touwen, 1976).

At birth, the infant – like the fetus (De Vries et al., 1984) – shows locomotor-like behaviour in the form of neonatal stepping movements (McGraw, 1943; Prechtl, 1977). These movements are probably generated by spinal pattern generators analogous to the locomotion in the hindlimbs of kittens after a transection of the thoracic cord (Forssberg et al., 1980) or in spinal lampreys (Grillner et al., 1995). It is still a matter of discussion whether humans have a similar hierarchical organization of neural networks for locomotion as quadrupeds, or whether supraspinal circuits have taken over some of the control functions. But recent evidence suggests that monoaminergic drugs can induce locomotion in non-human primates (Hultborn et al., 1993) and several groups have been able to induce locomotion in humans after incomplete spinal lesions (Fung et al., 1990). The infant stepping movements are rather primitive in character and differ largely from the flexible plantigrade gait of adulthood (Forssberg, 1985). The non-goal-directed neonatal stepping is characterized by a lack of segment-specific movements, implying that the legs tend to flex and extend as a single unit (Forssberg, 1985; Thelen, 1985), by a lacking heel strike, a variable muscle activation with a high degree of antagonistic coactivation, and by short latency EMG bursts at the foot contact due to segmental reflex activity (Forssberg, 1985). In the absence of specific training, the stepping movements can no longer be elicited after the age of 2–3 months (Touwen, 1976). A period of locomotor silence follows, which is succeeded in the third quarter of the first postnatal year by goal-directed progression in the form of crawling and supported locomotion. When the neonatal stepping is trained daily, the stepping response can be elicited until it is replaced by supported locomotion (Zelazo, 1983). This is perhaps not so surprising in the light of the fact that the locomotor pattern of supported locomotion is reminiscent of that of neonatal stepping – both lacking the determinants of plantigrade gait (Forssberg, 1985). Also the milestone transition into independent walking is not associated with a major change in specific locomotor activity. This indicates that the emergence of independent locomotion is not primarily induced by changes in the locomotor networks. Presumably, the development of independent walking is largely dependent on the development of postural control (Forssberg & Dietz, 1997; Van der Fits et al., 1999c).

Motor development during childhood

Postinfancy motor development is characterized by a gradual increase in agility, adaptability and the ability to make complex movement sequences. It is the phase of secondary variability, during which maturational processes, in continuous interaction with experience, produce highly adaptive secondary neuronal repertoires (Edelman, 1989; Touwen, 1993; Hadders-Algra et al., 1998b). The creation of the secondary repertoires is associated with extensive synapse rearrangement, the net result of synapse formation and synapse elimination (Huttenlocher et al., 1982; Purves, 1994). It is facilitated by increasingly shorter processing times which can be attributed in part to ongoing myelination (Müller et al., 1994).

Difficulties with the maintenance of balance dominate the picture of early locomotion. Postural control at toddler age is achieved by an activation of all direction specific leg-, trunk- and neck muscles and a rather high amount of antagonistic co-activation (Hadders-Algra et al., 1998b). This 'muscular corset strategy', which explains the stick-like locomotor behaviour of the toddler, can be regarded as a smart initial solution of the nervous system to master the large degrees of freedom of the upright moving body (cf., Bernstein, 1935). But this energy consuming strategy is only used during the so-called transient toddling phase, which ends at 2½–3 years (Hadders-Algra et al., 1998b). Thereafter, postural adjustments consist of a variable activation of direction-specific agonistic and antagonistic postural muscles. Further refinements of postural adjustments during (pre)school-age consist of increasingly shorter latencies until postural response onset (Haas et al., 1986), a decreasing reliance on visual input (Woollacott et al., 1987), and a better ability to deal with conflicting information from different afferent sources (Forssberg & Nashner, 1982). In addition, postural control during walking changes from a control which starts with the stabilization of the pelvis in space to a control which takes the stabilization of the head in space as a starting point (Assaiante, 1998). The age-related improvements in postural control are reflected in the development of skills like tandem gait, and standing and hopping on one leg, which emerge between 4–5 years and can be performed appropriately at 7–8 years (Sutherland et al., 1988).

Locomotion obtains its plantigrade characteristics slowly in the period between 1 and 5 years (Forssberg & Dietz, 1997). The coactivation of the tibialis anterior and gastrocnemius muscles decreases from about 2 years onwards, owing to a later occurrence of calf muscle activity in relation to tibialis activity. As a result, the heel strike develops. During this age period, the movements of the ankle get out of phase with those of the proximal joints. After 4 years of age, the reflex EMG-activity at foot contact disappears, suggesting that walking is getting controlled by increasingly complex polysynaptic circuitries (Berger et al., 1984).

During the postinfancy years, manual activities become increasingly complex. For instance, children learn to use eating utensils, to button their clothes and to tie their shoe-laces (Gesell & Armatruda, 1947). The coordination of the precision grip changes significantly (Gordon & Forssberg, 1997). When the precision grip emerges, it lacks the adult in parallel coordination of the 'lifting load' force and the 'squeezing grip' forces. Instead, 1-year-old children start with the generation of the squeezing grip force, while they simultaneously produce a negative load force by pressing the object to the support surface. More parallel force production emerges in the second half of the second year, but it is not until puberty that the perfect in parallel force coordination of the adult is accomplished. With increasing age, the ability to adapt grip forces to the slipperiness of the object develops. Also the ability to use anticipatory control mechanisms allowing the immediate scaling of grip forces to the known weight and the visually estimated size of an object is not immediately present. This ability emerges between 2 (known weight) and 3 years (visually estimated size; Gordon & Forssberg, 1997).

Early damage of the brain and recovery of function

The young brain shows substantial plasticity (Rosenzweig & Bennett, 1996). This plasticity explains why functional recovery after lesion of the brain in the neonatal period is in general larger than after similar lesions acquired during adulthood (Kennard, 1944; Armand & Kably, 1992). The functional recovery at an early age is mediated by considerable anatomical reorganization in the form of, for instance, excessive sprouting of fibres – including the development of an aberrant ipsilateral corticospinal tract (Kalil & Reh, 1982), increased dendritic arborization, maintenance of exuberant projections and lesion-induced synaptogenesis (Kolb & Whishaw, 1989). The extent of the recovery depends on a number of factors, such as the size and the site of the lesion (Passingham et al., 1983; Kolb & Whishaw, 1989), the species (recovery of function after a neonatal lesion of the sensorimotor cortex in cats is substantially larger than that in rhesus monkeys; Passingham et al., 1983; Armand & Kably, 1992), and the age of the brain at the insult. The Kennard principle (1944) stating 'the younger the age at insult, the better the outcome' is not always true. For instance, Villablanca and colleagues reported that lesions of the frontal cortex in fetal kittens resulted in neocortical dysgenesis and considerable sensorimotor deficits, whereas similar lesions acquired during the neonatal period were only followed by minimal functional deficits in the absence of gross structural anomalies (Villablanca et al., 1993). Comparable results were found in rats: the negative impact of cortical lesions (Kolb & Whishaw, 1989) and of cerebellar hemispherectomy (Gramsbergen, 1993) was larger when the rats acquired the lesion during the first postnatal days than when they were lesioned at postnatal day 20–30. It is conceivable that lesions at a very early age interfere with basic developmental processes in the brain, and consequently impede sensorimotor development to a larger extent, than do similar lesions occurring after the completion of these basic formative processes – but still at a time that the nervous system is plastic and young. This could explain the increase of severe disability among children with cerebral palsy (CP), which, according to the prevalence statistics of CP, is related to the larger number of survivors with a perinatal insult before 32 weeks of gestational age (Hagberg & Hagberg, 1996).

Animal experiments indicate that the age-dependent reorganizational events occurring after an insult to the brain at early age can enhance, but also hamper, functional recovery (Schneider, 1979). Possibly the same holds true for the effect of reorganization after early damage of the human brain. Carr and colleagues, for instance, who studied motor responses after transcranial magnetic stimulation of the motor cortex in children with hemiplegic CP, reported that independent finger movements were spared to some extent in children who presented with (hindering) mirror movements and in whom the stimulation experiments pointed to the presence of an abnormal bilateral projection of corticospinal axons to the spinal cord. Additional evidence suggested that the insult to the brain in these children had occurred before 29 weeks of gestation (Carr et al., 1993). Also Brouwer and coworkers found indications that the reorganization after brain lesion at early age could add to later motor dysfunction. They studied the projections of cortical neurons activated by transcranial magnetic stimulation to the motoneurons of the lower limb muscles in children with CP, and concluded that the abnormal projections from the motor cortex to the spinal motoneurons in the children with CP could contribute to the impairment in voluntary motility (Brouwer & Ashby, 1991).

Other factors which (seemingly) affect recovery of function after brain lesion at an early age are training and the age at which function is evaluated. Animal experiments indicate that specific training and enriched environments promote developmental outcome after brain lesion at an early age (Kolb & Whishaw, 1989). In addition, specific training can assist the suppression of abnormal behaviour due to anomalous, reorganizational connections (Schneider, 1979). With respect to age, it should be kept in mind that it can take considerable time before specific functions, such as the precision grip, are fully developed. Consequently, it can be equally long before certain dysfunctions become apparent (cf. Passingham et al., 1983; Hadders-Algra & Touwen, 2000).

Abnormal motor development

Early phases of abnormal motor development

The plasticity and developmental changes of the young brain hamper long-term prediction of motor outcome after brain lesions at early age. On the one hand, an early acquired brain lesion may not result in a motor disorder, on the other hand, it can take some time before a motor dysfunction can be expressed. In this respect, it is striking that the quality of spontaneous motility at a young age, i.e. the quality of GMs, does have substantial power to predict motor outcome. The quality of GMs can be classified as normal, mildly abnormal and definitely abnormal. Normal GMs are characterized by fluency, variation and complexity (Prechtl, 1990). The muscle coordination patterns of these movements are characterized by variation: variation in the muscles which participate, and in the timing and the quantity of the muscle activation (Fig. 21.3; Hadders-Algra et al., 1992, 1997). Despite this variation, muscle activity is not at random. Normal GMs show, for instance, during 70–85% of movement time a pattern of antagonistic coactivation. Mildly abnormal GMs lack fluency, but do show some movement complexity and variation. The corresponding variable EMG patterns exhibit abnormalities in the temporal and quantitative scaling of phasic muscle activity, suggesting dysfunction of the monoaminergic systems (Fig. 21.3; Hadders-Algra et al., 1997; Hadders-Algra & Groothuis, 1999). Definitely abnormal GMs lack fluency, complexity and variation altogether. This is reflected by the absence of variation in muscle coordination: the patterns consist either of a stereotyped synchronous activation of most participating muscles, or a stereotyped pattern of reciprocal activity (Fig. 21.3; Hadders-Algra et al., 1997). The persistent presence of definitely abnormal GMs despite transitions to the following GM-phases puts an infant at high risk (70–80%) for the development of CP (Ferrari et al., 1990). But, in a considerable number of infants, movement quality is not stable over age. The majority of changes occur at the transition periods at 36–38 weeks PMA and 6–8 weeks post-term (Fig. 21.4). This means, for instance, that definitely abnormal movements occurring before 36–38 weeks can change into mildly abnormal ones later on, and mildly abnormal movements into definitely abnormal ones. Consequently, GM quality during the final GM phase – the phase of 'fidgety' GMs – has the best predictive power. Definitely abnormal GMs at 'fidgety age' are associated with a high risk ($\pm$70%) for the development of CP (Hadders-Algra et al., 1997; Prechtl et al., 1997) with the remaining 30% of children developing minor neurological dysfunction (MND). Mildly abnormal GMs are associated with a minimal chance for CP and a 50% chance of the development of MND, whereas normal 'fidgety' GMs bear a favourable prognosis: no CP and about 10% chance of the development of MND at school-age (Hadders-Algra & Groothuis, 1999). The power of GM assessment to predict CP is

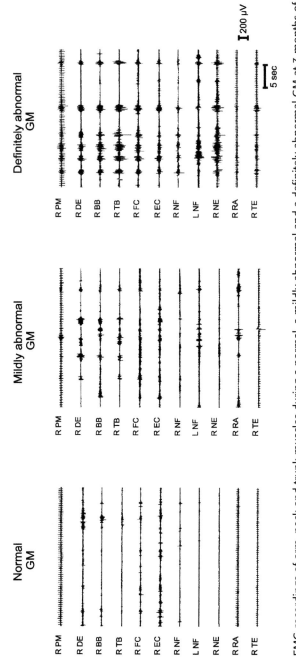

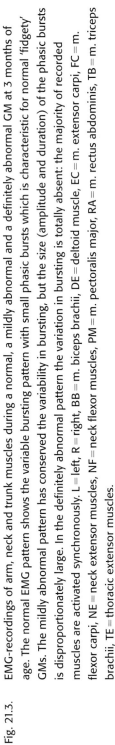

Fig. 21.3. EMG-recordings of arm, neck and trunk muscles during a normal, a mildly abnormal and a definitely abnormal GM at 3 months of age. The normal EMG pattern shows the variable bursting pattern with small phasic bursts which is characteristic for normal 'fidgety' GMs. The mildly abnormal pattern has conserved the variability in bursting, but the size (amplitude and duration) of the phasic bursts is disproportionately large. In the definitely abnormal pattern the variation in bursting is totally absent: the majority of recorded muscles are activated synchronously. L = left, R = right, BB = m. biceps brachii, DE = deltoid muscle, EC = m. extensor carpi, FC = m. flexor carpi, NE = neck extensor muscles, NF = neck flexor muscles, PM = m. pectoralis major, RA = m. rectus abdominis, TB = m. triceps brachii; TE = thoracic extensor muscles.

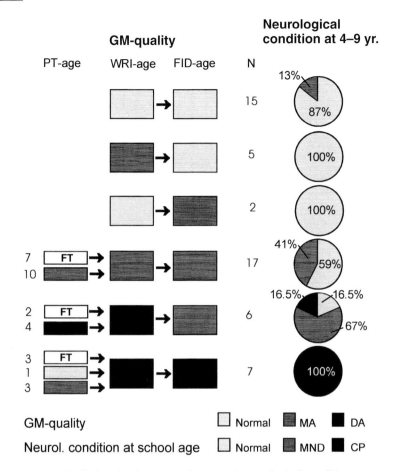

Fig. 21.4.   GM quality during the three GM phases and neurological condition at 4–9 years in a mixed group of low- and high-risk infants. The figure displays developmental trajectories in groups of children. For example, at the bottom row the development of 7 children is illustrated, who showed definitely abnormal GMs during the 'writhing' and the ' fidgety' GM-phases and who developed a CP. Three of those 7 were born at term (FT) and 4 preterm. Three of the preterm infants had shown mildly abnormal GMs during the 'preterm' GM-phase and one had shown normal GMs (the sudden and unusual change from normal to definitely abnormal GMs being due to a streptococcal meningitis at week 36). PT-age = phase of 'preterm' GMs, <37 weeks PMA; WRI-age = phase of 'writhing' GMs, 38–47 weeks PMA; FID-age = phase of 'fidgety' GMs, >47 weeks PMA. GM-quality: MA = mildly abnormal, DA = definitely abnormal. (Adapted from Hadders-Algra & Groothuis, 1999.)

higher than that of the traditional neurological examination at an early age, due to the fact that some infants with CP do show abnormal GMs, but no traditional neurological signs, such as abnormalities in muscle tone or head balance (Cioni et al., 1997).

Motor problems in cerebral palsies

The cerebral palsies are a group of serious motor disorders due to damage of the immature brain, affecting 1 out of 500 infants (Hagberg & Hagberg, 1996). The development of CP during infancy is primarily characterized by the lack of variation (Touwen, 1978, 1993). The lack of variation can be expressed as stereotyped motility and stereotyped postures, such a stereotyped flexion of the arms, fisting of the hands, extension of the legs, clawing of the toes, dominant ATNR (asymmetrical tonic neck reflex) posturing, hyperextension of neck and trunk, or stereotyped asymmetries (Touwen, 1978; Amiel-Tison & Grenier, 1986). Other frequently occurring signs are a poor head balance, abnormalities in muscle tone, visuo-motor signs, and persisting infantile reactions (Amiel-Tison & Grenier, 1986). The motor dysfunctions are often associated with a delay in motor development.

Deficits in postural control play a dominant role in the motor problems of CP. This holds especially true for children with severe spastic tetraplegia and severe athetosis, who do not develop an adequate head balance and an ability to sit without help. Two recent studies suggested that these profound postural deficits can be attributed to the absence of direction specific postural activity, i.e. the basic form of postural coordination (Hadders-Algra et al., 1999a,b). In children with less severe forms of CP, the basic level of postural organization is intact (Brogren et al., 1996; Woollacott et al., 1998). The postural adjustments of these children in response to external perturbations are less variable than those of healthy children (Hadders-Algra et al., 1999a), whereas those accompanying reaching movements are excessively variable (Hadders-Algra et al., 1999b). This might point to a deficient selection of the appropriate adjustment out of a limited repertoire of postural muscle activation patterns during goal-directed motor behaviour. The deficient selection could, in part, be due to an impaired processing of sensory information (Evans et al., 1991; Yekutiel et al., 1994). Children with spastic diplegia and spastic hemiplegia also show deficits in the ability to modulate muscle activity (EMG amplitude) with respect to specific conditions such as the pelvis position during sitting and arm movement velocity (Hadders-Algra et al., 1999a,b). This means that these children show deficits in their secondary, adaptive variability. Remarkably, a recent study showed that 18-month-old infants with spastic hemiplegia were able to modulate postural activity with respect to arm movement velocity when the moving arm was loaded with additional weight. This might imply that, in children with a spastic hemiplegia, more explicit afferent information can facilitate the task-specific modulation of postural adjustments during reaching (Hadders-Algra et al., 1999b).

Independent walking in children with CP is not only hampered by postural deficits, but also by specific locomotor dysfunctions. The locomotor pattern of children with CP, who are able to walk (with help), is characterized by features mimicking immaturity, such as the persistence of coactivation of antagonistic leg muscles during the stance-phase of gait, and a non-plantigrade gait (Berger et al., 1984; Leonard et al., 1991). The phasic EMG amplitude is reduced, which probably reflects the clinical sign of paresis. In children with spastic forms of CP, spasticity (the velocity-dependent increase of muscle response to imposed stretch) and secondary changes in the properties of the muscles contribute to the locomotor problems (Crenna, 1998).

Children with severe forms of CP do not develop a precision grip, but children with milder forms do (Ingram, 1966). In the latter group, the force coordination during precision grip is inappropriately organized (Eliasson et al., 1991). The children employ an excessively large squeezing grip force during the static 'in air' phase at the end of the object lifting movement. Grip forces are poorly adjusted to the slipperiness of the surface of the object and anticipatory control mechanisms are lacking. The latter suggests that children with CP have a diminished capability to build appropriate internal representations (Gordon & Forssberg, 1997).

Motor problems in the clumsy child

Clumsiness is an umbrella term covering a heterogenous group of motor disorders. It affects about 5–10% of children (Hadders-Algra, 2001). Clumsy children lack dexterity, and ease and grace in their movements. They are unskilful in gross and/or fine motor actions. During the last decades clumsy children have been labelled as 'minimal brain dysfunction', 'sensory integrative dysfunction' and 'developmental coordination disorders' (American Psychiatric Association, 1994). In 1994, an international consensus meeting was held (Polatajko et al., 1995), in which it was agreed to use the term developmental coordination disorder (DCD; American Psychiatric Association, 1994). Clumsiness (or DCD) may, or may not, be associated with minor neurological dysfunction (MND). In clumsy children without MND the poor motor competence probably can be attributed to social disadvantage or physical characteristics. Most likely, the motor functioning of these children will improve by motivation and motor training.

In other children, clumsiness is related to the presence of neurological dysfunction, such as mild hypotonia, choreiform dyskinesia, mild coordination problems or mild dysfunctions in fine manipulative ability. Early precursors can be – but not necessarily are – a delay in the achievement of motor milestones (Cermak, 2001), mildly abnormal GMs, and transient neurological abnormalities during infancy, such as 'transient dystonia' (Drillien et al., 1980). It should be realized, however, that a considerable proportion (40–50%) of clumsy children are not detected prior to school-age (Lindahl et al., 1988).

Clumsiness and MND are strongly age dependent, with the age-related prevalences being best described for MND. The rate of MND at toddler age is low. During the following years, the prevalence of MND shows a steady increase, to reach its peak shortly before the emergence of puberty (Hadders-Algra & Touwen, 2001). The age-dependent increase in minor neurological dysfunction runs parallel to – and is presumably related to – the age-dependent increase in the complexity of brain function. The onset of puberty induces a dramatic decline in the rate of MND. Possibly this decline is mediated by the hormonal changes occurring during this transformational phase of life (Soorani-Lunsing et al., 1993). The age-dependent changes in MND are accompanied by changing relationships with antecedent risk factors and concomitant cognitive problems and behavioural difficulties. During prepubertal school-age, the quantity of neurological signs matters; after the onset of puberty, the quality of neurological dysfunction. Apparently, the process of puberty converts the aspecific expression of dysfunction of the prepubertal nervous system into a specific and possibly more adult-like display of brain dysfunction (Hadders-Algra & Touwen, 2001). Notwithstanding the age-related changes in MND, two distinct categories of MND can be distinguished: simple MND and complex MND (Hadders-Algra & Touwen, 2001). The simple form occurs twice as often as the complex form. During the prepubertal period children with simple MND are characterized by the presence of one or two dysfunctions, such as hypotonia, choreiform dyskinesia, mild problems in coordination or fine manipulation; after the onset of puberty simple MND is denoted by the presence of either choreiform dyskinesia or hypotonia. In many instances of this type of MND, there is no apparent perinatal etiology. It is conceivable that this type of MND reflects the lower tail of the normal distribution of the quality of non-pathological brain function, i.e. a normal, but non-optimal brain function. In line with this hypothesis is the finding that simple MND is associated with a moderately increased risk for learning and behavioural problems (Hadders-Algra & Touwen, 2001). It is conceivable that this type of MND is mainly (epi)genetically determined. Another source of origin of this type of MND might be intercurrent diseases interfering with brain development during (pre) school-age (Hadders-Algra & Touwen, 2001). Children with complex MND present before the onset of puberty with at least three dysfunctions, and after the onset of puberty with problems in fine manipulation or coordination. Perinatal adversities, such as preterm birth and severe intrauterine growth retardation, play an evident etiological role in the development of this type of MND (Hadders-Algra & Touwen, 2001). Part of the adversities take place during the last trimester of pregnancy, a period during which high developmental activity is found in the cerebellum and periventricular regions. Consequently, dysfunction of fine manipulation and coordination may reflect dysfunction of the cortico-striato-thalamo-cortical and cerebello-thalamo-cortical pathways. These circuitries do not only play a role in sensorimotor aspects of motor programming, movement planning, program selection and motor memory, but also in cognitive tasks involved in learning (Alexander & Crutcher, 1990). This could explain the strong association of complex MND with cognitive and attentional difficulties (Hadders-Algra & Touwen, 2001).

Little is known about the pathophysiological mechanisms underlying clumsiness, probably due to the heterogeneity of the children evaluated at school-age. Deficits in the processing of sensory information can play a role. Problems in visual–spatial processing are most frequently reported, and deficits in visuoperceptual and visual memory ability and in kinaesthetic perception less often (Wilson & McKenzie, 1998). The data on motor organization are also diverse. Two characteristics are mentioned frequently: clumsy children often move slowly and with more variability than non-clumsy controls (Hadders-Algra, 2001). Recent studies on postural control indicate that children with MND lack the ability to adapt postural activity to task-specific conditions (Hadders-Algra et al., 1999a; Van der Fits et al., 1999a). The elegant study of Lundy-Ekman and coworkers (1991) on hand motor control in clumsy children, demonstrated that an increased variation in the timing of motor events was specific for clumsy children with mild coordination problems, whereas an increased variation in force output was characteristic of children with minor neurological signs suggestive of basal ganglia dysfunction, such as the presence of choreiform or athetotiform movements. The Lundy–Ekman paper underscores the notion that studies on motor mechanisms in children with DCD should take into account the type of the child's motor dysfunction.

Concluding remarks

It has gradually become clear that variation and selection are fundamental features of normal motor development. Damage of the brain at early age can result in reduced variation of the primary neural repertoires and it can hamper the selection of the appropriate motor strategies, thereby interfering with the adaptation of motor behaviour to task-specific conditions. Knowledge on the exact nature of the motor dysfunctions is still lacking. But, such knowledge is urgently needed, as it offers the basis for therapeutic intervention.

REFERENCES

Alexander, G. E. & Crutcher, M. D. (1990). Functional architecture of basal ganglia circuits: neural substrates of parallel processing. *Trends in Neurosciences*, **13**, 266–71.

American Psychiatric Association (1994). *Diagnostic and Statistical Manual of Mental Disorders*, 4th Ed. Washington DC: American Psychiatric Association.

Amiel-Tison, C. & Grenier, A. (1986). *Neurological Assessment During the First Year of Life*. Oxford: Oxford University Press.

Armand, J. & Kably, B. (1992). Behavioural and anatomical correlates of postlesion plasticity of the pyramidal tract during development of the cat. In *Tutorials in Motor Behavior II*, ed. G. E. Stelmach & J. Requin, pp. 845–59. Amsterdam: Elsevier Science Publishers.

Assaiante, C. (1998). Development of locomotor balance control in healthy children. *Neuroscience and Biobehavioral Reviews*, **22**, 527–32.

Atkinson, J. & Braddick, O. (1989). Development of basic visual functions. In *Infant Development*, ed. A. Slater & G. Bremner, pp. 7–41. London: Lawrence Erlbaum Associates.

Berger, W., Altenmüller, E. & Dietz, V. (1984). Normal and impaired development of children's gait. *Human Neurobiology*, **3**, 163–70.

Bernstein, N. (1935, 1984). The problem of the interrelation of co-ordination and localization. In *Human Motor Actions. Bernstein Reassessed*, ed. H. T. A. Whiting, pp. 77–119. Amsterdam: Elsevier Science Publishers B.V.

Brogren, E., Hadders-Algra, M. & Forssberg, H. (1996). Postural control in children with spastic diplegia: muscle activity during perturbations in sitting. *Developmental Medicine and Child Neurology*, **38**, 379–88.

Brouwer, B. & Ashby, P. (1991). Altered corticospinal projections to lower limb motoneurons in subjects with cerebral palsy. *Brain*, **114**, 1395–407.

Carr, L. J., Harrison, L. M., Evans, A. L. & Stephens, J. A. (1993). Patterns of central motor reorganization in hemiplegic cerebral palsy. *Brain*, **116**, 1223–47.

Cermak, S. A. (2001). Developmental dyspraxia and clumsiness in children. *Developmental Neuropsychology*, in press.

Changeux, J-P. & Danchin, A. (1976). Selective stabilisation of developing synapses as a mechanism for the specification of neuronal networks. *Nature*, **264**, 705–12.

Cioni, G. & Prechtl, H. F. R. (1990). Preterm and early postterm motor behaviour in low-risk premature infants. *Early Human Development*, **23**, 159–91.

Cioni, G., Ferrari, F., Einspieler, C., Paolicelli, P., Barbani, M. T. & Prechtl, H. F. R. (1997). Comparison between observation of spontaneous movements and neurological examination in preterm infants. *Journal of Pediatrics*, **130**, 704–11.

Coghill, G. E. (1929). *Anatomy and the Problem of Behaviour*. Cambridge: Cambridge University Press.

Crenna, P. (1998). Spasticity and 'spastic' gait in children with cerebral palsy. *Neuroscience and Biobehavioral Reviews*, **22**, 571–8.

De Vries, J. I. P., Visser, G. H. A., & Prechtl, H. F. R. (1982). The emergence of fetal behaviour. I. Qualitative aspects. *Early Human Development*, **7**, 301–22.

De Vries, J. I. P., Visser, G. H. A. & Prechtl, H. F. R. (1984). Fetal motility in the first half of pregnancy. In *Continuity of Neural Functions From Prenatal to Postnatal Life*, ed. H. F. R. Prechtl, *Clinics in Developmental Medicine*, No. 94, pp. 46–64. Oxford: Blackwell Scientific Publications.

De Vries, J. I. P., Visser, G. H. A., Mulder, E. J. H. & Prechtl, H. F. R. (1987). Diurnal and other variations in fetal movement and heart rate patterns at 20 to 22 weeks. *Early Human Development*, **15**, 333–48.

Drillien, C. M., Thomson, A. J. M. & Burgoyne, K. (1980). Low-birthweight children at early school-age: a longitudinal study. *Developmental Medicine and Child Neurology*, **22**, 26–47.

Droge, M. H., Gros, G. W., Hightower, M. H. & Czisny, L. E. (1986). Multi-electrode analysis of coordinated, multisite, rhythmic bursting in cultured CNS monolayer networks. *Journal of Neuroscience*, **6**, 1583–92.

Edelman, G. M. (1989). *Neural Darwinism. The Theory of Neuronal Group Selection.* Oxford: Oxford University Press.

Eliasson, A. C., Gordon, A. M. & Forssberg, H. (1991). Basic coordination of manipulative forces of children with cerebral palsy. *Developmental Medicine and Child Neurology*, **33**, 661–70.

Evans, A. L., Harrison, L. M. & Stephens, J. A. (1991). Cutaneomuscular reflexes recorded from the first dorsal interosseous muscle of children with cerebral palsy. *Developmental Medicine and Child Neurology*, **33**, 541–51.

Eviatar, L, Eviatar, A. & Naray, I. (1974). Maturation of neuro-vestibular responses in infants. *Developmental Medicine & Child Neurology*, **16**, 435–46.

Ferrari, F., Cioni, G. & Prechtl, H. F. R. (1990). Qualitative changes of general movements in preterm infants with brain lesions. *Early Human Development*, **23**, 193–231.

Forssberg, H. (1985). Ontogeny of human locomotor control. I. Infant stepping, supported locomotion and transition to independent locomotion. *Experimental Brain Research*, **57**, 480–93.

Forssberg, H. & Dietz, V. (1997). Neurobiology of normal and impaired locomotor development. In *Neurophysiology and Neuropsychology of Motor Development*, ed. K. J. Connolly & H. Forssberg, *Clinics in Developmental Medicine*, No. 143/144, pp. 78–100. London: MacKeith Press.

Forssberg, H. & Nashner, L. M. (1982). Ontogenetic development of postural control in man: adaptation to altered support and visual conditions. *Journal of Neuroscience*, **2**, 545–52.

Forssberg, H., Grillner, S. & Halbertsma, J. (1980). The locomotion of the low spinal cat. I. Coordination within a hindlimb. *Acta Physiologica Scandinavica*, **108**, 269–81.

Fung, G. D. & Feldman, J. L. (1995). Generation of respiratory rhythm and pattern in mammals: insights from developmental studies. *Current Opinion in Neurobiology*, **5**, 778–85.

Fung, J., Stewart, J. E. & Barbeau, H. (1990). The combined effects of clonidine and cyproheptadine with interactive training on the modulation of locomotion in spinal cord injured subjects. *Journal of Neurological Sciences*, **100**, 85–93.

Gesell, A. & Amatruda C.S. (1947). *Developmental Diagnosis. Normal and Abnormal Child Development*, 2nd. edn. New York: Harper & Row.

Gordon, A. M. & Forssberg, H. (1997). Development of neural mechanisms underlying grasping in children. In *Neurophysiology and Neuropsychology of Motor Development*, ed. K. J. Connolly & H. Forssberg, *Clinics in Developmental Medicine*, No. 143/4, pp. 214–31. London: MacKeith Press.

Gottlieb, G. (1991). Experiential canalization of behavioral development: theory. *Developmental Psychology*, **27**, 4–13.

Gramsbergen, A. (1993). Consequences of cerebellar lesions at early and later ages: clinical relevance of animal experiments. *Early Human Development*, **34**, 79–87.

Grillner, S., Deliagina, T., Ekeberg, Ö. et al. (1995). Neural networks that co-ordinate locomotion and body orientation in lamprey. *Trends in Neurosciences*, **18**, 270–9.

Haas, G., Diener, H. C., Bacher, M. & Dichgans, J. (1986). Development of postural control in children: short-, medium- and long latency EMG responses of leg muscles after perturbation of stance. *Experimental Brain Research*, **64**, 127–32.

Hadders-Algra, M. (2001). The clumsy child – at the border of cerebral palsy? In *Cerebral Palsy*, ed. M. Velcikovic Perat & B. Neville. Amsterdam: Elsevier Science Publ., in press.

Hadders-Algra, M. & Groothuis, A. M. C. (1999). An abnormal quality of general movements in infancy is related to the development of neurological dysfunction, attention deficit hyperactivity disorder and aggressive behaviour. *Developmental Medicine and Child Neurology*, **41**, 381–91.

Hadders-Algra, M. & Prechtl, H. F. R. (1992). Developmental course of general movements in early infancy. I: Descriptive analysis of change in form. *Early Human Development*, **28**, 201–14.

Hadders-Algra, M. & Touwen, B. C. L. (2001). Perinatal events and soft neurological signs in neurobehavioral outcome studies. *Developmental Neuropsychology*, in press.

Hadders-Algra, M., Van Eykern, L. A., Klip-van den Nieuwendijk, A. W. J. & Prechtl, H. F. R. (1992). Developmental course of general movements in early infancy. II. EMG correlates. *Early Human Development*, **28**, 231–52.

Hadders-Algra, M., Nakae, Y., Van Eykern, L. A., Klip-Van den Nieuwendijk, A. W. J. & Prechtl, H. F. R. (1993). The effect of behavioural state on general movements in healthy full-term newborns. A polymyographic study. *Early Human Development*, **35**, 63–79.

Hadders-Algra, M., Brogren, E. & Forssberg, H. (1996a). Ontogeny of postural adjustments during sitting in infancy: variation, selection and modulation. *Journal of Physiolology*, **493**, 273–88.

Hadders-Algra, M., Brogren, E. & Forssberg, H. (1996b). Training affects the development of postural adjustments in sitting infants. *Journal of Physiology*, **493**, 289–98.

Hadders-Algra, M., Klip-Van den Nieuwendijk, A. W. J., Martijn, A. & Van Eykern, L. A. (1997). Assessment of general movements: towards a better understanding of a sensitive method to evaluate brain function in young infants. *Developmental Medicine and Child Neurology*, **39**, 88–98.

Hadders-Algra, M., Brogren, E. & Forssberg, H. (1998a). Development of postural control – differences between ventral and dorsal muscles? *Neuroscience and Biobehavioral Reviews*, **22**, 501–6.

Hadders-Algra, M., Brogren, E. & Forssberg, H. (1998b). Postural adjustments during sitting at pre-school age: the presence of a transient toddling phase. *Developmental Medicine and Child Neurology*, **40**, 436–47.

Hadders-Algra, M., Brogren, E., Katz-Salamon, M. & Forssberg, H. (1999a). Periventricular leukomalacia and preterm birth have a different detrimental effect on postural adjustments. *Brain*, **122**, 727–40.

Hadders-Algra, M., Van der Fits, I. B. M., Stremmelaar, E. F. & Touwen, B. C. L. (1999b). Development of postural adjustments during reaching in infants with cerebral palsy. *Developmental Medicine and Child Neurology*, 41, 766–76.

Hagberg, B. & Hagberg, G. (1996). The changing panorama of cerebral palsy – bilateral spastic forms in particular. *Acta Paediatrica*, Suppl. 416, 48–52.

Hakamada, S., Hayakawa, F., Kuno, K. & Tanaka, R. (1988). Development of the monosynaptic reflex pathway in the human spinal cord. *Developmental Brain Research*, 42, 239–46.

Hall, W. G. & Oppenheim, R. W. (1987). Developmental psychobiology: prenatal, perinatal, and early postnatal aspects of behavioral development. *Annual Reviews of Psychology*, 38, 91–128.

Hamburger, V., Wenger, E. & Oppenheim, R. W. (1966). Motility in the chick and embryo in the absence of sensory input. *Journal of Experimental Zoology*, 162, 133–60.

Hebb, D. O. (1949). *The Organization of Behaviour*. New York: Wiley.

Hultborn, H., Petersen, N., Brownstone, R., & Nielsen, J. (1993). Evidence of fictive spinallocomotion in the marmoset (*Callitreix jacchus*). *Society of Neuroscience Abstracts*, 19, 539.

Humphrey, T. (1969). Postnatal repetition of human prenatal activity sequences with some suggestion of their neuroanatomical basis. In *Brain and Early Behavior*, ed. R. J. Robinson, pp. 43–71. New York, London: Academic Press.

Huttenlocher, P. R., DeCourten, C., Garey, L. J. & Van der Loos, H. (1982). Synaptogenesis in human visual cortex – evidence for synapse elimination during normal development. *Neuroscience Letters*, 33, 247–52.

Ianniruberto, A. & Tajani, E. (1981). Ultrasonographic study of fetal movements. *Seminars in Perinatology*, 5, 175–81.

Ingram, T. T. S. (1966). The neurology of cerebral palsy. *Archives of Disease in Childhood*, 41, 337–57.

Kalil, K. & Reh, T. (1982). A light and electron microscopic study of regrowing pyramidal tract fibres. *Journal of Comparative Neurology*, 211, 265–75.

Kennard, M. A. (1944). Reactions of monkeys of various ages to partial and complete decortication. *Journal of Neuropathology and Experimental Neurology*, 3, 289–310.

Kolb, B. & Whishaw, I. Q. (1989). Plasticity in the neocortex: mechanisms underlying recovery from early brain damage. *Progress in Neurobiology*, 32, 235–76.

Konczak, J., Borutta, M., Topka, H. & Dichgans, J. (1995). The development of goal-directed reaching in infants: hand trajectory formation and joint torque control. *Experimental Brain Research*, 106, 156–68.

Kugler, P. N. & Turvey, M. T. (1987). *Information, Natural Law, and the Self-assembly of Rhythmic Movement*. Hillsdale, NJ: Erlbaum.

Lawrence, D. G. & Hopkins, D. A. (1976). The development of motor control in the rhesus monkey: evidence concerning the role of corticomotoneuronal connections. *Brain*, 99, 235–54.

Leonard, C. T., Hirschfeld, H. & Forssberg, H. (1991). The development of independent walking in children with cerebral palsy. *Developmental Medicine and Child Neurology*, 33, 567–77.

Lindahl, E., Michelsson, K. & Donner, M. (1988). Prediction of early school-age problems by a preschool neurodevelopmental examination of children at risk neonatally. *Developmental Medicine and Child Neurology*, 30, 723–34.

Lundy-Ekman, L., Irvy, R., Keele, S. & Woollacott, M. (1991). Timing and force control deficits in clumsy children. *Journal of Cognitive Neurosciences*, **3**, 367–76.

McGraw, M. (1939). Later development of children specially trained during infancy, Johnny and Jimmy at school age. *Child Development*, **10**, 1–19.

McGraw, M. B. (1943). *The Neuromuscular Maturation of the Human Infant.* Reprinted (1989). *Classics in Developmental Medicine*, No. 4, London: MacKeith Press.

Massion, J. (1998). Postural control systems in a developmental perspective. *Neuroscience and Biobehavioural Reviews*, **22**, 465–72.

Müller, K., Ebner, B. & Hömberg, V. (1994). Maturation of fastest afferent and efferent central and peripheral pathways: no evidence for a constancy of central conduction delay. *Neuroscience Letters*, **166**, 9–12.

Nelson, P. G., Fields R. D., Yu, C. & Liu, Y. (1993). Synapse elimination from the mouse neuro-muscular junction *in vitro*: a non-Hebbian activity dependent process. *Journal of Neurobiology*, **24**, 1517–30.

Nijhuis, J. G., Prechtl, H. F. R., Martin, C. B. & Bots, R. S. G. M. (1982). Are there behavioural states in the human fetus? *Early Human Development*, **6**, 177–95.

Okada, A., Furber, S., Okado, N., Homma, S. & Oppenheim, R. W. (1989). Cell death of moto-neurons in the chick embryo spinal cord. X. Synapse formation in motoneurons following the reduction of cell death by neuromuscular blockade. *Journal of Neurobiology*, **20**, 219–33.

Okado, N. & Kojima, T. (1984). Ontogeny of the central nervous system: neurogenesis, fibre con-nection , synaptogenesis and myelination in the spinal cord. In: *Continuity of Neural Functions From Prenatal to Postnatal Life,* ed. H. F. R. Prechtl, *Clinics in Developmental Medicine*, No. 94, pp. 31–45. Oxford: Blackwell Scientific Publications.

Oppenheim, R. W. (1984). Ontogenetic adaptations in neural development; toward a more 'eco-logical' developmental psychobiology. In *Continuity of Neural Functions From Prenatal to Postnatal Life*, ed. H. F. R. Prechtl, *Clinics in Developmental Medicine*, No. 94, pp. 16–30. Oxford: Blackwell Scientific Publications.

Oppenheim, R. W., Pittman, R., Gray, M. & Maderdrut, J. L. (1978). Embryonic behavior, hatch-ing and neuromuscular development in the chick following a transient reduction of sponta-neous motility and sensory input by neuromuscular blocking agents. *Journal of Comparative Neurology*, **179**, 619–40.

Passingham, R. E., Perry, V. H. & Wilkinson F. (1983). The long-term effect of removal of sen-sorimotor cortex in infant and adult rhesus monkeys. *Brain*, **106**, 675–705.

Peiper, A. (1963). *Cerebral Function in Infancy and Childhood.* 3rd edn. New York: Consultants Bureau.

Polatajko, H., Fox, M. & Missiuna, C. (1995). An international consensus on children with devel-opmental coordination disorder. *Canadian Journal of Occupational Therapy*, **62**, 3–6.

Prechtl, H. F. R. (1977). *The Neurological Examination of the Full-term Newborn Infant.* 2nd edn. *Clinics in Developmental Medicine*, No. 63. London: Heinemann Medical Books.

Prechtl, H. F. R. (1981). The study of neural development as a perspective of clinical problems. In *Maturation and Development: Biological and Psychological Perspectives*, ed. K. J. Connolly & H. F. R. Prechtl, *Clinics in Developmental Medicine*, No. 77–78, pp. 189–215. London: Heinemann Medical Books.

Prechtl, H. F. R. (1984). Continuity and change in early neural development. In *Continuity of Neural Functions From Prenatal to Postnatal Life*, ed. H. F. R. Prechtl, *Clinics in Developmental Medicine*, No. 94, pp. 1–15. Oxford: Blackwell Scientific Publications.

Prechtl, H. F. R. (1990). Qualitative changes of spontaneous movements in fetus and preterm infant are a marker of neurological dysfunction. *Early Human Development*, 23, 151–8.

Prechtl, H. F. R. & Nolte, R. (1984). Motor behaviour of preterm infants. In *Continuity of Neural Functions From Prenatal to Postnatal Life*, ed. H. F. R. Prechtl, *Clinics in Developmental Medicine*, No. 94, pp. 79–92. Oxford: Blackwell Scientific Publications.

Prechtl, H. F. R., Fargel, J. W., Weinmann, H. M. & Bakker, H. H. (1979). Postures, motility and respiration of low-risk preterm infants. *Developmental Medicine and Child Neurology*, 21, 3–27.

Prechtl, H. F. R., Einspieler, C., Cioni, G., Bos, A., Ferrari, F. & Sontheimer, D. (1997). An early marker of developing neurological handicap after perinatal brain lesions. *Lancet*, 339, 1361–3.

Purves, D. (1994). *Neural Activity and the Growth of the Brain.* Cambridge: Cambridge University Press.

Roodenburg, P. J., Wladimiroff, J. W., Van Es, A. & Prechtl, H. F. R. (1991). Classification and quantitative aspects of fetal movements during the second half of normal pregnancy. *Early Human Development*, 25, 19–35.

Rosenzweig, M. R. & Bennett, E. L. (1996). Psychobiology of plasticity: effects of training and experience on brain and behavior. *Behavioural Brain Research*, 78, 57–65.

Rubinstein, M., Denays, R., Ham, H. R. et al. (1989). Functional imaging of brain maturation in humans using Iodine-123 Iodoamphetamine and SPECT. *Journal of Nuclear Medicine*, 30, 1982–5.

Saint-Anne Dargassies, S. (1974). *Le Développement Neurologique du Nouveau-né à Terme et Prématuré.* Paris: Masson et cie.

Schneider, G. E. (1979). Is it really better to have your brain lesion early? A revision of the 'Kennard principle'. *Neuropsychologia*, 7, 557–83.

Selverston, A.I. & Moulin, M. (1987). *The Crustacean Stomatogastric System.* Berlin: Springer Verlag.

Simmers, J., Meyran, P. & Moulins, M. (1995). Modulation and dynamic specification of motor rhythm-generating circuits in crustacea. *Journal of Physiology, Paris*, 89, 195–208.

Soorani-Lunsing, R. J., Hadders-Algra, M., Olinga, A. A., Huisjes, H. J. & Touwen, B. C. L. (1993). Minor neurological dysfunction after the onset of puberty: association with perinatal events. *Early Human Development*, 33, 71–80.

Sporns, O. & Edelman, G. M. (1993). Solving Bernstein's problem: a proposal for the development of coordinated movement by selection. *Child Development*, 64, 960–81.

Sutherland, D. H., Olshen, R. A., Biden, E. N. & Wyatt, M. P. (1988). *The Development of Mature Walking, Clinics in Developmental Medicine*, No. 104/105. Oxford: Blackwell Scientific Publications.

Ten Hof, J. & Nijhuis, I. J. M. (1998). Development of Fetal Heart Rate and Behaviour. PhD-Thesis, University of Utrecht, the Netherlands.

Thelen, E. (1985). Developmental origins of motor coordination: leg movements in human infants. *Developmental Psychobiology*, 18, 1–22.

Thelen, E. (1995). Motor development. A new synthesis. *American Psychologist*, **50**, 79–95.

Touwen, B. C. L. (1976). *Neurological Development in Infancy, Clinics in Developmental Medicine*, No. 58. London: Heinemann Medical Books.

Touwen, B. C. L. (1978). Variability and stereotypy in normal and deviant development. In *Care of the Handicapped Child*, ed. J. Apley, *Clinics in Developmental Medicine*, No. 67, pp. 99–110. London: Heinemann Medical Books.

Touwen, B. C. L. (1981). The preterm infant in the extrauterine environment. Implications for neurology. *Early Human Development*, **3/4**, 287–300.

Touwen, B. C. L. (1984). Primitive reflexes – conceptional or semantic problem? In *Continuity of Neural Functions From Prenatal to Postnatal Life*, ed. H. F. R. Prechtl, *Clinics in Developmental Medicine*, No. 94, pp. 115–25. Oxford: Blackwell Scientific Publications.

Touwen, B. C. L. (1993). How normal is variable, or how variable is normal? *Early Human Development*, **34**, 1–12.

Ulrich, B. D. (1997). Dynamic systems theory and skill development in infants and children. In *Neurophysiology and Neuropsychology of Motor Development*, ed. K. J. Connolly & H. Forssberg, *Clinics in Developmental Medicine*, No. 143–4, pp. 319–45. London: MacKeith Press.

Van der Fits, I. B. M., Flikweert, E. R., Stremmelaar, E. F., Martijn, A. & Hadders-Algra, M. (1999a). Development of postural adjustments during reaching in preterm infants. *Pediatric Research*, **46**, 1–7.

Van der Fits, I. B. M., Klip, A. W. J., Van Eykern, L. A. & Hadders-Algra, M. (1999b). Postural adjustments during spontaneous and goal-directed arm movements in the first half year of life. *Behavioural Brain Research*, **106**, 75–90.

Van der Fits, I. B. M., Otten, E., Klip, A. W. J., Van Eykern, L. A. & Hadders-Algra, M. (1999c). The development of postural adjustments during reaching in 6 to 18 months old infants: evidence for two transitions. *Experimental Brain Research*, **126**, 517–28.

Van Wulfften Palthe, T. & Hopkins, B. (1984). Development of the infant's social competence during early face-to-face interaction: a longitudinal study. In *Continuity of Neural Functions From Prenatal to Postnatal Life*, ed. H. F. R. Prechtl, *Clinics in Developmental Medicine*, No. 94, pp. 198–219. Oxford: Blackwell Scientific Publications

Ververs, I. A. P., De Vries, J. I. P., Van Geijn, H. P & Hopkins, B. (1994). Prenatal head position form 12–38 weeks. I. Developmental aspects. *Early Human Development*, **39**, 83–91.

Ververs, I. A. P., Van Gelder-Hasker, M. R., De Vries, J. I. P., Hopkins, B. & Van Geijn, H. P. (1998). Prenatal development of arm posture. *Early Human Development*, **51**, 61–70.

Villablanca, J. R., Hovda, D. A., Jackson, G. F. & Gayek, R. (1993). Neurological and behavioral effects of unilateral frontal cortical lesions in fetal kittens. I. Brain morphology, movement, posture, and sensorimotor tests. *Behavioural Brain Research*, **57**, 63–77.

Vles, J. S. H., Kingma, H., Caberg, H., Daniels, H. & Casaer, P. (1989). Posture of low-risk preterm infants between 32 and 36 weeks postmenstrual age. *Developmental Medicine and Child Neurology*, **31**, 191–5.

Von Hofsten, C. (1979). Development of visually directed reaching: the approach phase. *Journal of Human Movement Studies*, **5**, 160–78.

Von Hofsten, C. (1982). Eye-hand coordination in the newborn. *Developmental Psychology*, **18**, 450–61.

Von Hofsten, C. & Fazel-Zandy, S. (1984). Development of visually guided hand orientation in reaching. *Journal of Experimental Child Psychology*, **38**, 208–19.

Waddington, C. H. (1962). *New Patterns in Genetics and Development*. New York, London: Columbia University Press.

Wennergren, G., Milerad, J., Lagercrantz, H. et al. (1987). The epidemiology of SIDS and attack of lifelessness in Sweden. *Acta Paediatrica Scandinavica*, **76**, 898–906.

Wilson, P. H. & McKenzie, B. E. (1998). Information processing deficits associated with developmental coordination disorder: a meta-analysis of research findings. *Journal of Child Psychiatry*, **6**, 829–40.

Wolff, P. H. (1984). Discontinuous changes in human wakefulness around the end of the second month of life: a developmental perspective. In *Continuity of Neural Functions: From Prenatal to Postnatal Life*, ed. H. F. R. Prechtl, *Clinics in Developmental Medicine*, No. 94, pp. 144–58. Oxford: Blackwell Scientific Publications.

Woollacott, M., Debû, B. & Mowatt, M. (1987). Neuromuscular control of posture in the infant and child: is vision dominant? *Journal of Motor Behavior*, **19**, 167–86.

Woollacott, M., Burtner, P., Jensen, J., Jasiewicz-Roncesvalles, N. & Sveistrup, H. (1998). Development of postural responses during standing in healthy children and children with spastic diplegia. *Neuroscience and Biobehavioral Reviews*, **22**, 583–90.

Yekutiel, M., Jariwalda, M. & Stretch, P. (1994). Sensory deficit in the hands of children with cerebral palsy: a new look at assessment and prevalence. *Developmental Medicine and Child Neurology*, **36**, 619–24.

Zelazo, P. R. (1983). The development of walking: new findings and old assumptions. *Journal of Motor Behavior*, **2**, 99–137.

22

Antenatal glucocorticoids and programming of the developing brain

Stephen G. Matthews

Department of Physiology, Faculty of Medicine, University of Toronto, Canada

Introduction

Glucocorticoids (GCs; cortisol in humans and most mammals, and corticosterone in rats, mice and other lower vertebrates) are essential for normal brain development. They exert a wide spectrum of effects in most regions of the developing brain, ranging from subcellular reorganization to neuron–neuron and neuron–glial interaction. However, sustained elevation in, or removal of these hormones from, the fetal brain is detrimental to these processes, and can permanently modify the structure and function of the brain (Bohn, 1984).

The pioneering work of Liggins and Howie in the early 1970s has led to the widespread use of synthetic GCs to treat fetuses at risk of preterm delivery (Liggins & Howie, 1972). Preterm delivery occurs in approximately 7–10% of all births in North America and is responsible for about 75% of neonatal deaths (NIH Consensus Development Conference, 1995). In these cases, neonatal morbidity is high in surviving preterm infants and complications such as respiratory distress syndrome, intraventricular hemorrhage and necrotizing enterocolitis are common. Prenatal GC therapy reduces the frequency of the complications associated with preterm delivery. As a result, in 1994 the National Institute of Health Consensus Development Conference recommended antenatal treatment of all women at risk of preterm delivery, between 24 and 34 weeks of gestation, with GCs (NIH Consensus Development Conference, 1995). However, the Consensus Report highlighted the requirement for further research into the effects of antenatal GCs on brain development and function after birth. This review will explore the current state of knowledge in this area. Although there is a growing literature on the impact of prenatal GC exposure on cardiovascular and metabolic function after birth (Dodic et al., 1999), this aspect of programming will not be considered in detail in this review.

In addition to use in cases of preterm labour, synthetic GCs are also administered

This chapter is modified from two prior reviews published in *Pediatric Research* (2000), **47**, 291–300.

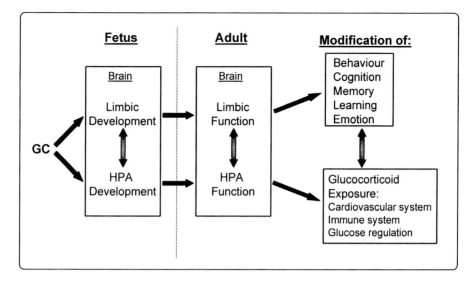

Fig. 22.1.   Diagrammatic representation of the routes by which prenatal glucocorticoid exposure programs adult behaviour and neuroendocrine function. The fetal limbic system (primarily the hippocampus), hypothalamus and anterior pituitary express high levels of corticosteroid receptors, and are sensitive to glucocorticoids. Exposure to exogenous glucocorticoid at this time will alter development and subsequent function of both the limbic system and the hypothalamo-pituitary-adrenal (HPA) axis. The hippocampus regulates HPA function, and endogenous glucocorticoids (the end product of HPA activation) modify many aspects of limbic function. The grey arrows indicate this close functional association. In the periphery, the overall effect of programming during development will be altered exposure to endogenous glucocorticoid throughout life. Increased exposure will predispose to a number of neurological, metabolic and cardiovascular diseases, while reduced exposure may act to protect against these pathologies. (See text for further details.)

to pregnant women in other clinical situations including congenital adrenal hyperplasia. Often, these treatments occur in early pregnancy and in some cases throughout gestation (Lajic et al., 1998). There is currently very little information as to the impact of such treatment regimes on brain and neuroendocrine development. However, some of the long-term effects discussed in this review may also occur in these clinical situations.

Development of the brain and neuroendocrine systems

Within the developing brain, the limbic system (primarily the hippocampus) is particularly sensitive to endogenous and exogenous GC during development (Weinstock, 1997; De Kloet et al., 1998). The hippocampus has a myriad of complex functions within the brain. These include cognition, behaviour, memory, co-ordination of autonomic activity and regulation of a number of endocrine systems (De Kloet et al., 1998; Beggs et al., 1999; Jacobson & Sapolsky, 1991). Given the wide spectrum of regulatory roles, programming of limbic function during development will have a profound impact in postnatal and adult life (see Fig. 22.1).

It has been known for four decades that hypothalamo-pituitary-adrenocortical (HPA) function can be permanently programmed during development, although the mechanisms have remained unclear. The HPA axis is modulated by efferent outflow from the limbic system (Jacobson & Sapolsky, 1991; Herman et al., 1996) (see Fig. 22.2). Glucocorticoids act at multiple loci within the body to maintain homeostasis, but also act in the CNS to modify behaviour and learning (Lupien & McEwen, 1997). Modification of systems that regulate HPA function during development will have major consequences on behaviour and other higher centre function, as well as on the long-term health of the individual (see Fig. 22.1).

The timing of maturation of the HPA axis relative to birth is highly species specific, and is closely linked to landmarks of brain development (Dobbing & Sands, 1979). In animals that give birth to mature young (sheep, guinea pigs and primates) maximal brain growth and a large proportion of neuroendocrine maturation (including corticosteroid receptor development) takes place in utero (Matthews & Challis, 1996; Matthews, 1998; Mesiano & Jaffe, 1997). In contrast, in species that give birth to immature young (rats, rabbits and mice), much neuroendocrine development occurs in the postnatal period (Sapolsky & Meaney, 1986). Therefore, maternal GC treatment in late gestation will impact on different stages of brain and HPA development depending on the species studied. Another important consideration when extrapolating between studies and species is that of receptor sensitivity. In this connection, mice and rats are corticosensitive (high receptor affinity for GCs) compared to other species such as guinea pigs and primates, which are considered corticoresistant (Claman, 1972).

Under normal circumstances, and in all species studied, access of maternal endogenous GCs (cortisol and corticosterone) to the fetus is low. This is due, in part, to the expression of 11β-hydroxysteroid dehydrogenase (11β-HSD) in the placenta (Seckl, 1997). Briefly, 11β-HSD interconverts cortisol and corticosterone to inactive products (cortisone, 11-dehydrocorticosterone). There are two known isoforms, 11β-HSD type 1 which is bidirectional and, type 2 which is unidirectional (cortisol to cortisone). The efficiency of placental 11β-HSD2 varies considerably amongst species; however it is generally accepted that placental 11β-HSD2 is of primary importance in excluding maternal glucocorticoid from the fetus (Seckl, 1997). 11β-HSD2 has a low affinity for synthetic GCs, and so dexamethasone and betamethasone pass rapidly from mother to fetus.

This review will focus on the impact of synthetic GCs in the developing brain, and resultant changes in neuroendocrine function and behaviour. However, studies that have utilized endogenous GCs will be cited where no information using synthetic GCs is available.

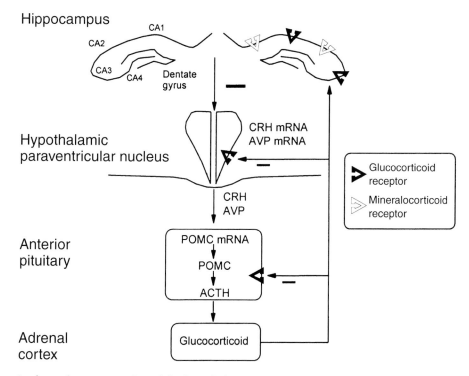

Fig. 22.2.   A schematic representation of the hypothalamo-pituitary-adrenal (HPA) axis. The hypothalamic paraventricular nucleus (PVN) controls pituitary-adrenocortical activity (Plotsky, 1991). The limbic system, primarily via the hippocampus, forms a major inhibitory input to the PVN (Jacobson & Sapolsky, 1991). There are few direct connections between the hippocampus and the PVN, but many indirect links via the bed nucleus of the stria terminalis and the ventromedial hypothalamus (Jacobson & Sapolsky, 1991; Herman et al., 1996). Parvocellular neurons in the PVN synthesize corticotrophin-releasing hormone (CRH) and vasopressin (AVP), which are then released into the hypophyseal portal circulation (Plotsky, 1991). CRH and AVP stimulate adrenocorticotrophin (ACTH) synthesis and release from corticotrophs in the anterior pituitary gland. ACTH then initiates the synthesis and secretion of cortisol from the adrenal cortex (Miller & Tyrrell, 1995). Due to the damaging effects of extended tissue exposure to GCs, the HPA axis is tightly regulated (Miller & Tyrrell, 1995). Glucocorticoids feedback, via glucocorticoid (GR) and mineralocorticoid receptors (MR), at several sites to inhibit further HPA activity (De Kloet et al., 1998). Synthetic GCs bind predominantly to the GR, and the effects on development following prenatal synthetic GC administration are probably mediated at the level of this receptor.

Prenatal glucocorticoid and adult HPA function

In the rat, fetal exposure to synthetic GC (0.1mg/kg) over the last week of gestation resulted in elevated basal plasma corticosterone levels in adult male offspring. This increase in corticosterone was associated with an increase in adult blood pressure. There was also a dexamethasone-induced reduction in birthweight, but no effect on gestation length (Levitt et al., 1996). In another study, maternal dexamethasone treatment (0.05mg/kg) on gestational day 17, 18 and 19, resulted in adult male offspring that mounted a greater corticosterone response to stress (Muneoka et al., 1997). In contrast, dexamethasone (0.4mg/kg) treatment on gestational day 17 and 19 failed to alter basal HPA function in prepubertal offspring. However, there was a significant difference in the ratio of vasopressin (AVP) and corticotropin-releasing hormone (CRH) in the external zone of the median eminence in young rats (Bakker et al., 1995), indicating that there were subtle long-term effects on HPA regulation. These studies clearly demonstrate that dexamethasone-exposure in utero, can program adult HPA function, but that the nature of the modification is dependent on dose and timing of exposure.

Administration of dexamethasone to pregnant guinea pigs on gestational day 50 and 51 (75% of gestation), resulted in prepubertal male, but not female, offspring with dramatically elevated basal plasma cortisol concentrations (Dean et al., 2001). There was no effect of GC administration on fetal, term or juvenile body or organ weights, although there was a significant increase in gestation length (Dean et al., 2001; Dean & Matthews, 1999). A single study has been undertaken to establish the long-term effects of fetal exposure to synthetic GCs on HPA function in the primate (Uno et al., 1994). Pregnant rhesus monkeys were treated daily with dexamethasone (4×1.25mg/kg) commencing on 132 days of gestation. Basal and stress-stimulated cortisol levels were elevated in the offspring (10 months of age) born to dexamethasone-treated mothers (Uno et al., 1994). Taken together, these studies demonstrate that short-term fetal exposure to synthetic GCs can program HPA function in species that give birth to neuroanatomically mature young (primates and guinea pigs). To date, no studies have assessed HPA function in school-age children or young adults who were exposed to antenatal GC during fetal life.

In summary, available evidence in animals indicates that prenatal exposure to GCs leads to offspring with elevated HPA activity. There is currently no information as to how programmed changes in pituitary–adrenocortical activity are modified with age. Increased HPA tone throughout life, will have a considerable impact on adult health, due to elevated tissue exposure to GCs. In humans, elevated levels of cortisol have been associated with increased atherosclerosis, cholesterol levels, incidence of diabetes, immunosuppression and cognitive impairment (Brindley & Rolland, 1989; Lupien & McEwen, 1997). Animal studies have found similar effects of chronically elevated HPA activity (Ader & Grota, 1973). Taken together, these data would indicate that chronically elevated HPA function leads to accelerated aging. In contrast, life-long exposure to reduced HPA activity may tend to slow down the onset of age-related pathologies.

Prenatal glucocorticoid and adult behaviour

Altered hippocampal development will have considerable effects on adult behaviour. This effect may be direct or indirect, via alterations in HPA function. In rats, treatment of pregnant dams with corticosterone (endogenous GC) resulted in sex-specific alterations in spontaneous and apomorphine-induced motor activity in adult offspring. In adult male offspring exposed to corticosterone as fetuses, exploratory activity was increased, while in females spontaneous locomotion was increased, but there was no effect on exploratory activity. In adult female offspring, there was an interaction between apomorphine-induced motor activity and prenatal GC exposure, indicating GC-induced alterations in central dopamine systems (Diaz et al., 1997). Daily dexamethasone treatment (0.1 mg/kg) over the last week of gestation had significant detrimental effects on sexual behaviour, such that male offspring became demasculinized and feminized (Holson et al., 1995).

In mice, maternal treatment with prednisone resulted in offspring with delayed development of eye opening, lifting, walking and gripping, indicating a retardation of muscular and motor development (Gandelman & Rosenthal, 1981). In another series of studies, either single (Rayburn et al., 1997) or repeat doses (Rayburn et al., 1998) of dexamethasone or betamethasone (0.1–0.2 mg/kg) were administered to pregnant mice over the last week of gestation. Following a single injection of GC on gestational day 14, there were specific differences in anxiety, memory and socialization when compared to control. However, there was no effect of GC on sensory, motor, motivation and learning performance (Rayburn et al., 1997). Together, these studies would suggest that prenatal GC exposure has significant but subtle effects on the behaviour of adult rodent offspring and that these effects are sex specific.

In rhesus monkeys, there was no effect of prenatal dexamethasone treatment (1.25 mg/kg/day for 4 days) at approximately 0.75 of gestation on physical development or locomotor behaviour in young primates, though there were dramatic differences in hippocampal structure (Uno et al., 1994). In humans, a number of studies have been undertaken to establish the long-term effects of prenatal GC exposure on learning, behaviour and intelligence. However, these have been undertaken in children who were born preterm, and therefore already at risk of delayed neurological development (McCarton et al., 1996). In these studies, there was no overall neurological delay or impairment in children who were exposed to synthetic GCs in late gestation (Salokorpi et al., 1997; MacArthur et al., 1982). However, in

6-year old children, antenatal GC exposure was associated with subtle effects on neurological function, including reduced visual closure and visual memory (MacArthur et al., 1982). A single study has considered the impact of GC on cognitive and behavioural development in children who were exposed to repeated antenatal GC treatment, but that were not born preterm (Trautman et al., 1995). Children exposed to dexamethasone in early pregnancy, due to increased risk of congenital adrenal hyperplasia, showed significant increases in emotionality, unsociability, avoidance and behavioural problems. Although no cognitive changes were noted, examination was carried out at an age (6 months to 5.5 years) when differences in cognitive function are difficult to discern. A recent study has shown that repeated courses of GC (each course; 2×11.4 mg, 12 to 24 h apart) in pregnant women at increased risk of delivering preterm, resulted in children with reduced head circumference (French et al., 1999). Further studies are required to establish the impact of repeated antenatal GC treatment, in late gestation, on behavioural outcome in children born at term.

Mechanisms of programming

Developmental and functional considerations

The impact of fetal GC exposure is dependent on the expression of corticosteroid receptors in the developing brain at the time of exposure. A number of studies have shown that levels of glucocorticoid receptors (GR) and mineralocorticoid receptors (MR) in the rat brain are low through gestation, but increase rapidly after birth. This would be consistent with the postnatal nature of brain and HPA development in this species. However, more detailed analysis has revealed that there is a distinct ontogenic pattern for GR and MR in the fetal rat brain (Diaz et al., 1998). GR mRNA is present in the anterior hypothalamus, hippocampus and pituitary by gestational day 13, and mRNA levels increase around term. In contrast, MR mRNA is not present in the hippocampus until gestational day 16 and the hypothalamus until day 17 (Diaz et al., 1998). It is unclear how fetal levels compare to those in the neonate and adult.

In the fetal guinea pig, GR and MR mRNA are present in the cortex and all regions of the hippocampus and dentate gyrus by gestational day 40 and then throughout the remainder of gestation (see Fig. 22.3 in colour plate section). Between gestational day 40 and gestational day 50, there is a dramatic increase in GR mRNA levels, but a decrease in MR mRNA abundance (Matthews, 1998), indicating differential developmental regulation of the two receptors in the hippocampus. Hippocampal GR mRNA levels increase to a peak near term, but there is little change in MR mRNA which remains low. In contrast, in the PVN, GR mRNA levels are higher at gestational day 40 than at any other stage of fetal or postnatal life.

There is a dramatic decrease (50%) in GR mRNA near term (Matthews, 1998). This likely represents a decrease in GC feedback in the PVN, allowing ACTH and cortisol to increase simultaneously at this time (Matthews, 1998). A similar reduction in GR mRNA in the PVN has been noted in the fetal sheep near term (Andrews & Matthews, 2000). In summary, these studies indicate that the development of GR and MR expression is highly species specific. Differences in receptor number probably account for the inconsistent outcomes observed following varied treatment regimes, as well as for the differences observed between species.

In the brain, MR has a higher affinity than GR for GC, and at basal concentrations of cortisol, MR are occupied while the GR remains largely unoccupied (De Kloet et al., 1998). However, during periods of elevated plasma cortisol, i.e. during stress, there is increased occupation of the GR (Dallman et al., 1994). It has been proposed that the hippocampal MR is primarily involved in feedback regulation during basal secretion, while the GR becomes important during periods of increased GC secretion, though this remains somewhat controversial. Synthetic GCs bind predominantly to the GR, and the effects on development following prenatal GC administration are likely to be mediated at the level of this receptor. In addition to binding to classic GR, synthetic glucocorticoids such as dexamethasone may also bind to neurosteroid receptors in the brain (Kliewer et al., 1998). This would represent a novel route of signal transduction and clearly warrants further investigation.

Glucocorticoids and central neurotransmitter systems

The catecholamines, epinephrine and norepinephrine, stimulate HPA function via alpha 1 adrenergic receptors (Herman et al., 1996). Catecholaminergic innervation of the parvocellular paraventricular nucleus (PVN) is derived principally from the caudal medulla. Brainstem catecholaminergic systems are also implicated in hippocampal function. Stress increases norepinephrine turnover in the hippocampus and prefrontal cortex (Herman et al., 1996), and norepinephrine has been shown to modulate hippocampal corticosteroid receptor activity (Yau & Seckl, 1992).

Dexamethasone exposure in the last week of gestation results in adult offspring with reduced norepinephrine turnover in the cerebellum and forebrain (Slotkin et al., 1992) and reduced norepinephrine content in the hippocampus and neocortex (Muneoka et al., 1997). However, longitudinal studies have shown that antenatal GC exposure results in premature maturation of norepinephrine systems in the brainstem, forebrain and cerebellum (Slotkin et al., 1992), and induces overexpression of the norepinephrine transporter. Unfortunately, norepinephrine levels and turnover, and norepinephrine transporter levels have not been measured in the hypothalami of offspring that were exposed to GCs as fetuses. No effect of prenatal dexamethasone on adrenergic receptors has been detected (Slotkin et al., 1992).

Without further measurements in the hypothalamus, it is unclear how dexamethasone-induced modification of adult brain norepinephrine systems relates to the increase in HPA function. However, it has been shown that alterations in hippocampal norepinephrine can induce changes in corticosteroid receptor levels (Barbazanges et al., 1996), and therefore modify GC-negative feedback. Antenatal GC have also been shown to promote early maturation of dopamine systems in the forebrain (Slotkin et al., 1992), and this is likely to be associated with subtle changes in behaviours, noted in these animals.

Ascending serotonergic neurons project directly to the parvocellular PVN and increase activity of CRH-containing neurons, stimulating CRH and adrenocorticotropin (ACTH) secretion into the hypophysial portal blood (Herman et al., 1996). There is also a rich serotonergic innervation of the hippocampus (Hayashi et al., 1998). Prenatal exposure to dexamethasone in the last week of gestation leads to male offspring with increased hypothalamic and medullary serotonin levels, but reduced hippocampal serotonin turnover (Muneoka et al., 1997). Prenatal GC exposure also promoted brainstem serotonin transporter development, and resulted in increased transporter activity throughout the life of the animal (Slotkin et al., 1996a). Measurement of transporter activity was only undertaken in the brainstem, and potential GC-induced changes in the hippocampus and hypothalamus remain to be determined. Alterations in serotonergic transporter function and increased hypothalamic serotonin levels are likely responsible, in part, for the elevation of HPA activity observed in adult offspring. The effect of serotonin on HPA function is not confined to the PVN as serotonin tonically inhibits the expression of hippocampal MR in adult male rats (Semont et al., 1999).

Glucocorticoids and central corticosteroid receptors

In the rat, dexamethasone (0.1 mg/kg) administered over the last week of gestation resulted in adult male offspring with reduced levels of GR mRNA and MR mRNA in the hippocampus (Levitt et al., 1996). There was no difference in GR or MR expression in the hypothalamus or in brainstem structures. Until recently, it was thought that occupation of the hippocampal MR and GR is associated with suppression of HPA activity (Jacobson & Sapolsky, 1991). Therefore, a reduction in expression would be associated with an increase in pituitary–adrenocortical activity. However, this view has recently been challenged, and it has been suggested that occupation of the hippocampal GR can, under certain circumstances, act to potentiate activated HPA function, while occupation of the MR suppresses activity (De Kloet et al., 1998). The reduction of hippocampal MR mRNA in animals that were exposed to GCs is consistent with increased basal and activated HPA activity (i.e. reduced GC feedback) in this model. However, the functional role of the decrease in hippocampal GR mRNA is less clear, and requires further study.

In the guinea-pig, it has recently been demonstrated that prenatal GC exposure, during the phase of rapid brain growth (gestational day 50 and 51), results in juvenile offspring with an altered hippocampal corticosteroid receptor compliment. This effect is highly sex specific. Male offspring exhibit increased GR mRNA levels in the cingulate cortex and hippocampal CA3, while females exhibit reduced GR mRNA in the hippocampus (CA3 and CA4), dentate gyrus and cingulate cortex (Dean et al., 2001). There was no effect of prenatal GC on levels of GR mRNA in the hypothalamus and anterior pituitary. Whether the hippocampal differences are maintained into adulthood remains to be determined.

There are a number of additional, and as yet uninvestigated, levels at which changes in central GC sensitivity may be mediated. It is possible that prenatal GC may have long-term influences on: (i) intracellular hormone availability, (ii) interactions between receptor and heat-shock protein, (iii) receptor phosphorylation, (iv) nuclear translocation and, (v) DNA binding and interaction (Bamberger et al., 1996). Further studies are required to verify these possibilities.

Mechanisms of corticosteroid receptor programming

In both the rat and guinea-pig, there are rapid changes in the expression of GR and MR around the time of maximal brain growth (guinea-pig gestational day 50; rat postnatal day 8; Dobbing & Sands, 1979). It is possible that GCs exposure can have permanent effects on the trajectory of GR and MR development at this time, such that the hippocampal receptor complement is permanently altered. Very little is known about the mechanisms by which GCs modulate developing GR and MR populations. Likely, mechanisms include autoregulation and/or modification by brain biogenic amines. High levels of GC in the brain may act to reduce (autoregulate) corticosteroid receptor expression. This area has been reviewed in detail (Bamberger et al., 1996). Briefly, it has been shown that synthetic GCs downregulate GR mRNA by 50–80% in a variety of cell types (Webster & Cidlowski, 1994). Of particular relevance to this discussion, extended exposure of HeLa cells to dexamethasone resulted in irreversible downregulation of GR mRNA, a consequence of conformational change in the GR promoter (Silva et al., 1994).

Only one study has investigated the immediate impact of synthetic GCs on hippocampal corticosteroid receptor levels in the fetus (Dean & Matthews, 1999). In the guinea-pig, injection of dexamethasone on gestational day 50 and 51 increased GR and MR in the CA1 region of the hippocampus in female fetuses. Day 50 of gestation is a time of rapid brain growth and very low plasma cortisol concentrations in the fetal guinea pig (Matthews, 1998). In rats, Kalinyak and colleagues found no change in total brain GR mRNA 6h. after a single dexamethasone injection, in pups less than a week of age, and daily injections of corticosterone for 5 days were found to cause only small decreases in hippocampal dexamethasone binding in rat pups

(Meaney et al., 1985). Together, these studies would suggest that autoregulation by high doses of synthetic GC does not occur during periods of low adrenocortical activity during development. However, this does not preclude the possibility that autoregulation (i.e. reduced receptor number) by GCs may occur earlier in development, prior to the animal's entry into the adrenal hyporesponsive period. It is also unclear whether the effects of the prenatal treatment on corticosteroid receptors observed in young animals will reflect the receptor compliment in the adult hippocampus. Emerging evidence from our laboratory would suggest that this may not be the case. In female guinea-pig fetuses, dexamethasone exposure increased hippocampal MR and GR mRNA(Dean & Matthews, 1999), but the same fetal treatment resulted in prepubertal female offspring with reduced hippocampal GR mRNA (Dean et al., 2001). Currently, there is very little information on the influence of exogenous GC on neurotransmitter activity in the fetal brain or on the impact of neurotransmitter levels on corticosteroid receptors in the fetal brain.

Meaney and colleagues have recently demonstrated that serotonin regulates GR in primary hippocampal cultures derived from fetal rat brain (Mitchell et al., 1990b). Serotonin treatment resulted in an increase in GR binding, and this effect was mediated via high affinity serotonin ($5\text{-}HT_2$) receptors. Further, the effect was permanent, as increased levels of GR were maintained for 60 days, in the absence of further serotonin exposure. This group also demonstrated that serotonin was responsible for the upregulation of hippocampal GR, previously demonstrated in adult rats that were handled as neonates (Meaney et al., 1994). Handling has been shown to increase thyroid activity in the neonate (Meaney et al., 1994). Further, neonatal thyroid hormone administration mimics the effects of handling on GR binding in adulthood. Subsequent studies demonstrated that both neonatal handling and thyroid hormone administration resulted in increased serotonin turnover in the hippocampus (Mitchell et al., 1990a). As a result, it has been suggested that the ascending serotonin neurons are stimulated by thyroid hormones to increase hippocampal serotonin and thence GR expression (Meaney et al., 1994). Prenatal GC exposure has also been shown to advance maturation of the serotonin transporter system in the developing rat brain (Slotkin et al., 1996a, b). In the fetal guinea-pig, exposure to dexamethasone resulted in an increase in fetal thyroid hormone and an up-regulation of GR mRNA (Dean & Matthews, 1999). Together, these data indicate that an increase in central serotonin levels may mediate the dexamethasone-induced increases in hippocampal GR mRNA in the fetus, although further work is required to confirm this possibility.

Prenatal glucocorticoid and brain structure

The effects of GC are not restricted to central changes in neurotransmitter levels and receptor numbers, but may also include modification of brain structure.

Several studies in young animals and adults have demonstrated that stress and increased GC can have a major impact on hippocampal structure (De Kloet et al., 1998). Perhaps the most striking of these are the observations that stressful experience or exposure to chronically elevated GC results in significant reductions in hippocampal volume (Sapolsky, 1999; Sheline et al., 1996; Bremner et al., 1995; Stein et al., 1997).

An elegant series of studies carried out in the rhesus monkey have considered the impact of short periods of fetal GC exposure during late gestation on structural development of the limbic system (Uno et al., 1990, 1994). The effect of single injections of dexamethasone (0.5, 5 and 10 mg/kg) at 132 days of gestation (term = 185 days) was assessed on gestational day 135. There was considerable dose-dependent neuronal degeneration in the CA1 to CA3 hippocampal pyramidal neurons, shrinkage and condensation of neuron soma and dendritic branches, depletion of the number of neurons, and disintegration of mossy fibre endings in the zona lucidum (Uno et al., 1990). Fetuses receiving multiple injections of lower doses (0.125 × 4, 1.25 × 4 and 2.5 mg/kg × 4) showed more severe damage than those receiving a single larger injection. This would be more analogous to the treatment regime in pregnant women, and the lower dose would be similar to that prescribed for suspected preterm labour (NIH Consensus Development Conference, 1995).

Another group of fetuses was studied 30 days after exposure, and though the acute neurodegenerative changes seen in the brains of the day 135 fetuses had subsided, the size of the perkaryonic soma of the pyramidal neurons was small and their dendritic branches with the mossy fibre endings in the CA3 regions were poorly developed, compared to normal age-matched controls (Uno et al., 1990). In the dentate gyrus, the density of the granular neurons was less and the individual neurons were smaller. Overall, the number of hippocampal neurons at day 162 was approximately 30% reduced in the dexamethasone-treated fetuses, and the size of the whole hippocampal formation was reduced (Uno et al., 1990). In a further experiment involving dexamethasone-treated fetal monkeys, the hippocampal volume was analysed at 20 months of age, by magnetic resonance imaging (MRI). This revealed an approximate 30% reduction in hippocampal volume in offspring exposed to dexamethasone (4 × 1.25 mg/kg) at day 132 of gestation (Uno et al., 1994).

Human and animal studies have demonstrated that morphological changes in the hippocampus are associated with a number of functional consequences (Sapolsky, 1999). Bremner et al. (1995) showed that male combat veterans with post-traumatic stress disorder had reduced MRI-derived right sided hippocampal volume compared to control subjects (Bremner et al., 1995), and that certain aspects of their memory deficit were correlated with hippocampal volume (Sheline et al., 1996). More recent studies have demonstrated a reduction in hippocampal volume in women victimized by childhood sexual abuse, and that the severity of psychiatric complications was correlated to reduction in hippocampal volume (Stein et al., 1997). It is therefore, likely that GC-induced changes in hippocampal structure during development have long-term behavioural and neuroendocrine consequences.

The mechanisms by which GC-induced damage to the hippocampus takes place are not well understood. It is generally accepted that GCs promote differentiation over proliferation (De Kloet et al., 1998). Animal studies have demonstrated that GCs interfere with normal rates of cell birth and death that occur during development (Gould et al., 1991). However, it is also known that GC exposure can indirectly damage mature neurons (Sapolsky, 1996). It has been shown that GCs block the uptake of glucose into neurons. Under resting conditions, GCs do not reduce energy metabolism sufficiently to kill neurons; however, during situations such as ischemia or glucose insufficiency, GCs decrease energy metabolism, making neurons more vulnerable to challenge. It is thought that glutamate, which is released during episodes of hypoxia and hypoglycemia, is responsible for inducing damage in compromised neurons (Sapolsky, 1996). Glucocorticoids have also been shown to increase extracellular glutamate levels in the hippocampus, by preventing glutamate reuptake, and therefore further exacerbating damage. This damage is consistent with that described in fetal primates exposed to GC.

Other aspects of CNS development are also affected by prenatal GC exposure. A recent study in the sheep has shown that repeated fetal exposure to GCs delays myelination of optic axons (Dunlop et al., 1997). In rats, fetal dexamethasone exposure tends to promote the replacement of neurons with glia in the forebrain (Carlos et al., 1992), and has sustained effects on the formation of polyamines (Carlos et al., 1991). The latter are major regulators of neural cell replication and differentiation. Glucocorticoids also regulate the expression of the neuronal cell adhesion molecule (Rodriguez et al., 1998), which is important in maturation and synaptic stabilization. A recent study, has shown that a single low dose of dexamethasone (0.05 mg/kg), can cause profound perturbation of nuclear transcription factors in the fetal rat brain (Slotkin et al., 1998). Indeed, low doses of dexamethasone caused changes in fetal brain c-fos expression and AP-1 binding proteins of the same or larger magnitude than those associated with GC-induced teratogenesis (Slotkin et al., 1996b), suggesting that the brain is especially vulnerable to GC exposure in late gestation.

Neurotrophic factors are essential for development of interneuronal and neuronal–glial interactions (Lindsay et al., 1994). Both stress and GCs affect the expression of neurotrophic factors in limbic and hypothalamic structures in the adult brain (Smith et al., 1995). Several neurotrophic factors exist in the developing brain although virtually nothing is known of the functional regulation of neurotrophic factors during development. It is highly likely that neurotrophic factors play a role in prenatal GC programming of hippocampal and hypothalamic function by modifying neuron–neuron and neuron–glial interaction, within and between these structures.

It is possible that compromise (i.e. reduction of pyramidal neurons or alterations in axonal/dendritic processes and synaptogenesis) in the developing hippocampus, may decrease the age at which hippocampal deficits are first noted. Prenatally programmed increases in HPA function may exacerbate this hippocampal deficit (Sapolsky, 1996, 1999), and in turn will lead to further increases in HPA function (due to reduced GC negative feedback). In this connection, ageing humans tend to undergo a decrease in HPA resiliency (ability to switch off the HPA response), and it has been suggested that this deficit is linked to increased life-long exposure to GCs (Seeman & Robbins, 1994). For these reasons, follow-up studies in humans and animal models, to investigate the impact of prenatal GC exposure, may fail to observe significant hippocampal deficits until adulthood or early old age.

Summary and conclusions

In most of the studies cited in this review, the doses and regimen of synthetic GC administration were not dissimilar from those administered to pregnant women at risk of delivering preterm. In a recent study, a very low dose of GCs in late gestation has been shown to have dramatic effects on transcription factor expression in the developing brain (Slotkin et al., 1998). An important consideration when extrapolating between studies and species is that of receptor sensitivity. In this connection, mice and rats are corticosensitive (i.e. high receptor affinity for GCs) compared to guinea-pigs and primates (including humans), which are considered corticoresistant (Claman, 1972). Current evidence indicates that prenatal GC exposure can program brain and neuroendocrine function in both corticosensitive and corticoresistant animals. The magnitude of effect will also depend on the corticosteroid receptor compliment within the brain at the time of treatment as well as the sex of the fetus. This is highly species and brain region specific. Recent studies have indicated that maturation of the GR and MR systems is advanced in species where rapid brain development occurs, in utero (guinea-pigs and sheep), and this is likely also the case in primates.

The preceding evidence has led many investigators to suggest that alterations in hippocampal corticosteroid receptor regulation are responsible for the programming of HPA and alterations in adult behaviour (see Fig. 22.4). However, fundamental questions that remain are: (i) at which point in development are these receptor systems susceptible to programming; (ii) in the fetus, are the effects of excess GCs mediated directly at the hippocampal receptor and/or are the effects mediated via

Adult brain

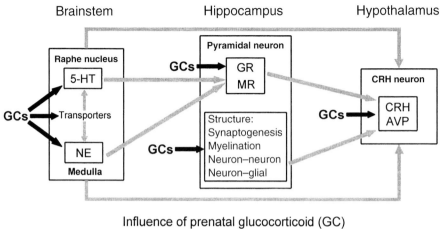

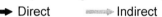

Influence of prenatal glucocorticoid (GC)

→ Direct   ⇢ Indirect

Fig. 22.4.   Diagram illustrating the potential routes by which prenatal glucocorticoid exposure leads to alterations in behavior and hypothalamo-pituitary-adrenal (HPA) activity in adulthood. During development, fetal exposure to glucocorticoids directly affects (i) development and subsequent function of neurotransmitter systems (and their transporter mechanisms) in the brainstem, (ii) development of corticosteroid receptor expression and structural components in the hippocampus and (iii) development and subsequent function of parvocellular neurons (CRH/AVP). Since the brainstem neurotransmitter systems project directly to the hippocampus and paraventricular nucleus (PVN), GC-induced changes in neurotransmitter and transporter systems will indirectly impact on function of the hippocampus and PVN. Also, given the important role of the hippocampus in regulating HPA function, any direct effects of GCs on the hippocampus will indirectly impact on PVN function. See text for further details. Serotonin (5-HT), norepinephrine (NE), glucocorticoid receptor (GR), mineralocorticoid receptor (MR), corticotropin-releasing hormone (CRH), vasopressin (AVP).

indirect routes (i.e. changes in neurotransmitter systems or structural interactions); (iii) does programming of receptor number occur solely during early development or do other changes in early life (i.e. permanent changes in neurotransmitter systems) lead to persistent alterations in GR and MR regulation in adulthood; (iv) what proportion of the programming effect is not associated with changes in corticosteroid receptors, but rather changes in other prenatally programmed systems, and (v) what are the mechanisms involved in the sex-specificity of HPA programming? Though not considered in detail in this review, it should also be noted that there are likely to be other indirect routes by which prenatal GC exposure alters fetal brain development. For example, treatment with antenatal GCs results in an increase in placental CRH production in humans (Marinoni et al., 1998). Placental CRH may enter the fetus and activate the HPA axis, however it may also have direct effects on blood flow within the placenta (Clifton et al., 1995). Significant research is required to further delineate the complex mechanisms by which GCs impact on the developing fetus.

In conclusion, there is no doubt that prenatal GC treatment affords great benefit to the preterm infant. However, animal studies, now carried out in many species, indicate that there may be some long-term physiological consequences of early exposure to excess GC, and that these may be sex specific. Further, the effects may not become apparent until later life. Given the dynamics of corticosteroid receptor systems in late gestation, it is likely that there are critical windows of development when specific regions of the brain are more sensitive to the influence of exogenous GC. Once such windows have been identified it will be possible to target prenatal treatments, so as to maximize benefit and reduce risk of long-term effects. Notwithstanding, the data reviewed above indicate that some caution should be exercised in the use of multiple course GC therapy during pregnancy.

Acknowledgements

The author's studies cited herein were supported by the Medical Research Council of Canada (MT-14691) and the Natural Sciences and Engineering Council of Canada.

REFERENCES

Ader, R. & Grota, L. J. (1973). Adrenocortical mediation of the effects of early life experiences. *Progress in Brain Research*, **39**, 395–406.

Andrews, M. H. & Matthews, S. G. (2000). Regulation of glucocorticoid receptor mRNA and heat shock protein 70 mRNA in the developing sheep brain. *Brain Research*, **878**, 174–82.

Bakker, J. M., Schmidt, E. D., Kroes, H. et al. (1995). Effects of short-term dexamethasone treatment during pregnancy on the development of the immune system and the hypothalamo-pituitary adrenal axis in the rat. *Journal of Neuroimmunology*, **63**, 183–91.

Bamberger, C. M., Schulte, H. M. & Chrousos, G. P. (1996). Molecular determinants of gluco-corticoid receptor function and tissue sensitivity to glucocorticoids. *Endocrine Review*, **17**, 245–61.

Barbazanges, A., Piazza, P. V., Le Moal, M. & Maccari, S. (1996). Maternal glucocorticoid secretion mediates long-term effects of prenatal stress. *Journal of Neuroscience*, **16**, 3943–9.

Beggs, J. M., Brown, T. H., Byrne, J. H. et al. (1999). Learning and memory: basic mechanisms. In *Fundamental Neuroscience*, ed. M. J. Zigmond, F. E. Bloom, S. C. Landis, J. L. Roberts & L. R. Squire, pp. 1411–54. San Diego: Academic Press.

Bohn, M. C. (1984). Glucocorticoid induced teratologies of the nervous system. In *Neurobehavorial Teratology*, ed. J. Yanai, pp. 365–87. New York: Elsevier Science Publishers.

Bremner, J. D., Randall, P., Scott, T. M. et al. (1995). MRI-based measurement of hippocampal volume in patients with combat-related posttraumatic stress disorder. *American Journal of Psychiatry*, **152**, 973–81.

Brindley, D. N. & Rolland, Y. (1989). Possible connections between stress, diabetes, obesity, hypertension and altered lipoprotein metabolism that may result in atherosclerosis. *Clinical Science*, **77**, 453–61.

Carlos, R. Q., Seidler, F. J., Lappi, S. E. & Slotkin, T. A. (1991). Fetal dexamethasone exposure affects basal ornithine decarboxylase activity in developing rat brain regions and alters acute responses to hypoxia and maternal separation. *Biology of the Neonate*, **59**, 69–77.

Carlos, R. Q., Seidler, F. J. & Slotkin, T.A. (1992). Fetal dexamethasone exposure alters macromolecular characteristics of rat brain development: a critical period for regionally selective alterations? *Teratology*, **46**, 45–59.

Claman, H. N. (1972). Corticosteroids and lymphoid cells. *New England Journal of Medicine*, **287**, 388–97.

Clifton, V. L., Owens, P. C., Robinson, P. J. & Smith, R. (1995). Identification and characterization of a corticotrophin-releasing hormone receptor in human placenta. *European Journal of Endocrinology*, **133**, 591–7.

Dallman, M. F., Akana, S. F., Levin, N. et al. (1994). Corticosteroids and the control of function in the hypothalamo-pituitary-adrenal (HPA) axis. *Annals of the New York Academy of Sciences*, **746**, 22–32.

De Kloet, E. R., Vreugdenhil, E., Oitzl, M. S. & Joels, M. (1998). Brain corticosteroid receptor balance in health and disease. *Endocrine Reviews*, **19**, 269–301.

Dean, F. & Matthews, S. G. (1999). Maternal dexamethasone treatment in late gestation alters glucocorticoid and mineralocorticoid receptor mRNA in the fetal guinea pig brain. *Brain Research*, **846**, 253–9.

Dean, F., Yu, C., Lingas, R. & Matthews, S. G. (2001). Prenatal glucocorticoid modifies hypothalamo pituitary–adrenal regulation in prepubertal guinea pigs. *Neuroendocrinology*, **73**(3), 194–202.

Diaz, R., Fuxe, K. & Ögren, S. O. (1997). Prenatal corticosterone treatment induces long-term changes in spontaneous and apomorphine-mediated motor activity in male and female rats. *Neuroscience*, **81**, 129–40.

Diaz, R., Brown, R. W. & Seckl, J. R. (1998). Distinct ontogeny of glucocorticoid and mineralocorticoid receptor and 11β-hydroxysteroid dehydrogenase types I and II mRNAs in the fetal rat brain suggest a complex control of glucocorticoid actions. *Journal of Neuroscience*, **18**, 2570–80.

Dobbing, J. & Sands, J. (1979). Comparative aspects of the brain growth spurt. *Early Human Development*, **3**, 79–83.

Dodic, M., Peers, A., Coghlan, J. P. & Wintour, M. (1999). Can excess glucocorticoid, in utero, predispose to cardiovascular and metabolic disease in middle age? *Trends in Endocrinology and Metabolism*, **10**, 86–91.

Dunlop, S. A., Archer, M. A., Quinlivan, J. A., Beazley, L. D. & Newnham, J. P. (1997). Repeated prenatal corticosteroids delay myelination in the ovine central nervous system. *Journal of Maternal–Fetal Medicine*, **6**, 309–13.

French, N. P., Hagan, R., Evans, S. F., Godfrey, M. & Newnham, J. P. (1999). Repeated antenatal corticosteroids: size at birth and subsequent development. *American Journal of Obstetrics and Gynecology*, **180**, 114–21.

Gandelman, R. & Rosenthal, C. (1981). Deleterious effects of prenatal prednisolone exposure upon morphological and behavioral development of mice. *Teratology*, **24**, 293–301.

Gould, E., Woolley, C. S. & McEwen, B. S. (1991). Adrenal steroids regulate postnatal development of the rat dentate gyrus: I. Effects of glucocorticoids on cell death. *Journal of Comparative Neurology*, **313**, 479–85.

Hayashi, A., Nagaoka, M., Yamada, K., Ichitani, Y., Miake, Y. & Okado, N. (1998). Maternal stress induces synaptic loss and developmental disabilities of offspring. *International Journal of Developmental Neuroscience*, **16**, 209–16.

Herman, J. P., Prewitt, C. M. & Cullinan, W. E. (1996). Neuronal circuit regulation of the hypothalamo-pituitary-adrenocortical stress axis. *Critical Reviews in Neurobiology*, **10**, 371–94.

Holson, R. R., Gough, B., Sullivan, P., Badger, T. & Sheehan, D. M. (1995). Prenatal dexamethasone or stress but not ACTH or corticosterone alter sexual behavior in male rats. *Neurotoxicology and Teratology*, **17**, 393–401.

Jacobson, L. & Sapolsky, R. (1991). The role of the hippocampus in feedback regulation of the hypothalamic-pituitary-adrenocortical axis. *Endocrine Reviews*, **12**, 118–34.

Kliewer, S. A., Moore, J. T., Wade, L. et al. (1998). An orphan nuclear receptor activated by pregnancy defines a novel steroid signalling pathway. *Cell*, **92**, 73–82.

Lajic, S., Wedell, A., Bui, T. H., Ritzen, E. M. & Holst, M. (1998). Long-term somatic follow-up of prenatally treated children with congenital adrenal hyperplasia. *Journal of Clinical Endocrinology and Metabolism*, **83**, 3872–80.

Levitt, N. S., Lindsay, R. S., Holmes, M. C. & Seckl, J. R. (1996). Dexamethasone in the last week of pregnancy attenuates hippocampal glucocorticoid receptor gene expression and elevates blood pressure in the adult offspring in the rat. *Neuroendocrinology*, **64**, 412–18.

Liggins, G. C. & Howie, R. N. (1972). A controlled trial of antepartum glucocorticoid treatment for the prevention of the respiratory distress syndrome in premature infants. *Pediatrics*, **50**, 515–23.

Lindsay, R. M., Wiegand, S. J., Altar, C. A. & DiStefano, P. S. (1994). Neurotropic factors: from molecule to man. *Trends in Neurosciences*, **17**, 182–90.

Lupien, S. J. & McEwen, B. S. (1997). The acute effects of corticosteroids on cognition: integration of animal and human model studies. *Brain Research and Brain Research Review*, **24**, 1–27.

MacArthur, B. A., Howie, R. N., Dezoete, J. A. & Elkins, J. (1982). School progress and cognitive development of 6-year-old children whose mothers were treated antenatally with betamethasone. *Pediatrics*, **70**, 99–105.

McCarton, C. M., Wallace, I. F., Divon, M. & Vaughan, H. G. Jr. (1996). Cognitive and neurologic development of the premature, small for gestational age infant through age 6:
Comparison by birthweight and gestational age. *Pediatrics*, **98**, 1167–78.

Marinoni, E., Korebrits, C., Di Iorio, R., Cosmi, E. V. & Challis, J. R. (1998). Effect of betamethasone in vivo on placental corticotropin-releasing hormone in human pregnancy. *American
Journal of Obstetrics and Gynecology*, **178**, 770–8.

Matthews, S. G. (1998). Dynamic changes in glucocorticoid and mineralocorticoid receptor
mRNA in the developing guinea pig brain. *Developmental Brain Research*, **107**, 123–32.

Matthews, S. G. & Challis, J. R. G. (1996). Regulation of the hypothalamo-pituitary-adrenocortical axis in fetal sheep. *Trends in Endocrinology and Metabolism*, 7, 239–46.

Meaney, M. J., Sapolsky, R. M. & McEwen, B. S. (1985). The development of the glucocorticoid
receptor system in the rat limbic brain I. Ontogeny and Autoregulation. *Developmental Brain
Research*, **18**, 159–64.

Meaney, M. J., Diorio, J., Francis, D. et al. (1994). Environmental regulation of the development
of glucocorticoid receptor systems in the rat forebrain: the role of serotonin. *Annals of the New
York Academy of Sciences*, **746**, 260–74.

Mesiano, S. & Jaffe, R. B. (1997). Developmental and functional biology of the primate fetal
adrenal cortex. *Endocrine Reviews*, **18**, 378–403.

Miller, W. L. & Tyrrell, J. B. (1995). The adrenal cortex. In *Endocrinology and Metabolism*, ed. P.
Felig, J. D. Baxter & L. A. Frohman, pp. 555–711. New York: McGraw Hill.

Mitchell, J. B., Iny, L. J. & Meaney, M. J. (1990a). The role of serotonin in the development and
environmental regulation of type II corticosteroid receptor binding in rat hippocampus.
Developmental Brain Research, **55**, 231–5.

Mitchell, J. B., Rowe, W., Boksa, P. & Meaney, M. J. (1990b). Serotonin regulates type II corticosteroid receptor binding in hippocampal cell cultures. *Journal of Neuroscience*, **10**, 1745–52.

Muneoka, K., Mikuni, M., Ogawa, T. et al. (1997). Prenatal dexamethasone exposure alters brain
monoamine metabolism and adrenocortical response in rat offspring. *American Journal of
Physiology*, **273**, R1669–75

NIH Consensus Development Conference (1995). Effect of corticosteroids for fetal maturation
and perinatal outcomes. *American Journal of Obstetrics and Gynecology*, **173**, 253–344.

Plotsky, P. M. (1991). Pathways to the secretion of adrenocorticotropin: a view from the portal.
Journal of Neuroendocrinology, **3**, 1–9.

Rayburn, W. F., Christensen, H. D. & Gonzalez, C. L. (1997). A placebo-controlled comparison
between betamethasone and dexamethasone for fetal maturation: Differences in neurobehavioral development of mice offspring. *American Journal of Obstetrics and Gynecology*, **176**,
842–50.

Rayburn, W. F., Christensen, H. D., Gonzalez, C. L., Rayburn, L. A. & Stewart, J. D. (1998). Effect
of in utero exposure to betamethasone on motivation/anxiety testing in mice offspring.
Neurotoxicology and Teratology, **20**, 475–81.

Rodriguez, J. J., Montaron, M. F., Petry, K. G. et al. (1998). Complex regulation of the expression
of the polysialylated form of the neuronal cell adhesion molecule by glucocorticoids in the rat
hippocampus. *European Journal of Neuroscience*, **10**, 2994–3006.

Salokorpi, T., Sajaniemi, N., Hällback, H., Kari, A., Rita, H. & Von Wendt, L. (1997). Randomized study of the effect of antenatal dexamethasone on growth and development of premature children at the corrected age of 2 years. *Acta Paediatrica*, **86**, 294–8.

Sapolsky, R. M. (1996). Stress, glucocorticoids, and damage to the nervous system: The current state of confusion. *Stress*, **1**, 1–19.

Sapolsky, R. M. (1999). Why stress is bad for your brain. *Science*, **273**, 749–50.

Sapolsky, R. M. & Meaney, M. J. (1986). Maturation of the adrenocortical stress response: Neuroendocrine control mechanisms and the stress hyporesponsive period. *Brain Research*, **396**, 64–76.

Seckl, J.R. (1997). Glucocorticoids, feto-placental 11β-hydroxysteroid dehydrogenase type 2, and the early life origins of adult disease. *Steroids*, **62**, 89–94.

Seeman, T. E. & Robbins, R. J. (1994). Aging and hypothalamic-pituitary-adrenal response to challenge in humans. *Endocrine Reviews*, **15**, 233–60.

Semont, A., Fache, M. P., Ouafik, L., Hery, M., Faudon, M. & Hery, F. (1999). Effect of serotonin inhibition on glucocorticoid and mineralocorticoid expression in various brain structures. *Neuroendocrinology*, **69**, 121–8.

Sheline, Y. I., Wang, P. W., Gado, M. H., Csernansky, J. G. & Vannier, M. W. (1996). Hippocampal atrophy in recurrent major depression. *Proceedings of the National Academy of Sciences, USA*, **93**, 3908–13.

Silva, C. M., Powell-Oliver, F., Jewell, C. M., Sar, M., Allgood, V. E. & Cidlowski, J. A. (1994). Regulation of the human glucocorticoid receptor by long-term and chronic treatment with glucocorticoid. *Steroids*, **59**, 436–42.

Slotkin, T. A., Lappi, S. E., McCook, E. C., Tayyeb, M. I., Eylers, J. P. & Seidler, F. J. (1992). Glucocorticoids and the development of neuronal function: effects of prenatal dexamethasone exposure on central noradrenergic activity. *Biology of the Neonate*, **61**, 326–36.

Slotkin, T. A., Barnes, G. A., McCook, E. C. & Seidler, F. J. (1996a). Programming of brainstem serotonin transporter development by prenatal glucocorticoids. *Developmental Brain Research*, **93**, 155–61.

Slotkin, T. A., Lau, C., Lappi, F. J. & Seidler, F. J. (1996b). Can intracellular signalling pathways predict developmental abnormalities? Sensitivity of the adenyl cyclase/c-fos protooncogene cascade to β-adrenergic agonists and glucocorticoids in the fetal rat. *Biomarkers*, **1**, 115–22.

Slotkin, T. A., Zhang, J., McCook, E. C. & Seidler, F. J. (1998). Glucocorticoid administration alters nuclear transcription factors in fetal rat brain: implications for the use of antenatal steroids. *Developmental Brain Research*, **111**, 11–24.

Smith, M. A., Makino, S., Kvetnansky, R. & Post, R. M. (1995). Stress and glucocorticoids affect the expression of brain-derived neurotrophic factor and neurotrophin-3 mRNAs in the hippocampus. *Journal of Neuroscience*, **15**, 1768–77.

Stein, M. B., Koverola, C., Hanna, C., Torchia, M. G. & McClarty, B. (1997). Hippocampal volume in women victimized by childhood sexual abuse. *Psychological Medicine*, **27**, 951–9.

Trautman, P. D., Meyer-Bahlburg, H. F. L., Postelnek, J. & New, M. I. (1995). Effects of early prenatal dexamethasone on the cognitive and behavioural development of young children: results of a pilot study. *Psychoneuroendocrinology*, **20**, 439–49.

Uno, H., Lohmiller, L., Thieme, C. et al. (1990). Brain damage induced by prenatal exposure to dexamethasone in fetal rhesus macaques. I. Hippocampus. *Developmental Brain Research*, **53**, 157–67.

Uno, H., Eisele, S., Sakai, A. et al. (1994). Neurotoxicity of glucocorticoids in the primate brain. *Hormones and Behavior*, **28**, 336–48.

Webster, J. C. & Cidlowski, J. A. (1994). Downregulation of the glucocorticoid receptor: A mechanism for physiological adaptation to hormones. *Annals of the New York Academy of Sciences*, **746**, 216–20.

Weinstock, M. (1997). Does prenatal stress impair coping and regulation of hypothalamic–pituitary–adrenal axis. *Neuroscience and Biobehavioral Reviews*, **21**, 1–10.

Yau, J. L. W. & Seckl, J. R. (1992). Central 6-hydroxydopamine lesions decrease mineralocorticoid, but not glucocorticoid receptor gene expression in the rat hippocampus. *Neuroscience Letters*, **142**, 159–62.

Index

References to figures are indicated by 'f' and references to tables by 't' when they fall on a page not covered by the text reference.